Exercise and the Heart in Health and Disease

FUNDAMENTAL AND CLINICAL CARDIOLOGY

Editor-in-Chief

Samuel Z. Goldhaber, M.D.

*Harvard Medical School
and Brigham and Women's Hospital
Boston, Massachusetts*

Associate Editor, Europe

Henri Bounameaux, M.D.

*University Hospital of Geneva
Geneva, Switzerland*

1. *Drug Treatment of Hyperlipidemia*, edited by Basil M. Rifkind
2. *Cardiotonic Drugs: A Clinical Review, Second Edition, Revised and Expanded*, edited by Carl V. Leier
3. *Complications of Coronary Angioplasty*, edited by Alexander J. R. Black, H. Vernon Anderson, and Stephen G. Ellis
4. *Unstable Angina*, edited by John D. Rutherford
5. *Beta-Blockers and Cardiac Arrhythmias*, edited by Prakash C. Deedwania
6. *Exercise and the Heart in Health and Disease*, edited by Roy J. Shephard and Henry S. Miller, Jr.
7. *Cardiopulmonary Physiology in Critical Care*, edited by Steven M. Scharf
8. *Atherosclerotic Cardiovascular Disease, Hemostasis, and Endothelial Function*, edited by Robert Boyer Francis, Jr.
9. *Coronary Heart Disease Prevention*, edited by Frank G. Yanowitz
10. *Thrombolysis and Adjunctive Therapy for Acute Myocardial Infarction*, edited by Eric R. Bates
11. *Stunned Myocardium: Properties, Mechanisms, and Clinical Manifestations*, edited by Robert A. Kloner and Karin Przyklenk
12. *Prevention of Venous Thromboembolism*, edited by Samuel Z. Goldhaber
13. *Silent Myocardial Ischemia and Infarction: Third Edition*, Peter F. Cohn
14. *Congestive Cardiac Failure: Pathophysiology and Treatment*, edited by David B. Barnett, Hubert Pouleur, and Gary S. Francis
15. *Heart Failure: Basic Science and Clinical Aspects*, edited by Judith K. Gwathmey, G. Maurice Briggs, and Paul D. Allen

Exercise and the Heart in Health and Disease

Second Edition, Revised and Expanded

edited by

Roy J. Shephard
University of Toronto
Toronto, Ontario, Canada

Henry S. Miller, Jr.
Wake Forest University School of Medicine
Winston-Salem, North Carolina

MARCEL DEKKER, INC.   NEW YORK · BASEL

ISBN: 0-8247-0227-1

This book is printed on acid-free paper.

Headquarters
Marcel Dekker, Inc.
270 Madison Avenue, New York, NY 10016
tel: 212-696-9000; fax: 212-685-4540

Eastern Hemisphere Distribution
Marcel Dekker AG
Hutgasse 4, Postfach 812, CH-4001 Basel, Switzerland
tel: 44-61-261-8482; fax: 44-61-261-8896

World Wide Web
http://www.dekker.com

The publisher offers discounts on this book when ordered in bulk quantities. For more
information, write to Special Sales/Professional Marketing at the headquarters address
above.

Current printing (last digit):
10 9 8 7 6 5 4 3 2 1

PRINTED IN THE UNITED STATES OF AMERICA

CMH

Series Introduction

Marcel Dekker, Inc., has focused on the development of various series of beautifully produced books in different branches of medicine. These series have facilitated the integration of rapidly advancing information for both the clinical specialist and the researcher.

My goal as editor-in-chief of the Fundamental and Clinical Cardiology series is to assemble the talents of world-renowned authorities to discuss virtually every area of cardiovascular medicine. In the current monograph, Roy J. Shephard and Henry S. Miller, Jr., have edited a much-needed and timely book. They have thoroughly updated and expanded upon their highly successful first edition by focusing on exercise throughout the cycle of life, from children to octogenarians. They devote special emphasis to women's health and exercise. In addition, they prescribe training programs for a wide spectrum of cardiovascular disorders. Their text is thorough and informative. As a general clinical cardiologist, I will keep *Exercise and the Heart in Health and Disease* within arm's reach in my office.

Samuel Z. Goldhaber, M.D.

Preface

The first edition of this book appeared in 1992, in response to the rapidly growing interest in exercise as a means to health, particularly cardiac health. Exercise was being embraced enthusiastically, not only by clinically healthy individuals of all ages, but also by individuals with various types of cardiac disorder, to the point that patients were completing marathon runs after both myocardial infarction and cardiac transplant operations. It was thus thought important to weigh carefully the evidence supporting such a practice, and to examine details of the frequency, duration, intensity, and type of physical activity appropriate to different ages of individual, different environmental conditions, and various types of cardiovascular disorder.

The past seven years has seen the accumulation of much solid evidence supporting the recommendation that both healthy individuals and clinical patients enhance their level of physical activity. There has also been a major shift in prescribing practice. For the general population, the emphasis has shifted from deliberate exercise sessions in a specialized facility to the incorporation of physical activity into ordinary daily life—the approach of "active living." It has increasingly been recognized that much of the potential health benefit associated with vigorous exercise can be realized through quite modest levels of physical activity, distributed over several relatively brief bouts on most days of the week. This approach, reflected throughout the new edition, seems much more likely to appeal to that substantial fraction of patients who express little interest in the traditional regimented type of exercise prescription.

A second issue that has emerged strongly since preparation of the first edition is the need to consider issues specific to the female patient. Topics explored in two chapters on this theme include the patterns of activity followed by women, the manifestations of cardiac disease in female patients, and possible gender differences in access to various types of treatment, including exercise and rehabilitation programs.

A third concern specifically addressed in the new edition is the issue of overtraining. Is it possible to induce a dangerous hypertrophy of the myocardium by excessive training? How prevalent is the risk of hypertrophic cardiomyopathy? Is there value in undertaking detailed laboratory examination of the heart prior to participation in a sports program, or is this merely an unnecessary barrier to participation?

The ability of regular physical activity to moderate stress and thus diminish the autonomic reactivity of the heart is a fourth area of growing interest. A new chapter focuses on this important question.

All other chapters in the book have been thoroughly updated, in some cases with new authors and/or coauthors. The book thus continues to provide physicians with an authoritative source of information on the prescription of exercise for both the clinically healthy person and the patient with cardiac disease. Detailed and specific information is given on the appropriate frequency, duration, intensity, and type of physical activity to be pursued in various environments. The issue of exercise-induced death is confronted, and safety is contrasted for the regular exerciser and the occasional weekend athlete. Modifications of exercise prescriptions are discussed that accommodate the needs of the young child, the middle-aged, the frail elderly, and the person with spinal injury. The likely benefits of regular physical activity are critically appraised in both health and disease, and the likely impact of cardioactive medications is carefully examined. These are a few of the important issues on which we have sought answers from a worldwide panel of experts.

Roy J. Shephard
Henry S. Miller, Jr.

Contents

Contributors

Gary J. Balady, M.D.   Professor, Director of Preventive Cardiology, Boston University Medical Center, Boston, Massachusetts

R. James Barnard, Ph.D.   Professor, Department of Physiological Science and Medicine, University of California, Los Angeles, California

David S. Braden, M.D.   Pediatric Cardiologist, Department of Pediatrics, Portsmouth Naval Hospital, Portsmouth, Virginia

Peter H. Brubaker, Ph.D.   Associate Professor, Department of Health and Exercise Science, Wake Forest University, Winston-Salem, North Carolina

Carl Foster, Ph.D.   Director, Department of Clinical Physiology, Milwaukee Heart Institute, Milwaukee, Wisconsin

Jason L. Fox, M.S.   Laboratory Coordinator, Cardiac Rehabilitation Program, Wake Forest University School of Medicine, Winston-Salem, North Carolina

Roger M. Glaser, Ph.D.†   Director, Institute for Rehabilitation Research and Medicine, Professor and Acting Chair, Department of Rehabilitation Medicine and Restorative Care, and Professor, Department of Physiology and Biophysics, Wright State University School of Medicine, Dayton, Ohio

Jack M. Goodman, Ph.D.   Associate Professor, Faculty of Physical Education and Health, University of Toronto, Ontario, Canada

---

† Deceased

Lisa L. Hector, M.S.   Clinical Physiologist, Department of Cardiac Rehabilitation, Memorial Hospital at Oconomowoc, Oconomowoc, Wisconsin

Thomas W. J. Janssen, Ph.D.   Acting Director, Institute for Rehabilitation Research and Medicine, and Research Assistant Professor, Department of Rehabilitation Medicine and Restorative Care, Wright State University School of Medicine, Dayton, Ohio

Terence Kavanagh, M.D.   Associate Professor, Department of Medicine, University of Toronto, and Medical Director, Toronto Rehabilitation Centre, Toronto, Ontario, Canada

Lori D. Kirwan, M.Sc., R.N.   Graduate Program in Exercise, Faculty of Physical Education and Health, University of Toronto, Toronto, Ontario, Canada

Arthur S. Leon, M.S., M.D., F.A.C.S.M.   Henry L. Taylor Professor, Division of Kinesiology, University of Minnesota, Minneapolis, Minnesota

Katharina Meyer, Ph.D.   Clinical Physiologist, Department of Cardiac Rehabilitation, Herz-Zentrum, Bad Krozingen, Germany

Henry S. Miller, Jr., M.D., F.A.C.C., F.A.C.S.M.   Professor, Department of Internal Medicine/Cardiology, Wake Forest University School of Medicine, Winston-Salem, North Carolina

Ralph S. Paffenbarger, Jr., M.D., Ph.D.   Professor, Division of Epidemiology, Department of Health Research and Policy, Stanford University School of Medicine, Stanford, California

Roy J. Shephard, M.D., Ph.D., D.P.E., F.A.C.S.M.*   Professor Emeritus, Faculty of Physical Education and Health, University of Toronto, Toronto, Ontario, Canada

Debra L. Sherman, M.D.   Instructor of Medicine, Division of Cardiology, Boston University Medical Center, Boston, Massachusetts

David B. Shuster, M.D.   Medical Director, Rehabilitation Institute of Ohio, Miami Valley Hospital, Dayton, Ohio

L. Kent Smith, M.D., M.P.H.   Director, Cardiac Rehabilitation and Drug Research, Arizona Heart Institute, Phoenix, Arizona

Wayne M. Sotile, Ph.D.   Sotile Psychological Associates, Winston-Salem, North Carolina

---

* Present address: P.O. Box 521, Brackendale, BC V0N 1H0, Canada.

Charles M. Tipton, Ph.D., F.A.C.S.M.   Professor, Department of Physiology, University of Arizona, Tucson, Arizona

Nanette Kass Wenger, M.D.   Professor, Department of Medicine, Emory University School of Medicine, Atlanta, Georgia

Linda D. Zwiren, Ed.D., F.A.C.S.M.   Professor, Department of Health and Physical Education and Department of Biology, Hofstra University, Hempstead, New York

Exercise and the Heart in Health and Disease

1

Physiological, Biochemical, and Psychological Responses to Exercise and Physical Activity

ROY J. SHEPHARD
University of Toronto
Toronto, Ontario, Canada

INTRODUCTION

In this first chapter, we explore in general terms the various factors determining physiological, biochemical, and psychological responses to exercise and physical activity in both health and disease. The terms *exercise* and *physical activity* are first defined. Acute responses to a single bout of exercise are then contrasted with the chronic reactions to training, and we examine the influence of intensity, duration, and frequency of activity on the training response. We consider also variations in response that depend on the type of physical activity undertaken as well as on environmental factors. The postulated medical and psychological benefits of regular physical activity are summarized, and a final section discusses the strengths and weaknesses of current evidence concerning these effects.

DEFINITIONS OF EXERCISE, PHYSICAL FITNESS, AND SPORT

Exercise

Exercise implies the voluntary performance of one or more bouts of physical activity with some deliberate objective, such as improving fitness, physical performance, or health (31,37).

Physical Fitness

Physical fitness may be considered the ability to perform physically demanding occupational or leisure activities satisfactorily. An increase of physical fitness is the normal consequence of regularly repeated bouts of exercise or vigorous daily physical activity. In part, it is specific to the mode of activity that has been practiced, but there is generally a carryover into other areas of fitness and health. A proportion of the variance in most physiological indices of fitness reflects social and genetic inheritance rather than the patterns of physical activity that have been adopted in recent months (128,172,173,208).

Sport

In some European countries, all types of exercise are described as ''sport''; but in North America, sport is a variant of exercise, where the primary motivation is found in such factors as the excitement of competition, the thrills of rapid body movement and danger, or an increase of opportunities for social contacts (116) rather than the improvement of health.

Physical Activity

Physical activity encompasses all forms of movement, whether undertaken voluntarily (exercise and sport), unavoidably (occupational and domestic chores), or deliberately (adoption of an active lifestyle).

Secular Trends

In the past, occupational and domestic responsibilities involved considerable physical activity; but with the automation of developed societies, such pursuits no longer provide sufficient physical activity to sustain an individual's physical condition (142,258). Two decades of promotional efforts by various western governments have had little influence on participation in either exercise or sport. Health authorities in the United States and Canada are therefore encouraging a return to ''active living,'' fostering the incorporation of such activities as walking, cycling, and stair climbing into the daily routine (258). Whereas the formal exercise sessions of the last two decades were prescribed fairly rigorously, the recommendation of active living generally involves lower intensities of activity, and there is a corresponding decrease in the need for close medical screening and supervision.

ACUTE RESPONSES TO PHYSICAL ACTIVITY

Duration

The duration of an acute bout of physical activity can vary from a few seconds (for instance, a 50-m dash), to an athletic event lasting 24 h or more (for example, a 100-km run). The responses of the body show a corresponding gradation. Although the average intensity of effort may be higher during a brief bout of activity, the disturbance of normal physiological, biochemical, and psychological functions is more profound and more long-lasting with a sustained increase in energy expenditure (Table 1).

Very Brief Activity

Physiological responses to a very brief (5–10 s) and exhausting bout of rhythmic physical activity are limited largely to a depletion of high-energy phosphate reserves (adenosine triphosphate and creatine phosphate within the active muscles). These ''phosphagen stores'' are rapidly replenished following activity, the halftime of the recuperative process averaging 22 s in a young, healthy adult (49, 210).

Brief Activity

If physical activity continues for somewhat longer (1–2 min), there is a substantial accumulation of lactate, and the associated hydrogen ions progressively inhibit the rate-limiting enzymes of glycolysis. At exhaustion, the intramuscular concentration of lactate may reach 30 mmol/L (90). The blood lactate also rises during brief, exhausting exercise and for 1–3 min following it. After a large-muscle activity such as running, young adults reach a limiting value of 10–12 mmol/L (208,210). Recovery requires 15–30 min and is speeded if blood flow to the active part is sustained by continued moderate activity (e.g., 40% of maximal oxygen intake).

Endurance Activity

If the period of all-out physical activity is further extended (as in an endurance event 5–10 min in duration), the exerciser usually reaches a plateau of oxygen

TABLE 1 Factors Limiting Exercise in Relation to the Duration of Activity

0–10 s	10–60 s	1–60 min	60–120 min	2–5 h	>5 h
		Motivation, release of inhibition, arousal			
Anaerobic power	Anaerobic capacity	Aerobic power	Fluid and mineral loss	Glycogen stores	Fat mobilization
Reaction time	Strength	Strength	Heat elimination	Fluid and mineral loss	Fat stores
Strength	Skill		Aerobic capacity	Heat elimination	Food intake
Skill				Fat mobilization	Protein reserves
Flexibility				Aerobic capacity	Bone and joint strength

intake [the peak oxygen intake for that task, a value 10–12 times the resting oxygen consumption when a young adult engages in a large-muscle exercise such as uphill treadmill running or pedaling a cycle ergometer (208)].

Associated with this aerobic response, there is a large increase of cardiac output (from a resting value of 5–6 L/min to a maximum of 25–30 L/min in a young man) and an even greater augmentation of respiratory minute volume [from perhaps 7 L/min to 90–120 L/min (210)]. If the intensity of effort is such that the accumulation of lactate in the bloodstream exceeds its rate of clearance [the so-called ventilatory threshold, around 70% of maximal oxygen intake (32, 264)], then the ventilation becomes disproportionate to oxygen consumption.

There are also increments of blood catecholamine levels (68,211,258, 260)—larger for exciting sports than for equivalent intensities of laboratory exercise.

Sustained Aerobic Activity

Traditional exercise prescriptions have called for bouts of aerobic exercise 30–60 min in duration. If physical activity is sustained for 30 min or longer, the intensity must be reduced to a level where there is little accumulation of lactate; the peak oxygen transport that can be sustained over this time frame is sometimes described as the *aerobic capacity.*

Depending on the person's choice of clothing and the environmental conditions, the local temperature within the active tissues rises by 1–4°C over the first 5 min of vigorous physical activity. The core temperature of the body also tends to stabilize, 1–4°C above its resting value, over 15–30 min of vigorous activity (10,101,246). Sweating is induced with a lag of a few minutes relative to the onset of exercise. Under adverse thermal conditions, a vigorous bout of physical activity can stimulate a flow of up to 2 L of sweat per hour (2,246). The corresponding tendency to depletion of fluid and mineral reserves (137,210) is less than in passive heat exposure, being partially offset by the liberation of up to 1.5 L of "bound" water as glycogen is metabolized.

The blood levels of many hormones increase during and following exercise (211,258). For instance, there is an increased output of cortisol (an index of stress), growth hormone [probably to facilitate fat mobilization (68,229,236)], and the hormones concerned with mineral and fluid balance (68,211). These changes depend in part on the rise in core temperature and are minimized if body temperature is "clamped"—for example, by exercising in cool water (43a).

Prolonged Physical Activity

Muscle glycogen stores vary with the extent of the training that has been undertaken, the recent diet of the individual, and the proportion of slow-twitch fibers in the body muscles (102,103). The average adult can exhaust carbohydrate reserves by about 100 min of exercise at 75% of maximal oxygen intake (the typical intensity adopted in prolonged bouts of an aerobic pursuit such as cross-country skiing or marathon running). Replenishment of glycogen stores proceeds relatively slowly, even given an optimal high-carbohydrate diet. Maximal levels are not reached for about 48 h following the activity, suggesting the value of restricting very prolonged bouts of exercise to alternate days.

Exercise bouts of 1 h and longer tend to cause a secretion of β-endorphins, with a corresponding elevation of mood (87,187). If the exercise bout is both prolonged and intense, local muscle microtrauma leads to a leakage of key proteins from the active skeletal muscles (and to a lesser extent from the myocardium). Such leakage is readily detected as increases in the serum concentrations of creatine kinase and lactate dehydrogenase (8). This response must be carefully distinguished from the increased serum enzyme levels that accompany myocardial infarction—for instance, by a study of isozyme patterns or the use of more specific markers of cardiac damage such as an increased blood level of cardiac troponin (44).

Microinjury is particularly marked if the activity calls for eccentric muscle contraction (for example, running downhill). The resulting inflammation has a negative influence upon a number of aspects of immune function (224,228). Often, normal immune function is regained within a few hours, but sometimes the disturbance may persist for as long as a week, and this may increase susceptibility to viral infections, at least temporarily (31a,151a).

Very Prolonged Physical Activity

Occasionally, people perform very prolonged bouts of exercise—for example, the woman who recently ran across Canada for a total of 112 days (138). Key factors in such circumstances are the ability to sustain a high level of food intake while exercising; the extent of initial fat and protein reserves; and the resistance of bones, joints, and tendons to severe repetitive stresses.

Type of Exercise

All of the patterns of physical activity discussed above are rhythmic in character. Contractions approach the isotonic condition, with little resistance opposing muscle shortening. This type of exercise is optimal in terms of developing cardiorespiratory function, but it does little to enhance muscle strength.

Resisted exercise (weight lifting and isometrics) was once criticized by cardiac specialists on the basis that it led to a large increase in systolic blood pressure and thus cardiac work rate. High pressures are eventually reached, but if the duration of individual contractions is limited to a few seconds and the individual is careful not to exhale against a closed glottis during the contraction, the rise of blood pressure may be no greater than in sustained endurance exercise (130).

Psychological Reactions

The immediate psychological response to a bout of vigorous exercise depends on the individual's initial psychological state and the environment in which the activity is performed. If the exerciser initially feels bored or depressed, then vigorous exercise (particularly with loud music or competitive excitement) may serve as an arousing stimulus (136,278), relieving these sensations. Perhaps for this reason, many people comment that exercise "makes them feel better."

On the other hand, if a person is initially anxious or overaroused, such activity is likely to increase anxiety; he or she needs a gentler, rhythmic type of activity, such as walking in pleasant and quiet surroundings (225). Those interested in the psychological benefits of physical activity are increasingly recommending moderate rather than all-out effort (121).

Physical activity influences sleep patterns in part because of direct influences upon neural arousal and in part because it stimulates the secretion of various hormones and cytokines (35,224). If moderate exercise is taken early in the day, it appears to facilitate sleep, enhancing the slow-wave component of the electroencephalogram (52). However, if vigorous exercise is taken too late at night, it has an arousing effect, making sleep difficult.

CHRONIC RESPONSES TO PHYSICAL ACTIVITY

Overall Effects of Training

If a subject repeats a given bout of exercise on a regular basis, then the body undergoes a progressive adaptation to the particular pattern of stress that has been imposed. Among functional consequences are (a) an increase in the ability to undertake that particular form of activity (that is, a higher peak rate of working becomes possible), (b) a progressive reduction in the disturbance of body function associated with a given intensity and duration of physical activity, and (c) a speedier rate of recovery following exercise (219).

Because the intensity of activity is usually lower and the duration often shorter, active living produces much smaller changes in physiological function than deliberate exercise, although there are claims that it provides almost as great benefit in terms of many aspects of health (23,258).

Specificity of Training

The adaptation of body function tends to be specific to the type of training that has been practiced. For example, there is little cross-transfer between cardiorespiratory and muscular training; indeed, very vigorous cardiorespiratory training may impede muscular development, possibly because of competing energy demands. Likewise, training of the arm muscles on a device such as an arm ergometer has little effect on performance when the subject is using the legs (127), although some 50% of the training effects developed by regular leg exercise can be transferred to the subsequent performance of aerobic work by the arms (42).

There also seems to be a specificity with respect to the intensity of activity, brief periods of intense exercise enhancing maximal performance and longer periods of more moderate exercise having a greater effect upon responses to submaximal effort.

Effects from Habituation and Learning

The earliest adaptations to repeated bouts of physical activity are cerebral in type, arising largely in the prefrontal cortex (72). Over the first few days, the body becomes "habituated" to a particular exercise situation (as do those who are supervising the activity), so that performance of what is becoming a familiar task induces less arousal (206). This type of adaptation is particularly important in the sedentary person who has not exercised for many years and who becomes anxious in response to the sensations associated with vigorous physical activity. As habituation proceeds, there is a parallel decrease in such physiological markers of arousal as the increment of heart rate and the rise of blood pressure observed at any given intensity of effort.

Some activities, such as walking, are already familiar to most adults; but if a program involves the acquisition of new skills, considerable learning can occur. As the task becomes more automatic, control is shifted from the special senses and the motor cortex to the cerebellum. Mechanical efficiency also improves, with a corresponding decrease in the loading of the respiratory system. The oxygen cost of a simple task such as treadmill walking may diminish by 10% over several days, and much larger changes are seen with the repeated performance of more complex activities such as swimming.

Functional Adjustments to Training

One group of training responses are functional in type: an improvement in the function of various organs without gross structural change.

Cardiovascular Function

The total blood volume and the tone of the peripheral veins are both increased by habitual physical activity, so that the stroke volume is better sustained during vigorous effort and the peak cardiac output is augmented (80,99,201,219).

At the same time, the distribution of the available blood flow becomes more effective from the viewpoint of performing physical work, so that the maximum arteriovenous oxygen difference is increased (108). In a trained individual, the circulation to inactive tissues shows a greater than normal reduction during physical activity, whereas there is an increase of flow to the active tissues (and to the skin in a hot climate) (190,237,238). In consequence, the maximal arteriovenous oxygen difference is larger in a trained than in an untrained person (108,237, 238).

Muscle Function

The muscles also appear stronger after training. This reflects an increased synchronization of neural firing, the mobilization of an increased fraction of the total motoneuron pool, and possibly a greater relaxation of antagonists (65). There are quite rapid increases of enzyme activity in the muscles as training continues (219, 272), although the precise balance of change between aerobic and anaerobic enzyme systems is somewhat specific to the type of exercise that has been pursued (77,98). Moreover, the ''purpose'' of any increase in aerobic enzyme activity seems to be to increase the proportion of fat metabolized rather than to facilitate the transport of oxygen to the working muscles (219,271).

Structural Changes Induced by Training

If the training is both protracted and vigorous, structural alterations eventually appear in a number of body systems.

Cardiovascular System

If the emphasis has been upon endurance training, there may be a progressive concentric hypertrophy of the left ventricular wall (43,95,122,191,222); Chapter 6); this reduces unit work per sarcomere in the ventricular wall (85) and facilitates maintenance of the ejection fraction and cardiac stroke volume at high work rates (219,248), with the development of a large maximal cardiac output. There have also been some claims of increases in either the dimensions coronary arteries or the collateral blood supply (97,109,254) and of an increase in the ventricular fibrillation threshold (153).

Respiratory System

Likewise, a strengthening of the respiratory muscles allows the subject to develop and sustain a larger maximal voluntary ventilation (185). Although ventilation rarely poses an absolute limit to oxygen transport, the effort tolerance of sedentary subjects is often limited by the sensation of breathlessness, and a strengthening of the respiratory muscles may raise the tolerated ceiling of ventilation. Benefit may be particularly large in asthma and chronic obstructive lung disease; in such patients, stronger muscles allow a rapid inspiration and a slow expiration, avoiding expiratory collapse of the airways (218).

Musculoskeletal System

If the emphasis of the training regimen has been upon isometric and isotonic muscle-building exercises, there will be an increase of muscle bulk in those body parts that have been active (61,65). In consequence, a given task can be performed at a smaller fraction of maximal voluntary force, with a smaller rise of blood pressure and less danger for the cardiovascular system.

The flexibility of the exercised joints is also increased, tendons and articular cartilages are strengthened (136a), and the density of bones subjected to gravitational or muscular forces is increased (39,51,244,269).

Metabolic System

If food intake remains unchanged, a further consequence of repeated, prolonged, moderate bouts of activity will be a progressive replacement of fat by lean tissue (216,236a), sometimes without any net change of body mass. For the person who is moderately obese, exercise offers a more effective remedy than dieting because it counters depression, conserves lean tissue, and may cause a small increase rather than a decrease in resting metabolic rate (14,139).

In general, hormonal reactions to a given intensity of exercise are reduced after training. For instance, there is a lesser secretion of catecholamines at any given rate of working (68,260). A given bout of exercise is usually perceived as less stressful (27), and—depending upon initial reactions—there may be an increase or decrease in the secretion of cortisol (229).

At any given intensity of effort, the tendency to subclinical muscle damage is also reduced with training. In consequence, there is a lesser release of enzymes such as creatine kinase (CK) and lactate dehydrogenase (LDH) into the circulation (8). Immune reactions are also less marked, but some features of the immune defenses, such as the resting count of natural killer cells, are increased (224).

Psychological Responses to Training

Psychological responses to a training program vary with the initial status of the individual. Little change is likely in the person with a well-balanced personality and a favorable mood state (121). However, in those who are initially anxious or depressed (for instance, as a consequence of a recent myocardial infarction), a more normal mood state is apparently restored by regular participation in an endurance training program (112). Perhaps because of the mood changes induced by endorphin secretion, there is some evidence that people can become addicted to prolonged bouts of exercise.

Time Course of Training and Detraining

The time course of the various physiological, biochemical, immunological, and psychological adaptations to the onset or cessation of training varies with the health of the individual, the pattern of conditioning (a progressively increasing load or a fixed-intensity program), and its intensity.

Much of the advantage of physical condition normally enjoyed by an endurance athlete is lost through 2–3 weeks of enforced bed rest or loss of normal gravitational stimuli (as in space travel) (197,250). Conversely, most of the physical condition that is lost during bed rest can be regained over a few weeks of renewed training (197) (Fig. 1). Hickson and associates (94) suggested that with

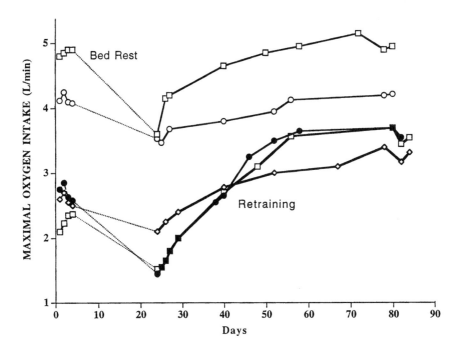

FIGURE 1   Decrease of maximal oxygen intake over 21 days of bed rest and time course of recovery with resumption of training. Data for three sedentary and two active young men. [Redrawn from Saltin, B., Blomqvist, B., Mitchell, J.H., Johnson, R.L., Wildenthal, K., and Chapman, C.B., Response to submaximal and maximal exercise after bed rest and training. *Circulation,* 38 (Suppl. 7): 1–68; used with permission.]

a constant training stimulus, the half-time for gains in maximal oxygen intake was as little as 10 days. However, critics of this work have pointed out that the normal training plan involves a progressive increase in both the intensity and the duration of effort rather than a constant training stimulus (110).

Given a progressive training plan, healthy 65-year-old subjects are still able to make large gains in their maximal oxygen intake over as little as 7 weeks of training (235). On the other hand, a person who has sustained a myocardial infarction either finds physical difficulty or lacks the confidence to exercise hard during the first few months following the clinical incident. In such patients (Fig. 2), the early training responses involve the peripheral rather than the central circulation (170), although after some 12 months of exercise at progressively increasing intensities, a small gain in cardiac stroke volume can be demonstrated (83, 170,182). The increase of maximal oxygen intake in "postcoronary" patients can continue slowly over several years provided that they are following a progressive training program (209).

Not all body systems respond in parallel. Saltin (194) drew attention to a discrepancy between tissue enzyme activity [which changes rapidly, over 7–10 days of training or detraining (93)] and maximal oxygen intake [which may con-

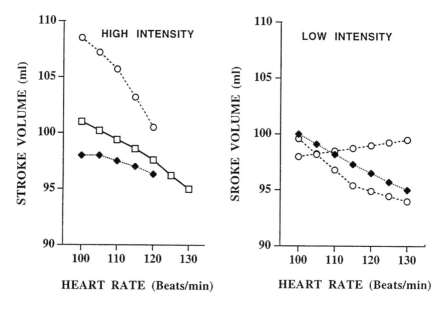

FIGURE 2   Influence of progressive endurance training on cardiac stroke volume. Data obtained on postcoronary patients following high-intensity or low-intensity exercise program for 6 and 12 months (Redrawn from Ref. 170; used with permission.)

tinue to increase over many weeks and months (209)]. In Saltin's view, this difference in time course suggests that the increase in maximal oxygen intake is due to central changes (particularly an increase of maximal cardiac output) rather than peripheral adaptations (enhanced enzyme activity and an increased extraction of oxygen from arterial blood). Smith and O'Donnell (242) noted that changes in ventilatory threshold developed faster than gains of maximal oxygen intake, which, in turn, changed faster than the heart rate response to submaximal exercise. In contrast, Rogers et al. (186) noted an improved response to submaximal exercise before gains in maximal oxygen intake. Possibly, such discrepancies reflect differences in the type or intensity of training.

The time course of psychological changes is known less precisely, since currently available tests of mood state and quality of life do not lend themselves to frequent repetition. We observed substantial improvements of affect in postcoronary patients when they were retested after a year of progressive training (112). In a sample with congestive heart failure, gains in quality of life were already present after four weeks of increased physical activity, and the response had only a moderate correlation with increases in aerobic power (234). Likewise, Stewart et al. (243) found an increase of self-efficacy after 12 weeks of training, but this bore little relation to gains in aerobic power.

EFFECTS OF INTENSITY, FREQUENCY, AND DURATION OF PHYSICAL ACTIVITY

The response to a training program is influenced by the intensity, frequency, and duration of physical activity relative to the initial fitness of the individual. Other variables influencing response include the type of activity performed, the age of the individual, fiber composition [those with a high proportion of slow-twitch fibers seem particularly susceptible to endurance training (193)], and other interindividual constitutional differences yet to be clarified (28).

Intensity

Need to Define Training Threshold

Whether the intent has been to develop cardiorespiratory performance, to enhance muscular strength, or to maintain good health and functional capacity, much of the classical literature on training has been built around the concept of a training threshold that must be reached in order to initiate a conditioning response.

Definition of the threshold has seemed important to the busy executive (who wishes to minimize personal investment of time and effort in fitness maintenance); to the international athlete (who wishes to maximize performance without

causing "staleness," tissue damage, immune dysfunction, and the negative psychological sequelae of "overtraining"); and to the older sedentary adult (who wishes to optimize health and function without provoking a heart attack). Recent position papers and consensus reports have substantially reduced the suggested threshold for many of the desired benefits of physical activity (5,23,258), but it still seems true that as a person becomes older, the margin between effective and dangerously intensive physical activity becomes narrower, with a corresponding need for greater sophistication in defining an appropriate program.

Need for Overloading

In physiological terms, some overloading of body systems must occur if there is to be a training response. If exercise is performed in an upright posture, cardiac stroke volume is not maximized until at least 50% of maximal oxygen intake is developed (12,56,237,238), (Table 2). The accompanying rise of systolic blood pressure (which offers an afterload to the ventricular muscle) is proportional to both the intensity of effort and its duration.

At the cellular level, the hypertrophy of skeletal and cardiac muscle is dependent on changes in both membrane permeability and the rate of protein transcription. Booth and Watson (26) found that in rats, muscle protein synthesis decreased during the first 30 min of exercise; but 7 h after activity, there was an increased net rate of protein formation. Potential triggers to the increase in protein synthesis included an increased intracellular concentration of amino acids brought

TABLE 2   Cardiovascular Responses to Arm (A) and to Leg (L) Exercise

Oxygen consumption (L/min STPD[a])	Stroke volume (ml)		Heart rate (beats/ min)		Cardiac output (L/min)		Arterio-venous oxygen difference (ml/L)	
	A	L	A	L	A	L	A	L
1.5	96	125	132	96	12.3	13.2	123	120
2.0	101	131	155	117	14.9	15.9	133	127
2.5	108	138	174	142	18.5	18.5	139	135
Maximal (2.79, A; 3.70, L)	103	138	178	179	18.3	24.7	144	150

[a]STPD: Standard temperature and pressure, dry gas.
Note: In both forms of activity, the stroke volume of the heart shows a small increase to more than 50% of the task-specific peak oxygen intake.
Source: From Ref. 238, used with permission.

about by a tension-induced degradation of protein, an increased influx of amino acids via the stretched sarcolemma of the loaded muscle, and an impact of decreasing intracellular adenosine triphosphate (ATP) and pH levels on Ca^{2+}-mediated stimulation of ribonucleic acid (RNA) transcription (26). Growth hormone and insulin-like growth factors (somatomedins) may also be involved (119), although a combination of such hormones and regular exercise seems essential for hypertrophy of either cardiac or skeletal muscle.

A moderate overload is also desirable from a psychological perspective. Sedentary people need to become accustomed to the sensations associated with vigorous exercise. Nevertheless, it is also important that they regard the suggested intensity of physical activity as appropriate to their personal training goals. Recruits will sometimes drop out of exercise classes, either because the required programs are perceived as not sufficiently challenging or (more commonly) because they seem beyond the capacity of the participant.

Dangers of Overloading

Excessive overloading may cause both local muscular lesions and systemic effects.

At the tissue level, local hypoxia and excessive changes in membrane permeability may allow a leakage of vital cellular constituents into the extracellular space, and frank microtrauma may give rise to an inflammatory response (9,131, 155), with delayed-onset muscle soreness and pain (15,44,224).

Prolonged and intensive cardiovascular effort may cause cardiac fatigue and pulmonary edema, even in a healthy young adult (36,183,265). The response is observed a few hours postexercise—too quickly to be attributed to muscle injury or a reaction analogous to the acute respiratory distress syndrome. It could be no more than an acute fluid overload (the ingestion of too much fluid or swimming in cold water) or a reaction to the inhalation of cold, dry, or polluted air; nevertheless, alterations of cardiac impedance in some instances have suggested a transient disturbance of myocardial function.

A small increase in cardiac preloading or afterloading is not critical, but an excessive rise of systolic pressure in a patient with coronary atherosclerosis can provoke myocardial ischemia, ventricular fibrillation, and even cardiac failure (167,209). Likewise, heavy preloading can provoke decompensation in a patient with a tendency to congestive heart failure.

In skeletal muscle also, it is necessary to develop an increase of tension for hypertrophy to occur, but an excessive loading during contraction (as in eccentric effort) can give rise to microscopic or gross muscular damage (133,134,155,157).

Classical Concept of the Cardiovascular Threshold

The classical concept of a cardiovascular training threshold is commonly attributed to Karvonen et al. (107), who studied training responses in male medical students. In some of the group, the speed of running yielded an average heart rate of 135 beats per minute; in these individuals, the cardiovascular responses to exercise remained unchanged. Other students exercised more vigorously, reaching a final heart rate of 160–180 beats per minute; in these individuals, it was necessary to increase the treadmill speed by 25–30% over a 4-week period in order to maintain a constant exercise heart rate.

Subsequent authors have sought to apply the findings of Karvonen et al. (107) to subjects of all ages, regardless of their initial physical condition. Some investigators have interpreted the cardiorespiratory training threshold as lying at 60% of the difference between resting and maximal heart rates (about 145 beats per minute in a young adult); others have inferred a threshold at 60% of maximal oxygen intake (about 135 beats per minute in a young adult); and a few authors have even suggested that the threshold lies at 60% of maximal heart rate (about 117 beats per minute). In fact, Karvonen et al. (107) did not define any universally generalizable threshold, although their data did show that if the stimulus was a brief period of treadmill exercise, a cardiovascular training response occurred at a heart rate of 170 beats per minute but not at 135 beats per minute.

The intensity of any threshold for the enhancement of cardiorespiratory function is probably modified by both the initial fitness of the individual and the duration of the activity. Certainly, there are some circumstances where training can occur at exercise heart rates of less than 160–180 beats per minute. Bouchard et al. (29) apparently produced some cardiovascular training at a heart rate of 130 beats per minute for no more than 10 min/day. Likewise, Durnin et al. (54) observed substantial improvement in the endurance fitness of young soldiers who walked 10–30 km/day at heart rates that are unlikely to have exceeded 120 beats per minute.

Oja (163) maintained that the physiological responses to walking matched those obtained with a jogging regimen, and others have since supported this view, at least for older individuals (226). One possible factor contributing to the effectiveness of walking programs for the middle aged and elderly is that fast walking brings many such individuals to 70% of their maximal oxygen intake (179). A further consideration is that a sedentary lifestyle has increases responsiveness to training. Restriction of recent activity is a particular feature of patients who have recently been hospitalized for myocardial infarction; among such individuals, there may be an initial cardiovascular training response to exercise heart rates as low as 110 beats per minute.

Empirical Assessments of Training Threshold

Multiple regression analysis of data from a series of treadmill experiments—where young, healthy male subjects were randomly allocated to laboratory-controlled training regimens differing in intensity, frequency, and duration (205)—

demonstrated that the intensity of effort relative to initial fitness was the most important determinant of cardiovascular response (Fig. 3).

Subsequent experiments, mainly with university-age males, have not greatly clarified determinants of the training response. Reports have claimed an effect of intensity (59); of intensity but not initial fitness (73); of both intensity and fitness (204), with intensity becoming insignificant after equating the total amount of work performed (203); of intensity despite equation of initial fitness and total amount of work performed (267); and of intensity and duration (47).

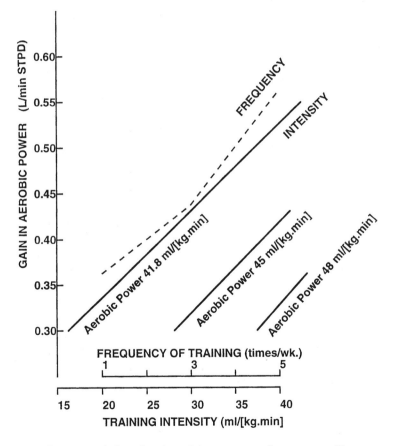

FIGURE 3   Factors influencing the training response of young men. The response to any given intensity of training varies inversely as the initial aerobic power of the group. If intensity and fitness are held constant, there is also a difference of response between one, three, and five training sessions per week. (Redrawn from Ref. 205; used by permission.)

Wenger and Bell (266) further claimed that the impact of a training program continued to increase with intensity of exercise up to loads demanding 90–100% of maximal oxygen intake.

The issues of initial physical condition and training intensity are particularly critical in comparing responses between young and elderly subjects. If the assessment of initial physical condition is based upon absolute figures rather than age-related standards, reactions may be compared (inappropriately) between a sedentary young adult and an extremely fit senior citizen. Likewise, if the intensity of training prescribed for a 65-year-old subject is equated with that of a young adult in terms of the absolute oxygen consumption developed during the required exercise program (198), the stimulus applied to the older person is much greater; in consequence, such a person may be judged as having a better training response than a younger individual. However, if the comparison is based upon programs demanding an equivalent fraction of the individual's maximal oxygen intake, then the training response depends much less strongly upon the age of the participant (226).

Classical wisdom set the optimal intensity of cardiorespiratory training for the average person at or just below a work rate where lactate began to accumulate (the so-called ventilatory or anaerobic threshold). This amounts to 60–70% of personal maximal oxygen intake in most sedentary individuals but may reach 75–80% of aerobic power in endurance competitors (3). An appropriate intensity of effort was then set for each individual in terms of a prescribed distance and pace (110). Alternatively, the subject was instructed to count the pulse rate during or immediately following a bout of exercise (25), although various circumstances (administration of β-blocking agents, cardiac transplantation, paraplegia) often precluded use of this index. Other options were to seek an intensity of exercise that initiates some sweating (118) and is perceived as moderate or somewhat hard while allowing continuation of a normal conversation (21,27,39,232).

Current Concepts of Training Threshold

During the last few years, there has been a growing realization that an intensity of exercise that is insufficient to alter cardiovascular physiology may nevertheless be sufficient to reduce other cardiovascular risk factors and thus diminish susceptibility to future cardiovascular disease.

Blair (23) has argued that the greatest improvement in cardiovascular prognosis is associated with progression from the lowest level of cardiorespiratory fitness [an aerobic power of 6 METs (MET-metabolic equivalent) to the next level (7 METs); although there are additional gains from a further improvement in physical condition.

On the basis of such arguments, the American College of Sports Medicine (5) and other organizations (169,258) have revised the recommendation downward, advocating 30 min of moderate-intensity activity (3–6 METs—for example, walking at 4.8–6.4 km/h) on most and preferably all days of the week. In contrast, Morris and associates (144,146) maintain that in Britain at least, activity must reach a *minimum* intensity of 31 kJ/min (7.5 kcal/min, 6 METs) in order to lead to any health benefit.

The issue remains to be resolved, but it seems reasonable to conclude that a little exercise is better than none and that more vigorous activity will carry greater dividends (166). Although some cardiac risk factors such as obesity are countered by quite light exercise, the slowing of exercise heart rate and reduction of blood pressure induced by more vigorous physical activity also make a valuable contribution to the enhancement of cardiovascular prognosis and functional ability. Inadequate strength and cardiovascular capacity are important causes of a decreasing quality of life in the frail elderly (Chap. 5).

Training Anaerobic Systems

Interval training offers a means of enhancing anaerobic power, anaerobic capacity, or aerobic power (11,55,89), depending on the length of exercise and recovery phases. Training of the anaerobic energy systems is facilitated if the effective body mass is increased during exercise sessions—for example, by carrying a backpack or wearing a 9–10 kg vest while training (192).

High intensities of effort are tolerated if intervals are brief (for instance, 10- to 30-s bouts of activity, followed by 10- to 30-s recovery periods). Such training leads to an increase of both glycogen stores and alkaline reserve in the active limbs, with increased local concentrations of ATP, myoglobin, and possibly of glycolytic enzymes (210). Longer intervals (1-min bouts of exercise followed by 1-min recovery periods) are particularly effective in enhancing the performance of patients when endurance activity would otherwise be halted by anginal pain (110).

Muscle-Training Threshold

The intensity of effort influences patterns of muscle fiber recruitment and thus the localization of training responses within the skeletal muscles. Moderate effort recruits predominantly slow-twitch fibers (1), selectively enhancing their function and increasing tolerance of fatiguing activity over several weeks. There are increases in the size, number, and complexity of mitochondria within the active fibers, with a corresponding increase in aerobic enzyme activity (98) (Fig. 4). The capillary/fiber ratio is also enhanced (251,95). However, there is little increase in the cross-section of individual muscle fibers. One consequence of these changes is that fat rather than glycogen is metabolized during prolonged bouts of activity (117,211) (Fig. 5).

More intensive resistance and isometric programs selectively recruit fast-

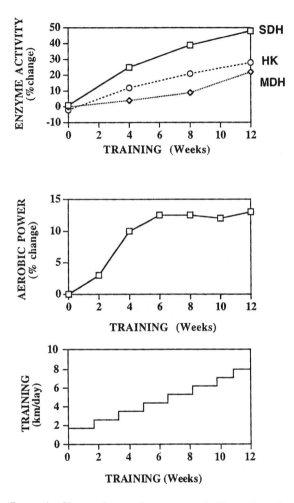

FIGURE 4 Changes in muscle enzyme activities and maximal oxygen intake in response to 12 weeks of swim training. SDH, HK, and MDH signify succinate dehydrogenase, hexokinase, and malate dehydrogenase, respectively. [Redrawn from Wilmore, J.H., and Costill, D.L., *Training for Sport and Physical Activity.* 3rd Ed. W.C. Brown. Dubuque, Iowa (1988); used with permission.]

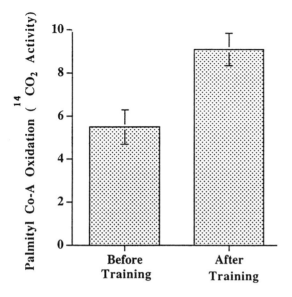

FIGURE 5   The effect of 8 weeks of endurance training upon the ability of skeletal muscle to oxidize fats. [From Wilmore, J.H., and Costill, D.L., *Training for Sport and Physical Activity.* 3rd Ed. W.C. Brown, Dubuque, Iowa, 1988, used with permission.]

twitch (type II) fibers. There is a hypertrophy (255) and sometimes a splitting of type II fibers (78), although it is still unclear if there is a true hyperplasia with the formation of new muscle fibers (240,250). Because of the increased amount of contractile protein within individual fibers, hypertrophy may cause some diminution in the volume density of the muscle mitochondria (129). The acute cellular response to functional overload is a slowing of protein synthesis within the muscle sarcoplasm; but within 24 h, supranormal rates of protein formation are observed. If the overload is too great, the muscles may become sore. There is then a disruption of connective tissue elements and an increase in the hydroxyproline/creatine ratio for the tissue (257), and the mitochondria may also show evidence of damage, particularly a swelling and destruction of their cristae (8,15,64).

Muscle training is usually associated with some change in the relative proportions of type IIa (fast oxidative glycolytic) and type IIb (fast glycolytic) fibers. Moreover, there is increasing evidence that high-intensity intermittent training may convert type I (slow-twitch) fibers into type II (50,100,239,253).

The appropriate intensity of effort for muscle-building exercises is usually set at a fraction of maximal voluntary force. Muscle endurance is developed by frequently repeated sets of contractions at 60% of maximal voluntary force, whereas strength is enhanced by higher-intensity contractions with only a limited number of repetitions (6a,81,86). During isometric effort, there also appears to be an interaction between the intensity and duration of contraction. Thus, Hettinger (92) observed a training response to maximal contractions that were held for 1–2 s; but if the intensity of effort was reduced to 67% of maximal force, then the minimal duration of contraction for a training response was 4–6 s. With further prolongation of the contraction, a training response was observed at forces as low as 40–50% of maximal voluntary effort.

Psychological Threshold

There is little objective information on an appropriate intensity of training from the viewpoint of inducing psychological gains. However, if the training program is to be perceived by the participant as achievable and yet effective, the optimal intensity is probably similar to that discussed in connection with physiological and biochemical gains. Most subjects perceive effort at the anaerobic threshold as moderately demanding.

Frequency

Relation to Recovery Processes

The optimal frequency of training has physiological, biochemical, immunological, psychological, and pathological connotations that can be related to the anticipated time course of both acute exercise responses and the speed of recovery processes.

The on-transient has been discussed above. The likely speed of recovery varies with the type, intensity, and duration of activity. Muscle phosphagen stores are replenished extremely rapidly (49), allowing a second burst of activity to draw upon such stores within a few seconds. Interval training designed to enhance anaerobic power may thus allow recovery periods as short as 10–60 s (273).

If activity continues long enough that lactate accumulates, muscle lactate concentrations fall substantially over the first 15–30 min of recovery. Thus, a second bout of effort is possible within an hour or so. Such training tends to maximize anaerobic capacity. Aerobic training can also be split into two or more sessions per day, apparently with little decrease in its effectiveness (5,169,258); this is a helpful tactic in the early stages of aerobic training for older adults.

If the main concerns are to permit an increase of protein synthesis, to restore glycogen reserves, and to repair muscle microtrauma while avoiding suppression of the immune system, then it may be desirable to carry out intensive training on every second day or at most to alternate "light" and "heavy" days of training. Glycogen stores peak 48 h after the last bout of exercise (196), and muscle soreness and abnormal blood levels of muscle-derived enzymes persist for several days after a very strenuous bout of exercise (9,44).

Empirical Data

Most empirical data sets have shown an increase in cardiovascular training as the frequency of exercise sessions is increased from one to five sessions per week (176,205,235), although not all studies have found this (16). One variable is probably the extent of overtraining that occurs during individual exercise sessions.

There may also be some interindividual variation. Thus Linden et al. (125a) found that some subjects could maintain their cardiovascular condition by as little as two bouts of exercise per week, but others needed daily training. The greater effectiveness of an increased frequency of training may be related to a consequent increase in the total amount of exercise that is taken (96). Plainly, many of the processes involved in training, from an increase of protein synthesis to the metabolism of excess body fat, must be related to the number of times a given stress is presented and/or the total quantity of work performed.

The current recommendation for those pursuing a moderate intensity of exercise is that this be pursued on "most" days of the week (5,169,258).

Psychological Considerations

The main psychological argument against recommending a low frequency of physical activity (such as one or two exercise sessions per week) is that the prescription is then easily forgotten by the patient. In contrast, sessions that are incorporated into the daily routine through encouragement of "active living" become much more automatic. Habit is an important determinant of exercise behavior (74) (Fig. 6), and activities such as walking or cycling to and from work (262) can form a valuable keystone of such a lifestyle.

If exercise sessions are infrequent, their intensity must be increased in order to obtain an adequate response. There is then a danger that the participant will become excessively fatigued. Attempts to meet a week's physical activity requirements in a single session may precipitate activity for which the individual is ill prepared, setting the stage for an exercise-induced cardiac catastrophe (220). Regular, moderate exercise is much less likely to cause myocardial infarction or cardiac arrest (261).

At the opposite extreme, if the frequency of the exercise makes excessive time demands, then the subject may complain of staleness, fatigue, boredom, or "lack of time," and there is a strong likelihood that the program will be abandoned. Psychological problems are particularly likely if the patient has pursued the activity to the point of excluding normal social contacts, if a further investment of time and effort does not appear to be yielding commensurate gains of

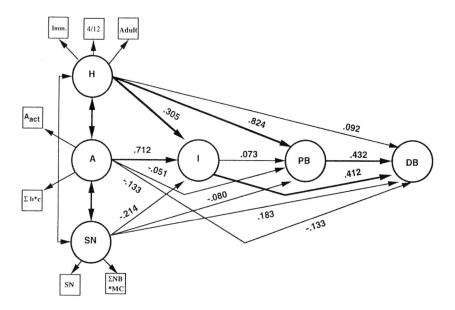

FIGURE 6   An empirical model illustrating the factors influencing exercise behavior. The technique of path analysis has been used to examine relationships between habit (H), attitude (A), subjective norms (SN), behavioral intentions (I), proximal behavior (PB), and distal behavior (DB). The strongest correlations are indicated by the heavier arrows. Thus, attitudes influence intention and distal behavior, whereas habits have a strong influence upon intention and proximal behavior. [Redrawn from Godin, G., Valois, P., Shephard, R.J., and Desharnais, R., Prediction of leisure-time exercise behavior: A path analysis (Lisrel V) model. *J. Behav. Med.,* 10: 145–158 (1987); used with permission.]

physical condition, or if muscle soreness, pain, and injuries have resulted from excessive amounts of exercise.

From the psychological viewpoint, the ideal program is thus sufficiently frequent to become habitual but such as to leave the participant ample opportunity for other pursuits.

Duration

The duration of an exercise bout influences the impact of a given intensity of exercise upon the training response. For example, sessions of at least 10 min are probably needed in order to induce aerobic training by moderate physical activity. However, because of acute adaptive reactions, two moderate-length bursts of activity may induce a training response as large as or even larger than a single bout of equivalent total duration.

This generalization is particularly true of neurological and psychological adaptations. For instance, the progressive decrease of exercise heart rate with habituation to a given form of physical activity depends more upon the number of times the activity has been attempted than on the duration of individual sessions.

If a primary intent of physical activity is to consume an excess of body fat, there is a roughly stoichiometric relationship between fat loss and the added energy cost of the exercise plus any postexercise stimulation of metabolism (139). However, prolonged bouts of exercise tend to induce a progressive increase in the metabolic response to a given rate of performance of external work (38). Moreover, because more fat and less carbohydrate are metabolized during low-intensity effort, prolonged slow walking may be a more effective method of inducing fat loss than an apparently equivalent energy expenditure that is developed by short bursts of more intensive activity. Optimization of the blood lipid profile requires an energy expenditure equivalent to that incurred by walking or jogging 18–20 km/week (113,270) (Fig. 7), again a measure of the quantity of exercise that is undertaken, rather than the frequency or duration of individual bouts.

On the other hand, some of the reactions to overload—for instance, the rise of blood pressure with sustained rhythmic or isometric exercise—are proportional to the duration of the individual bout of activity. A short period of vigorous exercise may provide a very valuable stimulus to both the cardiovascular system and the skeletal muscles, but if the effort is more prolonged, it may give rise to acute manifestations of myocardial ischemia or strain of the skeletal muscles. Biochemical (44), humoral (120), and immunological (115,224) evidence of overstrain is associated particularly with very prolonged bouts of exercise, whereas the development of gross musculoskeletal injuries can also be correlated with attempts to cover more than a specific jogging distance per week (177). For the average middle-aged person, a useful ceiling of effort is probably a weekly fast-walking or jogging distance of about 50 km; that is, 10 km/day, 5 days/week.

Empirical data show that although the duration of activity has some influence on the magnitude of the training response, the impact of this variable is less than that of intensity (47,205). Nevertheless, prolonged, moderate activity such as brisk walking may be a more practical form of training than shorter periods of more intensive effort, both for a person who wishes to exercise while commuting to a workplace that lacks shower facilities (262) and for an older individual who might be endangered by a more intensive bout of physical effort (261).

Effects of Type of Exercise

Endurance Training

Assuming that intensity, frequency, and duration of physical activity are controlled, does it matter what type of endurance activity is undertaken? In terms

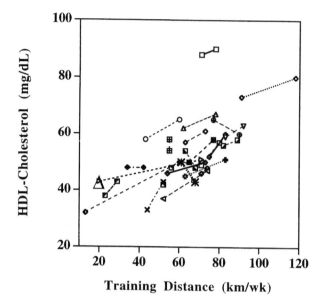

FIGURE 7   The influence of weekly jogging distance on serum levels of HDL cholesterol. Data for postcoronary patients. Each line joins observations on a single subject over a period of 1 year. During this period, some subjects increased and some decreased their weekly jogging distance, generally with a corresponding change in HDL cholesterol concentrations. The larger triangle indicates average values for patients who were content with a more modest exercise prescription. (Redrawn from Ref. 113; used with permission.)

of one criterion of cardiorespiratory response (the increment of maximal oxygen intake), Beaudet (18) found no difference in reactions to swimming, running, and cycling programs. Likewise, Milburn and Butts (140) reported that in terms of gains of oxygen transport, aerobic dance was just as effective as a jogging program.

Nevertheless, some specificity of the training response can be identified with respect to task learning, habituation, and local circulatory adaptations. Other important issues are the volume of muscle that is activated, the effects of adopting different postures while exercising, and subjective preferences.

Task Learning.   As a specific task is repeated, the various component movements become more automatic in type. Control is transferred progressively from the motor cortex to the cerebellum. At the same time, movements become mechanically more efficient; in consequence, the oxygen cost of working at any given speed is decreased (205). Such task learning affects the heart rate response and the perception of effort for a given task, but except in exceptional circumstances, there is little transfer from one task to another of the skills that are acquired.

Habituation.   Habituation is a form of negative conditioning that is peculiar to a given investigator and the conditions of a particular experiment (72,205). Initially, anxiety provoked by the investigator and the laboratory setting may cause a substantial cardiac response from about one subject in four. As a task is repeated and it becomes perceived as less threatening, the heart rate, blood pressure, ventilatory response, and humoral reactions all diminish. This type of adaptation depends on the integrity of the prefrontal cortex (72).

Much of the total habituation occurs over the first two or three exposures to an unfamiliar situation. A part of the process is highly task-specific, but there may also be a partial transfer of adaptations to similar tasks, particularly if the investigator and the general laboratory setting remain unchanged.

Local Circulatory Adaptations.   If training is undertaken by a relatively small group of muscles—for instance, when using an arm ergometer, a pulley system (82), or a swim bench (70)—many of the circulatory adaptations are local in type. The subject can develop a larger peak oxygen intake while using the arms, but little of this gain in performance is transferred to forms of exercise that use the legs (42,127,188). During maximal leg effort, such specificity of training seems more marked for the cycle ergometer than for the treadmill (probably because cycling is heavily dependent on quadriceps strength). However, during submaximal effort, the converse seems to be true, adaptations to the treadmill being more specific than those for a cycle ergometer (60); this may possibly reflect the perceived safety of the two forms of exercise.

The precise mechanisms responsible for specific improvements in performance are still debated. Conceivably, a local strengthening of the muscles allows them to contract at a smaller fraction of their maximal voluntary force (219), facilitating a better perfusion of the working limbs. However, in general, endurance training does not induce a major hypertrophy of skeletal muscle.

Alternatively, there may be a local increase of muscle capillarization (45, 184,202,247), with an increased activity of aerobic enzymes. Both of these changes would facilitate oxygen extraction by the active muscles (45). However, the intramuscular extraction of oxygen is fairly complete even prior to training (194), and it is hard to envisage how the muscular arteriovenous oxygen difference could undergo any major increase with conditioning. A third hypothesis is that training induces a greater neural traffic between local chemoreceptors in the exercised limb and cardiovascular centers in the brainstem; such a response might cause a local vasodilatation, facilitating the development of a larger peak oxygen intake.

If the training regimen involves large muscle groups, the condition of the central circulation usually improves, and the enhanced function is generalizable to other types of exercise (Fig. 8). Training may ultimately induce some cardiac hypertrophy, but immediate gains in cardiac output reflect an increased central blood volume (greater preloading), an increase of myocardial contractility, and a decrease of arterial blood pressure at a given work rate (decreased afterloading). Thus Wilmore et al. (272) found a transfer of training from cycling or jogging to treadmill performance, and White (268) reported that the trampoline was as effective a method of improving cardiorespiratory function as cycling or treadmill exercise. However, Daub et al. (46) noted that participation in ice hockey (a more intermittent and ''anaerobic'' type of activity) had no influence on the maximal oxygen intake that could be developed during skating or cycling, and Wilmore et al. (272) found no gains of treadmill performance after involvement in a 20-week tennis program.

It may finally be asked how far cardiovascular training interferes with muscular training or vice versa. It is possible to develop cardiovascular and muscular function simultaneously, but excessive endurance training hampers the development of muscular strength (53), particularly in parts of the body that are not actively involved in the aerobic program.

Volume of Active Muscle. The volume of active muscle influences the rise of systemic blood pressure, the extent of fatigue, and the magnitude of the training response.

Central cardiovascular training generally requires involvement of a sub-

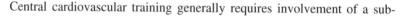
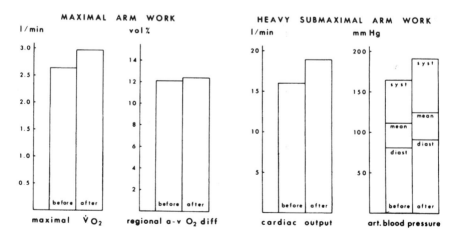

FIGURE 8 Findings during bouts of rhythmic arm exercise, performed before and after training of the legs on a cycle ergometer. Note that some of the training response is transferred from the legs to the arms [from Clausen, J. P. in Limiting Factors of Physical Performance, J. Keul ed. Thieme, Stuttgart, (1973); used with permission].

stantial muscle mass; the usual recommendation is to involve as much of the body musculature as possible. Appropriate activities include walking, jogging, running, vigorous swimming, cycling, and particularly cross-country skiing (110). However, attempts to increase the effectiveness of leg exercise by carrying hand-held weights have achieved only limited success (13,41). Negative features of arm loading include greater discomfort, greater impact stress while jogging, and a larger rise of systemic blood pressure [particularly in hypertensive patients (79)].

If a similar oxygen consumption is developed using a smaller muscle mass (for example, the arms rather than the legs), then increases in heart rate and blood pressure are greater, with a corresponding increase in cardiac work rate and associated risks of myocardial ischemia (154). A high-intensity circuit training program that involves extensive arm work can be very stressful, with a large secretion of epinephrine and norepinephrine (171). In general, the rise of blood pressure during muscular effort is proportional to the fraction of maximal voluntary force that is exerted (48), although very small muscles such as those involved in finger movements have a lesser impact on systemic blood pressure (75). A further variable is fiber type. Other factors being equal, the rise of systemic blood pressure is greater if the activated muscle has a high proportion of fast-twitch fibers (67).

The peak heart rate is generally lower with arm than with leg exercise (231, 237,238). This reflects a limitation of effort by peripheral muscular fatigue rather than cardiovascular performance. The rating of perceived exertion is approximately proportional to heart rate, but the muscular component of overall sensation is greater with small- than with large-muscle activities.

Deliberate training of small muscles is useful if a person's occupation calls for use of that particular group of muscles. If the muscles concerned have become weak through a period away from work (particularly immobilization or bed rest due to injury or a heart attack), such specific training may facilitate a return to normal or modified employment (65,66).

Posture.   Most forms of human endurance exercise are performed either standing or seated. Maintenance of the upright posture involves a large fraction of the body musculature but has the disadvantage that cardiac preloading is reduced, at least until the function of the muscle pump has overcome gravitational pooling in the capacity vessels of the lower half of the body. A somewhat larger cardiovascular response to training might be anticipated with the one form of exercise that is easily performed from a lying position—moderate-intensity swimming. In this situation, a combination of the horizontal posture, water pressure, and cooling of the superficial veins by the water increase the central blood volume and thus ventricular preloading.

Support of the body mass by immersion in water (123,213) or by sitting on a chair (132) can be particularly helpful to the frail elderly who wish to obtain some exercise despite degenerative changes in their knee joints or the lower part of the spine.

Certain postures where all or part of the body mass must be supported by prolonged isometric contraction place an additional strain on the circulation, particularly if the subject also performs a Valsalva maneuver in an attempt to increase muscular force. A rise of both systemic blood pressure and heart rate increases the cardiac work rate, and there is a corresponding increase in the risk of myocardial ischemia. An extended bout of "push-ups," for example, may be inadvisable for an older person with established cardiovascular disease.

Posture may finally be important in terms of sustaining bone mass. Some authors have argued that the prevention of osteoporosis is dependent on weight-bearing activity, suggesting that swimming would be a less desirable recommendation than rapid walking (51). Others have found benefit also from the action of vigorous muscle contractions, noting unusual bone development in the playing arm in tennis players (175).

Subjective Preferences.   If physiological responses to two possible types of physical activity are roughly comparable, much of the choice between alternatives should be based on the individual's motives for exercising, available skills, and available resources.

Many otherwise excellent exercise programs are ineffective because of poor patient compliance. Among possible techniques to increase participation, one obvious approach is to tailor the recommendation to subjective preferences. If the prime motivation of the individual is the enhancement of personal health, the meeting of an ascetic challenge, or stress relaxation (116), a solitary activity such as jogging or rapid distance walking may be an appropriate suggestion; but if the search is for competition, a vigorous individual or team sport may be more appropriate. If the desire is for increased social contacts, a gymnastic or social dance program may prove the optimal recommendation. Those with an "external locus of control" also have a greater need of external supervision and encouragement. Bassey et al. (17) found only limited gains of function when an unsupervised aerobics program was made available to factory workers. Kavanagh and Shephard (111) also commented that the physiological gains realized in a home exercise program were smaller than those achieved during a standard rehabilitation center–based cardiac program.

One important factor discouraging exercise is failure to reach a level of performance where the activity becomes enjoyable. There may also be defections because of inadequate cash reserves. Account should be taken of equipment already available to the patient, the availability of financial resources to purchase equipment essential to a particular type of pursuit, and opportunity costs involved in travel to and attendance at a specific fitness center (Chapter 22).

Finally, account must be taken of the negative impact of injuries. Injury is often associated with an excessive intensity and/or an excessive volume of physical activity. For instance, the incidence of injuries among joggers rises steeply above a weekly distance of 33–50 km/week (168,178,263). Some activities are more prone to cause injuries than others. For example, skipping seems a more frequent cause of damage than jogging (171), and—in Europe, at least—competitive sports are a frequent cause of injuries in young adults (150). Aerobic dance also has a bad reputation, probably due as much to program design (an excessive number of sessions per week) as to improper footwear or excessively hard floor surfaces (69,189). About 50% of aerobic dance participants and as many as 75% of instructors report injuries (189), although most of the complaints are relatively minor in nature (69).

Muscular Training

As with endurance training, there is some commonality of training response between different types of muscle-strengthening regimens. For example, Gettman et al. (71) found similar increments of lean mass in response to isotonic or isokinetic circuit training. Likewise, Manning et al. (135) found no difference in strength gains between variable- and constant-resistance isokinetic training.

However, there is also some specificity with respect to the velocity of contraction (84,106,188) and the joint angle tested. Those who train using rapid contractions increase their power during rapid movements, whereas those who train with slower movements increase mainly their ability to make slower contractions. Presumably, this reflects differences in the recruitment of muscle fibers during training. Isometric training is particularly liable to increase strength only at the specific joint angle involved in conditioning (92). This is partly a question of specific muscle development and partly an example of test learning, which can give a misleading impression of gains in strength in longitudinal experiments.

If training stops, muscle strength and power are conserved longer than aerobic power (62); indeed, no loss of function may be detectable over the first 4–6 weeks of detraining (149).

EFFECTS OF ENVIRONMENT

General Considerations

Training exposes the body to physical and sometimes psychological stress. An adverse environment heightens the intensity of stress for any given level of energy expenditure. The training response may be enhanced, but at the same time there is a danger of exceeding the optimal or "eu-stress" level to which adaptation is possible. Certainly, the risks of physical activity increase in extreme environments, and the individual's motivation and ability to train may also be reduced.

Hot Environments

Heat stress is not confined to tropical regions. If a radiant heat load of perhaps 100 W is imposed by exposure to bright sunlight (151), vigorous physical activity can cause serious heat stress over half an hour or less, even if the ambient temperature is only moderately warm. Thus, it is important to monitor the core temperatures of those who are undertaking prolonged bouts of strenuous exercise, even in supposedly temperate climates.

Dangers. Overexertion in the heat presents many dangers, ranging from skin rashes and infections to the major risks of heat exhaustion, heat collapse, hyperthermia, and heat stroke (101,125,210,246). The most vulnerable are individuals with a low maximal cardiac output—the unfit, the elderly, and particularly those with cardiac disease. Partly because of the increase in resting cardiac output and also because of the disturbances of mineral balance induced by prolonged sweating, hot weather increases cardiac mortality among such individuals (58,158,199).

Classical industrial studies have shown an increase in accidents as heat stress becomes excessive (259). A similar increase in the risk of physical injury seems likely if voluntary exercise is performed in a hot environment.

Heat increases cerebral arousal and thus augments the perception of exertion at any given fraction of an individual's maximal oxygen intake, invalidating exercise prescriptions set in a temperate environment (7,27,33). Partly for this reason, people take less voluntary activity in hot climates.

Finally, a heat-induced depletion of fluid and mineral reserves causes various long-term pathologies, including a feeling of neurasthenia and an irritability that interferes with participation in team activities (137,210,275).

Preventive Measures.   The primary means of avoiding exercise-induced heat problems (Table 3) is to change the locale or to moderate the intensity of physical activity when the wet bulb globe thermometer reading or other index of effective temperature (210) exceeds specified limits (3,4,252). The general population can often find appropriately cool conditions by use of a swimming pool or air-conditioned gymnasium or by a shift in the timing of activity sessions to the cooler parts of the day. Nevertheless, repeated bouts of heavy sweating can cause cumulative disturbances of mineral ion concentrations in plasma, and patients with known cardiac disease should be counseled to moderate the intensity of their physical activity and/or to seek further medical advice if they notice that hot weather is causing an increase in abnormal heart rhythms or an earlier onset of exercise-induced anginal pain.

TABLE 3   Prevention of Heat Injuries During Distance Running

Initial education
Runners should be taught how to recognize the early warning symptoms that precede heat injury (piloerection on the chest and arms, chilling, throbbing pressure in the head, unsteadiness, nausea, and a dry skin).

Medical preparations
Prior arrangements should be made with medical personnel for treatment of heat injury, with responsible and informed personnel at each "water station." Organizational personnel should reserve the right to stop runners who show signs of heat stroke or heat exhaustion.

Thermal limits
Distance races >16 km should not take place if the wet bulb/globe temperature (WB-GT) exceeds 28°C (WB-GT = 0.7 (WB) + 0.2 (GT) + 0.1 (DBT), where WB = wet bulb, GT = globe temperature, and DBT = dry bulb temperature). During periods of the year when daytime temperatures often exceed 27°C, distance races should be conducted before 9 A.M. or after 4 P.M.

Fluid replacement
Water stations should be provided at intervals of 3–4 km over races of 16 km and longer.

Recommendation of American College of Sports Medicine (1975):
　　　　<2.5% glucose, <10 mmol/L sodium, <5mmol/L potassium
400 to 500 ml 10–15 min before event; ingest "frequently" during competition.
Recommendation of American College of Sports Medicine (1984):
400 to 600 ml 15–20 min before event; ingest further 100–200 ml every 2–3 km.

Sources: American College of Sports Medicine (1975, 1984), and D. Minard, *Mil. Med.*, 126: 261 (1961).

Heat Acclimatization.   The long-term solution to a hot environment is heat acclimatization.

Certain parallels may be drawn between heat acclimatization and cardiovascular training. Both heat exposure and heavy exercise place a dynamic load on the circulation (although in the heat there is an increase in skin rather than in muscle blood flow). The deep body temperature rises progressively in both situations, with sweating and a progressive depletion of blood volume (7,137,210, 246). Moreover, as the individual becomes accustomed to either heat or exercise, there is a compensatory expansion of the resting blood volume (88), allowing peak cardiac output to be better sustained. With repetition of either heat exposure or exercise, the rise of core body temperature becomes smaller and sweating occurs earlier and in larger amounts (7,148,210,246).

It is not surprising that repeated exposure to one form of stress helps adaptation to the other (104), although for maximal adaptation, a hot environment and vigorous exercise must be presented simultaneously (7,276).

Cold Conditions

Cold exposure causes a peripheral venoconstriction. The resulting increase in central blood volume leads to a small immediate rise in maximal oxygen intake (34). However, exercise training has little influence on cold tolerance or acclimatization (200,217).

Cold Exposure and Fat Loss

A given amount of physical activity may metabolize more fat if the activity is performed in a cold environment (159–162,217) (Fig. 9). Reasons for the phenomenon are not fully understood.

Increases of energy expenditure due to the wearing of heavy clothing and

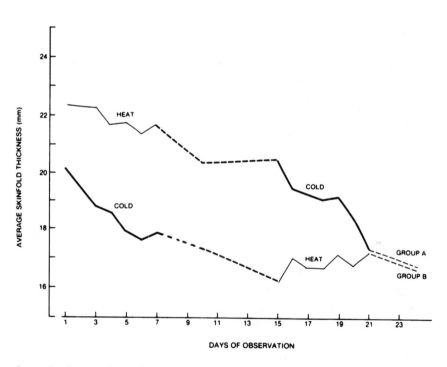

FIGURE 9   A comparison of the fat loss induced by a week of exercise in cold and warm environments. Crossover experiment involving two groups of young men (From Ref. 162; used with permission).

boots are largely offset by a reduction in peripheral body temperatures and thus a lower rate of basal metabolism. Possibly, catecholamine secretion and/or the sensitivity of catecholamine receptors is increased, augmenting "futile" metabolic cycles in brown fat or elsewhere (217). If so, each bout of activity might provoke a larger postexercise increase of metabolic rate than would be anticipated in a temperate climate. The mobilization of depot fat also provokes a ketosis, and energy is lost from the body as partially metabolized ketone bodies are excreted (159–162).

Cold-induced fat loss apparently occurs more readily in the obese than in thinner individuals (161) and (possibly because of a need to conserve the body reserves of fat for pregnancy and lactation) the phenomenon is less obvious in female than in male subjects (147).

General Hypothermia

Severe cold exposure can cause a fatal general hypothermia. Fat subjects might be thought less vulnerable than thinner individuals, but in fact much of the body's insulation depends on an active, neurally mediated reduction of blood flow to the superficial limb muscles rather than on passive protection from subcutaneous fat (217,241). Hypothermia is particularly likely if prolonged physical activity is performed in clothing that either lacks adequate insulation or has lost its insulation because of soaking by rain, mist, or sweat.

The ability to sustain shivering and to engage in prolonged, vigorous activity is an important protective measure depending on the extent of glycogen stores (105). Because unfit individuals have smaller initial reserves of glycogen and are less able to sustain vigorous physical activity, they are the usual victims of hypothermia in climbing accidents (181). The older members of the population are particularly vulnerable to hypothermia (20,76).

Local Hypothermia

Intensely cold conditions can also be dangerous from the viewpoint of provoking local hypothermia. Patients with a poor peripheral circulation are particularly vulnerable to frostbite. The risk of damage depends on the severity of the windchill factor and is exacerbated by any local disturbance of the film of air in immediate contact with the skin (for example, with the rapid movements of downhill skiing or speed skating).

Cold-induced peripheral vasoconstriction raises the systemic blood pressure, thus increasing the cardiac work rate. The resultant risk of myocardial ischemia is further augmented by the cold-induced secretion of catecholamines.

Exercise-Induced Bronchospasm

When a critical respiratory minute volume is reached (usually 30–40 L/min), most people start to breathe through their mouths as well as their noses (152).

This disturbs the normal mechanisms for warming, filtering, and humidifying the inspired air. The consequences include a provocation of bronchospasm—possibly with an associated reflex narrowing of the coronary vessels (the Bezold-Jarisch reflex) and an increased risk of myocardial ischemia.

Musculoskeletal Injuries

Older individuals with brittle bones and a deteriorating sense of balance are particularly vulnerable to falls under icy conditions.

Appropriate Patterns of Physical Activity

Moderate cold exposure generally encourages brisk movement. However, when the weather is extremely cold, there is a tendency to remain indoors and allow fitness to deteriorate.

One way to maintain physical condition during the winter months is to seek an indoor facility. Such a decision may provoke exercise-induced bronchospasm, because the air in gymnasiums often has a very low water content during the winter months. If the type of activity is modified, it is also necessary to reduce intensity, at least temporarily, in order to avoid overuse injuries.

A second option, particularly for younger adults, is to continue outdoor exercise. Activities such as cross-country skiing can be quite pleasant at ambient temperatures as low as −10 to −15°C given a calm, sunny day and appropriate clothing. Indeed, the change of recreational pursuit can add useful variety to a regimen. It is important to match the amount of clothing to the anticipated rate of metabolism. Failure to take this precaution may cause the protective garments to become soaked with sweat; the resulting loss of insulation then allows rapid cooling of the body when a rest pause is taken.

High Altitudes

Interest continues in the possibility of enhancing the response to cardiorespiratory training by exercising at altitude (141,207,210,217a,245).

The physiological effects of high altitudes include an increase of hemoglobin concentration (which develops progressively over several weeks, owing both to a steady increase in hemopoiesis and a reduction in plasma volume), a decrease of cerebrospinal fluid bicarbonate levels (developing within 12 h of exposure), and slower adjustments of acid/base balance, all of which normalize both blood and tissue pH over the course of the first weeks. However, any increase in cardiorespiratory endurance is short-lived, since the hemoglobin level reverts to normal within 2–3 weeks of a return to sea-level conditions (210,217a). The altitude-induced decrease of cerebrospinal fluid and serum bicarbonate concentrations has a negative impact on anaerobic performance, and the decrease of blood volume also reduces the ability to undertake sustained bouts of aerobic activity during the first few weeks at altitude.

From the viewpoint of safety, a number of hazards are specific to high altitudes, particularly if the person is unacclimatized to the new altitude. Specific dangers include acute mountain sickness and pulmonary edema (210,245). There is also some evidence that the risk of heart attacks is increased by exposure to high altitude, particularly in patients with a preexisting myocardial ischemia, although the elderly generally respond surprisingly well to such an environment (277).

High Ambient Pressures

Recreational diving is an increasingly popular form of physical activity; nevertheless, it presents both general dangers and risks specific to the cardiac patient.

General Dangers

Many of the general dangers of the diving-induced increase of ambient pressure and subsequent decompression are unrelated to the pattern of physical activity that is undertaken. However, the danger of exhaustion of gas supplies is proportional to both the intensity of effort and the depth of submersion. Likewise, the risks of nitrogen narcosis, oxygen poisoning, and decompression sickness all increase as the period under water is extended, and problems associated with an excessive work of breathing are particularly likely if intensive activity is attempted at substantial depths (57,210).

Specific Risks in the Patient with Cardiovascular Disease

The person with cardiovascular disease faces additional risks of cardiac arrest while submerged and of hypotension on leaving the water.

On first entering cold water, a reflex constriction of the cutaneous blood vessels caused by immersion of the face [the diving reflex (256)] and an augmented secretion of catecholamines increase the cardiac work rate and thus vulnerability to arrhythmias. Body temperatures drop progressively while the person is in the water; this furthers augment the secretion of catecholamines and the risk of cardiac arrest. Myocardial ischemia may develop in the later stages of a breath-hold dive. Finally, the development of pressure differentials between the peripheral veins and the interior of the thoracic cavity (a "pulmonary squeeze") augments preloading of the heart, adversely affecting the person with poor myocardial contractility. Even a brief loss of consciousness from any of these causes can be fatal under water.

The tone of the peripheral veins decreases progressively while a person is submerged, and the blood pressure may fall abruptly on climbing from the water.

Such hypotensive episodes and/or loss of consciousness are particularly likely in those who are unfit and/or are receiving hypotensive medication. Physical injury may result from a hypotensive attack.

Air Pollution

Catastrophic episodes of air pollution in London, England, during 1952 and 1956 (174) demonstrated that the very young and the frail elderly were especially vulnerable to the adverse effects of air contaminants. Advanced age and the presence of chronic cardiac or respiratory disease were particularly likely to lead to a fatal outcome.

Exercise increases exposure of the individual to air pollutants from several perspectives. First, there is often a two- to threefold gradient in the peak concentration of air contaminants from ambient air to the more protected environment inside a home with closed windows. Second, both particulate and gas-phase contaminants generally reach the body via the respiratory tract. Thus, an activity-induced increase in respiratory minute volume induces *at least* a proportionate increase in exposure to the toxic material. Finally, the proportion of soluble vapors absorbed in the trachea and larger bronchi diminishes as airflow increases, and if the intensity of activity is sufficient to induce mouth-breathing (above), the pulmonary exposure to air contaminants is increased about tenfold, because the normal scrubbing and filtering mechanisms of the nose are bypassed.

There are two broad categories of air pollution: reducing and oxidant smog.

Reducing Smog

Reducing smog is caused by an accumulation of the combustion products of fossil fuels (SO_2 SO_3, and soot particles). It was apparently responsible for the excess mortality in the London smog episodes of the 1950s.

At more normally encountered urban concentrations, the oxides of sulfur provoke a mild bronchospasm, with an increase of respiratory rate and a temporary paralysis of the tracheal ciliae; the respiratory tract more vulnerable to infecting microorganisms.

Oxidant Smog

Oxidant smog is the end result of an accumulation of automobile exhaust in bright sunlight. Constituents include carbon monoxide, ozone, and various oxides of nitrogen. Although the concentrations of oxidant pollutants depend heavily on traffic density, other critical determinants include atmospheric stability and the number of hours of recent sunshine.

Carbon Monoxide.   If carbon monoxide exposure is brief, the dose received varies with the individual's respiratory minute volume (and hence with the type and pattern of physical activity that is being undertaken) (Table 4). However, after several hours, the body and the environment reach an equilibrium that is independent of the level of ventilation.

Exposure to high concentrations of carbon monoxide can impair both oxygen transport and psychomotor function, but the most important health consequence is an exacerbation of preexisting cardiovascular disease (212). The time to onset of exercise-induced angina is shortened, and the risk of cardiac arrest is also increased. Carbon monoxide induces a tissue hypoxia, and its effects are exacerbated at high altitudes (where ambient carbon monoxide levels may also be high, because of narrow mountain valleys and car engines that are operating inefficiently).

Ozone.   Ozone is a respiratory irritant. At the concentrations sometimes encountered in urban air, it causes bronchospasm, with rapid shallow breathing and a decrease in maximal oxygen intake (62a,63). For the reasons noted above, the threshold for measurable effects drops from a concentration of about 0.75 ppm at rest to 0.1 ppm during vigorous physical activity.

Oxides of Nitrogen.   There has been less formal study of the nitrogen oxides, although they are known to cause pulmonary edema if concentrations are high. The likelihood of such a response is increased during vigorous physical activity,

TABLE 4   Influence of Atmospheric Partial Pressure of Carbon Monoxide, Duration of Exposure and Intensity of Physical Activity on Blood Carboxyhemoglobin Levels (%)

Partial pressure of carbon monoxide (Pa)	Duration of exposure, intensity of activity and COHb%								
	15 min			60 min			480 min		
	S	M	H	S	M	H	S	M	H
0.5	0.5	0.5	0.6	0.6	0.6	0.7	0.9	0.9	0.9
1.0	0.6	0.6	0.7	0.7	0.9	1.1	1.5	1.7	1.7
2.5	0.7	0.8	1.0	1.1	1.7	2.2	3.3	4.1	4.2
5.0	0.8	1.2	1.6	1.7	3.0	4.1	6.4	8.0	8.3
20.0	1.8	3.5	5.2	5.4	11.0	15.5	24.5	31.7	32.9

Predictions for sedentary subjects (S), subjects undertaking moderate physical activity (M) and subjects undertaking activity sufficient to induce a respiratory minute volume of 30 L/min (H). Based on model of Coburn et al., *J. Clin. Invest.,* 44: 1899–1910 (1965) and calculations of the World Health Organization (*Health Aspects Related to Indoor Air Quality,* WHO Regional Office for Europe, Copenhagen, 1979).
Source: Shephard, R.J., *Carbon Monoxide: The Silent Killer.* Charles C Thomas, Springfield, Illinois (1983); used with permission.

partly because the inhaled dose is larger, partly because the toxic gas is drawn deeper into the lungs, and partly because prolonged exercise itself predisposes to pulmonary edema.

Psychological Stress

The level of psychological stress encountered during exercise varies enormously from one situation to another. This is probably important in terms of the cardiovascular risks associated with physical activity (209,220).

Dangers of Stress

In some instances, a person may bring the pressures of time, perceived hostility, and other stressors from the home or office to the gymnasium or exercise site. If abnormalities of heart rhythm are to be avoided in such a situation, it is wise to moderate the intensity of an exercise prescription, since the emotional disturbances increase the heart rate, blood pressure, and catecholamine secretion for any given energy expenditure (Fig. 10). A change in the type of exercise may be helpful; for example, a peaceful walk in the countryside may do more to relieve occupational and domestic pressures than a game of squash that the individual is determined to win.

Excitement and competition can provide motivation for some people, but they are significant sources of additional cardiovascular stress. Thus, Blimkie et al. (24) observed that catecholamine levels were much higher in young men when

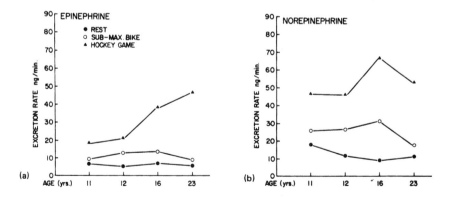

FIGURE 10 Urinary excretion of epinephrine and norepinephrine in males aged 11, 12, 16, and 23 years. Samples collected at rest, immediately after a game of ice hockey, and immediately after submaximal cycle ergometer exercise of comparable metabolic intensity (From Ref. 15; used with permission).

they had been playing a game of ice hockey than when they had undertaken metabolically equivalent exercise on a cycle ergometer (Fig. 10). Cardiovascular problems are particularly likely to arise if the intensity of competition is severe or seems beyond the capacity of the participant. Whereas a patient with a relaxed, "type B" personality may accept defeat graciously, those with the hostile and competitive behavioral traits typical of "type A" often remain determined to win even when they are conscious of physical exhaustion.

Reducing Stress by Habituation

Any unfamiliar situation can be a source of psychological stress. About 25% of patients are very anxious the first time they are tested in the exercise laboratory. The increase of heart rate, blood pressure, and ventilation induced by such anxiety not only tends to invalidate test results but also reduces the margin of safety for any procedure that is being carried out.

Ideally, patients should be habituated to the general environment of the test laboratory by one or more preliminary visits (206). Care should also be taken to explain all the intended procedures in a calm and reassuring manner, allowing the patient to experiment with unfamiliar devices before beginning a definitive test.

The claim is sometimes made that the effects of psychological stress are restricted to low intensities of effort. Some familiarization is undoubtedly possible during the course of a progressive exercise test, and in percentage terms the effect of an anxiety-induced increase in heart rate of 10 beats per minute is larger at rest than during vigorous physical activity. However, in our experience, the psychological impact of a first test does not abate as maximal effort is approached. Indeed, impending exhaustion may increase the level of anxiety and thus augment increases of heart rate and blood pressure.

POSTULATED HEALTH BENEFITS OF REGULAR PHYSICAL ACTIVITY

The acute health benefits of regular physical activity include an improvement of overall lifestyle, gains in perceived health, an improved mood state (Chapter 5), and possibly an enhancement of immune function (224). Many chronic health benefits have also been postulated (30,31), including a decreased risk of ischemic heart disease and hypertension; the control of obesity, maturity-onset diabetes, and cholecystitis; a strengthening of muscles, ligaments, cartilage, and bone structure; and a reduced incidence of certain forms of malignant disease. In some cases, the postulated gains are substantial, but for reasons discussed below, it is difficult to obtain categoric proof of benefit.

Improvement of lifestyle

Participation in regular physical activity may encourage other favorable changes of lifestyle, such as a more careful consideration of diet or the cessation of smoking (214). However, most studies to date have been cross-sectional in nature, so that it has been difficult to determine whether physical activity is the cause or the consequence of a favorable overall lifestyle. Moreover, several aspects of a favorable lifestyle have a common basis in such factors as a high socioeconomic status and a good level of education (227).

Empirical Data

An early uncontrolled study of master's athletes suggested that involvement in long-distance running had encouraged a high percentage of successful smoking withdrawals (143). Further study of master's competitors (114,233) indicated that in many instances smoking withdrawal had antedated master's competition, suggesting that the competitors had a primary interest in health. Nevertheless, a proportion of competitors also stated that running had helped them substantially to escape from a cigarette addiction (233).

Controlled trials of worksite exercise programs have also demonstrated a favorable impact upon obesity, cigarette and alcohol consumption, and overall health knowledge (22,221,230).

Likely Mechanisms

If regular physical activity has a beneficial effect on overall lifestyle, one might anticipate maximal benefit from those forms of physical activity that are perceived as health-related. There is some evidence that a low prevalence of cigarette smoking is linked with participation in endurance activity but not with social types of sport (156).

It may be helpful if the proposed regimen is well matched to the fitness and skills of the participant, so that participation enhances self-image and feelings of self-efficacy; motivation is then gained to fight against other adverse and addictive types of behavior such as smoking, overconsumption of alcohol, and overeating.

Other potential interactions between lifestyle and physical activity may be hypothesized. The vigorous breathing of a bout of endurance exercise may bring to light the dyspnea that is caused by smoking, encouraging the withdrawal process. An exercise-induced increase in cerebral arousal may counter the depression that often underlies an alcohol addiction. Finally, the compulsive eater may be dissuaded from unnecessary eating if the blood sugar is raised temporarily by a bout of intensive exercise, although more prolonged sessions of moderate physical activity are needed to establish a good long-term balance between food intake and energy consumption.

Perceived Health

The World Health Organization (274) has stressed the importance of a positive approach to health. Physicians should seek not merely to treat disease but also to optimize human potential with the building of complete social, psychological, and mental well-being. Many people suggest that the main reason they exercise is in order to "feel better." In essence, this comment reflects an improvement in perceived health. Each person operates along a continuum that extends from overt disease to optimal health (6,91), and one important benefit of involvement in regular physical activity is a displacement of perceptions along this continuum toward optimal health. Such a change probably explains the sharp reduction in demand for medical services that follows the introduction of a moderate exercise program (Chapter 22).

The type of activity likely to maximize wellness is relatively specific to a given individual. In some people, the arousal induced by a few minutes of vigorous exercise creates a sensation of optimal health: in others, the key factor may be the stress relaxation associated with a longer period of more gentle activity.

Some individuals may respond positively to an enhancement of their body image and the feeling of self-efficacy associated with a trim figure or well-toned muscles, whereas others react to the lessening of fatigue during their daily tasks as endurance fitness improves. A few may describe the euphoria associated with the increased output of β-endorphins in very prolonged exercise.

STRENGTHS AND WEAKNESSES OF CURRENT EVIDENCE

Where possible, important hypotheses should be tested by randomized, controlled experiments. However, there are substantial obstacles in applying such an approach to an evaluation of the long-term health benefits of an increase in physical activity.

Humans are well aware when they have engaged in a training program. Reactions are thus colored by their attitudes—whether positive or negative—toward the required physical activity. Moreover, many exercise classes offer close medical supervision, and regular contact with a medical team can in itself provide emotional support, advice on lifestyle, and a closer monitoring of clinical condition than that available to the control group. If subjects are randomly assigned between experimental and control conditions, there is a selective loss of subjects from the treatment group (those of lower socioeconomic class, with a poor life-

TABLE 5   To Illustrate the Disparate Data Sometimes Included in Meta-Analyses—
Controlled Trials of Exercise in Tertiary Prevention (Postcoronary Rehabilitation)

Authors	Sample size	Entry postinfarct	Follow-up period	Treatment
Kentala (1972)	298 (165)[a]	6–8 wk	1 yr	Individually supervised exercise 2–3/wk
Kallio (1981)	375 (74 F, 301 M)	2 wk	3 yr	Exercise + health education
Kallio et al. (1988)[b]	375	2 wk	10 yr	Exercise + health education (3 yr)
Hamalainen et al. (1988)[b,c]	456	2 wk	6 yr	Exercise + health education (3 months)
Palatsi (1976)	380[d]	2–3 months	29 months	Daily home program (1 yr)

[a]Numbers judged suitable for long-term follow-up.
[b]Coronary deaths, assuming 4-years follow-up of all subjects.
[c]Controls received community-based program.
[d]Nonrandomized allocation of subjects.
Note: For details of references, see Shephard, Ref. 215.

style and an above-average likelihood of clinical disorders). Those assigned to the control group are likely to be contaminated by an increased interest in physical activity (the most susceptible are health-conscious individuals from the higher socioeconomic strata). In investigating issues like the prevention of ischemic heart disease, it is finally necessary to recruit and retain a large sample (5000–10,000 subjects). Even if several major university centers agree to cooperate in such a venture, the numbers are difficult to obtain and even more difficult to retain.

Investigators have thus attempted to accumulate sufficient evidence by pooling results from all large trials of adequate quality [the technique of meta-analysis (19,164,180,215)]. Unfortunately, policies at individual centers tend to vary with respect to diagnostic criteria, time of entry into the exercise program, details of the regimen and ancillary treatment, duration of observation, and diagnostic endpoints. Although meta-analyses allow differences between experimental and control groups to reach conventional levels of statistical significance, it remains uncertain what hypothesis has been proven by the manipulation of such disparate data (Table 5).

An alternative approach is to draw inferences from epidemiological data (19,180), comparing the health experience of groups that supposedly differ in their levels of habitual physical activity. The criteria proposed by the eminent statistician Bradford Hill can then be applied to examine whether the observed associations between physical activity and health are causal or casual in type.

Strength of the Association

The strength of the association between regular physical activity and the prevention of cardiovascular disease is relatively weak. For example, there is a 25–50% reduction in the risk of fatal myocardial infarctions between active and sedentary individuals, compared with the nine- to tenfold increase in the risk of bronchial carcinoma seen when a lifelong nonsmoker is compared with a heavy cigarette smoker.

Consistency of the Association

Consistency of the association between an active lifestyle and the prevention of disease is generally good, but there are occasional anomalies. For instance, athletes may be quite active and yet remain vulnerable to cardiovascular disease because an adverse body build is also a criterion for success in the sport under consideration. Likewise, laborers who undertake hard physical work may fail to show the anticipated protection against cardiovascular disease because a low socioeconomic status encourages other bad habits such as smoking.

An Appropriate Lag Period

Some favorable responses to an increase of physical activity develop almost immediately, but others become apparent only if the activity is maintained consistently over a long period. Relatively few epidemiological studies have accumulated convincing data on long-term patterns of physical activity. Nevertheless, available information suggests development of protection after an appropriate lag period.

Biological Gradient

The studies of Paffenbarger (165,166) provide some evidence of a biological gradient linking the magnitude of weekly leisure-time energy expenditures with the extent of protection against ischemic heart disease. Unfortunately, the response appears to be nonlinear, and the optimum intensity may well decrease as a person grows older.

Plausibility

If an association is causal, it should have theoretical plausibility. There are plainly many reasonable mechanisms whereby an increase in habitual physical activity could reduce susceptibility to cardiovascular disease. Some are relatively independent of the intensity of the regimen—for example, companionship, mutual support, joie de vivre, and the incidental advice on lifestyle gained through membership in a fitness class. Benefits such as the metabolizing of excess fat and cholesterol and the lowering of resting blood sugar require the weekly expenditure of substantial additional amounts of energy. Other benefits depend on regular, moderate endurance activity—for instance, the lowering of the exercise heart rate, blood pressure, and cardiac work rate; an increase of plasma volume and total hemoglobin; and an increased secretion of fat-mobilizing hormones (growth hormone and cortisol). Finally, a few benefits probably require intensive bursts of activity; among these last items are habituation to the sensations of vigorous effort and a decreased secretion of catecholamines during maximal exertion.

Specificity

There is a long lag period before the clinical symptoms of ischemic heart disease become apparent. Moreover, there are many situational factors that help to determine whether the disease will progress to the point of producing clinical manifestations.

For example, a given degree of coronary narrowing may cause a myocardial infarction, but it may also remain silent because the person never exercises hard enough to provoke myocardial ischemia. There may thus seem to be a lack of specificity between physical inactivity and the onset of disease. However, the association becomes more specific and consistent if, for instance, the prevalence of myocardial ischemia is correlated with patterns of physical activity.

A further factor contributing to lack of specificity is the multifactorial nature of disease. For example, some people are unusually vulnerable to ischemic heart disease despite a lifetime of vigorous physical activity because they have inherited a severe disorder of lipid metabolism.

Coherence

Ideally, a causal relationship should explain all observable facts. It could be argued that the exercise hypothesis fails to satisfy this criterion. For instance, in the study of London bus workers, the incidence of angina was higher in what was presumed to be the more active group (the conductors) than in the sedentary comparison group (the drivers) (145). Possibly, the added physical demands made on the conductors brought to light subclinical disease that would have passed unnoticed in the drivers.

Likewise, in some instances, vigorous exercise increases the immediate risk of a heart attack (220,261).

Experimental Verification

Any hypothesis must ultimately be verified experimentally. We have already noted some of the obstacles in designing a controlled experiment to test the effect of increased physical activity on ischemic heart disease. Observations on experimental animals are not very satisfactory. The restricted diet and cramped living quarters of the average laboratory animal are not typical of normal life, and it is surprisingly difficult to persuade many species to undertake regular vigorous physical activity in a laboratory.

Further, there are no good animal models of atherosclerosis. Arterial lesions can be produced only by the constraints of providing a high fat diet to rigorously caged animals. Finally, the long lag period that precedes the appearance of clinical disease makes any experiments that *are* conducted very costly to complete.

Analogous Mechanisms

Epidemiologists hope to find analogous mechanisms as evidence to support a causal hypothesis. For example, it is hypothesized that if carcinomatous tars cause cancer in the smoker, then it should be possible to induce carcinomatous changes by painting the skin or treating isolated cells with the tars formed during the combustion of cigarettes.

There is little analogous evidence concerning the beneficial effects of exercise on cardiovascular disease. The recurrence of fatal myocardial infarction is reduced by the regular administration of β-blocking drugs (209), pointing to a possible analogy with the training-induced reduction in catecholamine secretion at a given power output. Likewise, if blood cholesterol levels are reduced by a regular daily dose of cholestyramine, there is some reduction in the incidence of fatal heart attacks among individuals with a high risk of cardiovascular disease (126), supporting the benefit of an exercise-induced amelioration of the blood lipid profile.

SUMMARY

In summary, there is much evidence suggesting the benefit of increased physical activity in the secondary and tertiary prevention of cardiovascular disease. However, for various technical reasons, it is difficult to mount conclusive double-blind, randomized, controlled experiments.

Not all of Bradford Hill's criteria of a causal linkage between regular physical activity and good cardiovascular health are fully satisfied. Nevertheless, the benefits of enhanced physical activity generally seem to outweigh any disadvantages. An increase in habitual physical activity can be commended not only in terms of the probable control of chronic disease but also (and perhaps more importantly) as a means of enhancing the quality of a person's remaining years of life.

REFERENCES

1. Abernethy, P.J., Thayer, R., and Taylor, A.W., *Sports Med.,* 10: 365–389 (1990).
2. Adams, W.C., Fox, R.H., Fry, A.J., and MacDonald, I.C., *J. Appl. Physiol.,* 38: 1030–1037 (1975).
3. American College of Sports Medicine, *Med. Sci. Sports,* 7: 7 (1975).
4. American College of Sports Medicine, *Med. Sci. Sports Exerc.,* 16: ix–xiv (1984).
5. American College of Sports Medicine, *Guidelines for Graded Exercise Testing and Exercise Prescription,* 5th Ed. Lea & Febiger, Philadelphia (1995).
6. Andersson, G., The importance of Exercise for Sick Leave and Perceived Health. Ph.D. dissertation, Linköping University, Sweden (1987).
6a. Anderson, T., and Kerney, J.T., *Res. Q.,* 53: 1–7 (1982).
7. Aoyagi, Y., McLellan, T.M., and Shephard, R.J., *Sports Med.,* 23: 173–210.
8. Armstrong, R.B., *Sports Med.,* 3: 370–381 (1986).
9. Armstrong, R.B., Warren, G.L., and Warren, G.A., *Sports Med.,* 12: 184–207 (1991).
10. Asmussen, E., and Bøje, O., *Acta Physiol. Scand.,* 10: 1–22 (1945).
11. Åstrand, I., Åstrand, P-O., Christensen, E.H., and Hedman, R., *Acta Physiol. Scand.,* 48: 448–453 (1960).
12. Åstrand, P.O., Cuddy, T.E., Saltin, B., and Stenberg, J., *J. Appl. Physiol.,* 19: 268–274 (1964).
13. Auble, T.E., Schwartz, L., and Robertson, J., *Phys. Sportsmed.,* 15(6): 133–140 (1987).
14. Ballor, D.L., and Keesey, R.E., *Int. J. Obes.,* 15: 717–726 (1991).
15. Banister, E.W., in *Frontiers of Fitness* (R.J. Shephard, ed.). Charles C Thomas, Springfield, Illinois, pp. 5–36 (1971).
16. Bartels, R., Billings, C.E., Fox, E.L., Mathews, D.K., O'Brien, R., Tauz, D. and Webb, W., *Abstracts, AAHPER Convention,* p. 13 (cited by Pollock, 1973) (1968).
17. Bassey, E.J., Patrick, J.M., Irving, J.M., Blecher, A., and Fentem, P.H., *Eur. J. Appl. Physiol.,* 52: 120–125 (1983).
18. Beaudet, S.M., *Ergonomics,* 27: 955–957 (1984).
19. Berlin, J.A., and Coldlitz, G.A., *Am. J. Epidemiol.,* 132: 612–628 (1990).
20. Besdine, R.W., and Harris, T.B., in *Principles of Geriatric Medicine* (R. Andres, E.L. Bierman, and W.R. Hazzard, eds.). McGraw-Hill, New York, pp. 209–217 (1985).
21. Birk, T.J., and Birk, C.A., *Sports Med.,* 4: 1–8 (1987).
22. Blair, S.N., Piserchia, P.V., Wilbur, C.S., and Crowder, J.H., *J.A.M.A.,* 255: 921–926 (1986).
23. Blair, S.N., in *Physical Activity, Fitness and Health* (C. Bouchard, R.J. Shephard, and T. Stephens, eds.), Human Kinetics Publications, Champaign, Illinois, pp. 579–590 (1994).

24. Blimkie, C.J., Cunningham, D.A., and Leung, F.Y., in *Frontiers of Activity and Child Health* (H. Lavallée and R.J. Shephard, eds.). Editions du Pélican, Québec City, pp. 313–321 (1977).

25. Boone, T., and Edwards, C.A., *Ann. Sports Med.,* 4: 29–31 (1988).

26. Booth, F.W., and Watson, P.A., *Fed. Proc.,* 44: 2293–2300 (1985).

27. Borg, G., in *Frontiers of Fitness* (R.J. Shephard, ed.) Charles C Thomas, Springfield, Illinois, pp. 280–294 (1971).

28. Bouchard, C., in *Endurance in Sport* (R.J. Shephard and P.-O. Åstrand, eds.). Blackwell Scientific Publications, Oxford, England, pp. 149–162 (1992).

29. Bouchard, C., Hollmann, W., Venrath, H., Herkenrath, G., and Schlussel, H., *Sportarzt Sportmed.,* 7: 348–357 (1966).

30. Bouchard, C., Shephard, R.J., Stephens, T., Sutton, J., and McPherson, B., *Exercise, Fitness and Health.* Human Kinetics Publications, Champaign, Illinois (1990).

31. Bouchard, C., Shephard, R.J., and Stephens, T., *Physical Activity, Fitness and Health.* Human Kinetics Publications, Champaign, Illinois (1994).

31a. Brenner, I.K.M., Shephard, R.J., and Shek, P.N., *Sports Med.,* 17: 86–107 (1994).

32. Brooks, G.A., Fahey, T.D., and White, T.P., *Exercise Physiology: Human Bioenergetics and its Applications,* 2nd Ed. Mayfield Publishing Company, Mountain View, California (1996).

33. Brück, K., and Olschewski, H., *Can. J. Physiol. Pharmacol.,* 65: 1274–1280 (1987).

34. Bryan, C., *Can. Med. Assoc. J.,* 96: 804 (1967).

35. Buguet, A., Rhind, S.G., Fidier, N., Gannon, G., Severs, Y., Gil, V., Brenner, I.K.M., Shek, P.N., Shephard, R.J., and Radomski, M.W., *Rapport de mission au Defence and Civil Institute of Environmental Medicine du 6 au 23 Octobre, 1996.* Rapport technique 7CRSSA/FH/PV. CRSSA, La Tronche, France.

36. Caillaud, C.F., Anseline, F.M., and Préfaut, C.G., *Eur. J. Appl. Physiol.,* 74: 141–147 (1996).

37. Caspersen, C.J., Powell, K.E., and Christenson, G.M., *Public Health Rep.,* 100: 126–131 (1985).

38. Chad, K.E., and Wenger, H.A., *Can. J. Sport Sci.,* 13: 204–207 (1989).

39. Chow, R.J. and Wilmore, J.H., *J. Cardiac Rehab.,* 4: 382–387 (1984).

40. Chow, R.K., Harrison, J.E., Sturtridge, W., Josse, R., Murray, T.M., Bayley, A., Dornan, J., and Hammond, T., *Clin. Invest. Med.,* 10: 59–63 (1987).

41. Claremont, A.D., and Hall, S.J., *Med. Sci. Sports Exerc.,* 20: 167–171 (1988).

42. Clausen, J.P., *Physiol. Rev.,* 57: 779–815 (1977).

43. Cox, M.L., Bennett, J.B., and Dudley, G.A., *J. Appl. Physiol.,* 61: 926–931 (1986).

43a. Cross, M.C., Radomski, M.W., Van Helder, W., Rhind, S.G., and Shephard, R.J., *J. Appl. Physiol.,* 81: 822–829 (1996).

44. Cummins, P., Young, A., Auckland, M.L., Michie, C.A., Stone, P.C.W., and Shepstone, B.J., *Eur. J. Clin. Invest.,* 17: 317–324 (1987).

45. Daub, W.D., Green, H.J., Houston, M.E., Thomson, J.A., Fraser, I.G., and Ranney, D.A., *Can. J. Physiol.,* 60: 628–633 (1982).

46. Daub, W.D., Green, H.J., Houston, M.E., Thomson, J.A., Fraser, I.G., and Ranney, D.A., *Med. Sci. Sports Exerc.,* 15: 290–294 (1983).

47. Davies, C.T.M., and Knibbs, A.V., *Int. Z. Angew. Physiol.,* 29: 299–305 (1971).

48. Davies, C.T.M., and Starkie, D.W., *Eur. J. Appl. Physiol.*, 53: 359–363 (1985).
49. DiPrampero, P.E., in *Frontiers of Fitness* (R.J. Shephard, ed.). Charles C Thomas, Springfield, Illinois, pp. 155–173 (1971).
50. Donselaar, Y., Eerbeek, O., Kernell, D., and Verhey, B.A., *J. Physiol.*, 382: 237–254 (1987).
51. Drinkwater, B., in *Physical Activity, Fitness and Health* (C. Bouchard, R.J. Shephard, and T. Stephens, eds.), Human Kinetics Publications, Champaign, Illinois, pp. 724–736 (1994).
52. Driver, H.S., Meintjes, A.F., Rogers, C.C., and Shapiro, C.M., *Acta Physiol. Scand.*, 133 (Suppl. 574): 8–13 (1988).
53. Dudley, G.A., and Fleck, S.J., *Sports Med.*, 4: 79–85 (1987).
54. Durnin, J.V.G.A., Brockway, J.M., and Whitcher, H.W., *J. Appl. Physiol.*, 15: 161–165 (1960).
55. Edwards, R.H.T., Ekelund, L.G., Harris, R.C., Hesser, C.M., Hultman, E., Melcher, A., and Wigertz, O., *J. Physiol.*, 234: 481–497 (1973).
56. Ekblöm, B., and Hermansen, L., *J. Appl. Physiol.*, 25: 619–625 (1968).
57. Elliott, D.H., in *Oxford Textbook of Sports Medicine* (M. Harries, C. Williams, W. Stanish, and L.M. Micheli, eds.). Oxford University Press, New York, pp. 191–204 (1994).
58. Ellis, F.P., *Environ. Res.*, 5: 1–4 (1972).
59. Faria, I.E., *Res. Q.* 41: 44–50 (1970).
60. Fernhall, B., and Kohrt, W. *Med. Sci. Sports Exerc.*, 17: 225 (1985).
61. Fiatarone, M.A., O'Neill, E.F., Ryan. N.D., Clements, K.M., Solares, G.R., Nelson, M.E., Roberts, S.B., Kehayias, J.J., Lipsitz, L.A., and Evans, W.J., *N. Engl. J. Med.*, 330: 1769–1775 (1994).
62. Fleck, S.J., and Kraemer, W.J., *Designing Resistance Training Programs.* Human Kinetics Publications, Champaign, Illinois (1987).
62a. Folinsbee, L., in *Endurance in Sport* (R.J. Shephard and P-O. Åstrand, eds.). Blackwell Scientific Publications, Oxford, England, pp. 479–486 (1992).
63. Folinsbee, L., Shephard, R.J., and Silverman, F., *J. Appl. Physiol.*, 42: 531–536 (1977).
64. Friden, J., *Int. J. Sports Med.*, 5: 57–66 (1984).
65. Fried, T., and Shephard, R.J., *Can. Med. Assoc. J.*, 100: 831–837 (1969).
66. Fried, T., and Shephard, R.J., *Can. Med. Assoc. J.*, 103: 260–266 (1970).
67. Frisk-Holmberg, M., Essén, B., Fredrickson, M., Ström, G., and Wibell, L., *Acta Med. Scand.*, 213: 21–26 (1983).
68. Galbø, H., in *Endurance in Sport* (R.J. Shephard and P.O. Åstrand, eds.). Blackwell Scientific Publications, Oxford, England pp. 116–126 (1992).
69. Garrick, J.G., Gillien, D.M., and Whiteside, P., *Am. J. Sports Med.*, 14: 67–72 (1986).
70. Gergley, T., McArdle, W., DeJesus, P., Toner, M., Jacobwitz, S., and Spina, R., *Med. Sci. Sports Exerc.*, 16: 125 (1984).
71. Gettman, L.R., Culter, L.A., and Strathman, T.A., *J. Sports Med. Phys. Fitness*, 20: 265–274 (1980).
72. Glaser, E.M. *The Physiological Basis of Habituation*, Oxford University Press, Oxford, UK, (1966).

73. Gledhill, N., and Eynon, R.B., in *Training: Scientific Basis and Application* (A.W. Taylor, ed.). Charles C Thomas, Springfield, Illinois, pp. 97–102 (1972).

74. Godin, G., and Shephard, R.J., *Sports Med.,* 10: 103–121 (1990).

75. Going, S.B., Ball, T.E., and Massey, B.M., *Med. Sci. Sports Exerc.,* 15: 163 (Abstr.) (1983).

76. Goldman, A., Exton-Smith, A.N., Francis, G. et al., *J. R. Coll. Phys. (Lond.),* 11: 291–306 (1977).

77. Gollnick, P., and Hermansen, L., *Exerc. Sport Sci. Rev.,* 1: 1–43 (1973).

78. Gonyea, W., Ericsson, G.C., and Bonde-Peterson F., *Acta Physiol. Scand.,* 99: 105–109 (1977).

79. Graves, J.E., Pollock, M.L., Montain, S.J., Jackson, A.S. and O'Keefe, J.M., *Med. Sci. Sports Exerc.,* 19: 260–265 (1987).

80. Green, H.J., Jones, L.L., and Painter, D.C., *Med. Sci. Sports Exerc.,* 22: 488–493 (1990).

81. Grimby, G., *Sports Med.,* 2: 309–315 (1985).

82. Grogan, J.W., and Kelly, J.M., *Med. Sci. Sports Exerc.,* 17: 268–269 (1985).

83. Grover, R.F., Weil, J.V., and Reeves, J.T., *Exerc. Sports Sci. Rev.,* 14: 269–302 (1986).

83a. Hagberg, J.M., Ehsani, A.A., and Holloszy, J.O., *Circulation,* 67: 1194–1197 (1983).

84. Hakkinen, K., and Komi, P.V., *Eur. J. Appl. Physiol.,* 55: 147–155 (1986).

85. Hamrell, B.B., and Hultgren, P.B., *Fed. Proc.,* 45: 2591–2596 (1986).

86. Hansen, J.W., *Int. Z. Angew. Physiol.,* 23: 367–370 (1967).

87. Harber, V.J., and Sutton, J.S., *Sports Med.,* 1: 154–171 (1984).

88. Harrison, M.H., *Sports Med.,* 3: 214–223 (1986).

89. Heinritze, J., Weltman, A., Schurrer, R.L., and Barlow, K. *Eur. J. Appl. Physiol.,* 54: 84–88 (1985).

90. Hermansen, L., in *Muscle Metabolism During Exercise* (B. Pernow and B. Saltin, eds.). Plenum Press, New York, pp. 401–408 (1971).

91. Herzlich, C., *Health and Illness.* Academic Press, London (1973).

92. Hettinger, T., *Physiology of Strength.* Charles C Thomas, Springfield, Illinois (1961).

93. Hickson, R.C., and Rosenkoetter, M.A., *Am. J. Physiol.,* 241: C140–C144 (1981).

94. Hickson, R.C., Hagberg, J.M., Ehsani, A.A., and Holloszy, J.O., *Med. Sci. Sports Exerc.,* 13: 17–20 (1981).

95. Hickson, R.C., Kanakis, C., Davis, J.R., Moore, A.M., and Rich, S., *J. Appl. Physiol.,* 53: 225–229 (1982).

96. Hill, J.S., Wearing, G.A., and Eynon, R.B., *Med. Sci. Sports* 3: k (1971).

97. Ho, K.W., Roy, R.R., Taylor, J.F., Heusner, W.W., and Van Huss, W.D., *Med. Sci. Sports Exerc.,* 15: 472–477 (1983).

98. Holloszy, J.O., and Booth, F.W., *Annu. Rev. Physiol.,* 38: 273–291 (1976).

99. Holmgren, A., *Can. Med. Assoc. J.,* 96: 697–702 (1967).

100. Howald, H., *Int. J. Sports Med.,* 3: 1–12 (1982).

101. Hughson, R., in *Endurance in Sport* (R.J. Shephard and P.O. Åstrand, eds.). Blackwell Scientific, Oxford, England, pp. 458–470 (1992).

102. Hultman, E., in *Frontiers of Fitness* (R.J. Shephard, ed.). Charles C Thomas, Springfield, Illinois, pp. 37–60 (1971).
103. Hultman, E., and Greenhaff, P.L., in *Endurance in Sport* (R.J. Shephard and P.O. Åstrand, eds.). Blackwell Scientific Publications, Oxford, England, pp. 127–135 (1992).
104. Inbar, O., Gutin, B., Dotan, R., and Bar-Or, O., *Med. Sci. Sports,* 10: 62 (1978).
105. Jacobs, I., Romet, T., and Kerrigan-Brown, D., *Eur. J. Appl. Physiol,* 54: 35–39 (1985).
106. Kanehisa, H., and Miyashita, M., *Eur. J. Appl. Physiol.,* 52: 104–106 (1983).
107. Karvonen, M.J., Kentaka, E., and Mustala, O., *Ann. Med. Exp. Fenn.,* 35: 307–315 (1957).
108. Katz, A., Sharp, R.L., Armstrong, L.E., and King, D.S., *Can. J. Appl. Spt. Sci.,* 9: 11–15 (1984).
109. Kavanagh, T., *Phys. Sportsmed.,* 17(1): 96–114 (1988).
110. Kavanagh, T., *Heart Attack? Counter-attack.* Van Nostrand, Toronto (1992).
110a. Kavanagh, T., and Shephard, R.J., *Arch. Phys. Med. Rehabil.,* 56: 72–76 (1975).
111. Kavanagh, T., and Shephard, R.J., *Arch. Phys. Med. Rehabil.,* 61: 114–118 (1980).
112. Kavanagh, T., Shephard, R.J., Tuck, J.A., and Qureshi, S., *Ann. N.Y. Acad. Sci.,* 301: 1029–1038 (1977).
113. Kavanagh, T., Shephard, R.J., Lindley, L.J., and Pieper, M., *Arteriosclerosis,* 3: 249–259 (1983).
114. Kavanagh, T., Lindley, L.J., Shephard, R.J., and Campbell, R., *Ann. Sports Med.,* 4: 55–64 (1988).
115. Keast, D., Cameron, K. and Morton, A.R., *Sports Med.* 5: 248–267 (1988).
116. Kenyon, G.S., *Res. Q.,* 39: 566–574 (1968).
117. Kiens, B., Essen-Gustavsson, B., Christensen, N.J., and Saltin, B., *J. Physiol.,* 469: 459–478 (1993).
118. Kohl, H.W., Blair, S.N., Paffenbarger, R.S., Macera, C.A., and Kronenfeld, J.J., *Am. J. Epidemiol.,* 127: 1228–1239 (1988).
119. Kraemer, W.J., in *Strength and Power in Sport* (P.V. Komi, ed.). Blackwell Scientific Publications, Oxford, England, pp. 64–76 (1992).
120. Kuipers, H., and Keizer, H.A., *Sports Med.,* 6: 79–92 (1988).
121. Landers, D.M., and Petruzello, S.J., in *Physical Activity, Fitness and Health* (C. Bouchard, R.J. Shephard, and T. Stephens, eds.). Human Kinetics Publications, Champaign, Illinois, pp. 868–882 (1994).
122. Landry, F., Bouchard, C., and Dumesnil, J., *J.A.M.A.,* 254: 77–80 (1985).
123. Lawrence, G., *Aqua-fitness for Women.* Personal Library Publishers, Toronto (1981).
124. Leatt, P., and Jacobs, I., *Can. J. Sport Sci.,* 14: 112–116 (1989).
125. Lee-Chiong, T.L., and Stitt, J.T., *Postgrad Med. J.,* 98: 26–28, 31–33, 36 (1995).
125a. Linden, R.J., Mary, D.A.S.G., and Winter, C., *J. Physiol.* 357: 100P (1984).
126. Lipid Research Clinics, *J.A.M.A.,* 251: 351–364; 365–374 (1984).
127. Loftin, M., Boileau, R., Massey, B.H., and Lohman, T.G., *Med. Sci. Sports Exerc.,* 20: 136–141 (1988).
128. Lortie, G., Bouchard, C., LeBlanc, C., Tremblay, A., Simoneau, J.A., Thériault, G., and Savoie, J-P., *Hum. Biol.,* 54: 801–812 (1982).

129. MacDougall, J.D., Sale, D.G., Moroz, J.R., Elder, G.C.B., Sutton, J.R., and Howald, H., *Med. Sci. Sports,* 11: 164–166 (1979).

130. MacDougall, J.D., Tuxen, D., Sale, D.G., Moroz, J.R, and Sutton, J.R., *J. Appl. Physiol.,* 58: 785–790 (1985).

131. MacIntyre, D.L., Reid, W.D., and McKenzie, D.C., *Sports Med.,* 20: 24–40 (1995).

132. McNamara, P.S., Otto, R.M., and Smith, T.K., *Med. Sci. Sports Exerc.,* 17: 266 (Abstr.) (1985).

133. Maier, A., Gambke, B., and Pette, D., *Cell Tissue Res.,* 244: 635–643 (1986).

134. Mair, J., Koller, A., Artner-Dworzak, E., Haid, C., Wicke, K., Judmaier, W., and Puschendorf, B., *J. Appl. Physiol.,* 72: 656–663 (1992).

135. Manning, R.J., Graves, J.E., Carpenter, D.M., Leggett, S.H., and Pollock, M.L., *Med. Sci. Sports Exerc.,* 22: 397–401 (1990).

136. Martens, R., *Ex. Sport Sci. Rev.,* 2: 155–188 (1974).

136a. Matsuda, J.J., and Vailas, A.C., *Med. Sci. Sports Exerc.,* 16: 120 (1984).

137. Maughan, R.J., in *Oxford Textbook of Sports Medicine* (M. Harries, C. Williams, W.D. Stanish, and L.J. Micheli, eds.). Oxford University Press, New York, pp. 82–93 (1994).

138. Mertens, D., Rhind, S., Berkhoff, F., Dugmore, D., Shek, P.N., and Shephard, R.J., *J. Sports Med. Phys. Fitness,* 36: 132–138 (1996).

139. Mertens, D.J., Kavanagh, T., and Shephard, R.J., *J. Sports Med. Phys. Fitness* (1998). In press.

140. Milburn, S. and Butts, N.K., *Med. Sci. Sports Exerc.,* 15: 510–513 (1983).

141. Milledge, J.S., in *Oxford Textbook of Sports Medicine* (M. Harries, C. Williams, W. Stanish, and L. Micheli, eds.). Oxford University Press, New York, pp. 217–230 (1994).

142. Montoye, H.J., *Physical Activity and Health: An Epidemiological Study of an Entire Community.* Prentice Hall, Englewood Cliffs, N.J. (1975).

143. Morgan, P., Gildiner, M., and Wright, G.R., *CAHPER J.,* 42(5): 39–43 (1976).

144. Morris, J.N., *Res. Q.* 67: 216–220 (1996).

145. Morris, J.N., and Crawford, M.D., *Lancet,* 2: 1053–1057, 111–1120 (1958).

146. Morris, J.N., Clayton, D.G., Everitt, M.G., Semmence, A.M., and Burgess, E.H. *Br. Heart J.,* 63: 325–334 (1990).

147. Murray, S.J., Shephard, R.J., Greaves, S., Allen, C., and Radomski, M.W., *Eur. J. Appl. Physiol.,* 55: 610–618 (1986).

148. Nadel, J., *Problems with Temperature Regulation during Exercise.* Academic Press, New York (1977).

149. Neufer, P.D., Costill, D.L., Fielding, R.A., Flynn, M.G., and Kirwan, J.P., *Med. Sci. Sports Exerc.,* 19: 486–490 (1987).

150. Nicholl, J.P., Coleman, P., and Williams, P.T. *Injuries in Sport and Exercise.* British Sports Council, London (1993).

151. Nielsen, B., Kassow, K., and Aschengreen, F.E., *Eur. J. Appl. Physiol.,* 58: 189–196 (1988).

151a. Nieman, D.C., Johanssen, L.M., Lee, J.W. and Arabatzis, K., *J. Sports Med. Phys. Fitness,* 30: 316–328 (1990).

152. Niinimaa, V., Cole, P., Mintz, S. and Shephard, R.J., *Respir. Physiol.,* 43: 69–75 (1980).

153. Noakes, T.D., Higginson, L., and Opie, L.H., *Circulation*, 67: 24–30 (1983).
154. Noble, B.J., Kraemer, W.J., Clark, M.J., and Culver, B.W., *Med. Sci. Sports Exerc.*, 16: 146 (Abstr.) (1984).
155. Northoff, H., Enkel, S., and Weinstock, C., *Ex. Immunol. Rev.*, 1: 1–25 (1995).
156. Norwegian Confederation of Sports, *Physical Activity in Norway, 1983* (1984).
157. Nosaka, K., and Clarkson, P.M., *Med. Sci. Sports Exerc.*, 28: 953–961 (1996).
158. Oeschli, F.W., and Buechley, R.W., *Environ. Res.*, 3: 277–284 (1970).
159. O'Hara, W.J., Allen, C., and Shephard, R.J., *Eur. J. Appl. Physiol.*, 37: 205–218 (1977).
160. O'Hara, W.J., Allen, C., and Shephard, R.J., *Can. J. Physiol.*, 55: 1235–1241 (1977).
161. O'Hara, W.J., Allen, C., and Shephard, R.J., *Can. Med. Assoc. J.* 117: 773–779 (1977).
162. O'Hara, W.J., Allen, C., Shephard, R.J., and Allen, G., *J. Appl. Physiol.*, 46: 872–877 (1979).
163. Oja, P., *Finn. Spts. Exerc. Med.*, 2: 62–71 (1983).
164. Oja, P., Vuori, I., Nieminen, R., Kukkonen-Harjula, K., and Niittymaki, S., *Med. Sci. Sports Exerc.*, 17: 270 (1985).
165. Paffenbarger, R., *Med. Sci. Sports Exerc.*, 20: 426–438 (1988).
166. Paffenbarger, R.S., and Lee, I.M., *Res. Q.* 67 (Suppl. 3): S11–S28 (1996).
167. Parker, J.O., DiGiorgi, S., and West, R.O., *Am. J. Cardiol.* 17: 470–483 (1966).
168. Pate, R., and Macera, C.A., in *Physical Activity, Fitness and Health* (C. Bouchard, R.J. Shephard, and T. Stephens, eds.). Human Kinetics Publications, Champaign, Illinois, pp. 1008–1018 (1994).
169. Pate, R.R., Pratt, M., Blair, S.N., Haskell, W.L., Macera, C.A., Bouchard, C., Buchner, D., Ettinger, W., Heath, G.W., King, A.C., Kriska, A., Leon, A.S., Marcus, B.H., Morris, J., Paffenbarger, R.S., Patrick, K., Pollock, M.L., Rippe, J.M., Sallis, J., and Wilmore, J.H., *J.A.M.A.*, 273: 402–407 (1995).
170. Paterson, D.H., Shephard, R.J., Cunningham, D., Jones, N.L., and Andrew, G., *J. Appl. Physiol.*, 47: 482–489 (1979).
171. Pels, A.E., Pollock, M.L., Dohmeier, T.E., Lemberger, K.A., and Dehrlein, B.F., *Med. Sci. Sports Exerc.*, 19: 66–70 (1987).
172. Pérusse, L., Lortie, G., LeBlanc, C., Tremblay, A., Thériault, G., and Bouchard, C. *Ann. Hum. Biol.* 14: 425–434 (1987).
173. Pérusse, L., LeBlanc, C., and Bouchard, C., *Can. J. Sport Sci.*, 13: 8–14 (1988).
174. Phair, J., Carey, G.C.R., and Shephard, R.J., *Measuring Human Reactions to Air Pollution: Monograph 4*. Franklin Institute, Washington (1958).
175. Pirnay, F., Bodeux, M., Crielaard, J.M., and Franchimont, P., *Int. J. Sports Med.*, 8: 331–335 (1987).
176. Pollock, M.L., *Exerc. Sports Sci. Rev.*, 1: 155–188 (1973).
177. Pollock, M.L., Miller, H.S., Linnerud, A.C., and Cooper, K.H., *Arch. Phys. Med. Rehabil.*, 56: 141–145 (1975).
178. Pollock, M.L., Gettman, L.R., Milesis, C.A., Bah, M.D., Durstine, L., and Johnson, R.B., *Med. Sci. Sports*, 9: 31–36 (1977).

179. Porcari, J., McCarron, R., Kline, G., Freedson, P.F., Ward, A., Ross, J.A., and Rippe, J.M., *Phys. Sportsmed.,* 15(2): 119–129 (1987).
180. Powell, K.E., Thompson, P.D., Caspersen, C.J., and Kendrick, J.S., *Annu. Rev. Public Health,* 8: 253–287 (1987).
181. Pugh, L.G.C.E., in *Environmental Effects on Work Performance* (G.R. Cumming, D. Snidal, and A.W. Taylor, eds.). Canadian Association of Sport Sciences, Ottawa (1972).
182. Quaglietti, S., and Frohlicher, V.F., in *Physical Activity, Fitness and Health* (C. Bouchard, R.J. Shephard, and T. Stephens, eds.). Human Kinetics Publications, Champaign, Illinois, pp. 591–608 (1994).
183. Rasmussen, B.S., Elkjaer, P., and Juhl, B., *J. Sports Sci.,* 6: 219–228, 1988.
184. Reading, J.L., Goodman, J., Plyley, M., Floras, J., Liu, P., McLaughlin, P.R., and Shephard, R.J., *J. Appl. Physiol.,* 74: 567–573 (1993).
185. Robinson, E.P., and Kjellgard, J.M., *J. Appl. Physiol.,* 52: 1400–1406 (1982).
186. Rogers, M.A., Yamamoto, C., Hagberg, J.M. Martin, W.H., Ehsani, A.A., and Holloszy, J.O., *Med. Sci. Sports Exerc.,* 20: 260–264 (1988).
187. Rosch, P.J., in *Psychomatic Cardiovascular Disorders—When and How to Treat* (P. Kielholz, W. Siegenthaler, P. Taggart, and A. Zanxhetti, eds.). Huber, Bern (1981).
188. Rösler, K., Conley, K.E., Howald, H., Gerber, C., and Hoppeler, H., *J. Appl. Physiol., 61:* 30–36 (1986).
189. Rothenberger, L.A., Chang, J.I., and Cable, T.A., *Am. J. Sports Med.,* 16: 403–407 (1988).
190. Rowell, L.B., in *Handbook of Physiology,* Vol. 27. American Physiological Society, Washington, D.C., pp. 967–1023 (1985).
191. Rubal, B.J., Al Muhailani, A.R., and Rosentwieg, J., *Med. Sci. Sports Exerc.,* 19: 423–429 (1987).
192. Rusko, H., and Bosco, C., *Eur. J. Appl. Physiol.,* 56: 412–418 (1987).
193. Rusko H., and Rahkila, P., *J. Sports Sci.,* 1: 185–194 (1983).
194. Saltin, B., in *Limiting Factors of Physical Performance* (J. Keul, ed.). Thieme, Stuttgart, pp. 235–252 (1973).
195. Saltin, B. *Res. Q.* 67 (Suppl. 3): S1–S10 (1996).
196. Saltin, B., and Hermansen, L., in *Nutrition and Physical Activity* (G. Blix, ed.). Almqvist and Wiksell, Uppsala, p. 32 (1967).
197. Saltin, B., Blomqvist, G., Mitchell, J.H., Johnson, R.L., Wildenthal, K., and Chapman, C.B., *Am. Heart Assoc. Monogr. 23:* 1–68 (1968).
198. Saltin, B., Hartley, L.H., Kilbom, Å., and Åstrand, I., *Scand. J. Clin. Lab. Invest.,* 24: 323–334 (1969).
199. Schuman, S.H., *Environ. Res.,* 5: 59–75 (1972).
200. Schwartz, E., Glick, Z. and Magazanik, A., *Aviat. Space Environ. Med.,* 48: 254–260 (1977).
201. Seals, D.R., Hagberg, J.M., Spina, R.J., Rogers, M.A., Schectman, K.B., and Ehsani, A.A., *Circulation,* 89: 198–205 (1994).
202. Sexton, W.L., Korthuis, R.J., and Laughlin, M.H. *Am. J. Physiol.,* 254: H274–H278 (1988).
203. Sharkey, B.J., *Med. Sci. Sports,* 2: 197–202 (1970).

204. Sharkey, B.J., and Holleman, J.P., *Res. Q.,* 38: 698–704 (1967).
205. Shephard, R.J., *Int. Z. Angew. Physiol.,* 26: 272–278 (1968).
206. Shephard, R.J., *Int. Z. Angew. Physiol.,* 28: 38–48 (1969).
207. Shephard, R.J., *Br. J. Sports Med.,* 8: 38–45 (1974).
208. Shephard, R.J., *Human Physiological Work Capacity.* Cambridge University Press, London (1978).
209. Shephard, R.J., *Ischemic Heart Disease and Exercise.* Croom-Helm Publishing, London (1981).
210. Shephard, R.J., *Physiology and Biochemistry of Exercise.* Praeger Publications, New York (1982).
211. Shephard, R.J., *Biochemistry of Exercise.* Charles C Thomas, Springfield, Illinois, 1983.
212. Shephard, R.J., *Carbon Monoxide—The Silent Killer.* Charles C Thomas, Springfield, Illinois (1983).
213. Shephard, R.J., *CAHPER J.,* 50(6): 2–5, 20 (1985).
214. Shephard, R.J., *Br. J. Sports Med.,* 23: 11–22 (1989).
215. Shephard, R.J., *Can. J. Sports Sci.,* 14: 74–84 (1989).
216. Shephard, R.J., *Body Composition in Biological Anthropology.* Cambridge University Press, London (1989).
217. Shephard, R.J., *Can. J. Sport Sci.,* 17: 83–90 (1992).
217a. Shephard, R.J., in *Endurance in Sport* (R.J. Shephard and P.-O. Åstrand, eds.). Blackwell Scientific Publications, Oxford, England, pp. 471–478 (1992).
218. Shephard, R.J., *J. Aging Phys. Activity,* 1: 59–83 (1993).
219. Shephard, R.J., *Aerobic Fitness and Health.* Human Kinetics Publications, Champaign, Illinois (1994).
220. Shephard, R.J., *Sports Sci. Rev.,* 4: 1–13 (1995).
221. Shephard, R.J., *Am. J. Health Prom.,* 10: 436–452 (1996).
222. Shephard, R.J., *Br. J. Sports Med.,* 30: 5–10 (1996).
223. Shephard, R.J., *Br. J. Sports Med.,* 31: 277–284 (1997).
224. Shephard, R.J., *Physical Activity, Immune Function and Health.* Cooper Publishing, Carmel, Indiana (1997).
225. Shephard, R.J., Physical activity and stress relaxation. *Sports Med.,* (1997). 23: 211–217.
226. Shephard, R.J., *Physical Activity Aging and Health.* Human Kinetics Publications, Champaign, Illinois (1997).
227. Shephard, R.J., and Bouchard, C., *J. Sports Med. Phys. Fitness,* 35: 149–158 (1995).
228. Shephard, R.J., and Shek, P.N., *Can. J. Physiol.,* 22: 95–116 (1997).
229. Shephard, R.J., and Sidney, K.H., *Exerc. Sport Sci. Rev.,* 3: 1–30 (1975).
230. Shephard, R.J., Corey, P., and Cox, M., *Can. J. Publ. Health* 73: 183–187, (1982).
231. Shephard, R.J., Bouhlel, E., Vandewalle, H., and Monod, H., *J. Appl. Physiol.,* 64: 1472–1479 (1988).
232. Shephard, R.J., Kavanagh, T., Mertens, D.J., and Yacoub, M., *Br. J. Sports Med.* 30: 116–121 (1996).
233. Shephard, R.J., Kavanagh, T., Mertens, D.J., Qureshi, S., and Clark, M., *Br. J. Sports Med.* 29: 35–40 (1995).

234. Shephard, R.J., Kavanagh, T., and Mertens, D.J., *J. Cardiopulm. Rehabil.* 18: 45–51 (1998).
235. Sidney, K.H. and Shephard, R.J., *Med. Sci. Sports Exerc.*, 10: 125–131 (1978).
236. Sidney, K.H., and Shephard, R.J., *Can. J. Appl. Spt. Sci.*, 2: 189–194 (1978).
236a. Sidney, K.H., Shephard, R.J., and Harrison, J., *Am. J. Clin. Nutr.*, 30: 326–333 (1977).
237. Simmons, R., and Shephard, R.J., *Int. Z. Angew. Physiol.*, 30: 73–84 (1971).
238. Simmons, R., and Shephard, R.J., *Int. Z. Angew. Physiol.*, 29: 159–172 (1971).
239. Simoneau, J.A., Lortie, G., Boulay, M.R., Marcotte, M., Thibault, M.C., and Bouchard, C., *Eur. J. Appl. Physiol.*, 54: 250–253 (1985).
240. Sjöström, M., Lexell, J., Eriksson, A. and Taylor, C.C., *Eur. J. Appl. Physiol.*, 62: 301–304 (1991).
241. Sloan, E.R.G. and Keatinge, W.R., *J. Appl. Physiol.*, 16: 167–169 (1973).
242. Smith, D.A., and O'Donnell, T.V., *Clin. Sci.*, 67: 229–236 (1984).
243. Stewart, K.H., Kelemen, M.H., and Ewart, C.K., *J. Cardiopulm. Rehabil.*, 14: 35–42 (1994).
244. Stillman, R.J., Lohman, T.G., Slaughter, M.H., and Massey, B.H., *Med. Sci. Sports Exerc.*, 18: 576–580 (1986).
245. Sutton, J.R., in *Exercise, Fitness and Health* (C. Bouchard, R.J. Shephard, T. Stephens, J. Sutton and B. McPherson, eds.). Human Kinetics Publications, Champaign, Illinois (1990).
246. Sutton, J.R., in *Oxford Textbook of Sports Medicine* (M. Harries, C. Williams, W.D. Stanish, and L. Micheli, eds.). Oxford Medical Publications, New York, pp. 231–238 (1994).
247. Tamaki, N., *Eur. J. Appl. Physiol.*, 56: 127–131 (1987).
248. Tanaka, K., Yoshimura, T., Sumida, S., Mitszono, R., Tanaka, S., Konishi, Y., Watanabe, H., Yamada, T., and Maeda, K., *Eur. J. Appl. Physiol.*, 55: 356–361 (1986).
249. Taylor, H.L., Henschel, A., Brozek, J., and Keys, A., *J. Appl. Physiol.*, 2: 223–239 (1949).
250. Taylor, N.A.S., and Wilkinson, J.G., *Sports Med.*, 3: 190–200 (1986).
251. Terjung, R.L., *Sports Sci. Exch.*, 8: 1–4 (1995).
252. Terrados, N., and Maughan, R.J., *J. Sports Sci.*, 13: 55S–62S (1995).
253. Tesch, P., Karlsson, J., and Sjödin, B., in *Exercise and Sport Biology* (P.V. Komi, ed.). Human Kinetics Publications, Champaign, Illinois, pp. 79–83 (1982).
254. Thomas, D.P., *Med. Sci. Sports Exerc.*, 17: 546–553 (1985).
255. Thorstensson., A. *Acta Physiol. Scand.*, 443 (Suppl.): 1–45 (1976).
256. Tipton, M.J., and Golden, F., in *Oxford Textbook of Sports Medicine* (M. Harries, C. Williams, W. Stanish, and L. Micheli, eds.). Oxford University Press, New York, pp. 205–216 (1994).
257. Turto, H., Lindy, S., and Haline, J., *Am. J. Physiol.*, 226: 63–65 (1974).
258. U.S. Surgeon General, *Physical Activity and Health.* Dept. of Health and Human Services, Washington, D.C. (1996).
259. Vernon, H.M., Bedford, T., and Karner, C.F., *Rep. Industr. Fatigue Res. Bd. (Lond.)*, 39. His Majesty's Stationery Office, London (1927).
260. Von Euler, U.S., *Med. Sci. Sport*, 6: 165–173 (1974).

261. Vuori, I.M., *Sport Sci. Rev.*, 4: 46–84 (1995).
262. Vuori, I.M., Oja, P., and Paronen, M., *Med. Sci. Sports Exerc.*, 26: 844–850 (1994).
263. Walter, S.D., Hart, L.E., McIntosh, J.M., and Sutton, J.R., *Arch. Intern. Med.*, 149: 2561–2564 (1989).
264. Wasserman, K., Whipp, B.J., Koyal, S.N., and Beaver, W.L., *J. Appl. Physiol.*, 35: 236–243 (1973).
265. Weiler-Ravell, D., Sheipak, A., Goldenberg, I., Halpern, P., Shoshani, O., Hirschorn, G. and Margolis, A., *Br. Med. J.*, 311: 361–362 (1995).
266. Wenger, H., and Bell, G.J., *Sports Med.*, 3: 346–356 (1986).
267. Wenger, H., and Macnab, R.B.J., in *Applications of Science and Medicine in Sport* (A.W. Taylor, ed.). Charles C Thomas, Springfield, Illinois, pp. 212–221 (1972).
268. White, J.R., *Med. Sci. Sports,* 12: 103 (Abstr.) (1980).
269. Williams, J.A., Wagner, J., Wasnich, R., and Heilbrun, L., *Med. Sci. Sports Exerc.,* 16: 223–227 (1984).
270. Williams, P.T., Wood, P.D., Haskell, W.L., and Vranizan, K., *J.A.M.A.,* 247: 2672–2679 (1982).
271. Wilmore, J., and Costill, D.L., *Physiology of Sport and Exercise.* Human Kinetics Publications, Champaign, Illinois (1994).
272. Wilmore, J.H., Davis, J.A., O'Brien, R.S., Vodak, P.A., Walder, G.R., and Amsterdam, E.A., *Med. Sci. Sports,* 12: 1–8 (1980).
273. Wilt, F., in *Exercise Physiology* (H. Falls, ed.). Academic Press, New York, pp. 395–414 (1968).
274. World Health Organization, *Official Records,* #2. (1948).
275. Wyndham, C.H., and Strydom, N.B., in *Zentrale Themen der Sportmedizin* (W.R. Hollman, ed.). Springer-Verlag, Berlin, pp. 131–149 (1972).
276. Wyndham. C.H., Strydom, N.B., Benade, A.J.S., and Van Rensbury, A.J., *J. Appl. Physiol.,* 35: 454–458 (1973).
277. Yaron, M., Hultgren, H.M., and Alexander, J.K., *Wilderness Environ. Med.,* 6: 20–28 (1995).
278. Yerkes, R.M., and Dodson, J.D., *J. Comp. Neurol. Psychol.* 18: 459–482 (1908).

2
Assessment of Exercise Capacity and Principles of Exercise Prescription

JACK M. GOODMAN
University of Toronto
Toronto, Ontario, Canada

INTRODUCTION: ASSESSMENT OF CARDIOVASCULAR FITNESS

The general assessment of fitness should incorporate four basic components, including measured or estimated maximal oxygen consumption or aerobic power ($\dot{V}_{O_2max}$), muscular strength and endurance, flexibility, and body composition. There are a number of ways of assessing these components, with both the specificity and reproducibility dependent upon the sophistication of the instrumentation used. This chapter provides an overview of the basis for assessing each of these components and provides a physiological basis for the prescription of exercise to improve overall fitness.

Basic Principles

An increase in oxygen consumption ($\dot{V}_{O_2}$) is brought about by an increase in cardiac output and peripheral extraction of oxygen. Cardiac output is augmented by increases in both heart rate (HR) and stroke volume, the latter through two mechanisms: an increase in end-diastolic volume (EDV) via the Frank-Starling relationship and a reduction in end-diastolic volume (ESV) via an augmented contractile state. The increase in EDV may occur predominantly during exercise below the ventilatory threshold (VT) (1), whereas changes in ESV occur at all

59

intensities of exercise. Increased extraction of oxygen [a widened $C(a\text{-}\bar{v})_{O_2}$ difference] is achieved by maximizing both the arterial content of O_2 (Ca_{O_2}) and subsequent extraction of oxygen in the muscle capillaries. Factors determining maximal Ca_{O_2} include the arterial oxygen pressure Pa_{O_2} (affected by pulmonary ventilation and diffusion) and the hemoglobin concentration. Complete oxygen extraction, represented by the lowest possible venous oxygen content ($C\bar{v}_{O_2}$) is dependent on capillary density (affecting tissue diffusing capacity), aerobic enzyme function, and fiber type. The functional limit to oxygen consumption can therefore be expressed by the Fick equation for oxygen, where:

$$\dot{V}_{O_2} = (\text{cardiac output}) \times [C(a\text{-}\bar{v})_{O_2} \text{ difference}]$$

Maximal values of each component will provide a physiological limit to $\dot{V}_{O_2max}$, depicted during graded exercise as a plateau of oxygen consumption despite increasing work rates; this, in turn, defines functional capacity. The linear relationship between work rate and $\dot{V}_{O_2}$ provides the basis for submaximal predictions of aerobic power (see Fig. 1).

Direct gas-exchange measurements using rapid-response O_2 and CO_2 analyzers (see below) can provide accurate measures of $\dot{V}_{O_2max}$, VT, and other gas-exchange parameters that are useful in the clinical assessment of cardiopulmonary

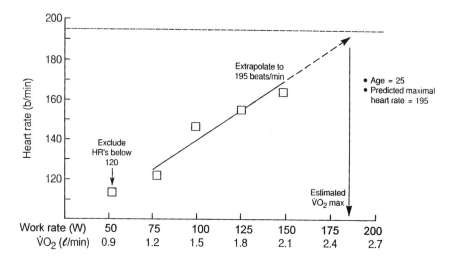

FIGURE I Pattern of $\dot{V}_{O_2}$ during progressive exercise on a cycle ergometer. A linear increase in $\dot{V}_{O_2}$ is observed during graded, submaximal exercise. The linear relationship allows extrapolation from submaximal levels of exercise to an age-predicted heart rate and corresponding oxygen consumption.

impairment, efficacy of pharmacologic intervention, or general fitness (Table 1). Clinical exercise testing now often includes measurement of oxygen consumption and other gas-exchange variables, since $\dot{V}_{O_2max}$ and the VT, versus traditional measures such as left ventricular ejection fraction alone may provide more objective information on both functional status and prognosis in certain cardiac disease states (2). When facilities for these determinations are unavailable, $\dot{V}_{O_2max}$ can be estimated by various methods employing submaximal predictions.

Submaximal Versus Maximal Exercise Testing

Prediction of maximal aerobic power ($\dot{V}_{O_2max}$) remains a common method to assess functional capacity during clinical exercise testing. Advantages over maximal, direct measures of $\dot{V}_{O_2max}$ include (a) short test duration (b) greater safety, (c) low cost (d) less equipment required, (e) less expertise required, and (f) possibility of group testing (3–6). Prediction requires establishment of a steady-state heart rate at a given work rate. The error of prediction ranges from 10–15%, for greater accuracy, a direct measure of maximal O_2 consumption is recommended. The formulas used to predict maximal heart rate (see "Exercise Prescription," below) provide estimates with a standard deviation of about 11 beats per minute (7). Consequently, maximal oxygen intake may be under- or overestimated.

Supine Versus Erect Exercise

Supine exercise tests are slowly been supplanted by upright protocols. However, many laboratories still use supine cycle ergometry for clinical assessment of left ventricular function. Supine testing offers the advantage of a greater likelihood of detecting of ST-segment abnormalities in myocardial ischemia (8). When the individual is supine, left ventricular end-diastolic volume is maximal, thereby increasing LV wall stress (and thus myocardial oxygen demand), with little change in stroke volume throughout a progressive exercise test. Measures of $\dot{V}_{O_2max}$ are typically 12–18% less during supine exercise testing; therefore results must be interpreted carefully relative to data obtained from upright protocols.

Choice of Ergometer and Protocol

Values for $\dot{V}_{O_2max}$ differ depending on the type of ergometer used for testing. Treadmill testing yields a "true" $\dot{V}_{O_2max}$ when subjects are properly motivated. It is therefore used as the gold standard for the assessment of functional capacity. Supine cycle ergometry will yield a $\dot{V}_{O_2max}$ 12–18% less than treadmill testing, and upright cycle ergometry produces values 90–96% of those obtained during maximal treadmill testing (9). Arm cranking yields a peak $\dot{V}_{O_2}$ 30–35% less than treadmill running. These discrepancies are due in part to differences in the muscle

TABLE 1   Common Gas-Exchange Measurements, Definitions, and Normal Ranges

Measurement	Definition	Normal Range
$\dot{V}_{O_2max}$	Upper limit for O_2 consumption obtained despite increase in work rate. Functional limit of cardiovascular system.	Male: 4.2−0.0032 (age) L/min (SD ± 0.4); 60−0.55 (age) ml/kg/min^{-1} (SD ± 7.5)[a] Female: 2.6−0.014 (age) L/min (SD ± 0.4); 48−0.37 (age) ml/kg/min^{-1} (SD ± 7.0)[a]
$\dot{V}_{O_2}$ slope ($\Delta\dot{V}_{O_2}/\Delta WR$)	Aerobic contribution to exercise; low slope implies greater anaerobic contribution to work.	8.6−12 ml/min/W
O_2 pulse ($\dot{V}_{O_2}/HR$)	Proportional to $C(a-\bar{v})_{O_2}$ difference when SV is constant. Varies with age, sex, height, and hemoglobin; higher in the endurance-trained. Can reflect changes in SV at maximum exercise if $C(a-\bar{v})_{O_2}$ is constant.	10−14 (males) 7−10 (female)
Ventilatory threshold (VT)	Noninvasive index of the nonlinear increase in blood lactate. Disproportionate increase in $\dot{V}_E$ versus $\dot{V}_{O_2}$ or other criteria (see text).	Absolute (%$\dot{V}_{O_2max}$): 45−65% Relative (ml/kg/min^{-1}): >25 ml/kg/min
$\dot{V}_E$/MVV (dyspnea index)	Index providing analysis of balance between demand and capacity of ventilatory system.	65−80%
HR_{max}	Maximal heart rate obtained during maximal-effort exercise test. Age-dependent.	$HR_{max} = 210 − 0.65$ age $= 220 −$ age
RER_{max} ($\dot{V}_{CO_2}/\dot{V}_{O_2}$)max	Indicates substrate utilization (1 = complete carbohydrate metabolism). Rest = 0.75−0.85.	Values >1.10−1.15 indicate maximal effort reached (when used in conjunction with other criteria—see text).
VD/VT	Physiological ratio of dead space/tidal volume. Indicates matching of ventilation to perfusion. Falls with exercise, high in obstructive lung disease.	25−40% at rest, 5−20 during exercise

Abbreviations: HR = heart rate; MVV = maximum voluntary ventilation; RER = respiratory gas exchange ratio; $\dot{V}_{O_2}$ = oxygen consumption; $\dot{V}_{CO_2}$ = carbon dioxide production; VD = dead space; $\dot{V}_E$ = ventilation; VT = tidal volume.
[a]Adapted from Ref. 21; used with permission.

mass involved and can be related directly to the cardiac output seen in each case. Each device has advantages and disadvantages (Table 2). Common ergometers include the step bench, treadmill, and cycle ergometer, as described briefly below. For clinical exercise testing, cycle ergometers are more popular in Europe, whereas in the United States, treadmills are the common modality (6). Step-bench ergometers have gained some popularity for submaximal testing but are not well suited for maximal exercise testing. They remain largely an option for screening healthy individuals prior to the prescription of exercise.

Whether the cycle or treadmill ergometer is used, the optimal test duration for eliciting a true $\dot{V}_{O_2max}$ is 8–10 min (6,10), with a 1- to 2-min low-load warm-up preceding the definitive exercise stress.

Three commonly used protocols are (a) intermittent incremental loading, where successive work rates are separated by short rest periods; (b) continuous-step incremental loading, where increasing work rates are applied continuously with individual stages lasting from 1–3 min—this method usually involves achieving a ''steady state'' heart rate and/or $\dot{V}_{O_2}$; and (c) continuous incremental or ''ramp'' loading.

TABLE 2   Comparison of Testing Ergometers—Advantages and Disadvantages

Ergometer	Advantages	Disadvantages
Step bench	Low cost	Maximal testing not possible
	Low maintenance	Ancillary measures difficult
	No calibration	Limited by anthropometric factors
	Habituation easy	
Treadmill	Yields a plateau in $\dot{V}_{O_2}$	Costly
	Effort is not self-paced	Noisy
	Common activity (walking)	Ancillary measures difficult
		Hazardous (running)
		Habituation difficult
Cycle ergometer	Ancillary measures easy	Pedaling frequency affects loading
	Habituation easy	Limited by muscle strength
	Reproducible work rates	Requires regular calibration (mechanically braked)
	High mechanical efficiency	Plateau in $\dot{V}_{O_2}$ not usually obtained in sedentary subjects
	Easily calibrated	
	Occupies little space	

Source: Modified from Ref. 9; used with permission.

Step-Bench Ergometer

The step bench is simple and inexpensive, requires little habituation, and is a low-maintenance device. However, it is not widely accepted for maximal testing (9). Power output is determined by body mass, frequency of stepping, and the height of the step or steps. The mechanical efficiency of stepping is relatively low and has a narrow range (15–19%). Stepping frequency (footplants) should not exceed 150 footplants per minute.

The Canadian Standard Test of Fitness uses a two-step configuration. Although it was designed primarily as a motivational tool, scores can yield a moderately accurate submaximal prediction of $\dot{V}_{O_2max}$ (11,12) in either a field or laboratory setting. Cadence is controlled by music speed, progressing every 3 min until 70% of predicted heart rate is obtained, with normative scores available for comparison.

Cycle Ergometers

Both mechanically and electrically braked cycle ergometers are widely used for clinical and laboratory exercise testing. Stable monitoring of blood pressure, facility of electrocardiographic (ECG) recording, and sampling for blood, easy habituation, and moderate cost make this type of ergometer popular. Furthermore, power output can easily be measured and reproduced. Because leg fatigue often limits performance on this modality, $\dot{V}_{O_2max}$ is commonly 8–10% lower than with the use of a treadmill (9). Pedaling frequencies used for testing range from 50 rpm (Åstrand-Ryhming test) to 90 rpm for well-trained cyclists.

Irma Åstrand (13) described a nomogram for estimating $\dot{V}_{O_2max}$ based on the linear relationship between $\dot{V}_{O_2}$ and heart rate, the final version of the nomogram providing a correction for age. The nomogram (Fig. 2) is based on the heart rate achieved at a single work rate performed for 6 min, sufficient to elicit a heart rate between 125 and 170 beats per minute. The Bannister-Legg nomogram (14) may be more accurate for less fit individuals (Fig. 2).

A modified YMCA protocol (15) uses the Åstrand and Ryhming nomogram (Fig. 2) and incremental work rates until subjects reach 70% of the age-predicted heart rate. An initial work rate of 25 W is used for females and males above 35 years of age, with males below age 35 beginning at 50 W. In each case, the work rate is increased by the initial amount every 2 min until 60–70% of the age-predicted heart rate is obtained. After this point, work rate is increased by 25 W and exercise continues for 2 min more. $\dot{V}_{O_2max}$ (L/min) is estimated by using the Åstrand nomogram and the age-correction equations provide below (15):

$$\text{Males: } \dot{V}_{O_2max} = 0.348 \, (X) - 0.035 \, (\text{age, years}) + 3.011$$

$$\text{Females: } \dot{V}_{O_2max} = 0.302 \, (X) - 0.019 \, (\text{age, years}) + 1.593$$

where X is the $\dot{V}_{O_2max}$ obtained from the Åstrand nomogram.

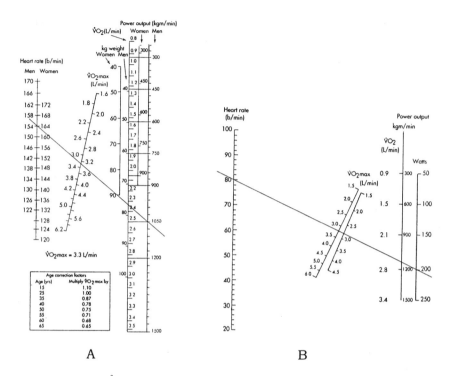

A   B

FIGURE 2   (A) The Åstrand and (B) Bannister-Legg nomogram for determination of maximal oxygen consumption during submaximal cycle ergometry or step testing. Heart rates at a given work rate correspond to an estimated $\dot{V}_{O_2 max}$. A line is connected from the work-rate scale to the observed pulse rate at that work rate, providing a predicted maximal oxygen uptake. Two examples are provided here (dashed lines), with work rates of 100 and 200 W achieved during a cycle ergometer test. In using the Åstrand nomogram, a correction factor for age should be applied if subjects are above 30 years of age, using the following equation: Corrected $\dot{V}_{O_2}$ = 1.189–0.0086 (age, years). If either age or maximal heart rate is known, the following table may be used.

Age	Factor	HR_{max}	Factor
15	1.1	210	1.12
25	1.0	200	1.00
35	0.87	190	0.93
40	0.83	180	0.83
45	0.78	170	0.75
50	0.75	160	0.69
55	0.71	150	0.64
60	0.68		
65	0.65		

Source: From Refs. 13 and 14.

Another submaximal protocol (16) uses an extrapolation technique, where $\dot{V}_{O_2}$ is estimated at three or more work rates and a line of best fit is extrapolated to an age-predicted maximal heart rate (Fig. 1). The choice of work rates is varied according to the activity level and body mass of the individual (Table 3), with step increments (e.g., every 3 min). The initial work rate should elicit a minimum heart rate of 120–125, since heart rate contributes more and stroke volume contributes less to increases in cardiac output, and hence $\dot{V}_{O_2}$, above this level.

Treadmill Testing

Functional capacity may be predicted in terms of either metabolic equivalents (METs), or $\dot{V}_{O_2}$. All protocols use step increments in work rate and therefore are not advised for determination of the VT; however, they are generally effective for ECG stress testing. The Bruce protocol (17) increases grade and speed every 3 min. Although treadmill testing is basically a walking protocol, running may be required in well-trained individuals who reach the final test stages. This test is usually completed rapidly and is widely used in clinical settings. The Balke and Ware (18) protocol was first designed to test military personnel and offers smaller increments of work rate (2% in the first minute and 1% each minute thereafter) at a set speed of 5.3 km/h. The disadvantage of this protocol is the length of time required to complete the testing of most subjects. A modified version uses greater increments in grade (5% every 3 min). Among other protocols (19), the Ellestad protocol begins at 2.7 km/h, increasing to 9.7 km/h and an initial grade of 10% and finishing at 15% by 11 min. The Naughton protocol uses a constant speed (3.2 and 5.3 km/h), with 2.5–3.5% grade increments every 3 min. Each work rate corresponds to an increase of 3.5 ml O_2/kg/min^{-1}.

Small but rapid increments in work rate are preferred when direct measurement of $\dot{V}_{O_2max}$ and the VT are desired. Weiner and Lourie (20) describe a widely used protocol in which subjects choose a comfortable running speed, with grade

TABLE 3 Cycle Ergometry Protocols and Selection of Power Output (W): American College of Sports Medicine Protocol

Protocol	Test stage, minutes			
	1 (1–2)	2 (3–4)	3 (5–6)	4 (7–8)
A	25	50	75	100
B	25	50	100	150
C	50	100	150	200

Key: A = body mass < 73 kg; inactive or active; 74–90 kg, inactive. B = body mass 74–90 kg, active; > 91 kg, not active. C = body mass > 91 kg, active.
Source: Modified from Ref. 16; used with permission.

increasing 2% every 2 min. Recommended running speeds are 11.3 km/h for average healthy females, 12.1 km/h for female runners, 12.9 km/h for average healthy males, and 13.7 km/h for male runners (5).

Direct Measurement of Maximal Oxygen Consumption

On-line computer-driven metabolic carts have made measurement of $\dot{V}_{O_2max}$ simple and expeditious. With proper calibration and careful maintenance, the test-retest reliability is 0.95, with a coefficient of variation of <3% (21). Equipment uses involves semiautomatic or fully automated systems, incorporating either a mixing chamber for time-average sampling of expired gases or breath-by-breath gas analysis. Breath-by-breath systems are costly and are not advised unless advanced measures of pulmonary/respiratory function are required.

Various gas-exchange data can be determined and, in conjunction with heart-rate data, can provide important information on cardiopulmonary status (Table 1) and factors potentially limiting exercise performance. Metabolic carts can generate graphic reports illustrating the HR and $\dot{V}_{O_2}$ response to exercise and identifying the VT (Fig. 3). Use of the VT and $\dot{V}_{O_2max}$ has gained popularity in the clinical evaluation of cardiovascular disease states (2). Concurrent radionuclide angiography (RNA) and gas-exchange measurements provide comprehensive information on cardiopulmonary status (1) (Table 1). In our protocol, upright cycle ergometry with graded exercise (15-W increments every minute) is performed in conjunction with first-pass RNA measurements. Gated RNA is performed at rest, during submaximal exercise (below the VT), and near peak exercise.

Criteria Used to Establish Attainment of $\dot{V}_{O_2max}$

A number of gas-exchange variables and ancillary data provide evidence of a true maximal effort. Failure to increase oxygen consumption despite an increase in work rate represents the functional limit of the cardiorespiratory system; further work can be performed anaerobically, but a test rarely proceeds more than 60–90 s beyond this point. Taylor et al. (22) first described acceptable criteria for a plateau of oxygen consumption during a progressive interrupted treadmill test: a rise in oxygen consumption of less less than 2.1 ml/kg/min^{-1} (150 ml/min) with an increase in work rate (2.5% grade at 11.3 km/h). Other criteria include the attainment of an age-predicted heart rate (see below), a respiratory gas-exchange ratio >1.10, and blood lactate >8 mmol/L (23).

In well-trained subjects, a plateau in $\dot{V}_{O_2}$ can be achieved in a high percentage of cases (>80%). However, only 50% of untrained individuals are likely to demonstrate a plateau.

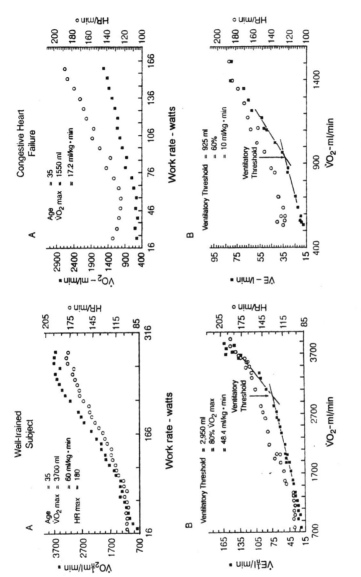

FIGURE 3 Ventilatory gas-exchange data obtained during graded exercise to maximum in well-trained subjects, and in patients with congestive heart failure. Data are averaged over 30 s, obtained from breath-by-breath sampling. In each example, graph A illustrates the heart rate/$\dot{V}_{O_2}$ response; graph B illustrates identification of the ventilatory threshold from $\dot{V}_E$ and $\dot{V}_{O_2}$ data. Highly deconditioned subjects or those with pathological conditions limiting cardiovascular function exhibit a lower $\dot{V}_{O_2max}$ and ventilatory threshold.

Field Tests to Assess Aerobic Power

The advantage of field testing is low cost, with data that show a relatively good correlation to $\dot{V}_{O_2max}$. Disadvantages include dependency on a high degree of motivation (since running tests require a "maximal" effort). Another limitation is imposed by interindividual differences in running economy, particularly in smaller children (4). The most widely used running test for determining aerobic power is Cooper's 12-min run (24) and the AAHPERD's 1.6-km (1-mi) walk/run. Walking tests have also yielded acceptable predictions of $\dot{V}_{O_2max}$ (25), particularly in older adults. In this example, subjects would walk as fast as possible for 1.6 km (1 mi), and $\dot{V}_{O_2max}$ could be estimated as follows:

$$\dot{V}_{O_2max} = 132.9 - 0.035 \text{ (wt)} - 0.388 \text{ (age)} + 6.32 \text{ (sex)}$$
$$- 3.26 \text{ (time)} - 0.157 \text{ (HR)}$$

where wt is body mass in kg, age is number of years, sex equals 0 for females and 1 for males, time is number of minutes and hundredths of minutes, and HR is measured during the last 0.4 km (0.25 mi) measured in beats per minute.

Classification of Aerobic Power

Maximal aerobic power depends on sex, age, genotype, and level of habitual activity. It can be altered acutely by drugs, anemia, ambient P_{O_2}, and other factors (3). Table 4 provides a general classification of $\dot{V}_{O_2max}$ for healthy individuals.

TABLE 4 Classification of Aerobic Power

| | $\dot{V}_{O_2max}$, ml/kg·min | | | | |
Age	Low	Fair	Average	Good	High
Men:					
20–29	<25	25–33	34–42	43–52	>53
30–39	<23	23–30	31–38	39–48	>49
40–49	<20	20–26	27–35	34–42	>43
50–69	<18	18–24	25–33	34–42	>43
60–69	<16	16–22	23–30	31–40	>41
Women:					
20–29	<24	24–30	31–37	38–48	>49
30–39	<20	20–27	28–33	34–44	>45
40–49	<17	17–23	24–30	31–41	>42
50–59	<15	15–20	21–27	28–37	>38
60–69	<13	13–17	18–23	24–34	>35

Source: Modified from Ref. 39.

Subjective means of classifying functional status in patients with heart failure, such as the New York Heart Association's levels 1–4, are now being replaced by more objective measures according to $\dot{V}_{O_2max}$ and the VT (Table 5) (2). Other gas-exchange variables that provide additional information on cardiopulmonary status are presented in Table 1. World-class endurance athletes have values for $\dot{V}_{O_2max}$ in excess of 70–80 ml/kg/min^{-1}, and some paraplegic athletes are capable of reaching figures of 60 ml/kg/min^{-1}. Such athletes may have stroke volumes in excess of 200 ml and maximal cardiac outputs greater than 40 L/min.

Equations can estimate maximal cardiac output and stroke volume (with heart-rate data) (21) from maximal oxygen consumption, where:

$$\text{Cardiac output}_{max}(\text{L/min}) = 5.31 + 4.6 \, (\dot{V}_{O_2max}\text{L/min})$$

Safety of Exercise Testing

The risks associated with maximal exercise testing are relatively low. The risk of death during an exercise test in apparently healthy individuals is approximately 0.5 per 10,000 tests (26). Pooled data from a number of cardiac laboratories suggest an overall risk of death, including a 4-day period following exercise testing of approximately 1 death per 10,000 tests (27). In non-clinical settings, risks are even lower. In testing those suspected of coronary disease, risks can be reduced through attendance of an experienced physician, pretest history and exam, resting 12-lead ECG, continuous ECG monitoring during and after exercise, ensuring the availability of emergency resuscitation and drug kits, and a full cool down prior to showering (6). In certain cases, the risks of exercise testing may outweigh the potential benefits, and unless unusual circumstances dictate, exercise testing should be avoided in such cases. Absolute and relative and contraindications for exercise testing are presented in Table 6.

TABLE 5   Classification of Functional Impairment

Class	Aerobic power, ($\dot{V}_{O_2max}$) ml/kg·min	Ventilatory threshold, ml/kg·min
A: Mild to none	>20	>14
B: Mild to moderate	16–20	11–14
C: Moderate to severe	10–16	8–11
D: Severe	6–10	5–8
E: Very severe	<6	<4

Source: From Ref. 2; used with permission.

TABLE 6   Contraindications to Exercise Testing

Absolute:
   Recent myocardial infarction
   Unstable angina
   Uncontrolled cardiac arrhythmias compromising LV function
   Severe heart failure
   Severe aortic stenosis
   Dissecting aortic aneurysm
   Recent systemic or pulmonary emboli or acute thrombophlebitis
   Acute pericarditis
   Acute infection or fever
Relative:
   Resting DBP > 120 mmHg; SBP > 200 mmHg
   Left main coronary artery disease obstruction
   Fixed-rate pacemakers
   Cardiomyopathies
   Dangerous LV irritability
   Ventricular aneurysm
   Moderate valve disease
   Conduction defects
   Uncontrolled metabolic diseases
   Neuromuscular or musculoskeletal limitations

Abbreviations: DBP = diastolic blood pressure; SBP = systolic blood pressure; LV = left ventricle.

The Electrocardiogram and Exercise Testing

Preparation and Lead Configuration

Reliable recording of the ECG during testing is assured by adequate skin preparation and appropriate choice of lead configuration. Typical problems include those caused by changes in body position and respiratory movements. Changes in body position alter the QRS axis and R-wave amplitude, whereas respiratory movements can alter Q waves, R-wave amplitude, baseline voltage, and T-wave orientation. Improvement of the signal-to-noise ratio and baseline drift is best achieved by abrading the skin surface to remove the dry surface keratin.

A standard 12-lead ECG should be performed prior to exercise. The ideal number of leads to monitor during exercise is still not agreed. The V_5 position has the greatest sensitivity for detecting ST-segment depression and is therefore routinely used, with Frank's X, Y, and Z leads advocated by some.

When testing athletes and those previously assessed as free of cardiovascular disease, the modified lead II or CM5 lead is preferred. The ECG signal should be obtained every minute during exercise and for a period of 5–10 min following exercise. Oscilloscopic monitoring allows for instantaneous waveform analysis.

If subjects are suspected of having coronary artery disease, sensitivity in detecting myocardial ischemia is enhanced by supine recovery. But in normal circumstances, recovery should be active (25–30% $\dot{V}_{O_2max}$) so QS to minimize orthostatic hypotension and cramping and to speed the removal of blood lactate. Systemic blood pressure should be measured concurrently with the ECG. If movement and noise prevents this, resting, peak exercise, and recovery measurements are essential.

Analysis of the Exercise Electrocardiogram

Analysis of the exercise ECG should include (a) rate, (b) rhythm, (c) P waves, (d) PR interval, (e) QRS complex, (f) ST segment, (g) T waves, (h) U waves, and (i) QT interval (19). Briefly, the normal response to exercise includes a reduction in the QT interval, an upsloping ST segment at the j point, superpositioning of the P and T waves, reduction in the R wave, and an increased amplitude of the Q and T waves. Common ECG criteria indicating myocardial ischemia during exercise testing include (a) ST-segment changes; (b) U-wave inversion; (c) changes in R- and Q-wave amplitude, and (d) T-wave changes (Table 7).

Responses must be assessed relative to the *sensitivity* and *specificity* of the test (Table 8). Sensitivity reflects the percentage of diseased patients who demonstrate positive test results; a large number of false-negative tests therefore reflects poor test sensitivity. Specificity reflects the ability of the test to rule out disease in a healthy population; false-positive tests reduce specificity.

Causes of false-positive and false-negative tests are presented in Table 9. Treadmill ECG testing provides an overall specificity of 90% and sensitivity of

TABLE 7 Ischemic Electrocardiographic Criteria

Segment or wave	Pattern
ST segment	1. Horizontal 0.1 mV > 80 ms
	2. Upsloping "ST-delay" > 0.1 mV > 80 ms
	3. Downsloping > 0.1 mV > 80 ms at J point
	4. Elevation > 0.1 mV above resting ST segment
T wave	Inversion
U wave	Inversion
R wave	Diminished amplitude

TABLE 8   Diagnostic Value of Testing—Calculations and Definition

Calculation		Definition
Specificity	$= \dfrac{TP}{TP + FN} \times 100$	• Percentage of normal (undiseased) subjects who show negative tests Reduced by FP test results
Sensitivity	$= \dfrac{TN}{FP + TN} \times 100$	• Percentage of patients with documented CAD who show positive test results Reduced by FN test results
Predictive value of abnormal test	$= \dfrac{TP}{TP + FP} \times 100$	• Percentage of individuals with an abnormal test who *have* disease
Relative value	$= \dfrac{TP(TP + FP)}{FN(TN + FN)}$	• Relative rate of occurrence of disease in groups with abnormal tests versus those with a normal test

Abbreviations: CAD = coronary artery disease; TP = true positive (positive test result and documented disease); FP = false positive (positive test result but no disease); TN = true negative (negative test result and no disease); FN = false negative (negative test result but disease present).
Source: From Ref. 8; used with permission.

70% (8), with details of test methodology contributing significantly to the wide range reported for each variable (specificity, 35–90%; sensitivity, 40–100%).

Atypical Electrocardiographic Responses in Healthy Subjects

Well-trained athletes often exhibit ECG abnormalities (including abnormal waveforms and dysrhythmias) during and after exercise, many of which mimic alterations found in disease. ECG abnormalities are common in the athletic population (Table 10). Rhythm disturbances are likely related to increased parasympathetic activity, and waveform abnormalities reflect various forms of cardiomegaly. Using proper diagnostic criteria, most training-induced irregularities can be differentiated from true pathological conditions (28).

Termination of an Exercise Test

Exercise tests should normally be terminated if maximal oxygen intake is achieved or if medical and/or safety factors compromise the subject's health (Table 11). Warnings of potential medical problems include mild to moderate myocardial ischemia and/or nonspecific abnormalities in the ECG. During treadmill testing, caution is necessary when subjects approach maximal effort. If subjects

TABLE 9 Causes of False-Positive and False-Negative Tests

False-negative tests:
    Inadequate work rate achieved
    Limited ECG leads
    Absence of ancillary data (blood pressure, heart rate)
    Single-vessel disease
    Adequate collateral circulation (CAD without ischemia)
    Other exercise limitations
    Observer or technical error
    Post–bypass surgery patients
False-positive tests:
    Female sex
    LV hypertrophy
    Digitalis
    Hypokalemia
    Preexisting ST-segment depression at rest
    Sudden intense exercise
    Valvular disease
    Anemia
    Cardiomyopathy
    Pectus cavatum
    Pericardial disease
    Vasoregulatory asthenia
    Conduction defects (Wolff-Parkinson-White syndrome/BBB)
    Hypertension
    Hyperventilation

Abbreviations: CAD = coronary artery disease; ECG = electrocardiogram; BBB = bundle branch block; LV = left ventricular.

are attached to a mouthpiece, a hand-signaling system should be established prior to exercise to indicate impending exhaustion (e.g., 1 min). This may not only prevent injury but also encourage the subject to complete a final work rate, yielding valuable data that might otherwise have been lost.

Assessment of Flexibility

Static flexibility is defined as the maximal range of motion at a single joint or a series of joints (29). *Dynamic flexibility* reflects the resistance of a joint to motion.

Flexibility is often an overlooked component of fitness, but in certain sports it is essential, and it is linked to both prevention of and recovery from various acute injuries. Factors that limit flexibility include joint structural characteristics (e.g., hinge, gliding, ball and socket, etc.), opposition of soft tissues, joint patholo-

TABLE 10   Common Electrocardiographic Abnormalities During Exercise in Well-Trained Athletes

Abnormality	Possible physiologic cause
Conduction and rhythm	Increased parasympathetic activity
Sinus bradycardia	
AV dissociation	
Wandering atrial pacemaker	
AV block	
Premature atrial contractions	
Premature ventricular contractions	
Supraventricular contractions	
Waveform	
↑ P-wave amplitude	Atrial dilation and/or hypertrophy
QRS criteria for hypertrophy	LVH, RVH
↑ QRS duration and notching	Conduction defects, bundle branch blocks
ST-segment elevation	Blocks
↑ T-wave amplitude, inversion, biphasic	Increased vagal tone, increased RV volume
↑ U-wave voltage	Bradycardia

Abbreviations: LVH = left ventricular hypertrophy; RV = right ventricle.

gies, and/or injuries. Joint rigidity is likely a function of joint capsule and muscle flexibility and is influenced to a lesser extent by tendons and ligaments.

Tests of flexibility include both *indirect* and *direct* methods. Indirect methods, while simple and expedient to administer, are limited by the confounding influence of anthropometric factors such as limb length, and the tests may involve muscle compartments not intended in a specific protocol. Direct methods are relatively precise but are more time-consuming and suffer from a paucity of normative scores.

Indirect Methods to Assess Flexibility

Cureton's Test of Minimal Flexibility

This test has two parts: first, the subject performs straight-legged toe-touching (males: fingers must reach floor; females: palms must touch floor). The second part involves a simple "sit and reach" procedure with the legs extended; the distance from the forehead to the floor is measured in inches.

Wells and Dillon

The Wells and Dillon sit-and-reach test for hamstring and upper and lower back flexibility uses a fixed scale mounted 30 cm above the ground. The subject is

TABLE 11 Reasons for Terminating an Exercise Test

Absolute:
  Severe angina or progressing angina (to 3+ on angina scale)
  Severe dyspnea
  Marked ST-segment depression (>4 mm)
  Multifocal PVC (couplets, triplets)
  Excessive increase in BP (SBP > 250 mmHg; DBP > 120 mmHg)
  Drop in SBP with increasing work rate
  Second- or third-degree block
  Sustained SVT
  Confusion, pallor, cyanosis, cold clammy skin
  Patient request
  Equipment failure
Relative:
  ECG abnormalities including ST-segment depression >2 mm
  Appearance of BBB or conduction abnormalities
  Hypertensive response
  SVT
  PVC (multifocal)
  Leg fatigue and/or cramps
  Increased chest pain

Abbreviations: DBP = diastolic blood pressure; SBP = systolic blood pressure; BP = blood pressure; BBB = bundle branch block; SVT = supraventricular tachycardia; PVC = premature ventricular contraction.

instructed to lean forward as far as possible along the scale, pointing the fingers. The Canadian Standardized Test of Fitness utilizes a modified Wells and Dillon flexometer to assess flexibility (12). The subject sits with legs fully extended, with the soles of the feet against the crossbars of the flexometer, which is adjusted vertically according to foot length. With legs fully extended, the subject reaches forward, sliding a marker along the measuring scale as far as possible. Maximal forward flexion is measured to the nearest centimeter and is compared to available normative scores (Table 12).

Shoulder Elevation and Trunk Extension

Shoulder elevation is tested with the subject prone and the arms extended a shoulder width apart. A measuring stick is raised while the chin remains on the floor.

Direct Methods to Assess Flexibility

Direct techniques are best for athletic populations when specific assessments of joint flexibility are required during training or rehabilitation.

TABLE 12   Modified Wells and Dillon Sit-and-Reach Scores

Age	Trunk flexion, cm				
	20–29	30–39	40–49	50–59	60–69
Male:					
Excellent	>39	>37	>34	>34	>32
Above average	34–39	33–37	29–34	28–34	25–32
Average	30–33	28–32	24–28	24–27	20–24
Below average	25–29	23–27	18–23	16–23	15–19
Poor	<25	<23	<18	<16	<15
Female:					
Excellent	>40	>40	>37	>38	>34
Above average	37–40	36–40	34–37	33–38	31–34
Average	33–36	32–35	30–33	30–32	27–30
Below average	28–32	27–31	25–29	25–29	23–26
Poor	<28	<27	<25	<25	<24

Source: Modified from Ref. 12; used with permission.

Goniometer

This involves the use of a protractor-like device. The arms of the instrument are placed along the limbs and the center of the goniometer is placed at the axis of rotation of the joint. The electrogoniometer uses a potentiometer in place of a protractor. It can assess joint mobility during physical activity. The problems associated with goniometric measurements include identification of the axis of rotation of the joint and precise positioning of the protractor arms along on the limbs (29).

Leighton Flexometer

The Leighton flexometer uses a device incorporating a rotating needle that is sensitive to gravity. The device is fixed to a limb and is capable of measuring the range of motion in several joints in various planes of orientation (30). This technique has a high test-retest reliability coefficient and provides a standardized starting position with direct quantification of joint flexibility (29). Furthermore, it can be used on a wide number of joints and is relatively inexpensive.

Assessment of Muscle Strength and Endurance

The method chosen for assessment of muscle strength and endurance depends on the type of strength (isometric, isotonic, isokinetic) and the *specificity* desired for assessment and performance. Simple yet practical field tests may provide a coarse measure of muscle strength, whereas laboratory tests can provide sophisticated data for athletes or for those undergoing neuromuscular and/or musculoskeletal rehabilitation. The test-retest variation of usual methods is around 10%, but the degree of specificity depends largely on the similarity of the test to the sport or activity under consideration (31).

Assessment of Isotonic Strength

Isotonic strength testing elicits a muscular contraction against a resistance while allowing muscle shortening. For instance, the investigator may measure the heaviest weight that can be lifted during a single attempt, known as a "1 RM," or repetition maximum. This method is still seen as the "gold standard" for determining strength (32). It requires an initial conservative estimate of the maximal weight (mass) that the individual is capable of lifting. Although many protocols for determining the 1 RM have been described (32), it is ideally found within three to five maximal efforts. Adequate rest is required between efforts for an accurate determination (2–4 min). Either free weights or lifting machinery (e.g., a universal gym) may be used. Upper and lower body strength could include the 1 RM bench press (upper body) and leg press (lower body) tests on the Universal™ gym. Scores are usually expressed as Newtons (N) but more typically as kilograms (kg) (31).

Calisthenic exercise testing has been widely employed, but strict procedures are essential if reliable data are to be obtained. Commonly used field tests include *sit-ups* and total *push-ups* (Table 13 and 14). Typically, the push-up test is administered differently for males and females. Males must lower the upper body to the height of a fist above the ground and must extend with straight arms. For females, the knees are bent and on the floor. Note is taken of the total number performed while maintaining the required position. The 1-min speed sit-up test requires the subject to perform the maximum number of bent-knee sit-ups possible in the allocated time (1 min), keeping the hands locked behind the head. The tester holds the ankles as the subject sits up, touching elbow to knee. Although this test can provide a simple measure of abdominal strength, repeated practice may lead to lower back pain unless the legs are bent, the feet are unrestrained, and the small of the lower back is well supported.

Assessment of Isometric Strength

Forearm isometric strength can be tested by using a handgrip dynamometer (Harpenden) adjusted for hand size. A combined right- and left-hand (age-specific) score is usually reported (Tables 13 and 14). Alternatively, calibrated force transducers or strain gauges can provide a record of force, rate of force development, and the force-time integral (31). True isometric movements are rare during physi-

TABLE 13   Normative Scores for Push-ups, Sit-ups, and Handgrip Tests of Strength: Males

	Age, years				
	20–29	30–39	40–49	50–59	60–69
Combined left and right hand grip (newtons)					
Excellent	>1129	>1120	>1083	>1000	>927
Above average	1037–1129	1037–1120	1010–1083	936–1000	854–927
Average	973–1028	963–1028	936–1000	881–927	789–845
Below average	890–964	890–955	863–927	799–872	725–780
Poor	<890	<890	<863	<799	<725
Push-ups (total performed)					
Excellent	>35	>29	>21	>20	>17
Above average	29–35	22–29	17–21	13–20	11–17
Average	22–28	17–21	13–16	10–12	8–10
Below average	17–21	12–16	10–12	7–9	5–7
Poor	<17	<12	<10	<7	<4
Sit-ups (total in 60 s)					
Excellent	>42	>35	>31	>26	>23
Above average	37–42	31–35	26–30	22–25	17–22
Average	33–36	27–30	22–25	18–21	12–16
Below average	29–32	22–26	17–21	16–17	7–11
Poor	<29	<22	<17	<13	<7

Note: 1 kg = 9.18 newtons.
Source: Modified from Ref. 12; used with permission.

TABLE 14   Normative Scores for Push-ups, Sit-ups, and Handgrip Tests of Strength: Females

	Age (years)					
	20–29	30–39	40–49	50–59	60–69
Combined left and right hand grip (newtons)					
Excellent	>643	>661	>661	>558	>542
Above average	579–643	606–661	597–661	542–588	496–542
Average	560–588	560–597	542–588	505–532	568–587
Below average	505–551	514–551	505–532	468–496	441–459
Poor	<514	<505	<505	<568	<441
Push-ups (total performed)					
Excellent	>29	>26	>23	>20	>16
Above average	21–29	20–26	15–23	11–20	12–16
Average	15–20	13–19	11–14	7–10	5–11
Below average	10–14	8–12	5–10	2–6	1–4
Poor	<10	<8	<5	<1	<1
Sit-ups (total in 60 s)					
Excellent	>35	>28	>24	>18	>15
Above average	31–35	24–28	20–24	12–18	12–15
Average	25–30	20–23	15–19	5–11	4–11
Below average	21–24	15–19	7–14	3–4	2–3

Note: 1 kg = 9.18 newtons.
Source: Modified from Ref. 12; used with permission.

cal activity, and the value of conclusions drawn from this test method is therefore limited. Endurance tests can be performed, holding a certain percentage of maximum voluntary force (e.g., 50–70%) for a fixed time (e.g., 1 min); a fatigue index (FI) is then determined as the percent decline in force.

Isokinetic Strength Assessment. Isokinetic ("constant velocity") strength testing is usually performed in a laboratory and is typically confined to elite athletes or those undergoing serial assessment during rehabilitation. Strength is usually measured during concentric muscle contraction and is expressed as peak torque (N/m). The advantages of isokinetic testing over isometric or isotonic testing are numerous, including the following: (a) The strength curve matches the range of motion for any specific movement and joint; therefore, maximal strength is measured throughout a specified range of movement. (b) Specific muscles are tested. (c) A range of angular velocities is easily assessed (e.g., 0 to 300°/s. (d) Eccentric strength testing is also possible using certain types of equipment (Biodex isokinetic dynamometer) (31).

Assessment of Body Composition

Indirect methods to assess lean mass and fat mass include hydrostatic weighing, soft tissue radiography, potassium (^{40}K) counting, total body water (TBW isotope dilution), photon absorptiometry, bioelectric impedance analysis (BIA), total-body electrical conductivity (TOBEC), ultrasound, and anthropometric techniques (4,33). Both BIA and ultrasound methods have become popular in recent years, but their reliability and accuracy remain questionable. Counting of 40 K, TBW, and TOBEC are costly techniques and are not practical in basic assessment of body composition. A new and reasonably accurate technology uses dual-energy x-ray absorptiometry (DEXA) to determine whole-body and regional lean tissue, bone, mineral, and fat content (4). Comparison between studies as yet remains limited because of a wide variation in the results provided by different software packages (34).

Hydrostatic Weighing

This technique uses Archimedes' principle of water displacement. At a specified temperature, the loss of weight of a submerged body is equal to the weight of water displaced and thus to body volume. Residual volume of the lungs must be measured (for instance, by helium dilution) or estimated using equations based on body mass, height, age, and sex (4). Most investigators assume a gastrointestinal air volume of 100 ml (35). Body fat (percent) is then calculated on the assumption that fat and lean tissue densities are constant throughout the general population (36). This technique is likely the best method but is usually impractical in clinical work.

Skinfold and Girth Measurements

These methods assess fat mass indirectly. Using calipers that exert a uniform pressure (10 g/mm^2), the thickness of the skinfold is determined in millimeters within 2 s of applying the caliper. All measurements are made on the right side of the body. A mathematical relationship is assumed between subcutaneous fat stores and body density. Generalized equations have been developed for men and women using various skinfold sites (37), with early reports suggesting a good correlation to the hydrostatic method. Common measurement sites include the triceps, biceps, suprailiac crest, subscapular, abdomen, and upper thigh folds. A logarithmic transformation of biceps, triceps, suprailiac and subscapular skinfolds is sometimes used to determine the percentage of body fat (38), whereas Jackson and Pollock (37) have developed generalized equations based on a quadratic sum of skinfolds. For women, triceps, suprailiac and thigh folds are measured; in men, chest, abdominal, and thigh skinfolds are used.

High interindividual variation in technique, poor identification of skinfold sites, and unreliable calipers compound weaknesses inherent in the basic assumptions of skinfold assessment.

Based upon body composition assessment, other indices can be calculated, such as absolute fat mass (percent fat/100 $\times$ body mass), lean body mass (body mass $-$ absolute fat mass), and desirable mass (lean body mass/1.00 $-$ desirable percent fat). There is a wide range of normality, but some suggest an ideal body fat range of 12–18% for men and 20–28% for women, depending on age. Standards of percent body fat (Table 15) and the sum of skinfolds (Table 16) provide a basis for monitoring weight-management programs, although it may be more

TABLE 15   Percentage Body Fat—Standard Values

Score	20–29	30–39	40–49	50–59	>60
Men:					
Excellent	<10	<11	<13	<14	<15
Good	11–13	12–14	14–16	15–17	16–18
Average	14–20	15–21	17–23	18–24	19–25
Fair	21–23	22–24	24–26	25–27	26–28
Poor	>24	>25	>27	>28	>29
Women:					
Excellent	<15	<16	<17	<18	<19
Good	16–19	17–20	18–21	19–22	20–23
Average	20–28	21–29	22–30	19–22	20–23
Fair	29–31	30–32	31–33	32–34	33–35
Poor	>32	>33	>34	>35	>36

Source: Adapted from Ref. 33; used with permission.

Table 16   Sum of Skinfolds—Percentile Scores

Percentile score	Age group									
	20–29		30–39		40–49		50–59		60–69	
	M	F	M	F	M	F	M	F	M	F
95	26	37	28	40	28	42	31	48	33	45
90	29	40	32	45	37	48	36	54	38	54
85	30	43	35	48	40	51	40	60	41	61
80	32	46	38	52	44	56	44	65	45	65
75	34	49	41	55	49	59	46	69	48	67
70	36	51	44	58	48	62	48	73	50	70
65	38	53	46	61	51	66	51	75	52	72
60	40	56	49	63	53	69	53	78	54	76
55	43	58	52	66	56	16	55	81	56	80
50	46	60	55	69	58	77	58	84	58	82
45	49	63	58	72	60	81	60	87	59	85
40	52	65	60	76	63	86	62	90	61	87
35	55	69	63	79	66	90	65	93	63	93
30	58	72	67	83	69	94	68	97	65	98
25	62	76	71	88	72	98	71	101	69	100
20	68	81	76	93	75	105	74	106	72	103
15	74	86	82	99	79	113	77	112	76	112
10	82	95	89	109	86	125	91	121	81	123
5	94	111	101	128	91	150	88	138	91	139

ᵃSum of: triceps + biceps + subscapular + iliac crest + medial calf (mm)
Source: Based on Canada Fitness Survey, 1981. Modified from Ref. 12; used with permission.

accurate simply to sum the skinfolds and use these measurements serially over time to assess changes in body composition. Use of nomograms describing body mass index (BMI) should be incorporated into such determinations.

PRESCRIPTION OF EXERCISE

Precautions

Large-scale trials have clearly shown that increased physical activity can significantly reduce mortality from cardiovascular diseases and all-cause mortality (39–43). Contraindications to an increase of physical activity and factors limiting training may be identified by various screening options. Self-administered questionnaires—such as the Par-Q (Fig. 4)—medical examination, and clinical stress testing are commonly used as screening devices prior to the writing of an exercise prescription. Medically supervised stress testing is not recommended for apparently healthy and "risk free" individuals. Such testing should be restricted to those with multiple primary risk factors and/or symptoms of coronary heart disease in addition to those in the coronary-prone age group (males, age 40–49) and/or those who are grossly overweight. Healthy patients should be encouraged

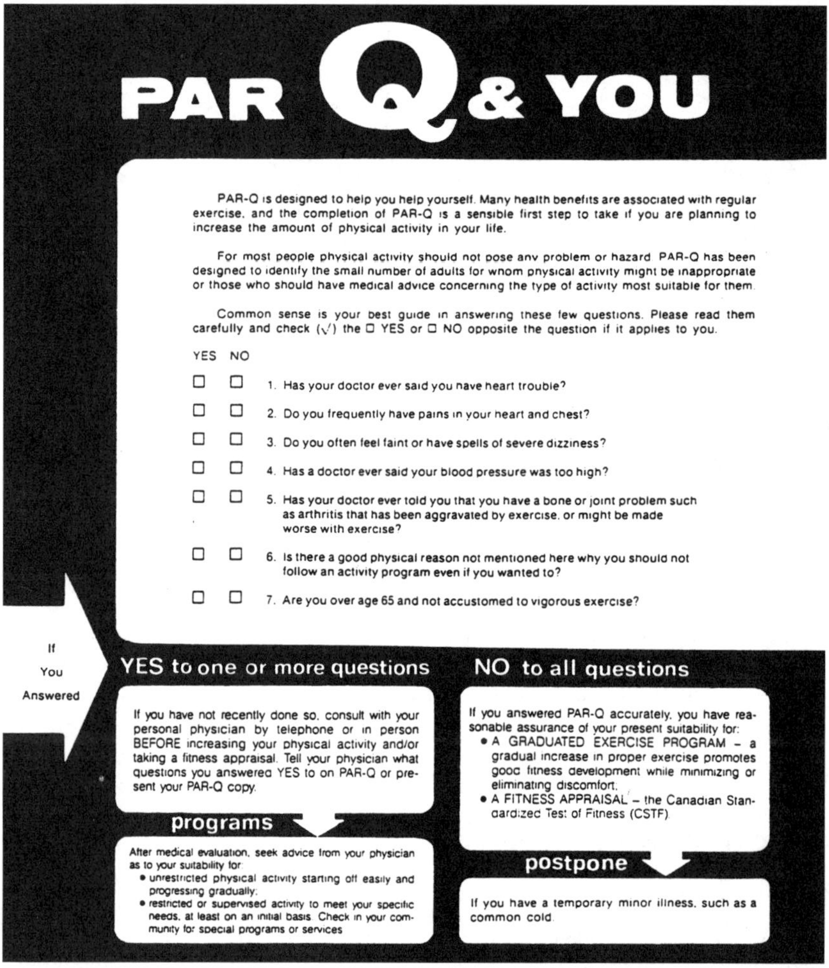

PAR Q & YOU

PAR-Q is designed to help you help yourself. Many health benefits are associated with regular exercise, and the completion of PAR-Q is a sensible first step to take if you are planning to increase the amount of physical activity in your life.

For most people physical activity should not pose any problem or hazard. PAR-Q has been designed to identify the small number of adults for whom physical activity might be inappropriate or those who should have medical advice concerning the type of activity most suitable for them.

Common sense is your best guide in answering these few questions. Please read them carefully and check ($\sqrt{}$) the ☐ YES or ☐ NO opposite the question if it applies to you.

YES NO

☐ ☐ 1. Has your doctor ever said you have heart trouble?

☐ ☐ 2. Do you frequently have pains in your heart and chest?

☐ ☐ 3. Do you often feel faint or have spells of severe dizziness?

☐ ☐ 4. Has a doctor ever said your blood pressure was too high?

☐ ☐ 5. Has your doctor ever told you that you have a bone or joint problem such as arthritis that has been aggravated by exercise, or might be made worse with exercise?

☐ ☐ 6. Is there a good physical reason not mentioned here why you should not follow an activity program even if you wanted to?

☐ ☐ 7. Are you over age 65 and not accustomed to vigorous exercise?

If You Answered

YES to one or more questions

If you have not recently done so, consult with your personal physician by telephone or in person BEFORE increasing your physical activity and/or taking a fitness appraisal. Tell your physician what questions you answered YES to on PAR-Q or present your PAR-Q copy.

programs

After medical evaluation, seek advice from your physician as to your suitability for:
- unrestricted physical activity starting off easily and progressing gradually;
- restricted or supervised activity to meet your specific needs, at least on an initial basis. Check in your community for special programs or services

NO to all questions

If you answered PAR-Q accurately, you have reasonable assurance of your present suitability for:
- A GRADUATED EXERCISE PROGRAM – a gradual increase in proper exercise development while minimizing or eliminating discomfort;
- A FITNESS APPRAISAL – the Canadian Standardized Test of Fitness (CSTF).

postpone

If you have a temporary minor illness, such as a common cold.

FIGURE 4   The Par-Q (Physical Activity Readiness Questionnaire), used for screening prior to exercise testing and participation in an exercise program.

to undergo submaximal exercise testing and generalized fitness assessment. Such evaluations provide valuable information for quantification of the exercise prescription and motivation toward program compliance.

Absolute contraindications for exercise training include conditions that seriously alter the normal cardiovascular response to exercise, thereby dangerously compromising the patient's health. "Relative" contraindications should also be considered when the potential benefits of exercise training relative to its risks are being weighed and when the necessary extent of control and monitoring is being decided. Patients in this category should undergo a supervised exercise test and enter a supervised program (Table 17).

Additional conditions, both medical and environmental, may merit caution in the prescription of exercise or a temporary moderation of activity (Table 18).

TABLE 17   Absolute and Relative Contraindications to Exercise Training

Absolute:
    1. Recent myocardial infarction (<6 weeks)
    2. Unstable angina at rest
    3. Severe sinus arrhythmias and conduction disturbances
    4. Congestive heart failure
    5. Aortic stenosis—severe
    6. Diagnosed or suspected aortic aneurysm
    7. Myocarditis or disease induced cardiomyopathy (recent)
    8. Thrombophlebitis, recent emboli (systemic or pulmonary)
    9. Fever
    10. Uncontrolled metabolic disorders
    11. Severe hypertension with exercise (SBP > 250 mmHg; DBP > 120 mmHg)
Relative:
    1. Frequent ectopic beats and/or uncontrolled supraventricular arrhythmias
    2. Pulmonary hypertension—untreated
    3. Moderate ventricular aneurysm and/or aortic stenosis
    4. Severe myocardial obstructive syndrome
    5. Mild cardiomyopathy
    6. Toxemia or complicated pregnancy
Conditions requiring a supervised program:
    1. Myocardial infarction; post–aortocoronary bypass surgery; documented CHD
    2. Pacemakers—fixed rate or demand
    3. Cardiac medication—chronotropic or inotropic
    4. Morbid obesity in conjunction with multiple risk factors
    5. ST-segment depression at rest
    6. Severe hypertension
    7. Intermittent claudication

Source: Adapted from Ref. 49; used with permission.

TABLE 18 Conditions Requiring Precaution in the Exercise Prescription
and Moderation of Activity

Conditions requiring precaution in exercise prescription:
1. Viral infection or cold
2. Chest pain
3. Irregular heartbeat
4. Exercise-induced asthma
5. Prolonged, unaccustomed physical activity
6. Conduction disturbances (left bundle branch block, complete AV block, biphasic block with or without first-degree block, rare conduction syndromes)

Conditions requiring moderation of activity:
1. Extreme heat and relative humidity
2. Extreme cold, especially when strong winds are present
3. Following heavy meals
4. Exposure to high altitudes (>1700 m)
5. Musculoskeletal injuries

Source: Adapted from Ref. 49; used with permission.

If activity is curtailed for a long time (>3–4 weeks), modification of the exercise prescription may be necessary.

Intensity of Aerobic Exercise

The intensity of exercise is the most important issue in prescribing exercise. A heart rate below a "target" level (Fig. 5) may be insufficient to elicit a training effect; the threshold commonly lies at 60% of the difference between maximal and resting heart rate, although the level can vary from 50–80% of $\dot{V}_{O_2max}$.

Typically, intensity is expressed as (a) a percentage of maximal heart rate or heart rate reserve (the maximum minus the resting value), or (b) functional capacity (percent of $\dot{V}_{O_2max}$ or metabolic equivalents or MET). The initial prescription is highly dependent on the initial level of fitness. Unconditioned patients have a low threshold for improvement in functional capacity, whereas conditioned patients require a high intensity. However, as the intensity of effort increases, the incidence of musculoskeletal injuries rises. The dose-response relationship that describes the required exercise training intensity relative to the adaptive response indicates a diminishing return once exercise intensity approaches a moderate level (Fig. 6). Therefore, recommendations should be phrased carefully to encourage an increased level of physical activity (41).

Determining Intensity by Heart Rate

Assuming a linear relationship between heart rate and $\dot{V}_{O_2}$, this technique provides an indirect method of expressing intensity as a percentage of functional capacity.

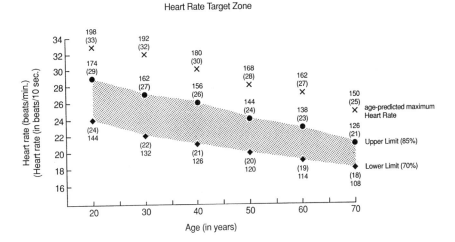

FIGURE 5   The "target zone" for exercise training. Pulse rates (per minute and per 10 s) are illustrated, showing the decline in maximal heart rate with age and the corresponding slope of optimal training intensity with increasing age.

Intensity is expressed as a percentage of maximal heart rate (HR_{max}), where HR_{max} = 220 − age or 210 − 0.65 (age). Thus, the absolute work rate varies with the individual's age. Intensities 60–75% of maximal heart rate ("target zone") are usually sufficient to induce a training effect; these correspond to approximately 65–85% of functional capacity (Fig. 5). Potential errors in the estimation of maximal heart rate can lead to significant errors in the prescription of exercise intensity. The submaximal heart rate can also be influenced by a number of factors (including eating prior to testing, body temperature, environmental temperature, humidity, and administration of various drugs) and can cause alteration in the heart rate/oxygen consumption relationship during exercise testing. This can lead to an error in the calculation of the training intensity (4). Consequently a conservative estimation of exercise intensity is recommended.

In the Karvonen method, the heart rate reserve (HRR) = HR_{max} − HR_{rest}, and the training heart rate (THR) is calculated as:

$$THR = (0.60 - 0.85) (HR_{max} - HR_{rest}) + HR_{rest}$$

where (0.60 − 0.85) represents a range of intensity. Intensity should begin at low levels (0.6), increasing gradually as fitness improves. This method accounts for training-induced bradycardia and is preferred over simple measures of maximal heart rate.

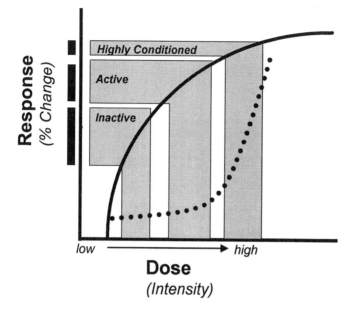

FIGURE 6   The dose-response relationship between training intensity (dosage), changes in cardiorespiratory fitness (response), and probability of musculoskeletal injury. Low dosage or stimulus is required at the initial stage of training, with smaller gains observed at high levels of conditioning. The stimulus requirements are lowest in deconditioned or pathological states and greatest in well-conditioned athletes. Lower intensity and duration will yield lower injury rates. (Modified from Ref. 41, with permission.)

Exercise Prescription Using METs

Intensity of exercise may be prescribed in MET units once functional capacity has been determined. This method allows for prescription of various activities with documented energy requirements. Expressing work output in METs (1 MET = 3.5 ml/kg · min) is comparable to expressing work output by heart rate, since the two variables tend to be linearly related. Prescriptions often utilize both units, with a range from 60–85% maximum METs (MMET), corresponding to low and peak conditioning intensities, respectively (16). An average training intensity may be calculated by (a) adding the MMET as a base value to 60%, (b) dividing this value by 100, and (c) multiplying by MMET. Thus, for an individual with a maximal functional capacity of 15 METs, the average conditioning intensity = $[(60 + 15)/100] \times$ MMETs = 11.25 METs. Since 1 MET = 4.19 kJ/kg/min^{-1} (1 kcal/kg · h), energy expenditure per activity session can also be determined. Hence a 70-kg male exercising at this intensity for 30 min would expend 1651 kJ (394 kcal).

Use of the Ventilatory Threshold

Exercise should be set well below the VT in untrained adults, since this intensity corresponds to a rapid increase in blood lactate, probably brought about by increased anaerobiosis. Those with greater aerobic power will have a higher relative threshold level (greater percent of $\dot{V}_{O_2max}$), with a correspondingly greater $\dot{V}_{O_2}$ intensity requirement. The prescribed exercise intensity is typically set at 5–15% below the threshold. The "breath test" is a good rule of thumb for prescribing the intensity: the participant should be able to maintain a light conversation while walking yet hear breathing sounds. This may closely reflect an exercise intensity just below the VT.

Duration of Exercise

Duration is the second most important factor in exercise prescription, with a minimum recommended energy expenditure of 1200–1300 kJ per session (300 kcal). Very short periods of exercise (5–10 min) are sufficient to induce a cardiovascular training effect even if they are performed at a high intensity (90–95% of functional capacity). However, at least 30 min of moderate to intense aerobic activity is ideal for conditioning and reducing the risk of coronary disease (41). Initially, the stimulus period should remain relatively short (15–20 min), but it can gradually be extended as cardiovascular endurance improves. Fat utilization increases significantly after approximately 20 min of light to moderate exercise (44), thereby enhancing weight control and fat loss. Favorable changes in the blood lipid profile, including a reduction in triglyceride, increases in high-density lipoprotein cholesterol (HDL-C), and the HDL-C:total cholesterol ratio are also associated with longer periods of exercise (3,4,40–43).

Frequency of Exercise Sessions

The optimal frequency of training depends on the intensity and duration of the exercise program. A training threshold of two sessions per week is required to improve aerobic power, but the exercise intensity must be relatively high for conditioning to occur (45). The recommended frequency for normal adults (3–10 METs functional capacity) is three sessions per week, with sessions scattered evenly through the week. This is optimal at the initial stage of an exercise program, as it allows for sufficient rest between exercise bouts for musculoskeletal adaptations to occur.

In obese subjects and adults with very low functional capacities (less than 3 METs), it may be more practical to recommend frequent (>4) and short (5 min) sessions daily. As functional capacity improves to 3–5 METs, there can be a transition to one to two daily sessions.

Five days per week is adequate to attain optimal fitness levels. Progression from 3 to 5 days per week should occur gradually over a 4-week period, and no more than three intense exercise sessions should occur per week. Activity on the remaining days should be of reduced intensity and duration. Exercising 7 days per week does not improve aerobic power further; any gains (at most, 1–2%) are relevant only for the competitive athlete.

If strength fitness or isotonic resistance training activities are to be incorporated into the regular aerobic exercise program, these should be undertaken no more than 2–3 days per week, as the recuperative period is longer for heavy resistance work than for lower-intensity aerobic activities.

Exercise Mode

Activities that utilize large muscle groups in a rhythmic and continuous manner are the preferred modes of aerobic exercise. Theoretically, there should be no difference between modalities in terms of their conditioning effect provided that the criteria of intensity, frequency, and duration are met (6). Most investigations have shown a similar cardiovascular training effect with jogging/running, swimming, bicycling, and cross-country skiing programs. Less intense activities (e.g., golf, bowling) offer little training stimulus, since heart rates rarely exceed 100 beats per minute, well below the "target" heart rate (Fig. 5). Certain indoor racquet sports (e.g., squash) involve rapid starts, thereby increasing systemic blood pressure and myocardial oxygen demand; they should thus be prescribed only in healthy, risk-free patients.

Sustained isometric (static) activities with heavy resistance are strongly discouraged in unconditioned, hypertensive, and/or coronary-prone patients. Little or no improvement in $\dot{V}_{O_2max}$ is observed using heavy weights. The mode of activity should be of sufficient intensity to elicit a cardiovascular training effect, minimizing both musculoskeletal strain and the blood pressure response.

Type of Exercise

Exercise training can include either continuous or intermittent (interval) exercise. The advantage of interval training (high intensity and short duration, with rest intervals) is that more energy expenditure is possible without a progressive accumulation of blood lactate. In the case of an athlete, increased speed is often the objective, whereas in highly deconditioned patients, total work can be accomplished with less physiological stress. Therefore, it may be advantageous to prescribe exercise on an alternating run-walk basis initially; as functional capacity improves, there may be a higher energy output on a more continuous basis. Activities that are continuous and elicit a constant heart-rate response (walking, jogging or running, cross-country skiing, swimming, and cycling) are preferred when both duration and control of the exercise intensity are desired.

Muscular Strength Activities

Enhancement of muscle strength through dynamic, high-resistance, low-repetition exercise is strongly discouraged for patients who are unconditioned, hypertensive, at risk for cardiovascular disease, or with documented cardiovascular disease. Dynamic and static strength exercises, especially when performed with the Valsalva manoeuver, may cause an excessive rise of systemic blood pressure, thereby reducing venous return and increasing ventricular afterload. Use of light weights, preferably in the form of a circuit training session, may be the optimal method of combining cardiorespiratory fitness and muscle strength training.

The Exercise Session

Each exercise session should include three components: a warm-up period, an endurance phase (stimulus period), and cool-down. The warm-up should be relatively short (5–10 min), consisting of light calisthenics, static stretching exercises, slow jogging, and walking. Such activities facilitate a favorable response to subsequent, more intensive exercise. Increases in muscle and general body temperature, as brought about by warming up, increase local muscle blood flow, reduce muscle viscosity, and enhance both oxygen dissociation and enzymatic reactions (law of Arrhenius). There is evidence that sudden bursts of intense exercise without a warm-up may precipitate ventricular fibrillation and that a warm-up reduces the likelihood of unfavorable electrocardiographic responses (Tables 7 and 10).

The definitive stimulus period, consisting of the specified intensity and duration of activity (see text), should be initiated slowly and should immediately follow the warm-up period.

A gradual cool-down of 5–10 min, utilizing exercises similar to those used during the warm-up period, is recommended. An abrupt cessation of exercise, particularly in a warm and humid environment, may cause orthostatic hypotension, precipitating myocardial ischemia in those with latent coronary disease. Thus, hot showers, saunas, and whirlpools are strongly discouraged until long after the cool-down period and are contraindicated in patients with coronary heart disease.

Monitoring Exercise

A 10-s pulse is taken immediately (within 5 s) following exercise. The first beat is counted as zero, and the observed value is compared to recommended ''target'' levels (see Fig. 5). As individuals become accustomed to perceiving an appropriate intensity of exercise, pulse rates can be counted once during and once after the stimulus period. In addition, Borg's linear or nonlinear rating of perceived exertion (RPE) scale (Table 19) can be used to monitor exercise intensity in selected patients. Scores of 12–16 on the old (nonlinear) scale represent the target-zone heart rate for most age groups (60–85% $\dot{V}_{O_2max}$). They provide reproducible self-ratings of effort (46).

Progression of Exercise Prescriptions

Intensity, frequency, and duration can be adjusted to a higher level over time, but the *rate* of progression is often difficult for the practitioner to determine. The individual patient and training environment must be considered in planning progression. Three phases can be identified (42). The initial stage covers the first to the fifth week of training. It concludes an introduction to stretching, light calisthenics, and low intensity aerobics. The duration of the aerobic session should be kept at 12–15 min, with an aim of achieving an energy expenditure of 830–850 kJ per session (200 kcal) during the first week of training and eventually 1200–1300 kJ per session (300 kcal). The inverse association between weekly energy expenditure and cardiovascular disease mortality suggests that

TABLE 19   Borg's Scales for Rating of Perceived Exertion

Original categoric scale		Linear (ratio) scale	
6		0	Nothing at all
7	Very, very light	0.5	Very, very weak
8		1	Very weak
9	Very light	2	Weak
10		3	Moderate
11	Fairly light	4	Somewhat strong
12		5	Strong
13	Somewhat hard	6	
14		7	Very strong
15	Hard	8	
16		9	
17	Very hard	10	Very, very strong
18		•	Maximal
19	Very, very hard		
20			

Source: From Ref. 46.

TABLE 20   Energy Costs of Various Activities

Activity		METs[a]	kJ/kg•min
Walking			
	4.8 km/h (81 m/min)	3.0	6.3
	6.4 km/h (107 m/min)	4.6	9.7
Running			
	7.5 min/km (134 m/min)	8.7	18.3
	6.2 min/km (161 m/min)	10.2	21.4
	5.0 min/km (201 m/min)	12.5	26.5
	3.7 min/km (268 m/min)	16.3	34.4
Cycling			
	50 W	3.7	7.8
	75 W	5.0	10.5
	100 W	6.0	12.6
	125 W	7.0	14.7
	150 W	8.5	17.9
	Pleasure	7–8+	14.7+
	16.1 km/h	7.0	114.7
Swimming (front crawl)			
	20 m/min	6.0	12.6
	40 m/min	12.0	25.2
Golf		5.1	10.7
Hiking		3–7	6.3–12.6
Cross-country skiing		6–12+	12.6–25.2+
Squash		8–14	16.8–25.2
Tennis		6–10	12.6–21

Note: 1 kcal = 4.19 kJ.
[a]MET = metabolic equivalent.

exercise demanding 2000 kcal/week provides the greatest reduction in risk for cardiovascular disease and is an optimal long-term goal (40, 41). Familiarization with the energy cost of various activities would therefore help those initiating a fitness program (Table 20).

Objective indications that the participant can progress to the next level include (a) a decrease of 3–8 beats per minute in heart rate during the aerobic phase of exercise, (b) a slightly faster voluntary jogging or walking pace, and (c) an improvement of functional capacity ($\dot{V}_{O_2max}$, steady-state $\dot{V}_{O_2}$, METs). Subjective measures include the level of fatigue, facial expression, breathing, RPE scores, and biomechanical form.

The second stage is where the most improvement is observed and can last from 6–24 weeks. It is characterized by the progression of intensity (from 60% in the first phase to 70–80%), duration, and frequency.

In certain individuals where functional capacity is low, the transition from walking to jogging might best be accomplished by initially using discontinuous walk/run aerobic exercise and progressing toward continuous steady-state exercise. Duration should be increased before increasing the intensity.

The third phase of progression is the maintenance stage. Participants should now be exercising at the full 70–80% of estimated functional capacity for at least 30–45 min four to five times per week.

Compliance with Exercise Programs

Compliance may be defined as the degree to which someone's behavior matches medical or health advice (47). It is a key factor in the long-term success of exercise programming. Willingness to adopt and comply with exercise on a regular basis typically ranges from 30–60% of a population. Some studies report that fewer than 50% of those who begin an exercise program will be complying sufficiently after 4 weeks. A number of factors that enhance compliance have been identified, including (a) convenience of sessions or proximity to the exercise facility; (b) spousal support and/or participation; (c) freedom from musculoskeletal injury, particularly early in the programs; (d) group exercise programs; and (e) desire to improve fitness (47).

The time course of adaptation (changes in $\dot{V}_{O_2max}$) is initially rapid. A 10- to 11-day half-time has been reported for improvement of $\dot{V}_{O_2max}$ (4,48). The initial improvement provides considerable motivation and can greatly influence compliance. Further improvements are less dramatic, and at this stage maintenance of fitness must be stressed. During the third phase, compliance-oriented goals become particularly important. New activities can be introduced to provide variety while holding the energy expenditure, duration, and intensity at the levels necessary to maintain aerobic fitness. Periodic reassessment of cardiovascular fitness will provide ongoing feedback and aid in sustaining compliant behavior.

EQUATIONS USED FOR CALCULATING EXERCISE INTENSITY

Intensity Based on Heart Rate

$$HR_{train} = HR_{rest} + 0.6 - 0.8(HR_{max} - HR_{rest})$$
$$HR_{max} = 210 - 0.65(age) \text{ or } = 220 - age$$

Walking, Jogging, and Running Speeds Using METs

METs to speed of walking or jogging at less than 6.4 km/h:

$$v = \frac{(\text{TMETs} - 1 \text{ MET})}{0.88} - 1.01$$

At 6.4–8.0 km/h:

$$v = \frac{(\text{TMETs} - 1 \text{ MET})}{3.37} + 8.51$$

At more than 8 km/h:

$$v = \frac{(\text{TMETs} - 1 \text{ MET})}{1.37} - 1.85$$

where v = speed (km/h) and TMETs = calculated training METs.

Walking or Jogging Speed Based on % $\dot{V}_{O_2max}$ (ml/kg · min)

$$\text{Jogging velocity (km/h)} = \frac{I(\dot{V}_{O_2max}\text{ml/kg/min}^{-1}) - 3.5}{8.63}$$

$$\text{Walking velocity (km/h)} = \frac{I(\dot{V}_{O_2max}\text{ml/kg/min}^{-1}) - 3.5}{4.31}$$

where I = desired training intensity.

Oxygen Costs of Walking, Jogging, and Running

$$\dot{V}_{O_2} = 2.97(v) + 6.57$$

where v = running speed (1.6–4.8 km/h).

$$\dot{V}_{O_2} = 7.36(v) - 29.8$$

where v = walk/jog speed (5.6–8 km/h).

$$\dot{V}_{O_2} = 1.94(v) + 3.5$$

where v = walking speed (8–16.1 km/h).

Cycle Ergometry

$$\dot{V}_{O_2} \text{ ml/min} = 10.7 \text{ (W)} + 300$$

$$\dot{V}_{O_2} \text{ ml/min} = (\text{W} \times 12 \text{ ml}) + 3.5 \text{ ml/kg/min} \times \text{kg (wt)}$$

REFERENCES

1. Goodman, J. M., Lefkowitz, C. A., Liu, P. P., Mclaughlin, P. R., and Plyley, M. J., Left ventricular functional response to moderate and intense exercise. *Can. J. Sport Sci.,* 16: 204–209 (1991).
2. Weber, K. T., Janicki, J. S., and McElroy, P. A., Cardiopulmonary exercise (cpx) testing. In *Cardiopulmonary Exercise Testing: Physiologic Principles and Clinical Applications* (K. T. Weber and J. S. Janicki, eds.). Saunders, Philadelphia, pp. 151–168 (1986).
3. Robergs, R. A., and Roberts, S. O., *Exercise Physiology: Exercise, Performance, and Clinical Applications.* Mosby–Year Book, Toronto (1997).
4. Powers, S. K., and Howley, E. T., *Exercise Physiology: Theory and Application to Fitness and Performance.* WCB McGraw-Hill, Dubuque, Iowa (1997).
5. Thoden, J. S., Wilson, B. A., and MacDougall, J. D., in *Physiological Testing of the High Performance Athlete* (J. D. MacDougall, H. A. Wenger, and H. J. Green, eds.) Human Kinetics, Champaign, Illinois, pp. 107–174 (1991).
6. Fardy, P. S., and Yanowotz, F. G., *Cardiac Rehabilitation, Adult Fitness, and Exercise Testing.* Williams & Wilkins, Philadelphia (1995).
7. Londeree, B. R., and Moeschberger, M. L., Influence of age and other factors on maximal heart rate. *J. Cardiac Rehab.,* 4: 44–49 (1984).
8. Froelicher, V. F., Myers, J., Follansbee, W. P., and Labovitz, A. J., *Exercise and the Heart.* Mosby–Yearbook, St. Louis (1993).
9. Plyley, M. J., in *Current Therapy in Sports Medicine,* 2nd Ed. (J. S. Torg, R. P. Welsh, and R. J. Shephard, eds.). B. C. Decker, Philadelphia, pp. 139–144 (1990).
10. Wasserman, K., Hanson, J. E., Sue, D. Y., Whipp, B. J., and Casaburi, R., *Principles of Exercise Testing and Interpretation.* Lea & Febiger, Philadelphia (1994).
11. Jette, M., Campbell, J., Mongeon, J., and Routhier, R., predicitor of aerobic capacity. *Can. Med. Assoc. J.,* 114: 680–683 (1976).
12. *Canadian Standardized Test of Fitness (CSTF) Operations Manual.* Minister of Supply and Services, Ottawa (1986).
13. Åstrand, P. O., and Rodahl, K., *Acta Physiol. Scand.,* 49: 169 (1960).
14. Legg, B. J., and Bannister, E. W., *J. Appl. Physiol.,* 61: 1203–1209 (1986).
15. Siconolfi, S. F., Cullinane, E. M., Carleton, R. A., and Thompson, P. D., *Med. Sci. Sports Exer.,* 14: 335–338 (1982).
16. American College of Sports Medicine, *ACSM's Guidelines for Exercise Testing and Prescription.* Williams & Wilkins, Baltimore (1995).
17. Bruce, R. A., in *Exercise Testing and Training of Apparently Healthy Individuals:*

A Handbook for Physicians. American Heart Association, New York, pp. 32–34 (1972).

18. Balke, B., and Ware, R., *U.S. Armed Forces Med. J.,* 10: 675–688 (1959).
19. Hanson, P., *Resource Manual for Guidelines for Exercise Testing and Prescription.* Lea & Febiger, Philadelphia (1988).
20. Weiner, J. S., and Lourie, J. A., *Practical Human Biology.* Academic Press, New York (1981).
21. Jones, N. L., *Clinical Exercise Testing.* W. B. Saunders, Toronto (1988).
22. Taylor, H. L., Buskirk, E., and Henschel, A., *J. Appl. Physiol.,* 8: 73–80 (1955).
23. Davis, J. A., in *Physiological Assessment of Human Fitness* (P. J. Maud and C. Foster, eds.) Human Kinetics, Champaign, Illinois, pp. 9–17 (1995).
24. Cooper, K. H., *The Aerobics Way.* Bantam, New York (1977).
25. Kline, G. M., Porcari, J. P., Hintermeister, R., Freedson, P. S., Ward, A., et al., *Med. Sci. Sports Exerc.,* 19: 253–259 (1987).
26. Rochmis, P., and Blackburn, H., *J.A.M.A.,* 217: 1061–1075 (1971).
27. Thompson, P. D., in *Resource Manual for Guidelines for Exercise Testing and Prescription* (S. N. Blair, P. Painter, R. R. Pate, L. K. Smith, and C. B. Taylor, eds.) Lea & Febiger, Philadelphia, pp. 273–277 (1988).
28. Rost, R., *Athletics and the Heart.* Yearbook, Chicago (1986).
29. Maud, P. J., and Cortez-Cooper, M. Y., in *Physiological Assessment of Human Fitness* (P. J. Maud and C. Foster, eds.), Human Kinetics, Champaign, Illinois, pp. 221–244 (1995).
30. Leighton, J. R., The Leighton flexometer and flexibility test. *Journal of the Association for Physical and Mental Rehabilitation* 20: 86–93.
31. Sale, D., in *Physiological Testing of the High Performance Athlete,* 2nd ed. (J. D. MacDougall, H. A. Wenger, and H. J. Green, eds.). Human Kinetics, Champaign, Illinois, pp. 21–106 (1991).
32. Kraemer, W. J., and Fry, A. C., in *Physiological Assessment of Human Fitness* (P. J. Maud and C. Foster, eds.). Human Kinetics, Champaign, Illinois, pp. 115–138 (1995).
33. Gettman, L. R., in *Resource Manual for Guidelines for Exercise Testing and Prescription* (S. N. Blair, P. Painter, R. R. Pate, L. K. Smith, and C. B. Taylor, eds.). Lea & Febiger, Philadelphia, pp. 161–170 (1988).
34. Van Loan, M. D., Keim, N. L., Berg, K., and Mayclin, P. L., *Med. Sci. Sports Exerc.,* 27: 587–591 (1995).
35. Lohman, T. G., *Advances in Body Composition Assessment.* Human Kinetics, Champaign, (1992).
36. Brozek, J., Grande, F., Anderson, J. T., and Keys, A., *Ann. N.Y. Acad. Sci.,* 110: 113–140 (1963).
37. Jackson, A. S., and Pollock, M. L., *Can. J. Appl. Sport Sci.,* 7: 189–196 (1982).
38. Durnin, J. V., and Womersley, J., *Br. J. Nutr.,* 32: 77–92 (1974).
39. American Heart Association, *Circulation* 86: 340–344 (1992).
40. Blair, S. N., Kohl, H. W. III, Paffenbarger, R. S., Clark, D. G., Cooper, K. H., et al., *J.A.M.A.,* 262: 2395–2401 (1989).
41. Pate, R. R., Pratt, M., Blair, S. N., Haskell, W. L., Macera, C. A., et al., *J.A.M.A.,* 273: 402–407 (1995).

42. American College of Sports Medicine, *Med. Sci. Sports Exerc.,* 22: 265–274 (1990).

43. American College of Sports Medicine, *Med. Sci. Sports Exerc.,* 25: i–x (1993).

44. Shephard, R. J., *Physiology and Biochemistry of Exercise.* Praeger Publishers, New York (1982).

45. Pollock, M. L., *Exerc. Sport Sci. Revi.,* 1: 155–188 (1973).

46. Borg, G. V., *Med. Sci. Sports Exerc.,* 14: 377–381 (1982).

47. Oldridge, N. B., *Med. Sci. Sports Exerc.,* 11: 373–375 (1979).

48. Hickson, R. C., Hagberg, J. M., Ehsani, A. A., and Holloszy, J. O., *Med. Sci. Sports Exerc.,* 13: 17–20 (1981).

49. Goodman, J., and Goodman, L., *Current Therapy in Sports Medicine.* B. C. Decker, Philadelphia (1985).

3

Children and Physical Activity

LINDA D. ZWIREN
Hofstra University
Hempstead, New York

INTRODUCTION

Physical inactivity has become widespread among children and adults. National surveillance studies (1,2) have reported that about one in four adults currently have sedentary lifestyles—i.e., no leisure-time physical activity. In addition, one out of three adults are not sufficiently active to attain health benefits or physical fitness. The prevalence of inactivity for all ages varies by gender, age, ethnicity, health status, physical ability, fitness status, and obesity (1). Data from the 1990 Youth Risk Behavior Survey (3) show that most teenagers in grades 9 through 12 are not performing regular vigorous activity. About 50% of high school students reported were not enrolled in physical education classes. Preadolescents, who are usually considered naturally active, were spending large amounts of time watching television, using the computer, and/or playing video games (4,5). Although an increasingly urbanized environment and an increasingly mechanized existence may be counteracting children's innate drive for physical activity, a case has been made that most children are active enough to maintain health (6,7).

Increased awareness of the health benefits of physical activity has led to a demand for initiatives that reduce sedentary lifestyles (2). Health professionals, schools, communities, and parents should be actively involved in promoting physical activity among children and adolescents, because many children and young adults already have risk factors for chronic disease associated with adult morbidity and mortality (2). Obesity is increasing among children and is related to physical inactivity. Data indicate that obese children and adolescents exhibit some coronary risk factors and have a high risk of becoming obese adults. Obesity in adults is highly related to coronary artery disease, hypertension, and non–

99

insulin dependent diabetes mellitus (NIDDM) (1). Thus the prevention of childhood obesity has the potential of reducing cardiovascular disease in adults significantly.

The chapter focuses on research on children inclusive of preadolescents and adolescents. *Adolescence* is defined as comprising ages 11 to 21 years, in accordance with the recent International Consensus Conference on Physical Activity Guidelines for Adolescents (8). In published research, older adolescents are often described as young adults. Although preadolescents (also described as children) are considered as below age 11 years, there is substantial interindividual variability in growth status and maturity level at any given chronological age, making the distinction between preadolescents and adolescents somewhat imprecise. Data on preadolescents are limited by the fact that many experimental procedures are not appropriate for use with children.

Although the terms *physical activity, physical fitness, exercise,* and *sport* are often used interchangeably, each term has a unique meaning and refers to a different concept. *Physical activity* is bodily movement produced by skeletal muscles, which increases energy expenditure above rest and produces progressive health benefits (1). Therefore, an increase in physical activity can be a result of walking, gardening, chopping wood, swimming, vacuuming, climbing stairs, riding a bicycle, etc. Physical activity can be performed at various intensity levels. To increase children's and adolescents' physical activity levels means to decrease the time children are lying down or sitting and to increase the time they are moving. Physical inactivity denotes a level of activity less than that needed to maintain good health (1).

Physical fitness refers to a set of physical attributes that an individual has and that can be improved by engaging in appropriate exercise programs. *Exercise* is defined as any physical activity that is planned, structured, repetitive, and purposeful in the sense that improvement or maintenance of one or more components of physical fitness or of sport skill attainment is an objective (9).

Improvement of a child's health-related physical fitness level would include increasing cardiovascular (endurance) fitness by way of large-muscle activities that significantly increase the amount of blood flowing throughout the body in 1 min. Activities like jogging or running, swimming, and roller blading would have to be performed within a given intensity zone (60–90% of the individual's maximal heart rate) for 20–60 min three to five times a week (10). Physical fitness should also be enhanced by using resistance training or calisthenics (e.g., curl-ups, pelvic tilts) to increase muscular strength, muscular endurance, and flexibility. Attaining and maintaining a reasonable and healthy body mass is a further component of health-related physical fitness.

Sports are activities that require specific skilled movements performed during organized game situations. To participate in sports, children need a certain level of motor fitness and the ability to perform the specific sport-skill movements.

This chapter first examines the existence of cardiovascular disease risk factors in children who are inactive and/or obese. Trends of physical activity in subpopulations of children are examined in further detail and research regarding the tracking of inactivity, obesity, and cardiovascular disease risk factors into adulthood is reported. Activity guidelines for increasing physical activity, aerobic fitness, and strength in preadolescents and adolescents developed by national agencies and professional organizations are discussed and interventions to increase physical activity and decrease obesity are reviewed. Finally, a short overview of pediatric exercise testing is given.

CARDIOVASCULAR DISEASE RISK FACTORS

The risk factors for coronary heart disease (CHD) in adults are listed in Table 1. Although the morbidity and mortality from cardiovascular disease is low in children, there is evidence of risk factors in children and adolescents. Rabbia and colleagues (11) examined 1413 adolescents aged 12–15 years and found that 41% of females ($n = 698$) had at least one risk factor (3% had hypertension, 9% obesity, and 29% a low physical activity level); likewise, 40% ($n = 705$) of males were affected (3% had hypertension, 16% were obese, and 21% were sedentary). Fatty streaks and fibrous plaques have been found in the arteries of children by 10 years of age, and the presence of such lipid deposits in the coronary arteries has been associated with adult atherosclerosis (12). The Bogalusa Heart Study examined CHD risk factors in black and white children from birth to 26 years of age between 1937 and 1982 (13,14). Using a combination of cross-sectional

TABLE I   Coronary Heart Disease Risk Factors in Adults

| Unmodifiable | Modifiable | |
	Blood profiles	Other factors
Age	↑Tot-C ↑LDL-C	Smoking
Ethnic/racial background	↓HDL-C ↓ApoA-I	Inactivity
Family history	↑ApoB ↑triglycerides	Hypertension
Gender	↑Homocysteine	Obesity (especially
	↑Fibrinogen level	abdominal)
	Impaired fibrinolysis	Poor dietary
	(due to ↑PAI-1	habits
	levels)	NIDDM
	Hyperactive platelets	Glucose intolerance

Sources: Risk factors obtained from Refs. 11, 14, 20, 35, and 36.

and longitudinal methods, data were collected on subsets of 5000 children. Measurements included anthropometric and demographic data, blood pressure, serum lipids and lipoproteins, nutrition, and behavior. The information gathered strongly substantiated the concept that atherosclerosis began in childhood, supporting pediatric approaches to the primary prevention of atherosclerotic CHD.

Hypertension

Resting systolic, diastolic, and mean systemic blood pressure rise progressively during childhood (15). The systolic pressure of children in the Bogalusa Heart Study increased by 2 mmHg/year, while the diastolic pressure increased by 1 mmHg/year except for 2- to 4-year-old children (16). Increases in blood pressure reflect mainly an increase in body size (particularly an increase in left ventricular size), although the influence of changes in factors affecting peripheral vascular resistance is largely unknown (15).

Blood pressure tracks somewhat into adulthood. In the Bogalusa Heart Study (16), a linear discriminant model was only moderately effective in distinguishing the characteristics of children who maintained a high blood pressure ranking from those who did not. The tracking was most persistent for those who had extremely high ranks in systolic pressure.

Lauer and colleagues (17) noted that many longitudinal studies of children have shown a degree of peer rank-order consistency for blood pressure. Although there is indeed some tracking of blood pressure, there is also a considerable lability of pressure rank over time. If a child maintains a persistent ranking above the 90th blood pressure percentile relative to age, height, and gender over a period of 6 to 12 months and the parents are hypertensive, such children are particularly likely to become hypertensive as adults (17,18).

In the Muscatine Study (19), 126 subjects at Tanner stage 1 (aged 7–12 years) had approximately a 64% greater probability of remaining in the extreme tertile for left ventricular mass and blood pressure when measured 2 years later. The children whose systolic pressure increased the most tended to be those who gained the most weight and body fat and whose physical fitness decreased.

Blood Lipid and Lipoprotein Profile

Various blood lipoproteins have been linked to an increased risk of cardiovascular disease in adults. Elevated serum total cholesterol, low-density lipoprotein cholesterol (LDL-C), very low density lipoprotein cholesterol (VLDL-C), triglycerides, and apoprotein B are atherogenic, but high levels of high-density lipoprotein cholesterol (HDL-C) and apoprotein A-I protect against atherosclerosis. The ratio of LDL-C to HDL-C or the ratio of Total-C to HDL-C is more closely related to coronary morbidity and mortality than is Total-C (20).

At birth, plasma Total-C, LDL-C, and triglycerides (TG) are very low, but there are sharp increases during the first year of life. After infancy, LDL-C, HDL-C, and TG levels remain relatively stable until puberty. The Bogalusa Heart Study (21) found that the mean Total-C was approximately 169 mg/dl from 2 years of age until the onset of sexual maturation (6). This finding did not differ with race or gender. LDL-C was the major component of Total-C at all ages. Therefore, youngsters with elevated Total-C usually had an elevated LDL-C as well. Both Total-C and LDL-C declined during adolescence but increased in later adolescence. There was a rise in the ratio of LDL-C to HDL-C, in VLDL-C, and in TG in white adolescent males, placing these individuals at an extremely high risk of premature CHD. This was related to the greater body fat content in white children of the Bogalusa region.

An 8-year follow-up study of lipid and lipoprotein levels (20) showed a high degree of tracking. Tracking of plasma lipid values into adulthood was most evident during and after puberty in those children with extreme plasma lipid values (16). The National Cholesterol Education Program (22) found that children who had high levels of cholesterol were almost three times more likely to have high cholesterol levels as adults. Other longitudinal studies on risk factors found that tracking persisted into adulthood for children in the extreme percentiles of Total-C, LDL-C, and body fat (23–25).

Physically fit and active youth have lower TG levels than unfit and inactive children. Total-C, LDL-C, HDL-C do not differ by activity level in children. However, there is considerable evidence that increased activity levels may increase HDL-C and reduce TG in young and older men and women, particularly if it is accompanied by loss of body fat (specifically visceral fat) (26). Suter and Howes (27) examined the relationships of physical activity and physical fitness to body fat, diet, and blood lipid profiles in 39 boys and 59 girls 10–15 years of age. In boys, a high level of physical activity was related to high concentrations of HDL-C, low concentrations of VLDL-C and TG, and a low ratio of Total-C to HDL-C. In girls, physical activity was positively related to HDL-C. Cardiovascular fitness was not significantly related to any of the blood lipid concentrations in either boys or girls. Subcutaneous fat thickness (as measured by the sum of 10 skinfolds) was inversely associated with apolipoprotein A-I (APO A-I) and HDL-C and positively associated with APO B in girls and with Total-C/HDL-C in boys.

Fasting Insulin Levels and Insulin Sensitivity

Plasma insulin levels are related to the risk of CHD. In nondiabetic men, fasting plasma insulin is a better predictor of CHD risk than the postglucose-load value (14).

Fasting plasma insulin levels increase from 5 to 17 years of age. Insulin sensitivity is higher in 5- to 10-year-olds than in adolescents and adults. A decrease in insulin sensitivity occurs in both boys and girls at puberty; in girls, the cause may be an increase in body fat, whereas in boys, the explanation seems to be an increase in free testosterone (28). There is a need for earlier recognition of those at risk for later diabetes or the syndrome of insulin resistance. Minimal investigation should include a complete family history and an estimate of insulin resistance, such as the fasting insulin: glucose ratio (29).

A high fasting plasma insulin level after 10 years of age may be a useful indicator of CHD risk, since insulin insensitivity is an important determinant of plasma lipoprotein levels (30). Puberty is associated with relative insulin resistance; insulin insensitivity and obesity are significant correlates of hypertension. Since adiposity exacerbates insulin hypersecretion, it is important to pay attention to the obese adolescent and to identify the specific classification of obesity in identifying those who need risk modification (16,28,29). Children have better glucose control if they are regularly active (31).

Obesity

It has been stated that obesity is ''the most prevalent chronic illness among children in North America and represents an immense public health challenge'' (32). Data from National Health and Nutrition Evaluation Survey (NHANES) and the Bogalusa Heart Studies show that the number of overweight children and adolescents has increased dramatically during the last decade (33,34). Obesity confers significant cardiovascular risk upon adolescents: abnormal glucose tolerance (35); hypertension (11,35); increased fibrinogen levels (36); and lipid profile abnormalities (35). Adverse cardiovascular risk factor profiles improve with weight loss (35,37).

Of greatest concern and potential public health effect is the risk that adolescent overweight will persist into adulthood. Longitudinal studies of children who have been followed into young adulthood suggest that overweight children become overweight adults, particularly if obesity is present in older children and adolescents (38,39). There is substantial evidence that obesity in childhood and in adolescence lays the metabolic groundwork for adult cardiovascular disease (40). As children progress from childhood into adulthood, a major predictor of acquiring risk factors for cardiovascular disease is excess weight (37,41,42). Overweight in late youth and extreme overweight in adolescence is associated with increased morbidity and mortality late in life (35,43). National Institutes of Health (NIH) (1) have placed major emphasis on the prevention of childhood obesity as a means of reducing cardiovascular disease in adults. The management of overweight in children should not be delayed until adulthood, when the pathophysiological changes associated with overweight are likely to be established and it is more difficult to change lifestyle (39).

Definition of Obesity.   Definitions of obesity that use the body dimensions of height and weight:

1. Weight-height ratios that are 20% or more above the upper limit of desirable weight as assessed by standard growth charts (31)
2. Children who have a body mass index (BMI) in the 85th or 95th percentile [BMI = mass divided by square of height (kg/m^2)] (33,39).

Such measures do not always reflect an increase in body fat. An elevated BMI may reflect a large-muscle mass rather than excessive adiposity in relation to height (15). The NHANES study (33) did not consider BMI a valid measure of fatness for children, especially when comparing across varying ages and degrees of maturity. The BMI changes dramatically with age through childhood, and a given BMI has different implications depending on age and maturity. The components that contribute to BMI change throughout youth. During growth and maturation, body mass, body proportions, and the ratio of lean to fat tissue change at differing rates. Therefore, caution is necessary when BMI is used as a measure of body fat. Ideally, some measure of body composition should be incorporated into the determination of obesity. The risk of cardiovascular disease is higher if excess fat is in the abdominal area, so some measure of where excess body fat is located is also needed (29).

Body composition is frequently conceived as a two-compartment system [fat-free mass (FFM) and fat mass (FM)] (Fig. 1). The term *lean body mass* (LBM) is often used interchangeably with FFM, although, by definition, LBM consists of fat-free mass plus essential body fat (i.e., structural fat as opposed to storage fat). Investigators have used both direct and indirect methods to determine the body composition of children.

Direct methods include densitometry (body volume being estimated by underwater weighing); hydrometry [total body water (TBW) determinations]; and newer methodologies using dual-energy x-ray absorptiometry (DEXA) and magnetic resonance imaging. Body density must be converted to estimates of FFM and FM using an equation assuming that FFM and FM have different but consistent densities. Determination of FFM from TBW depends on assumptions about tissue hydration. Bioelectrical impedance determines TBW from differences in the electrical conductivity of the two body components; it has appeal for researchers and clinicians working with children because of its testing simplicity (15). TBW is the principal conductor and TBW reflects FFM. The lower the resistance to electrical flow, the greater the FFM.

Indirect methods include the use of anthropometric measurements (such as skinfolds, circumferences, and bone diameters) to estimate body density from regression equations developed by direct methods. The majority of regression equations presently existing for children are based on densitometry. Lohman (44) has pointed out that children's body fat is often estimated inaccurately because

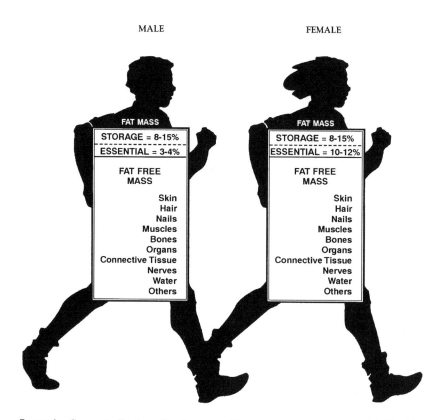

FIGURE 1 Conceptualization of body composition as a two-component model: Total body mass = (fat-free mass) + (fat mass).

prediction equations have been based on adult models. The child is ''chemically immature''; the densities of FFM and FM are not the same as in adults and are changing as the child matures. In addition, ''various populations of children with a particular activity history (e.g., different athletic groups), or particular physique (i.e., mesomorphic) or from a particular ethnic group (i.e., Hispanic), or with a history of a particular disease (i.e., congestive heart failure) may differ in their fat-free body density and may not provide exact estimates for various populations'' (44, p. 21).

Slaughter and colleagues (47) have developed equations that relate skinfold sums to percentage of body fat in children aged 7 to young adulthood, taking account of the changing relationship among body components. Equations for children below 7 years of age are lacking. Lohman (44) suggests that skinfold measurements should not be used to predict percentage of body fat in very young children. Instead, skinfolds should be interpreted in relation to national norms.

Malina (45) compiled body density data from 32 studies and TBW data from eight studies of children, youth, and young adults. To allow for the changing chemical composition of the FFM during growth, estimates of density and water content at different ages (44) were used to derive FFM and FM from body density and TBW values. Malina (45) found that FFM followed a growth pattern similar to those of stature and body mass. Girls tended to have a slightly higher FM and percent body fat than boys during prepubescence, and the gender difference became more clearly established during the adolescent growth spurt. For boys, the adolescent spurt reflected mainly gains in skeletal tissue and muscle mass, with fat mass remaining relatively stable at the time of peak height velocity (PHV). Girls did not experience as intense an increase in stature or muscle mass as boys, but they had a continuing rise in fat mass (46). Malina (45) estimated that from the ages of 10 to 18 years boys gain about 4.1 kg FFM but only 0.4 kg FM, so that there is a decrease of 0.3% fat per year. In contrast, girls gain about 2.2 kg FFM, 0.9 kg FM, and 0.6% fat per year. In late adolescence and young adulthood, males have, on average, an FFM that is about 1.5 times larger than that of females, while females have, on the average, about 1.5 to 2.0 times the FM of males.

FFM and FM are gross estimates and do not reflect fat distribution.

> Fat distribution refers to location of fat and not to the absolute or relative amount of fat. Adults with a more central distribution of fat, e.g., relatively more on the abdomen than on the extremities, are apparently more at risk for cardiovascular disease and non-insulin-dependent diabetes. . . . The proportional distribution of trunk and extremity subcutaneous fat is rather stable during childhood and similar in boys and girls. Subsequently, sex differences in subcutaneous fat distribution occur. Females appear to gain relatively more subcutaneous fat on the trunk during early adolescence, but later they gain fat on the trunk and extremities at a similar rate. Males, on the other hand, accumulate relatively more fat on the trunk during adolescence, which is accentuated by reduction in subcutaneous fat on the extremities at the time (45, p. 233).

The genetic influence on skinfold thickness, circumferences, and body mass is less than that on stature and bone dimensions. However, the pattern of fat distribution is strongly influenced by genetics (48).

Each method of determining body composition has some limitations. Table 2 summarizes the validity of testing methods in children. Lohman (44,49) provides more complete detail on body composition assessment in children.

Causes of Childhood Obesity.   Obesity is related to an energy imbalance (i.e., a food intake in excess of energy expenditure). Dietary data from NHANES II and NHANES III (33) suggest that a dramatic increase of energy intake *alone*

TABLE 2 Validity of Body Composition Methods for Estimating Percent Body Fat in Children

Method	Age, years			
	Infancy, 0–2	Preschool, 3–5	Child, 6–11	Youth, 12–17
Densitometry	NA	NA	G to VG 1.085[a]	G 1.092 ± .005[a]
Body water	G to VG	VG	VG	VG
Body mass index	F,U	F,U	F	F
Triceps skinfold	G[b]	G[b]	G	G
Sum of skinfolds	G[b]	G[b]	G	G
Circumference	U	U	G[c]	G[c]
Impedance	U	U	G[c]	G[c]

Key: VG = very good (2%); G = good (3%); F = fair (4–5%); P = poor (6%); U = uncertain; NA = not applicable.
[a]Needs new equation.
[b]Use percentiles from national norms.
[c]Vary fat-free body density with age.
Source: From Ref. 44.

does not explain the increased prevalence of overweight among children and adolescents. Although energy-dense foods are abundant and readily available in the United States, the percentage of energy intake from fat has continued on a downward trend since the mid-1960s (33). In addition, sequential cross-sectional studies suggest little change in total energy intake of children over many years (40). Many argue that a decrease in physical activity is the main reason for the increased prevalence of childhood obesity. Data for secular changes in the physical activity of children are lacking, but one study of high school students found that participation in physical education had declined from 1984 to 1990 (50). Issues of safety, poverty, parental work habits, television viewing, availability of video games, computers, and other cultural aspects of the environment have all decreased incentives for physical activity (33).

Bouchard (51) argues that a good portion of obesity is preventable. He states that the hereditary contribution to obesity and body fat content is at most moderate. The prevalence of overweight has increased steadily over the past 50 years, and this time period is too short for a change in the frequency of obesity genes. Bouchard believes that a more physically active lifestyle is likely the cornerstone of a prevention strategy aimed at decreasing the proportion of children and adults who are in positive energy balance.

Several studies have found that as adults, early-maturing females were fat-

ter than late-maturing females (52). The Amsterdam Growth and Health Longitudinal Study noted that rapid maturation of both boys and girls resulted in adult
obesity (53). X-ray measurements of the hand/wrist confirmed that early maturation coincided with higher adult fat mass in both sexes (52). Analyses of nutrient
intake and physical activity levels found ''that late maturation seems to coincide
with a higher energetic nutrient intake and a slightly higher activity pattern rather
than early maturation during adolescence'' (p. 238). The authors were surprised
to observe that early maturing subjects (EMs) of both sexes had a higher sum
of skinfolds than late maturers (LMs), although the energy intake of EMs was
less than that of LMs. The authors suggested that regulation of body weight was
ineffective at low physical activity levels and that inactivity resulted in overweight and obesity.

Precautions and Recommendations.   Unfortunately, societal ideals of slim-
ness may be perceived by vulnerable adolescents, who are susceptible to eating
disorders, as setting impossible standards (35). Preoccupation with body size and
weight, especially among adolescent females, makes careful recommendations
important for this age group; in particular, children and adolescents who are susceptible to eating disorders must be identified. Body perceptions are partly shaped
by unrealistic media images that create a false connection between the thinness
of a female and her success, attractiveness, and acceptance by peers. Athletes of
both sexes may also make an inappropriate association between ''leanness'' and
successful performance, so that energy intake is reduced to such an extent that
performance decreases, menstruation may be delayed or interrupted in females,
and there is a risk of severe bone loss. Physicians need to know what questions
to ask to determine if a patient is susceptible to disordered eating; manifestations
include extreme restriction of energy intake, excessive amounts of exercise, use
of laxatives or purging, and other unhealthy methods that may be adopted in
attempts to reduce body weight. (See Table 3 for danger signals of anorexia and
bulimia.)

Although the major problem in North America is the increase in fat levels
among children and adolescents, family members and health professionals may
unwittingly reinforce disordered eating behavior in normal-weight or slightly
overweight adolescents by the manner in which they counsel their patients regarding body weight. Therefore the following recommendations have been made:

1.   Avoid *specific weight* guidelines for children and adolescents, since
research is lacking to provide specific guidelines for body mass; marked changes
in fat distribution with age add uncertainty to interpretation of data. The absence
of longitudinal data during adolescence and analysis of weight and weight change
as continuous rather than discrete variables also preclude guidelines for the adolescent age group (35).

2.   When using BMI, the 95th percentile is the most appropriate criterion

TABLE 3   Danger Signals of Eating Disorders

Anorexia nervosa	Bulimia nervosa
Has lost a great deal of weight in a relatively short period	Binges regularly (eats large amounts of food, empties refrigerator; food disappears)
Continues to diet although already thin	
Reaches weight goal and immediately sets another goal for further weight loss	Purges regularly (uses diet pills, caffeine, water pills, diuretics)
Remains dissatisfied with appearance, claims to feel fat	Exercises often but retains or regains weight
Loses menstrual periods	Disappears into the bathroom for long periods of time
Develops eating rituals and eats small amounts of food (e.g., cuts food into tiny pieces or measures everything before eating extremely small amounts)	Appears depressed much of the time
Prefers to eat alone	
Becomes obsessive about exercising	
Appears unhappy much of the time	

Source: From Ref. 112.

of overweight for children and adolescents (33). Screening guidelines, including tables and norms for adolescents using the 95th percentile, have been presented in a couple of articles (39,55). A second-level screening for BMI that exceeds the 85th but not the 95th percentile includes family history, blood pressure, total serum cholesterol, and large previous increments in BMI (55). Even using the more conservative 95th percentile, approximately 4.7 million children and adolescents (aged 6–17 years) would be classified as overweight (33).

3.   Certain skinfold measures correlate well with determinations of adiposity by hydrodensity and with obesity-related morbidity. Consideration should thus be given to incorporating skinfold measurements (in particular subscapular and/or triceps) into clinical practice and epidemiological research (44,56).

4.   Short of specific guidelines, the focus should be on the prevention of childhood and adolescent obesity through an increase in physical activity, a decrease in the time spent in sedentary activity (see below) and better food choices (35). To improve compliance, the entire family should be involved in treatment. Emphasis should be placed on improving the entire family's health. To avoid stigmatizing the overweight child, the goal should be the maintenance of a normal growth pattern rather than weight loss (40). Must (35) estimates that 1 to 2 years of weight maintenance are required to counter each 20% increment in excess body weight.

5. The risk may be most "dramatic for the less active infants and older children who may happen to have inherited genes making them more susceptible to be in positive energy balance and to gain fat" (51, p. 129).

6. "The goals for dietary restriction should be tailored to the age of the child. As a general rule, if the child is young, not very obese, and has not reached his/her peak height velocity, then very moderate dietary restriction and an activity program should be sufficient to facilitate the child growing into his/her weight, thus altering body composition. This approach may be most effective for younger children, particularly those aged 2 through 6. This is a period when child BMI naturally decreases" (57, p. 432)

The major problem is clearly the increase in obesity among North American children. A decrease in opportunities for physical activity, safety issues, poverty, cultural aspects, and the advertising of high-energy, high-fat, low-nutrient foods are all factors contributing to childhood obesity. Therefore, while an approach targeting the individual is necessary, it may not be enough.

> It will be a daunting task to change the course of nations that have progressively become quite comfortable with [an] effortless lifestyle in which individual consumption is almost unlimited. It will require massive resources and an unprecedented level of coordinated effort among public health agencies and private organizations to begin reversing the trends that have emerged over the last decade (51, p. S130).

Kelly Brownell contends that we have failed to control increasing obesity by educational efforts aimed at proper nutrition by dieting and trying to change personal behavior, or by studying genetics, maintaining that "the true battle must be waged against an increasingly seductive environment" (58, p. A1). Brownell contends that the environment is the real cause of obesity and that what is needed is to lower the consumption of high-fat foods by barring commercials for unhealthy snack foods aimed at children (like the ban on cigarette and alcohol advertising). Foods with little nutrient value should be taxed and the revenues used to build public exercise facilities (58).

Physical Inactivity

The emphasis of childhood interventions, especially for prepubescents, has recently centered on increasing habitual daily physical activity rather than on prescribing exercise to improve cardiovascular or aerobic fitness. In adults, maximal aerobic power ($\dot{V}_{O_2max}$) serves as an indicator of cardiovascular efficiency and the ability to perform endurance-type work. In children, however, maximal aerobic power may not have the same implications (59). While physical fitness (of which aerobic fitness is a major component) and physical activity are interrelated and can influence each other, they are separate entities with differing guidelines. To reduce risks of disease, improve health status, and help control body weight, current guidelines concentrate on increasing the time spent in movement, decreasing the time spent in sedentary activities, increasing energy expenditure, and developing a habit of lifetime physical activity. Improvement in aerobic fitness necessitates engaging in vigorous physical activity for 20–60 min three to five times a week, an exercise prescription that may not be enjoyable for children.

Although many argue that levels of physical activity are decreasing among North American children; others contend that American youth are not nearly as inactive as many people think (7,60). Nevertheless, certain groups of children are experiencing very little activity. The ''Year 2000'' objectives (61) of the U.S. Public Health Service call for a decrease in sedentary behavior and an increase in regular physical activity as a means of reducing cardiovascular disease and controlling obesity (see Table 4).

As children grow into adolescents, vigorous physical activity becomes less frequent, particularly among girls. In 1992, the National Health Interview Survey—Youth Risk Behavior (NHIS-YRB) assessed the frequency of physical activity among U.S. youth in the preceding 7 days, based on 11 groupings that ranged from vigorous activity through walking or cycling for 30 min or more to housecleaning or yard work lasting 30 min or more (62). Some 60% of all male adolescents but only 47% of female youth engaged in *vigorous* activity three or

TABLE 4   Three-Year 2000 Objectives Pertaining to Activity Levels in Children and Adolescents

Number	Objective
1.3	Increase to at least 30% the proportion of people aged 6 and older who engage regularly, preferably daily, in light to moderate physical activity for at least 30 min per day. (Baseline: 22% of people aged 18 and older were active for at least 30 min five or more times per week and 12% were active seven or more times per week in 1985.)
1.4	Increase to at least 20% the proportion of people aged 18 and older and to at least 75% the proportion of children and adolescents aged 6 through 17 who engage in vigorous physical activity that promotes the development and maintenance of cardiorespiratory fitness 3 or more days per week for 20 or more minutes per occasion. (Baseline: 12% for people aged 18 and older in 1985; 66% for youth aged 10 through 17 in 1984.)
1.5	Reduce to no more than 15% the proportion of people aged 6 and older who engage in no leisure-time physical activity. (Baseline: 24% for people aged 18 and older in 1985.)

Source: From Ref. 61.

more times a week. The discrepancy between males and females was age-dependent. At 12 years of age, males and females showed a similar prevalence of vigorous physical activity (68%); but by age 21, levels were 42% for males and 30% for females. White, non-Latino females had higher levels of vigorous activity (49%) than did black, non-Latino, or Latina females (about 42%), whereas males had similar levels regardless of race/ethnicity.

The 1993 Youth Risk Behavior Survey (YRBS), a U.S. population-based survey, also found an inverse relationship between self-reported moderate to vigorous activity and age (i.e., higher activity levels in 9th grade than in 12th grade), with boys having a higher level of physical activity than girls (6).

In terms of moderate-intensity activity, however, the YCYFS and YRBS data support the view that in the representative population of U.S. youth surveyed, more than 80% of adolescents met the "Healthy People 2000" objective, undertaking 30 min or more of moderate-intensity physical activity on a daily basis (6). There remains a need to identify subgroups who are at a high risk for developing and maintaining an inactive lifestyle.

The amount of physical activity also varies with socioeconomic status (more affluence being associated with increased physical activity) (62). In addition, those who have a low physical fitness status and those who are obese tend to have low levels of physical activity (6).

Harsh economic conditions, prejudice, and institutional barriers have limited physical activity for many poor boys and girls, boys and girls of color, and children with disabilities. The educational system and society have failed to meet or accept the challenges of economic isolation and racism. Many poor children in inner cities and rural communities live in areas where underfunding, limited facilities, no interfacing of community resources, large safety issues, and few opportunities to engage in activity and sport are common (63). The persistence of social and economic barriers has a disproportionate effect on females. The cultural prominence of men's sports and a disproportionate lack of opportunity for girls to participate in school and community-based programs still shortchange girls in their pursuit of physical activity (54). There is a need to reshape public policy, gearing educational and community resources to help these underserved youth.

Persons with disabilities make up another subgroup whose participation in regular physical activity is low. In general, persons with disabilities are less active and have a lower physical work capacity than able-bodied individuals (64). Persons with disabilities comprise a very heterogeneous group, including those with orthopedic impairments, arthritis, spinal cord injuries, neurological diseases, amputations, and mental disability. The long-term effects of physical inactivity in this subgroup is an important public health issue. Besides increasing the risk of cardiovascular disease, non-insulin-dependent diabetes mellitus (NIDDM), hypertension, obesity, and osteroporosis, an inactive lifestyle decreases function and personal independence. The limited activity of the 38 million noninstitution-alized U.S. adults with disabilities (1992 data) may decrease their function to a point where they cannot undertake activities of daily living (ADLs) (64). Promot-ing increases in endurance, strength, and flexibility will increase their physical work capacity and decrease the severity of secondary complications—or even eliminate them—as well as decreasing the risk of chronic disease. "The under-standing of environmental and social barriers to physical activity among persons with disabilities needs further exploration . . . physical activity determinants re-search among persons with disabilities, including the role of assistive technology as well as maximizing the intrinsic capacity of functional anatomy and physiol-ogy, needs to be addressed" (64, p. 224).

Tracking into Adulthood.   Part of the assumption of encouraging an increase in the physical activity of children is that an active lifestyle will continue into adulthood. Not many longitudinal studies have been conducted to examine this assumption. Glenmark and colleagues (65) determined the activity levels of 16-year-olds (62 males and 43 females) by questionnaire, repeating the measure-ments 11 years later. There was a correlation of 0.64 for women and 0.48 for men between physical activity at ages 16 and 27. The data of Raitakari and col-leagues (66) also suggests that physical activity tracks significantly from adoles-cence to adulthood and that the habit of physical activity begun or maintained in childhood may carry over into adulthood.

ANATOMICAL AND PHYSIOLOGICAL ASPECTS

Major differences in physiological responses to exercise exist between preadoles-cents, adolescents, and adults. These differences and their implications for exer-cise are summarized in Table 5. Apart from a low economy of locomotion and a decreased tolerance of climatic extremes, no underlying *physiological* factors have been identified that would make preadolescents less suitable than adults for prolonged, continuous activities (67).

Preadolescents can perform exercise over a wide variety of intensities and durations, but they *spontaneously* prefer short-term intermittent activities with a high recreational component and variety relative to monotonous, prolonged activities. Physiologically, preadolescents may use oxygen more efficiently than adults, but they are less able to exploit anaerobic pathways. Therefore, preadoles-cent children have greater oxygen-dependent ATP generation and have a higher limiting pH during exercise. In accordance with their physiological profile and psychological aptitude, children are best suited to repeated activities of varying intensities that last a few seconds, interspersed with short rest periods. Short bursts of activity may optimize the anabolic effect of exercise in the growing

TABLE 5   Physiological Characteristics of the Exercising Child

Function	Comparison to adults	Implications for exercise prescription
METABOLIC		
Aerobic		
$\dot{V}O_{2_{peak}}$ (L/min)	Lower function of body mass.	
$\dot{V}O_{2_{peak}}$ (ml/kg/min)	Similar.	Can perform endurance tasks reasonably well.
Submaximal oxygen demand (economy)	Cycling: similar (18–30% mechanical efficiency); Walking and running: higher metabolic cost.	Greater fatigability in prolonged high-intensity tasks (running and walking); greater heat production in children at a given speed of walking or running.
$\dot{V}CO_2$	Time required to increase $\dot{V}CO_2$ at onset of activity and to return to baseline is markedly faster in preadolescents.	
Anaerobic		
Glycogen stores	Lower concentration and rate of utilization of muscle glycogen. Increase with age, similar to adult levels by about age 16.	
Phosphofructokinase (PFK concentration)	Glycolysis limited because of low level of PFK. For children aged 11–14 years, a variety of glycolytic enzymes are the same as in adults at maximal exercise.	Ability of preadolescent children to perform *intense* anaerobic tasks that last 10 to 90 s is distinctly lower than that of adults. Same ability to deal metabolically with very brief intense exercise.
Phosphagen stores	Stores and breakdown of ATP and creatine phosphate are the same.	Same ability to deal metabolically with very brief intense exercise.
Oxygen transient	Faster attainment of steady state than in adults. Shorter half-time of oxygen increase in children.	Preadolescent children reach metabolic steady state faster. Children contract a lower oxygen deficit. Faster recovery. Children therefore are well suited to intermittent activities.

TABLE 5   Continued

Function	Comparison to adults	Implications for exercise prescription
LA_{peak}	Lower blood lactate levels at $\dot{V}O_{2_{peak}}$, especially in prepubescent children.	Individual variability is wide.
LA_{submax}	Lower at a given percent of $\dot{V}O_{2_{peak}}$.	May be reason children perceive a given workload as easier.
Heart rate (HR) at lactate threshold (LT)	Higher.	Children are able to exercise closer to peak exercise levels than adults before LT is reached.
CARDIOVASCULAR		
Maximal cardiac output ($\dot{Q}_{max}$)	Lower due to size difference.	Immature cardiovascular system means child is limited in bringing internal heat to surface for dissipation when exercising intensely in the heat.
$\dot{Q}$ at a given $\dot{V}O_2$	Somewhat lower.	
Maximal stroke volume (SV_{max})	Lower due to difference in size and heart volume.	
SV at given $\dot{V}O_2$	Lower.	
Maximal heart rate (HR_{max})	Higher.	Up to maturity, HR_{max} is between 195 and 215 beats per minute.
HR at submaximal work	At given power output and at relative metabolic load, child has higher HR.	Higher HR compensates for lower SV.
Oxygen-carrying capacity	Blood volume, hemoglobin concentration, and total hemoglobin are lower in children.	
O_2 content in arterial and venous blood ($Ca_{O_2} - C\bar{v}_{O_2}$)	Somewhat higher.	Potential deficiency of peripheral blood supply during maximal exertion in hot climates.
Blood flow to active muscle	Higher.	
Systolic and diastolic pressures	Lower maximal and submaximal.	No known beneficial or detrimental effects on working capacity of child.

TABLE 5   Continued

Function	Comparison to adults	Implications for exercise prescription
PULMONARY RESPONSE		
Maximal minute ventilation $\dot{V}_{Emax}$ (L/min)	Smaller.	Early fatigability in tasks that require large respiratory minute volumes.
$\dot{V}_{Emax}$ (ml/kg/min)	Same as in adolescents and young adults.	
$\dot{V}_{Esubmax}$	$\dot{V}_E$ at any given $\dot{V}O_2$ is higher in children.	Less efficient ventilation would mean a greater oxygen cost of ventilation. May explain the relatively higher metabolic cost of submaximal exercise.
Respiratory frequency and tidal volume	Marked by higher rate of tachypnea and shallow breathing response.	Children's physiological dead space is smaller than that of adults; therefore alveolar ventilation is still adequate for gas exchange.
Ventilatory threshold (VT)	VT occurs at a higher percentage of $\dot{V}O_{2max}$ in children.	Additional indicators that children may rely more on aerobic metabolism to meet energy demands.
R_{max} ($\dot{V}CO_2/\dot{V}O_2$)	Lower in children.	
PERCEPTION		
RPE (rating of perceived exertion)	Exercising at a given physiological strain is perceived to be easier by children.	Implications for initial phase heat acclimatization.
THERMO-REGULATORY		
Surface area (SA)	Per unit mass is approximately 36% greater in children (percentage is variable, depends on size of child—i.e., SA per mass may be higher in younger children and lower in older).	Greater rate of heat exchange between skin and environment. In climatic extremes, children are at increased risk of stress.
Sweating rate	Lower absolute amount per unit of SA. Greater increase in core temperature required to start sweating.	Greater risk of heat-related illness on hot, humid days due to reduced capacity to evaporate sweat. Lower tolerance time in extreme heat.

(Table Continues)

Table 5 Continued

Function	Comparison to adults	Implications for exercise prescription
Acclimatization to heat	Slower physiologically; faster subjectively.	Children require a longer and more gradual program of acclimatization; special attention during early stages of acclimatization.
Body cooling in water	Faster cooling due to higher SA per heat-producing unit mass; lower thickness of subcutaneous fat.	Potential hypothermia.
Body core heating during dehydration	Greater.	Prolonged activity; hydrate well before and force fluid intake during activity.

Source: From Ref. 113.

child (68). The least suitable form of exercise for preadolescent children, from a physiological viewpoint, is highly intense activity lasting 10 to 90 s (69).

Adolescent children (identified by chronological ages 11 to 21 years) can be prepubescent, going through puberty, or postpubescent. Thus, it is hard to identify the specific physiological responses of the adolescent. The prepubescent would have a physiological profile similar to that of a preadolescent. The postpubescent child would respond to exercise like an adult. The precise physiological response of a child going through puberty, therefore, depends on his or her somatic and biological maturity.

Somatic Growth and Biological Maturation

It is important to keep children "naturally active." A child's physical activity level has a negative impact on somatic growth only if activity falls below a biological threshold (68). There does *not* seem to be any evidence that increasing levels of physical activity above this threshold will increase the age at peak height velocity, skeletal maturation, or sexual maturation (32). At the other extreme, however, there is evidence that excessive training may result in a reduction of growth potential (70).

Bone Mass

Although longitudinal studies regarding physical activity and the gaining of bone mass to one's greatest genetic potential are lacking, adolescence seems a crucial time in terms of maximizing bone density. Therefore, the International Consensus on Physical Activity Guidelines for Adolescents (71) supports the view that physical activity and exercise (especially weight bearing), including short bouts of intense daily activity and resistance training, are needed to maximize bone density. The positive effect of mechanical loading is seen only with an adequate intake of energy and calcium together with an appropriate hormonal status.

It is important to monitor the menstrual status of postmenarchal females, since amenorrhea can have severe consequences for bone density. *The American Academy of Pediatrics (AAP) recommends intervention after the onset of amenorrhea in physically active females in order to preserve normal bone development and to prevent skeletal demineralization* (72).

The current recommendation is that females be encouraged to engage in all intensities of activity. However, since disordered eating coupled with intense exercise can lead to amenorrhea (predisposing to loss of bone mass and osteoporosis), it is imperative that active adolescents eat a sufficient quantity of nutrient-dense foods (15). (See Table 3 for danger signs associated with eating disorders.)

Precautions When Exercising in Climatic Extremes

Because preadolescent children have a high metabolic rate at a given submaximal walking or running speed, children produce relatively more body heat than adults. This higher metabolic load—compounded by a poor sweating capacity, a large surface-to-mass ratio, and an immature cardiovascular system (Table 5)—reduce a child's tolerance of exercise in hot climates, increasing the susceptibility to heat stress (73). The AAP recommends that "Clothing should be lightweight, limited to one layer of absorbent material in order to facilitate evaporation of sweat and to expose as much skin as possible. Sweat-saturated garments should be replaced by dry ones. Rubberized sweat suits should never be used to produce loss of weight" (74).

Children have a poor tolerance of both extreme heat and extreme cold; however, they thermoregulate as effectively as adults when exercising in neutral or moderately warm climates (69,75). The AAP emphasizes that "heat related disorders are particularly pronounced in races that exceed 30 minutes in duration" (67). Activities lasting 30 min or more should be reduced whenever relative humidity and air temperature are above critical levels (Table 6).

Depending on the degree of maturation of sweat glands, the state of the cardiorespiratory organs, and mechanical efficiency, the postpubescent adolescent should have an exercise-heat tolerance similar to that of adults. Heat tolerance also depends on physical fitness and body composition (i.e., cardiovascular fitness increases and obesity decreases heat tolerance).

Preadolescent children have characteristics that *increase their risk of heat*

TABLE 6 Weather Guide for Prevention of Heat Illness

Air temperature, °F	Danger zone, % relative humidity	Critical zone, % relative humidity
70	80	100
75	70	100
80	50	80
85	40	68
90	30	55
95	20	40
100	10	30

Note: Table developed for adults. Children are at increased risk of stress in climatic extremes, especially on hot, humid days, due to reduced capacity to evaporate sweat.
Source: From Ref. 76.

illness, but it is not necessarily dangerous for children to work out in hot and humid environments. Preadolescent children are more likely to suffer from heat exhaustion than from other types of heat illness. Adolescents are more likely to be victims of heat stroke when competing in thermally stressful environments (75).

Acclimatization. Preadolescent children tend to lag behind adults in their rate of physiologic acclimatization; therefore, they should undertake a longer and more gradual program of adjustment to an adverse environment. The AAP recommends that "intensity and duration of exercise should be restrained initially and then gradually increased over a period of 10 to 14 days to accomplish acclimatization to the effects of heat" (74). Children can acclimate to some extent when they exercise in thermally neutral environments and when they rest in hot climates; however, they acclimatize subjectively faster than adults. Therefore, at an early stage of acclimatization, children may feel quite capable of performing physical exercise in the heat, despite a marked physiological heat stress (73,75).

Fluid Replacement. During continuous activity of more than 30 min duration, 100 to 150 ml of fluid should be drunk every 15 to 30 min, even when the child is not thirsty (69,74,76). In preadolescent children who are well hydrated, carbohydrate drinks (i.e., sports drinks) offer no advantages over water (77).

Overuse Injuries

The number of children experiencing overuse injuries is increasing (78). Overuse injuries are caused by repetitive musculoskeletal microtrauma (79). Risk factors include the following (78–80):

Significant changes in the intensity, duration, frequency, or type of training
Musculotendinous tautness in early adolescence
Imbalance in strength and flexibility
Anatomic malalignment of the lower extremities
Incorrect biomechanics
Improper footwear
Training on hard surfaces
Excessive loading of the back during growth spurts

It has been estimated that one-half of overuse injuries in children are preventable (80). Prevention involves (a) improvement in musculoskeletal fitness and sports-specific skills; (b) monitoring of growth rate to identify periods of accelerated growth, when vulnerability may be greatest and, therefore, training regimes should be modified; and (c) a gradual progression in training, with no more than a 10% increase in the amount of training time, amount of distance covered, or number of repetitions performed per week (80). The AAP recommends that pediatricians consider the risks of distance running in advising parents and children. However, unless new data become available, there is no reason to exclude children from distance running events (67).

EXERCISE PRESCRIPTIONS

Large-Muscle Activity

The recommendation for adults who seek to lower their risk of all-cause and coronary heart disease mortality is to develop an energy expenditure of 12.5 to 17 kJ/kg/day (3 to 4 kcal/kg/day; equivalent to about 30 min of brisk walking) (7). Health-related fitness (i.e., $\dot{V}O_{2max}$) is increased by engaging in repetitive large-muscle activity at 50–85% of maximal oxygen uptake for 20–60 min three to five times a week. Health-related fitness also includes resistance training to improve muscle strength and endurance as well as stretching exercises (10).

For preadolescent children, the recommendation is to accumulate 30 min to 1 h of activity per day (25 to 34 kJ per kilogram of body weight per day) to ensure that when they reach adulthood, they will meet the adult standard despite the present trend for adults to become less active as they grow older (81). Younger children usually do not enjoy prolonged exercise without rest periods; therefore, a prescription to undertake sustained large-muscle activity for a minimum of 20 min per session may be discouraging and interfere with the child's enjoyment of movement (82). Increased energy expenditure and appropriate eating habits are major components of multidisciplinary programs both for obese children and for the prevention of obesity (83).

For preadolescent children, the primary goal is to maintain activity, since children enjoy moving, and to develop lifelong activity habits. To accomplish these goals:

1.   Preadolescent children should be allowed to be naturally active and to control the intensity and duration of their activity (82); enjoyment of activity is paramount. In substituting physical activity for a sedentary behavior such as television watching, children are more likely to choose to be active if they are given a choice of several lifestyle activities rather than asked to engage in a specific structured exercise program (84).

2.   Reduce the access to sedentary activity. Children should be encouraged to go outside and get away from the television and the computer. Epstein and colleagues (84) found that obese children who were reinforced for reducing sedentary behaviors (rather than reinforcing exercise) tended to substitute higher expenditure activities.

3.   Emphasis should be placed on the gaining of basic motor and sport skills, since children who perceived themselves as competent are more likely to engage in moderate to vigorous physical activity (82). The individual who can play a variety of sports or who can dance well is more likely to remain active throughout life (32).

4.   Children need to be taught about the benefits of exercise and the risk factors for cardiovascular disease and diabetes (84).

5.   Parents/guardians and family members should support and encourage children to engage in physical activity and provide active role models. Parents' beliefs about the child's competency and attitudes toward engaging in extracurricular activities are major determinants of a child's activity level (85,86). However, peer influences become more powerful during adolescence (6).

6.   Multidisciplinary intervention programs should be implemented for those children who are sedentary, obese, or disabled. Girls may require more support to be physically active. Culturally appropriate activities and innovative techniques should be explored and supported to increase activity levels among ethnic minorities and children living in impoverished areas.

7.   Those children who are not physically fit should be identified. Although there is only a modest relationship ($R^2 = .25$) between the amount of physical activity in which a child engages and her or his physical fitness (87), childhood fitness values are relatively stable (37). Determining childhood fitness should help to identify future unfit adults and therefore individuals who will be at risk for coronary heart disease in their later years (37).

8.   Primary care providers can play a major role in the promotion of physical activity.

The Primary Care Provider's Role in the Promotion of Physical Activity.   In the United States, one of the ''Healthy People 2000'' goals is to increase to at least 50% the number of primary care providers who assess and counsel their patients appropriately about physical activity (61). There are several barriers to physician counseling about physical activity, including lack of time, lack of clear-cut recommendations, lack of knowledge, a belief that patient behavior cannot be changed, and negative personal beliefs and behaviors about the health value of physical activity (88).

Two programs have been successful in changing physician and patient behavior. The INSURE (Industrywide Network for Social, Urban, and Rural Efforts) project developed and tested a clinical model of preventive health services that included patient education as a primary medical care and insured benefit. Some 36% of patients receiving primary care counseling subsequently engaged in physical activity (89). This and similar projects indicate that, given appropriate training, primary care physicians can provide successful health promotion interventions affecting large numbers of patients (88,90).

Project Pace (Physician-Based Assessment and Counseling for Exercise) is a practical system of matching counseling with patient readiness for engaging in physical activity. It was developed to help physicians attain U.S. health promotion goals for the year 2000 (91). Physicians are trained (a) to identify and to intervene according to the patient's stage of readiness for physical activity (precontemplation, contemplation, preparation, action, and maintenance); (b) to provide a written activity description (a stage-of-readiness matched self-help manual); and (c) to support and maintain physical activity with follow-up phone calls and visits. Physicians were provided with assessment forms to identify their patients' current levels of physical activity and to determine the appropriate counseling protocol to use (forms found in Ref. 91).

Preliminary evidence suggests that PACE is a practical and effective method of increasing physical activity. Some 75% of providers rated the program as good or very good; more than 80% of the patients were also receptive to the intervention techniques, and over 70% reported that the counseling had been helpful. Moreover, 37% of the providers reported an increase in their own physical activity during the study. These results suggest that physician-based counseling for physical activity is effective in producing short-term increases in moderate physical activity among previously sedentary patients (88).

According to Patrick and colleagues (88, p. 240):

Evidence to date suggests that characteristics of successful interventions for physical activity based on health-care providers will induce the following:

Brevity: Short length of interaction with provider. Necessary for pragmatic reasons but, given adequate patient follow-up, this may be as effective as lengthy interactions.

Focus: Through either a stages-of-change or other "patient-centered" approach, messages given to patients should be tailored to their individual needs. Shotgun admonitions to "Just do it" are unlikely to produce meaningful change.

Follow-up and reinforcement: Follow-up prompting, via phone calls after the provider visit, has been used by PACE and others to encourage adoption of walking. As with other behavior interventions, it is likely that repeated attention during subsequent office visits will be necessary.

A systems approach: Interventions prompted by health-care providers must be embedded in a larger, supportive system of related activities that addresses predisposing, enabling, and reinforcing factors at the individual, organizational, and community levels.

Exercise Prescription in Adolescence

For adolescent children, acquisition of motor and sports skills should still be emphasized. The specific guidelines from the International Consensus Conference on Physical Activity Guidelines for Adolescents (92, pp. 307–308) are as follows:

Guideline 1: *All adolescents should be physically active daily, or nearly every day, as part of play, games, sports, work, transportation, recreation, physical education, or planned exercise, in the context of family, school, and community activities.* Adolescents should do a variety of physical activities as part of their daily lifestyles. These activities should be enjoyable, involve a variety of muscle groups and include some weight-bearing activities. The intensity or duration of the activity is probably less important than the fact that energy is expended and a habit of daily activity is established. Adolescents are encouraged to incorporate physical activity into their lifestyles by doing such things as walking up stairs, walking or riding a bicycle for errands, having conversation while walking with friends, parking at the far end of parking lots, and doing household chores.

Guideline 2: *Adolescents should engage in three or more sessions per week of activities that last 20 min or more at a time and that require moderate to vigorous levels of exertion.* Moderate to vigorous activities are those that require at least as much effort as brisk or fast walking. A diversity of activities that use large muscle groups are recommended as part of sports, recreation, chores, transportation, work, school, physical education, or planned exercise. Examples include brisk walking, jogging, stair climbing, basketball, racquet sports, soccer, dance, swimming laps, skating, strength (resistance) training, lawn mowing, strenuous housework, cross-country skiing, and cycling.

The promotion of an active lifestyle and the lowering of obesity prevalence depends also on community support and the availability of safe and accessible facilities, advertising, and socioeconomic and political factors. Therefore, it is imperative to look at the broader picture of activity promotion, especially for minorities, individuals with disabilities, and poorer individuals. Children with an illness or disability may require a modified exercise prescription (10,69,93,94). Specific prescriptions may also be advised for hypokinetic children and for those who have two or more risk factors for coronary artery disease.

Exercise Prescription to Improve Cardiovascular Fitness (Maximal Oxygen Intake)

One has to exercise above a certain threshold intensity for a minimum duration and frequency in order to improve cardiovascular fitness. For adults, an intensity between 50 and 85% of $\dot{V}O_{2max}$ must be maintained for 20–60 min three to five times per week (10). The intensity range is quite large. Individuals in poor or fair condition should exercise at the lower end of the range (50 to 65%), while those in good to excellent condition should exercise at the upper end (75 to 85%). In a practical setting, heart rate (HR), and/or rating of perceived exertion (RPE) may be used to determine whether one is exercising at an appropriate intensity. Exercise can also be prescribed using metabolic equivalents (METs) (10). Heart rate is measured either during exercise [using an electrocardiogram (ECG) or an HR monitor] or is palpated for 10 s immediately after stopping exercise. Two methods use HR to establish intensity. The Karvonen formula is based on HR reserve (HRR)—that is, maximal HR minus resting HR. Maximal HR is either determined from a graded exercise test or is predicted by subtracting the individual's age from the number 220. The intensity range is the same as for $\dot{V}O_{2max}$ (50 to 85%). The HR training zone is:

$$\%(HHR) + HR_{rest}$$

For example, the training zone for a 20-year-old who is in poor physical condition with a resting HR of 70 beats per minute would be 50–60%:

0.50 (200 − 70) + 70 = 65 + 70 = 135 beats per minute

0.60 (200 − 70) + 70 = 84.5 + 70 = 148 beats per minute

The alternative method calculates a percentage of HR_{max}. The intensity zone is then 60 to 90%, since the slope of the relationship between HR and HRR with $\dot{V}O_{2max}$ is different. Therefore, for the same 20-year-old individual, the target HR zone (using 60–70%) would be:

0.60 (200)* = 120 beats per minute

0.70 (200)* = 140 beats per minute

The same training-zone ranges established for adults have been used for adolescents and young adults. However, there is little information concerning the appropriate intensity, duration, and frequency needed for prepubescents to improve their aerobic power. As emphasized previously, activity guidelines for prepubescents should focus on keeping children active and maximizing energy expenditure rather than seeking to improve $\dot{V}O_{2max}$. Some evidence suggests that the intensity of work must be quite vigorous if prepubescent children are to increase their aerobic power (81). Rowland (81) argues that, to tax the oxygen delivery system appropriately, children must train at an intensity equal to the lactate threshold (LT—the intensity level of exercise where blood lactate concentration begins to increase). Therefore, the target HR for prepubescents should be set at 85% of maximal HR, which corresponds to the child's ventilatory anaerobic threshold.

Borg (95) developed two scales that could be used by individuals to rate their perception of the intensity of work. After being trained in how to use RPE or after using RPE as an adjunct to HR, adults can use RPE alone to establish whether they are exercising within their training intensity zone. The appropriate range of intensity is usually from a rating of 12 (somewhat hard) to 16 (hard) for asymptomatic individuals (10). RPE is not recommended in certain patient populations where precise knowledge of heart rate may be critical to the safety of the program, or where the relationship of HR to $\dot{V}O_2$ is altered (for example, cardiac transplantation).

Although research is somewhat limited, it appears that the Borg RPE scale is a valid psychophysical instrument to assess perceptions of exertion in normal and clinically involved children and adolescents (96). However, it is not agreed whether children aged 8 to 16 years can use the Borg RPE scale to assess their predetermined (target) exercise intensities accurately. Ward (97) and Williams (98) both reported that children 8–14 years old could use Borg's RPE scale correctly, but Bar-Or (99) reported that children under 16 years of age made less competent use of the Borg RPE scale than those 18 years of age or older.

Very young children are unable to match the full perceptual range correctly with various levels of exercise intensities (96). Williams (98) observed that children under age 11 years were cognitively unable to assign numbers to words or phrases that described exercise-related feelings and that very young children also had difficulty in interpreting certain verbal descriptors because they went beyond

---

* HR_{max} predicted from age.

their level of reading comprehension. Therefore, a developmentally indexed scale has been deviced to assess exertional perceptions in young children (98). The Children's Effort Rating Table (CERT) is a partitioned scale that has numerical categories ranging from 1 to 10, with verbal descriptors assigned to each category.

Strength Training

Strength is the maximal force or torque developed by a muscle or muscle group during one maximal voluntary contraction. *Muscle endurance* is the ability of a muscle or muscle group to exert force continuously (without producing movement) or repeatedly (while producing or resisting movement). *Power* is the rate at which work is performed. *Strength training* is the use of a variety of methods— including free weights, weight machines, and/or one's body weight—to increase the ability to exert or resist force (81,100). Strength training usually involves making a series of contractions against some resistance. The more repetitions (and, therefore, the lower the resistance), the more likely that training will improve muscle endurance; fewer repetitions with a higher resistance maximize strength gains (101). Strength (resistance) training is usually undertaken to increase fitness, enhance performance in a sport, or prevent injury. *Weight lifting* and *power lifting* are competitive sports in which maximal weight is lifted in a single attempt (102). *Body building* is a competitive sport in which the participants use various resistance methods to develop muscle size, symmetry, and definition (103).

Any consideration of the potential benefits of training (e.g., strength gains, injury protection, improved sports performance, psychological benefits, and learning of proper techniques) must be weighed against the potential risks (e.g., low back injury, growth plate injury in adolescents, and other acute and chronic musculoskeletal injuries; weight lifter's blackout; and hypertension) (104). Nevertheless, the benefits of participation generally outweigh risks when sessions are supervised by a well-trained adult and the child has the emotional maturity to follow directions (102–104).

Strength testing and training equipment should be adaptable to children (102). Field and laboratory tests of muscular strength and endurance are described in the literature (100). Recommendations for strength training in children are numerous and fairly consistent (10,93,102,104,105). Programs should be characterized by close and continuous supervision; adequate warm-up; a high number of repetitions per set (no less than six to eight repetitions per set); an adequate recovery time between sessions (a frequency of no more than 2 to 3 days a week); an emphasis on proper form; and inclusion of flexibility exercises (especially during adolescent growth spurts). In the early stages of a program, children can use their body weight as a resistance; specific lifts should be introduced using little or no load, with the emphasis on technique. Overload is initially achieved by increasing the number of repetitions, followed by increases in resistance. Children should *avoid* the practices of weight lifting, power lifting, or body building as well as the use of maximal amounts of weight in strength training programs until they have reached the Tanner stage 5 level of developmental maturity (103). Strength training should be one component of a child's program for increasing fitness or performance, but it should not be the sole component.

Strength gains can be realized with a minimal risk of injury in prepubescent and pubescent children (102). Preadolescents respond to similar resistance training programs with similar relative (percentage improvement) but smaller absolute strength gains than adolescents and young adults. As in adults, the gains depend on the training load. Training-induced strength gains are lost during detraining (104).

GRADED EXERCISE TESTING

Rationale for Exercise Testing

Reasons for exercise testing in pediatric diagnosis are listed in Table 7. Application of graded exercise testing (GXT) to specific diseases or problems is beyond the scope of this chapter, and we refer the reader to other sources of detailed information (106–108). In many cases, the GXT is used most successfully as an affirmation to the child and his or her parents that exercise can be performed at a high intensity with no ill effects. The legality and ethics of involving children in research projects should be considered carefully. Informed consent of both the parent and child should be sought whenever possible (109).

Ergometers

The same types of ergometers can be used with children and adults. Some test procedures (e.g., radionuclide imaging and echocardiography) are more conveniently determined on a cycle ergometer than on a treadmill (107); although, in general, children (especially those younger than age 7 years) are best tested on a treadmill. Premature local muscle fatigue and the inability to maintain a specific cadence prevent many children from reaching maximal values on a cycle ergometer. Most children must be taught how to use the ergometers correctly. Cardiorespiratory measurements must be assessed directly on the treadmill, since variations in efficiency of gait preclude prediction of maximal values from submaximal $\dot{V}O_2$ (69). Hand rails on the treadmill and the support system for gas-analysis equipment will need to be modified (110).

If a cycle ergometer is used, an electronically braked cycle ergometer is

TABLE 7   Rationale for Exercise Testing in Pediatric Diagnosis

Measurement of physical working capacity
1. To assess daily function—to establish whether a child's daily activities are within the child's physiological functioning level
2. To identify a deficiency in specific fitness component—muscular endurance and strength may limit daily performance rather than aerobic power (e.g., muscular dystrophy)
3. To establish a baseline before beginning an exercise program
4. To assess the effectiveness of an exercise prescription
5. To chart the course of a progressive disease (e.g., cystic fibrosis, Duchenne muscular dystrophy)

Exercise as a provocation test
1. To amplify pathophysiological changes
2. To trigger changes not seen in the resting child

Exercise as an adjunct diagnostic test
1. A noninvasive exercise test can be used to determine the need for an invasive test
2. To assess the severity of dysarrhythmias
3. To assess the functional success of surgery
4. To assess the adequacy of drug regimens at varying exercise intensities

Assessment and differentiation of symptoms: chest pains (asthma from myocardial infarction), breathlessness (bronchoconstriction from low physical capacity), coughing, easy fatigability

Instill confidence in child and parent

Motivation or compliance with exercise program

Source: From Ref. 114.

preferred, because power output is then less dependent on pedal rate. On mechanically braked ergometers, pedal rates of 50 to 60 revolutions per minute are recommended (69). If children under the age of 8 or 9 years are to be tested, special pediatric models should be used or existing cycle ergometers should be modified. The handlebars should be lengthened, the seat height must be adjusted so that the angle of the extended knee joint is no more than 15 degrees, and the pedal crank length should be reduced (0.13 m for age 6 years; 0.15 m for age 8 to 10 years) (69,107). Smaller work-rate increments are likely to be needed, and the cycle ergometer scale should be in 5-W gradations. Testing of children with diseases that involve the legs may require the use of arm ergometers.

Protocol

A variety of exercise protocols for children are available (69,106,107,111). Some are very similar to those used with adults, but others reduce the initial power output and subsequent increments of loading. The specific protocol selected depends on the question(s) to be answered, the measurements to be obtained, whether submaximal and/or maximal data are needed, and on the abilities and limitations of the patient. A GXT is not required in evaluating an asymptomatic child except for research purposes.

Supervisory Personnel

A physician with training in exercise testing and the performance of exercise tests by children with disorders of varying severity must assume responsibility for directing the laboratory during diagnostic exercise testing. The actual conduct of the test may be delegated to other qualified personnel (107). A physician should be actively involved in testing children with the following conditions (69,107):

Serious rhythm disorders
Aortic stenosis with anticipated gradients over 50 mmHg
Myocardial disease
Cyanotic heart disease
Advanced pulmonary vascular disease
Ventricular dysrhythmia with heart disease
Coronary arterial disease

"Maximal exercise testing of normal pediatric age volunteers for research purposes can safely be done by individuals with ACSM certification (or with equivalent training in pediatric exercise testing) without direct supervision of test procedures" (107, p. 2174).

Contraindications

In addition to the general contraindications listed in the ACSM guidelines (Table 8), specific contraindications for testing pediatric patients include the following (69,107):

1. An asthmatic child who is dyspneic at rest, or whose 1-s forced expiratory volume (FEV_1) or peak expiratory flow is less than 60% of the predicted value
2. Acute renal disease, hepatitis
3. An insulin-dependent diabetic who did not take the prescribed quantity of insulin or who is ketoacidotic
4. Acute rheumatic fever with carditis
5. Severe pulmonary vascular disease, poorly compensated congestive heart failure
6. Severe aortic or mitral stenosis; hypotrophic cardiomyopathy with syncope

TABLE 8   Contraindications to Exercise Testing for Adults

Absolute contraindications
1. A recent significant change in the resting ECG suggesting infarction or other acute cardiac event
2. Recent complicated myocardial infarction (unless patient is stable and pain-free)
3. Unstable angina
4. Uncontrolled ventricular arrhythmia
5. Uncontrolled atrial arrhythmia that compromises cardiac function
6. Third-degree AV heart block without pacemaker
7. Acute congestive heart failure
8. Severe aortic stenosis
9. Suspected or known dissecting aneurysm
10. Active or suspected myocarditis or pericarditis
11. Thrombophlebitis or intracardiac thrombi
12. Recent systemic or pulmonary embolus
13. Acute infections
14. Significant emotional distress (psychosis)

Relative Contraindications:
1. Resting diastolic blood pressure >115 mmHg or resting systolic blood pressure >200 mmHg
2. Moderate valvular heart disease
3. Known electrolyte abnormalities (hypokalemia, hypomagnesemia)
4. Fixed-rate pacemaker (rarely used)
5. Frequent or complex ventricular ectopy
6. Ventricular aneurysm
7. Uncontrolled metabolic disease (e.g., diabetes, thyrotoxicosis, or myxedema)
8. Chronic infectious disease (e.g., mononucleosis, hepatitis, AIDS)
9. Neuromuscular, musculoskeletal, or rheumatoid disorders that are exacerbated by exercise
10. Advanced or complicated pregnancy

Note: See text for additional contraindications for testing pediatric patients.
Source: From Ref. 10.

Criteria for Termination of an Exercise Test

Criteria for stopping an exercise are similar to those in adults, as shown in the ACSM guidelines (Table 9).

Attainment of Maximal Oxygen Consumption ($\dot{V}O_{2max}$).   A plateau in oxygen consumption ($\dot{V}O_2$) is often used as a criteria for a maximal test, however, children do not often reach a plateau (110). The value used as *peak* $\dot{V}O_2$ is the highest $\dot{V}O_2$ reached during an exercise test meeting established criteria for *peak effort*. Data on intraindividual variations in $\dot{V}O_{2max}$ indicate, however, that acceptable

TABLE 9   General Indications for Stopping an Exercise Test in Apparently Healthy Adults[a]

1. Onset of angina or angina-like symptoms
2. Significant drop (20 mmHg) in systolic blood pressure or a failure of the systolic blood pressure to rise with an increase in exercise intensity
3. Excessive rise in blood pressure: systolic pressure >260 mmHg or diastolic pressure >115 mmHg
4. Signs of poor perfusion: light-headedness, confusion, ataxia, pallor, cyanosis, nausea, or cold and clammy skin
5. Failure of heart rate to increase with increased exercise intensity
6. Noticeable change in heart rhythm
7. Subject requests to stop
8. Physical or verbal manifestations of severe fatigue
9. Failure of the testing equipment

[a]Assumes that testing is nondiagnostic and is being performed without direct physician involvement or electrocardiographic monitoring.
Source: From Ref. 10.

data can be obtained even if a plateau in $\dot{V}O_2$ is not reached (69,111). Therefore, $\dot{V}O_{2max}$ and $\dot{V}O_{2peak}$ are considered interchangeable terms.

Attainment of Maximal Heart Rate.   Children with weak or atrophied peripheral musculature (e.g., muscular dystrophy or cerebral palsy) are not able to generate enough power to reach the maximal heart rates anticipated in children of their age (10). Children with congenital heart block (and other congenital heart defects), anorexic children, and children receiving β-blocker therapy may also have reduced maximal heart rates (69). Young children attain a higher HR_{max} than adults (Table 4). Maximal heart rates usually do not change until after puberty, when a decrease of 0.7 or 0.8 beats per minute per year of age begins. Treadmill exercise results in a slightly higher HR_{max} than does cycle ergometry (107).

REFERENCES

1. National Institutes of Health, *N.I.H. Consensus Statement,* 13(3): 1–33 (1995).
2. Centers for Disease Control and Prevention (CDCP), *M.M.W.R.,* 46: 1–36 (1997).
3. Pate, R.R., Heath, G.W., Dowda, M., and Trost, S.G., *Am. J. Public Health,* 86: 1577–1581 (1996).
4. Groves, D., Is childhood obesity related to TV addiction? *Phys. Sports Med.,* 16(11): 117–122 (1988).

5. Ross, J.G., and Pate, R.R., *J. Phys. Educ. Rec. Dance,* 58(9): 51–56 (1987).
6. Pate, R.R., in *NIH: Physical Activity and Cardiovascular Health* (A.S. Leon, ed.). Human Kinetics, Champaign, Illinois, pp. 210–217 (1997).
7. Blair, S.N., Clarke, D.G., Cureton, K.J., and Powell, K.E., in *Exercise and Fitness in Childhood: Implications for a Lifetime of Health* (C.V. Gisolfi and D.R. Lamb, eds.). Benchmark Press, Indianapolis, pp. 401–422 (1989).
8. Sallis, J.F., Patrick, K., and Long, B.J., *Pediatr. Exerc. Sci.,* 6(4): 299–301 (1994).
9. Caspersen, C.J., Powell K.P., and Christenson, G.M., *Public Health Rep.,* 100(2): 126–131 (1985).
10. American College of Sports Medicine (ACSM), *ACSM's Guidelines for Exercise Testing and Prescription.* Williams & Wilkins, Baltimore (1995).
11. Rabbia, F., Veglio, F., Pinna, G., Olivia, S., Surgo, B., Rolando, B., Bessone, A., Melchio, R., and Chiandussi, L., *Prev. Med.,* 23: 809–815 (1994).
12. McGill, H.C., Jr., in *Childhood Prevention of Arteriosclerosis and Hypertension* (R.M. Lauer and R.R. Sheleke, eds.). Raven Press, New York, pp. 41–49 (1980).
13. Newman, W.P., III, Freedman, D.S., Voors, A.W., Gard, P.D., Srinivasay, S.R., and Cresanta, J.L., *N. Engl. J. Med.,* 314: 138–144 (1986).
14. Smoak, C.G., Burke, G.L., Webber, L.S., Harsha, D.W., Srinivasan, S.R., and Berenson, G.S., *Am. J. Epidemiol.,* 125: 364–372 (1987).
15. Rowland, T.W., *Developmental Exercise Physiology.* Human Kinetics, Champaign, Illinois (1996).
16. Webber, L.S., Cresanta, J.L., Voors, A.W., and Berenson, G.S., *J. Chronic Dis.,* 36: 647–660 (1983).
17. Lauer, R.M., Burns, T.L., Mahoney, L.T., and Tipton, C.M., in *Perspectives in Exercise Science and Sports Medicine: Youth, Exercise, and Sport* (C.V. Gisolfi and D.R. Lamb, eds.). Benchmark Press, Indianapolis, pp. 431–459 (1989).
18. Rocchini, A.P., *Pediatr. Clin. North Am.,* 31: 1259–1273 (1984).
19. Janz, K.F., Burns, T.L., and Mahoney, L.T., *Med. Sci. Sports Exerc.,* 27: 818–825 (1995).
20. Cresanta, J.L., Hyg, M.S., Burke, G.L., Downey, A.M., Freedman, D.S., and Berenson, G.S., *Pediatr. Clin. North Am.,* 33: 835–858 (1986).
21. Cresanta, J.L., Srinivasan, S.R., Webber, L.S., and Berenson, G.S., *Am. J. Dis. Child.,* 138: 379–387 (1984).
22. National Cholesterol Education Program (NCEP), NIH publication #91-2732. National Heart, Lung and Blood Institute, Bethesda, Maryland (1991).
23. Kemper, H.C.G., Suel, J., Verschuur, R., and Strom-Van Essen, L., *Prev. Med.,* 6: 642–655 (1990).
24. Mahoney, L.T., Lauer, R.M., Lee, J., and Clarke, W.R., *Ann. N.Y. Acad. Sci.,* 623: 120–132 (1991).
25. Porrka, K.V.K., Viikari, J.S.A., and Akerblom, H.K., *Prev. Med.,* 20: 713–724 (1991).
26. Stefanik, M.L., in *Physical Activity and Cardiovascular Health: A National Consensus* (A.S. Leon, ed.). Human Kinetics, Champaign, Illinois, pp. 98–104 (1997).
27. Suder, E., and Howes, M.R., *Med. Sci. Sports Exerc.,* 25: 748–754 (1993).
28. Desprès, J.P., Bouchard, C., and Malina, R.M., *Exercise Sports Science Review,* vol. 18. Macmillan, New York, pp. 243–262 (1990).

29. Sims, E.A.H., in *Child Health, Nutrition, and Physical Activity* (L.W.Y. Cheung and J.B. Richmond, eds.). Human Kinetics, Champaign, Illinois, pp. 171–178 (1995).
30. Burke, G.L., Webber, L.S., Srinivasan, S.R., Radhakrishramurthy, B., Freedman, D.S., and Berenson, G.S., *Metabolism,* 35: 441–446 (1986).
31. Freedson, P.S., and Bunker, L.K., in *President's Council on Physical Fitness and Sports Report: Physical Activity in Sport in the Lives of Girls.* PCPFS, Washington, D.C., pp. 1–16 (1997).
32. Bar-Or, O., and Malina, R.M., in *Child Health, Nutrition, and Physical Activity* (L.W.Y. Cheung and J.B. Richmond, eds.). Human Kinetics, Champaign, Illinois, pp. 79–124 (1995).
33. Troiano, R.P., Flegal, K., Kuczmarski, R.J., Campbell, S.M., and Johnson, C.J., *Arch. Pediatr. Adolesc. Med.,* 149: 1085–1091 (1995).
34. Webber, L.S., Wattingney, W.A., Srinivasan, A.R., and Berenson, G.S., *Am. J. Med. Sci.,* 310(Suppl): S53–S61 (1995).
35. Must, A., *Am. J. Clin. Nutr.,* 63(Suppl): 445S–447S (1996).
36. Eichner, E.R., in *Physical Activity and Cardiovascular Health* (A.S. Leon, ed.). Human Kinetics, Champaign, Illinois, pp. 120–126 (1997).
37. Janz, K.F., and Mahoney, L.T., *Pediatr. Exerc. Sci.,* 7: 364–378 (1995).
38. Serdula, M.K., Ivery, D., Coates, R.J., Freedman, D.S., Williamson, D.F., and Byers, T., *Prev. Med.,* 22: 167–177 (1993).
39. Guo, S.S., Rocke, A.F., Chumela, W.C., Gardner, J.D., and Sierugel, R.M., *Am. J. Clin. Nutr.,* 59: 810–819 (1994).
40. Gidding, S.S., Leibel, R.L., Daniels, S., Rosenbaum, M., Van Horn, L., and Marx, G.R., *Circulation,* 94: 3383–3387 (1996).
41. Lauer, R.M., Lee, J., and Clark, W.R., *Pediatrics,* 82: 577–582 (1988).
42. Malcolm, D.D., Burns, T.L., Mahoney, L.T., and Lauer, R.M., *Pediatrics,* 92: 703–709 (1993).
43. Nieto, F.J., Szklo, M., and Comstock, G.W., *Am. J. Epidemiol.,* 136: 201–213 (1992).
44. Lohman, T.G., *Pediatr. Exerc. Sci.,* 1: 19–30 (1989).
45. Malina, R.M., in *Perspectives in Exercise Science & Sports Medicine: Youth, Exercise, and Sport* (C.V. Gisolfi and D.R. Lamb, eds.). Benchmark Press, Indianapolis, pp. 223–265 (1989).
46. Buenen, G., and Malina, R.M., *Exerc. Sport Sci. Rev.,* 16: 503–540 (1988).
47. Slaughter, M.H., Lohman, T.G., Boileau, R.A., Horwill, C.A., Stillman, R.H., Van Loan, M.D., and Bemben, D.A., *Hum. Biol.,* 60: 709–723 (1988).
48. Malina, R.M., in *Advances in Pediatric Sport Sciences* (R.A. Boileau, ed.). Human Kinetics, Champaign, Illinois, pp. 59–84 (1984).
49. Lohman, T.G., *Advances in Body Composition Assessment.* Human Kinetics, Champaign, Illinois (1992).
50. Casperson, C.J., and Zack, M.M., in *NIH: Physical Activity and Cardiovascular Health: A National Consensus* (A.S. Leon, ed.). Human Kinetics, Champaign, Illinois, pp. 32–39 (1997).
51. Bouchard, C., *Nutr. Rev.,* 54: S125–S130 (1996).
52. Kemper, H.C.G., Post, C.B., and Twisk, J.W.R., *Int. Nutr.,* 7: 229–240 (1997).

53. vanLenthe, F.J., Kemper, H.C.G., and vanMechelen, W., Health Study. *Am. J. Clin. Nutr.,* 64: 18–24 (1996).

54. Sabo, D., in *President's Council on Physical Fitness and Sports Report: Physical Activity and Sport in the Lives of Girls, PCPFS.* U.S. Government Printing Office, Washington, D.C., pp. xix–xxvii (1997).

55. Himes, J.H., Dietz, W.H., *Am. J. Clin. Nutr.,* 59: 307–316 (1994).

56. Dietz, W.H., in *Child Health, Nutrition, and Physical Activity* (L.W.Y. Cheung and J.B. Richmond, eds.). Human Kinetics, Champaign, lllinois, pp. 155–169 (1995).

57. Epstein, L.H., Coleman, K.J., Meyers, M.D., *Med. Sci. Sports Exerc.,* 28: 428–435 (1996).

58. Brownell, K.D., *New York Times,* Dec. 15, p. A29 (1994).

59. Rowland, T.W., *Pediatr, Exerc, Sci.,* 1: 313–328 (1989).

60. Pate, R.R., in *Child Health, Nutrition, and Physical Activity* (L.W.Y. Cheung and J.B. Richmond, eds.). Human Kinetics, Champaign, Illinois, pp. 140–145 (1995).

61. U.S. Public Health Service, DHHS publication no. (PHS) 91-50212. Washington D.C., U.S. Department of Health and Human Services (1991).

62. Caspersen, C.J., and Zack, M.M., *NIH: Physical Activity and Cardiovascular Health: A National Consensus* (A.S. Leon, ed.). Human Kinetics, Champaign, Illinois, pp. 32–39 (1997).

63. Martinek, T.J., *Quest* 49(1): 3–7 (1997).

64. Heath, G.W., Fentem, P.H., *Exerc. Sports Sci. Rev.,* 25: 195–234 (1997).

65. Glenmark, B., Hadberg, G., and Jansson, E., *Eur. J. Appl. Physiol.,* 69: 530–538 (1994).

66. Raitakari, O.T., Porrka, K.V., Taimela, S., Telama, R., and Rasanen, L., *Am. J. Epidemiol.,* 140: 195–204 (1994).

67. American Academy of Pediatrics Committee on Sports Medicine, *Pediatrics,* 86: 656–657 (1990, reaffirmed, 1994).

68. Cooper, D.M., in *New Horizons in Pediatric Exercise Science* (C.J.R. Cameron and O. Bar-Or, eds.). Human Kinetics, Champaign Illinois, pp. 1–24 (1995).

69. Bar-Or, O., *Pediatric Sports Medicine for the Practitioner.* Springer-Verlag, New York, 1983.

70. Theintz, G.E., Howard, H., Weiss, V., and Sizonenko, P.C., *J. Pediatr.,* 122: 306–313 (1993).

71. Bailey, D.A., Martin, A.D., *Pediatr. Exerc. Sci.,* 6: 424–433 (1994).

72. American Academy of Pediatrics, AAP Committee on Sports Medicine, *Pediatrics* 84: 394–395 (1989).

73. Bar-Or, O., *Perspectives in Exercise Science and Sports* (C.V. Gisolfi and D.R. Lamb, eds.). Benchmark Press, Indianapolis, pp. 335–368 (1989).

74. American Academy of Pediatrics, *Phys. Sports Med.,* 11: 155–159 (1983).

75. Armstrong, L.E., and Maresh, C.M., *Pediatr. Exerc. Sci.,* 7: 239–252 (1995).

76. Haymes, E.M., and Wells, C.L., *Environment and Human Performance.* Human Kinetics, Champaign, Illinois (1986).

77. Meyer, F., Bar-Or, O., MacDougall, D., and Heighenhauser, G.J.F., *Med. Sci. Sports Exerc.,* 27: 882–887 (1995).

78. Macera, C.A., and Wooten, W. *Pediatr. Exerc. Sci.,* 6: 424–433 (1994).

79. American Academy of Pediatrics, Committee on Sports Medicine and Fitness,

Sports Medicine: Health Care for Young Athletes. American Academy of Pediatrics, Elk Grove Village, Illinois (1991).

80. American College of Sports Medicine, *Med. Sci. Sports Exerc.,* 25(8 Suppl): 1 (1993).

81. Rowland, T.W., *Exercise and Children's Health.* Human Kinetics, Champaign, Illinois (1990).

82. Pangrazi, A.F., Corbin, C.B., and Welk, G.J., *J Phys. Educ. Rec. Dance,* 67(4): 38–43 (1996).

83. Pate, R.R., *Contemp. Nutr.,* 18(2): 1–2 (1993).

84. Epstein, L.H., Valoski, A.M., Vara, L.S., McCurley, J.M., and Wisniewski, L., *Health Psychol.,* 14(2): 109–155 (1995).

85. Atsalakis, M., and Sleap, M., *Pediatr. Exerc. Sci.,* 8: 166–176 (1996).

86. Kimiecik, J.C., Horn, T.S., and Shurin, C.S., *Res. Q. Exerc. Sport,* 67: 324–336 (1996).

87. Pate, R.R., Dowda, M., and Ross, J.G., *Am. J. Dis. Child.,* 144: 1123–1129 (1990).

88. Patrick, K., Calfas, K.J., Wooten, W.J., Long, J.B., and Sallis, J.F., in *NIH: Physical Activity and Cardiovascular Health* (A.S. Leon, ed.). Human Kinetics, Champaign, Illinois, pp. 245–251 (1997).

89. Logsdon, D.N., Lazaro, M.A., and Meir, R.V., *Am. J. Prev. Med.,* 5: 249–256 (1989).

90. Lewis, B.S., and Lynch, W.D., *Prev. Med.,* 22: 110–121 (1993).

91. Patrick, K., Sallis, J.F., Long, B., Calfas, K.J., Wooten, W.J., Heath, G., and Pratt, M., *Phys. Sports Med.,* 22(11): 45–55, 1994.

92. Sallis J.F., Patrick, K., *Pediatr. Exerc. Sci.,* 6(4): 302–314 (1994).

93. Goldberg, B., *Sports and Exercise for Children with Chronic Health Conditions.* Human Kinetics, Champaign, Illinois (1995).

94. Small, E., and Bar-Or, O., The young athlete with chronic disease. *Clin Sports Med.,* 14: 709–726 (1995).

95. Borg, G., *Med. Sci. Sports Exerc.,* 14: 377–381 (1982).

96. Robertson, R.J., and Noble, B.J., in *Exercise and Sports Sciences Reviews,* vol. 25 (J.O. Holloszy, ed.). Williams & Wilkins, Baltimore, pp. 407–452 (1997).

97. Ward, D., Jackman, J., and Galiano, F., *Pediatr. Exerc. Sci.,* 3: 209–218 (1991).

98. Williams, J.G., Easton, R.G., and Stretch, C., *Pediatr. Exerc. Sci.,* 3: 21–27 (1991).

99. Bar-Or, O., in *Pediatric Sports Medicine for the Practitioner* (G. Ljunggren and S. Durne, eds.). Springer-Verlag, Berlin, pp. 105–113 (1989)

100. Gaul, C.A., in *Measurement in Pediatric Exercise Science* (D. Docherty, ed.). Human Kinetics, Champaign, Illinois, pp. 225–228 (1996).

101. Wathen, D., in *Essentials of Strength Training and Conditioning* (T.R. Baechle, ed.). Human Kinetics, Champaign, Illinois (1994).

102. National Strength and Conditioning Association (NSCA), *Natl. Strength Condi. Assoc. J.,* 7(4): 27–31 (1985).

103. American Academy of Pediatrics (AAP), Committee on sports medicine, *Pediatrics* 86: 801 (1990).

104. Blimkie, C.J., *Sports Med.,* 15: 389–407 (1993).

105. Freedson, P.S., Ward, A., and Rippe, J.M., in *Advances in Sports Medicine and*

Fitness (W.A. Grana, J.A. Lombardo, B.J. Sharkey, and J.A. Stone, eds.). Year Book Medical Publishers, Chicago, pp. 57–65 (1990).

106. Rowland, T.W., in *Pediatric Laboratory Exercise Testing: Clinical Guidelines* (T.W. Roland, ed.). Human Kinetics, Champaign, Illinois, pp. 19–41 (1993).

107. American Heart Association (AHA), *Circulation* 90: 2166–2179 (1994).

108. Tomassoni, T.L., *Med. Sci. Sports Exerc.,* 28: 403–405 (1996).

109. Armstrong, N., and Welsman, J.R., *Exerc. Sports. Sci. Rev.* 22: 435–476 (1994).

110. Docherty, D., in *Measurement in Pediatric Exercise Science* (D. Docherty, ed.). Human Kinetics, Windsor, Ontario, pp. 1–3 (1996).

111. Léger, L., in *Measurement in Pediatric Exercise Science* (D. Docherty, ed.). Human Kinetics, Windsor, Ontario, pp. 183–224 (1996).

112. Casper, R.C., in *Child Health, Nutrition, and Physical Activity* (L.W.Y. Cheung and J.B. Richmond, eds.). Human Kinetics, Champaign, Illinois, p. 226 (1995).

113. Zwiren, L.D., and Manos, T.M., in *Resource Manual for ACSM Guidelines for Exercise Testing and Prescription* (J.L. Roitman, ed.). Williams & Wilkins, Baltimore. (1998).

114. Bar-Or, O., *Scand. J. Sports Sci.,* 7: 35–39 (1985).

4

Exercise Testing and Training in the Middle-Aged

ROY J. SHEPHARD
University of Toronto
Toronto, Ontario, Canada

INTRODUCTION

This chapter discusses issues of exercise testing and prescription that have particular relevance for the late-middle-aged patient, whom we will arbitrarily define as having an age between 40 and 65 years. During this time, women pass through the menopause, and both sexes experience a major change in life roles. Children are becoming independent and taking physical activity separately from their parents. Women may be returning to paid employment after a period as full-time homemakers. Men have often reached a plateau in their careers and are beginning to seek other methods of self-actualization than working 12 h per day. Debts associated with education and house purchase have often been repaid, and many couples note a substantial increase in disposable income. Retirement is seen as a less distant prospect, and there is recognition of a need for interests and hobbies appropriate to a time of greater leisure.

At the same time, many people become conscious of declining physical abilities, particularly if they are still involved in competitive athletic pursuits (Table 1). Some are discouraged by slower swimming speeds or an increasing golfing handicap, and others note that domestic tasks that were once accomplished with ease are now becoming progressively more difficult.

Chronic diseases have often developed substantially relative to early adulthood. The typical individual has sustained a 10-kg increase in body mass, repre-

TABLE 1   Age-Related Decline in the World Record Performance of Selected Athletic Events

Event	Age, years					
	40–44	45–49	50–54	55–59	60–64	65–69
100-m run (s)	10.7	11.1	11.4	11.6	12.0	13.2
1500-m run (min: s)	3:52	4:03	4:14	4:20	4:53	4:59
Marathon run (min: s)	131:19	140:12	145:17	146:35	167:46	173:03
Long jump (m)	7.34	6.68	6.23	6.03	5.38	4.68

Source: Based on data accumulated by Stones, M.L., and Kozma, A., *Exp. Aging Res.*, 7: 274 (1981).

senting a 15-kg accumulation of fat and a 5-kg loss of lean tissue. Osteoporosis begins around 25–30 years of age (earlier in women than in men), and women show a major acceleration of bone calcium loss in the 5-year perimenopausal period. Perhaps 30% of an urban sample have smoked heavily for many years, with a cumulative deterioration in respiratory function; 5–10% of the sample have also become problem drinkers, with an associated cardiomyopathy. Coronary atherosclerosis is still typically silent, but in about one-fifth of patients, intravenous plaques are reaching the critical size (>70% of the intravascular lumen) where significant myocardial ischemia may be anticipated during vigorous exercise (67).

EVALUATION

Reasons for exercise testing in middle age include an individual's desire for a report on personal fitness or response to training, a wish to resume vigorous physical activity safely following a period of sedentary living, a need to evaluate obscure symptoms, work assessment following injury or in jobs with a bonafide occupational fitness requirement, and monitoring of the response to drugs and rehabilitation.

Brief comment is offered on stress testing, analysis of body composition, and the assessment of muscular strength.

Stress Testing

Submaximal tests of aerobic performance are of limited value, even in a young adult. In older individuals, such procedures offer a progressively less satisfactory estimate of peak power output. Aging leads not only to a decrease in average maximal heart rates but also to an increased interindividual variation about the average response (Fig. 1) (3,48).

A progressive test with the measurement of peak power output and/or peak oxygen consumption thus has increasing attraction as a method of assessing an individual's peak cardiorespiratory performance. The procedure is carried through to subjective exhaustion unless there are medical indications to halt the test at an earlier stage (Table 2). As the person becomes older, uphill treadmill walking becomes the preferred mode of exercise. If a cycle ergometer is used, quadriceps weakness may limit attainment of an oxygen consumption plateau (76,80). Stepping is a third possibility, particularly under field conditions, provided that there has been no loss of stability of the knee joints (34).

More specialized and specific equipment such as rowing ergometers and swim benches may be used for groups such as master athletes, although it is not always easy to select sport-specific equipment, since older competitors often engage in a variety of sports (42).

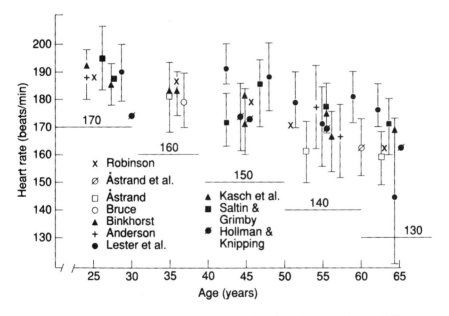

FIGURE 1   Decline in maximal heart rate with age (based on data from the world literature collected by S.M. Fox and W.L. Haskell and reproduced with permission from the authors, with a hypothetical line showing decline from a maximum of 195 beats per minute in a young adult to 170 beats per minute at age 65 years. (For details of original sources, see Ref. 24.)

Table 2   Medical Indications to Halt a Measurement of Maximal Oxygen Intake in the Laboratory

Increasing chest pain of anginal type
Severe dyspnea or fatigue
Faintness
Nausea or vomiting
Claudication
Signs of cerebral insufficiency (pallor, cold moist skin, cyanosis, staggering gait, light-
  headedness, confusion)
Excessive rise in blood pressure
Sudden fall in systolic blood pressure
ST segmental depression >0.2mV (horizontal or downsloping)
Premature ventricular contractions (more than three in 10s, polyfocal, R on T)
Paroxysmal ventricular or supraventricular dysrhythmia
Conduction disturbance other than slight atrioventricular block

Personal Interest

Where the test is conducted for personal interest, the scale of assessment is determined largely by the individual's financial commitment. A medically supervised maximal treadmill test, with electrocardiographic (ECG) monitoring and determination of maximal oxygen consumption, may involve an investment of several hundred dollars.

Resumption of Physical Activity

At one time, American physicians maintained that any patient over the age of 40 years who wished to begin an exercise program required a stress ECG (1, 15). However, Canadian authorities have always regarded this as an unwarranted expense for those who merely intended to begin the typical late-middle-age program of moderate walking and investment of a little more time in gardening and yard work (71,84). Rather, Canadian exercise scientists recommended that apparently healthy individuals should complete a simple physical activity readiness questionnaire (Table 3), either administering it themselves, or doing so in conjunction with an exercise specialist. The advice of a physician should be sought only if the results of the questionnaire are ambiguous. More recently, U.S. experts have moved closer to the Canadian viewpoint, noting the need to consider the initial fitness of the individual, the severity of the proposed activity, and the presence of other symptoms and cardiac risk factors (Tables 4 to 6) (2) before deciding on the need for detailed stress testing.

On the other hand, if a patient expresses a wish for a return to serious

TABLE 3   Physical Activity Readiness Questionnaire (Par-Q)—Modified Version

(C-R)

Physical Activity Readiness
Questionnaire - PAR-Q
(revised 1994)

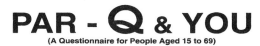

PAR - Q & YOU

(A Questionnaire for People Aged 15 to 69)

Regular physical activity is fun and healthy, and increasingly more people are starting to become more active every day. Being more active is very safe for most people. However, some people should check with their doctor before they start becoming much more physically active.

If you are planning to become much more physically active than you are now, start by answering the seven questions in the box below. If you are between the ages of 15 and 69, the PAR-Q will tell you if you should check with your doctor before you start. If you are over 69 years of age, and you are not used to being very active, check with your doctor.

Common sense is your best guide when you answer these questions. Please read the questions carefully and answer each one honestly: check YES or NO.

YES	NO		
☐	☐	1.	Has your doctor ever said that you have a heart condition <u>and</u> that you should only do physical activity recommended by a doctor?
☐	☐	2.	Do you feel pain in your chest when you do physical activity?
☐	☐	3.	In the past month, have you had chest pain when you were not doing physical activity?
☐	☐	4.	Do you lose your balance because of dizziness or do you ever lose consciousness?
☐	☐	5.	Do you have a bone or joint problem that could be made worse by a change in your physical activity?
☐	☐	6.	Is your doctor currently prescribing drugs (for example, water pills) for your blood pressure or heart condition?
☐	☐	7.	Do you know of <u>any other reason</u> why you should not do physical activity?

YES to one or more questions

If

you

answered

Talk with your doctor by phone or in person BEFORE you start becoming much more physically active or BEFORE you have a fitness appraisal. Tell your doctor about the PAR-Q and which questions you answered YES.

• You may be able to do any activity you want — as long as you start slowly and build up gradually. Or, you may need to restrict your activities to those which are safe for you. Talk with your doctor about the kinds of activities you wish to participate in and follow his/her advice.

• Find out which community programs are safe and helpful for you.

NO to all questions

If you answered NO honestly to <u>all</u> PAR-Q questions, you can be reasonably sure that you can:

• start becoming much more physically active — begin slowly and build up gradually. This is the safest and easiest way to go.

• take part in a fitness appraisal — this is an excellent way to determine your basic fitness so that you can plan the best way for you to live actively.

DELAY BECOMING MUCH MORE ACTIVE:

• if you are not feeling well because of a temporary illness such as a cold or a fever — wait until you feel better; or

• if you are or may be pregnant — talk to your doctor before you start becoming more active.

Please note: If your health changes so that you then answer YES to any of the above questions, tell your fitness or health professional. Ask whether you should change your physical activity plan.

Informed Use of the PAR-Q: The Canadian Society for Exercise Physiology, Health Canada, and their agents assume no liability for persons who undertake physical activity, and if in doubt after completing this questionnaire, consult your doctor prior to physical activity.

You are encouraged to copy the PAR-Q but only if you use the entire form

NOTE: If the PAR-Q is being given to a person before he or she participates in a physical activity program or a fitness appraisal, this section may be used for legal or administrative purposes.

I have read, understood and completed this questionnaire. Any questions I had were answered to my full satisfaction.

NAME _____

SIGNATURE _____   DATE _____

SIGNATURE OF PARENT _____   WITNESS _____
or GUARDIAN (for participants under the age of majority)

continued on other side...

© *Canadian Society for Exercise Physiology*
 Société canadienne de physiologie de l'exercice

Supported by: 🇨🇦   Health   Santé
 Canada   Canada

(Table continues)

TABLE 3 Continued

...continued from other side

PAR - Q & YOU

Physical Activity Readiness
Questionnaire - PAR-Q
(revised 1994)

We know that being physically active provides benefits for all of us. Not being physically active is recognized by the Heart and Stroke Foundation of Canada as one of the four modifiable primary risk factors for coronary heart disease (along with high blood pressure, high blood cholesterol, and smoking). People are physically active for many reasons — play, work, competition, health, creativity, enjoying the outdoors, being with friends. There are also as many ways of being active as there are reasons. What we choose to do depends on our own abilities and desires. No matter what the reason or type of activity, physical activity can improve our well-being and quality of life. Well-being can also be enhanced by integrating physical activity with enjoyable healthy eating and positive self and body image. Together, all three equal VITALITY. So take a fresh approach to living. Check out the VITALITY tips below!

Active Living:
- accumulate 30 minutes or more of moderate physical activity most days of the week
- take the stairs instead of an elevator
- get off the bus early and walk home
- join friends in a sport activity
- take the dog for a walk with the family
- follow a fitness program

Healthy Eating:
- follow Canada's Food Guide to Healthy Eating
- enjoy a variety of foods
- emphasize cereals, breads, other grain products, vegetables and fruit
- choose lower-fat dairy products, leaner meats and foods prepared with little or no fat
- achieve and maintain a healthy body weight by enjoying regular physical activity and healthy eating
- limit salt, alcohol and caffeine
- don't give up foods you enjoy — aim for moderation and variety

Positive Self and Body Image:
- accept who you are and how you look
- remember, a healthy weight range is one that is realistic for your own body make-up (body fat levels should neither be too high nor too low)
- try a new challenge
- compliment yourself
- reflect positively on your abilities
- laugh a lot

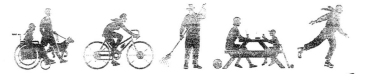

Enjoy eating well, being active and feeling good about yourself. That's VITALITY.

FITNESS AND HEALTH PROFESSIONALS MAY BE INTERESTED IN THE INFORMATION BELOW.

The following companion forms are available for doctors' use by contacting the Canadian Society for Exercise Physiology (address below):

The **Physical Activity Readiness Medical Examination (PARmed-X)** - to be used by doctors with people who answer YES to one or more questions on the PAR-Q.

The **Physical Activity Readiness Medical Examination for Pregnancy (PARmed-X for PREGNANCY)** - to be used by doctors with pregnant patients who wish to become more active.

References:
Arraix, G.A., Wigle, D.T., Mao, Y. (1992). Risk Assessment of Physical Activity and Physical Fitness in the Canada Health Survey Follow-Up Study. **J. Clin. Epidemiol.** 45:4 419-428.
Mottola, M., Wolfe, L.A. (1994). Active Living and Pregnancy, In: A. Quinney, L. Gauvin, T. Wall (eds.), **Toward Active Living: Proceedings of the International Conference on Physical Activity, Fitness and Health.** Champaign, IL: Human Kinetics.
PAR-Q Validation Report, British Columbia Ministry of Health, 1978.
Thomas, S., Reading, J., Shephard, R.J. (1992). Revision of the Physical Activity Readiness Questionnaire (PAR-Q). **Can. J. Spt. Sci.** 17:4 338-345.

To order multiple printed copies of the PAR-Q, please contact the

Canadian Society for Exercise Physiology
1600 James Naismith Dr., Suite 311
Gloucester, Ontario CANADA K1B 5N4
Tel. (613) 748-5768 FAX: (613) 748-5763

The original PAR-Q was developed by the British Columbia Ministry of Health. It has been revised by an Expert Advisory Committee assembled by the Canadian Society for Exercise Physiology and Fitness Canada (1994).

Disponible en français sous le titre «Questionnaire sur l'aptitude à l'activité physique - Q-AAP (revisé 1994)».

© *Canadian Society for Exercise Physiology*
Société canadienne de physiologie de l'exercice

Supported by: Health Santé
Canada Canada

Table 3   Continued

Adult Consent Form

I, the undersigned, do hereby acknowledge:

- my consent to perform a health-related fitness appraisal consisting of stepping on double 20 cm steps at speeds appropriate for my age and gender, measurements of standing height, weight, girths, and skinfolds, and tests of grip strength, push-ups, trunk forward flexion, curl-ups, and vertical jump, the results of which will assist in determining the type and amount of physical activity most appropriate for my level of fitness;

- my understanding that heart rate and blood pressure will be measured prior to and at the completion of the appraisal;

- my consent to answer questions concerning my physical activity participation and my lifestyle;

- my consent to the appraisal measures conducted by an appraiser who has been trained to administer the Canadian Physical Activity, Fitness, and Lifestyle Appraisal. I understand that the interpretation of results is limited to placing my scores in the appropriate Health Benefit Zones and providing information on physical activity participation and other healthy lifestyle topics.

- my understanding that there are potential risks; i.e., episodes of transient lightheadness, fainting, abnormal blood pressure, chest discomfort, leg cramps, and nausea, *and that I assume willfully those risks;*

- my obligation to immediately inform the appraiser of any pain, discomfort, fatigue, or any other symptoms that I *may suffer* during and immediately after the appraisal;

- my understanding that I may stop or delay any further testing if I so desire and that the appraisal may be terminated by the appraiser upon observation of any symptoms of undue distress or abnormal response;

- my understanding that I may ask any questions or request further explanation or information about the procedures at any time before, during, and after the appraisal;

- that I have read, understood, and completed the Physical Activity Readiness Questionnaire (PAR-Q) and answered NO to all the questions or received clearance to participate from my physician.

_____   _____

Signature   Date

_____   _____

Witness   Date

NOTE: This form must be completed, signed and submitted to the appraiser, along with the completed PAR-Q, at the time of testing. The form must also be witnessed at the time of signing and the witness must be of the age of majority and independent of the organization administering the appraisal.

(Table continues)

TABLE 3   Continued

Youth Consent Form

I, the undersigned, do hereby acknowledge:

- my consent for my dependent to perform a health-related fitness appraisal consisting of stepping on double 20 cm steps at speeds appropriate for my age and gender, measurements of standing height, weight, girths, and skinfolds, and tests of grip strength, push-ups, trunk forward flexion, curl-ups, and vertical jump, the results of which will assist in determining the type and amount of physical activity most appropriate for my dependent's level of fitness;

- my understanding that the heart rate and blood pressure of my dependent will be measured prior to and at the completion of the appraisal;

- my consent for my dependent to answer questions concerning his/her physical activity participation and lifestyle;

- my consent to the appraisal measures conducted by an appraiser who has been trained to administer the Canadian Physical Activity, Fitness, and Lifestyle Appraisal. I understand that the interpretation of results is limited to placing the scores of my dependent in the appropriate Health Benefit Zones and providing information on physical activity participation and other healthy lifestyle topics.

- my understanding that there are potential risks; i.e., episodes of transient lightheadness, fainting, abnormal blood pressure, chest discomfort, leg cramps, and nausea, *and that I, on behalf of my dependent, assume wilfully those risks;*

- the obligation of my dependent to immediately inform the appraiser of any pain, discomfort, fatigue, or any other symptoms that he/she *may suffer* during and immediately after the appraisal;

- my understanding that my dependent may stop or delay any further testing if he/she so desires and that the appraisal may be terminated by the appraiser upon observation of any symptoms of undue distress or abnormal response;

- my understanding that I and my dependent may ask any questions or request further explanation or information about the procedures at any time before, during, and after the appraisal;

- that I have read, understood, and completed the Physical Activity Readiness Questionnaire (PAR-Q) and answered NO to all the questions regarding my dependent or received clearance from my physician for my dependent to participate.

_____

Name of Dependent

_____   _____

Signature of Parent/Guardian   Date

_____   _____

Witness   Date

NOTE: This form must be completed, signed and submitted to the appraiser, along with the completed PAR-Q, at the time of testing. The form must also be witnessed at the time of signing and the witness must be of the age of majority and independent of the organization administering the appraisal.

Source: From Ref. 84.

TABLE 4   American College of Sports Medicine Guidelines for Graded Exercise
Testing and Participation

Recommendation	Apparently healthy		Higher-risk[a]		
	Younger[b]	Older	No symptoms	Symptoms	Disease[c]
Medical exam and diagnostic exercise test recommended prior to:					
Moderate exercise[d]	No[f]	No	No	Yes	Yes
Vigorous exercise[e]	No	Yes[g]	Yes	Yes	Yes
Physician supervision recommended during exercise test:					
Submaximal testing	No	No	No	Yes	Yes
Maximal testing	No	Yes	Yes	Yes	Yes

[a]Patients with two or more cardiac risk factors (Table 5) or symptoms (Table 6).
[b]Men <40 years and women <50 years of age.
[c]Patients with known cardiac, pulmonary, or metabolic disease.
[d]Exercise well within the patient's current capacity that can be performed comfortably for a prolonged period (e.g., 60 min); typically 40–60% of aerobic power, noncompetitive, and with slow progression.
[e]Exercise intense enough to present a substantial challenge to the patient, ordinarily producing fatigue within 20 min (typically >60% of aerobic power).
[f]"No" indicates that the test is not necessary, although this does not preclude its completion (e.g., for research purposes).
[g]"Yes" indicates that an item is recommended.
Source: From Ref. 2; reproduced with permission.

training and competition [for example, preparation for a marathon run or master's competition (41,42,60)], a careful evaluation of exercise performance is required. Particular features to note are (a) a poor overall peak performance, (b) the development of premature ventricular contractions (PVCs) and ST-segment depression (Fig. 2), (c) an excessive rise of blood pressure, (d) failure of blood pressure to show the anticipated rise, and (e) any unusual exercise-induced symptoms.

Poor Peak Performance.   A poor peak performance is always an indication for caution, since it implies that a given intensity of physical activity will impose a greater stress on the individual concerned, with a corresponding increase in the risks of an untoward event such as electrical failure of the heart and sudden death during exercise. Such patients usually show a poor left ventricular ejection

Table 5   Major Coronary Risk Factors (For Use with Table 4)

1. Diagnosed hypertension or systolic blood pressure >160 mmHg or diastolic blood pressure >90 mmHg on at least two separate occasions or on antihypertensive medication.
2. Serum cholesterol >6.2 mmol/L (>240 mg/dL)
3. Cigarette smoking
4. Diabetes mellitus[a]
5. Family history of coronary or other atherosclerotic disease in parents or siblings before age 55 years.

[a]Patients with insulin-dependent diabetes mellitus (IDDM) who are over 30 years of age or have had IDDM for more than 15 years and persons with non-insulin-dependent diabetes mellitus who are over 35 years of age should be classified as patients with disease and treated as such (Table 4).
Source: From Ref. 2; reproduced with permission.

Table 6   Major Symptoms or Signs Suggestive of Cardiopulmonary or Metabolic Disease (For Use in Context of Table 4)

1. Pain or discomfort in the chest or surrounding area that appears to be ischemic in nature
2. Unaccustomed shortness of breath or shortness of breath with mild exertion
3. Dizziness or syncope
4. Orthopnea and paroxysmal nocturnal dyspnea
5. Ankle edema
6. Palpitations or tachycardia
7. Claudication
8. Known heart murmur

Source: Based on recommendations of the American College of Sports Medicine (2).

fraction, due to such possible causes as exercise-induced myocardial ischemia, incompetent or stenotic valves, a previously undetected infarction, and/or a cardiomyopathy. Underlying pathologies can commonly be elucidated by further investigations, including echocardiography, scintigraphy, and angiography (26, 28,31,51,73).

Premature Ventricular Contractions.   Occasional premature ventricular contractions (PVCs) are observed in a person who has maintained a high level of cardiorespiratory training, with a corresponding augmentation of vagal tone and a slow resting heart rate. Indeed, as many as 44% of apparently healthy men show an occasional PVC during maximal testing (93). In a healthy person, the PVCs tend to become less frequent or disappear as the heart rate increases. In contrast, PVCs of ischemic etiology become more frequent as the intensity of

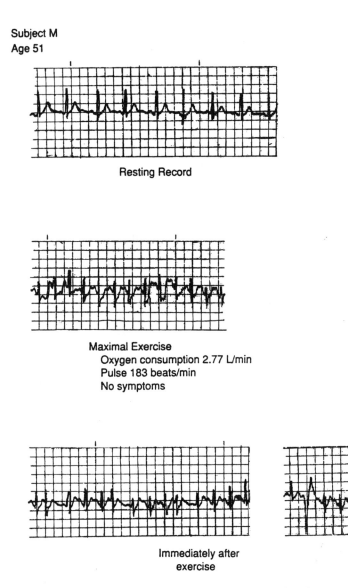

Subject M
Age 51

Resting Record

Maximal Exercise
    Oxygen consumption 2.77 L/min
    Pulse 183 beats/min
    No symptoms

Immediately after
exercise

FIGURE 2   Example of an electrocardiogram (CM5 lead) signaling an adverse prognosis. The individual in question died a few weeks later while running up a flight of stairs to attend to an emergency (a burst water pipe).

physical activity is increased (14,49,97). Adverse features of the ECG record are multiple PVCs (>3 in 10 s), associated symptoms (prolonged palpitations, dizziness, or loss of consciousness), runs or polyfocal PVCs, and the occurrence of PVCs early in the repolarization cycle [R-on-T phenomenon (73)].

ST-Segment Depression.   Many older adults show slight ST-segment depression during vigorous physical activity. True ischemic changes are horizontal or downsloping in type, rather than the more commonly encountered J-point depression with subsequent upward slope. A 1-mm (0.1-mV) horizontal depression of the ST segment during near maximal exercise is associated statistically with an increased risk of myocardial infarction (10,37), and it is commonly regarded as dangerous to allow an exercise test to continue if a 2-mm ST-segment depression is observed.

The difficulty in advising the individual patient is that although an abnormal exercise ECG implies a two- to threefold increase in the risk of a heart attack over the next quinquennium (40), this risk may not apply in every case since— if the person under evaluation is drawn from a middle-aged, symptom-free population—there is a two in three chance that an apparently positive test is a false-positive result (67) (Tables 7 and 8). Cynics have suggested that relative to the stress ECG, the toss of a coin is a more effective way of distinguishing vulnerable patients! Nevertheless, this may not be an entirely fair criticism, since in the same population a negative result is correct 99% of the time. Moreover, many of the false-positive results can be clarified at some cost to the patient (anxiety, medical expense, and a finite risk from angiography) by such techniques as two-dimensional echocardiography during exercise or dobutamine administration (26,63, 90), intravenous injection of thallium-201 with computed tomographic scanning (26,64), technetium-99 scintigraphy (26,65), and angiography (26).

Each new test result adds some independent information, increasing the likelihood of a correct diagnosis. Nevertheless, it remains controversial whether extensive investigation is cost-effective in the symptom-free middle-aged adult.

TABLE 7   False-Positive Results from Exercise Testing[a]

Test result	Ischemia		Test errors, % of category
	Absent	Present	
Positive	95 cases	40 cases	70.4
Negative	855 cases	10 cases	1.2

[a]This table illustrates the high incidence of false-positive test results obtained by the routine application of exercise electrocardiography to a symptom-free middle-aged population. The true incidence of "silent" myocardial ischemia is 50 cases per 1000.

TABLE 8   Common Causes of False-Positive and False-Negative Responses During Exercise ECG Testing

False positive
   Female gender
   Sudden exercise without warm-up
   Resting ST depression
   Hyperventilation
   Cigarette smoking
   Use of diuretics
   Potassium loss
   Glucose and carbohydrate loading
   Left ventricular hypertrophy
   Abnormal stress on left ventricle (hypertension, aortic stenosis or insufficiency,
      mitral valve prolapse, cardiomyopathy)
   Abnormal conduction path (e.g., left ventricular bundle-branch block, Wolff-
      Parkinson-White syndrome)
   Antidysrhythmic drugs (e.g., procainamide, quinidine)
   Other drugs (digitalis, antianxiety and antidepressant drugs)
   Anemia
   Hypoxia
False negative
   Insufficient exercise intensity
   Resting ST elevation
   Use of nitroglycerin and other coronary vasodilators
   Abnormalities of ventricular conduction

The advice offered to the patient (an improvement of overall lifestyle, a correction of modifiable cardiac risk factors, and a program of moderate physical activity, initiated progressively, with avoidance of prolonged isometric straining) is unlikely to be changed even if significant narrowing of the coronary vessels is confirmed. The best plan is simply to recommend an intensity of physical activity a little below the threshold where ECG abnormalities become marked.

In any event, an exercise-induced cardiac catastrophe is hard to avoid even with extensive testing. Neither regular training nor the absence of cardiac risk factors guarantees immunity, and one of the few fairly consistent warnings is provided by vague prodromal symptoms in the 24 h immediately preceding an attack (25,56,67).

There are nevertheless some situations where a more precise diagnosis is warranted. One indication is the development of symptoms suggestive of myocardial ischemia during exercise, and another is the patient's wish to return to vigorous competition. In such situations, it may be warranted to determine the extent of any vascular lesion and, if it is severe, to consider angioplasty or coronary artery bypass surgery.

Excessive Rise of Blood Pressure. Patients with a tendency to resting hypertension may show an even more abnormal pressure during exercise (Table 9); indeed, some authors have suggested that an excessive exercise-induced rise of blood pressure is a useful harbinger of future hypertension (38), although unfortunately some endurance competitors also show this characteristic.

The hypertension associated with physical activity has particular importance, since it can precipitate myocardial ischemia, cardiac failure, and (occasionally) vascular rupture. On the other hand, regular moderate physical activity is still appropriate for hypertensive subjects, since it reduces blood pressure both at rest and during exercise (19,66,95). Some investigators have argued that the long-term impact of training on blood pressure during exercise compares favorably with the response to hypotensive drugs (27). Moreover, exercise has fewer side effects and yields substantial additional benefits in other areas of health. The

TABLE 9   Rise of Blood Pressure with Aging

Systolic pressure (kPa)[a] in Relation to Age and Work Rate (METS = ratio of exercise to resting oxygen consumption).

Age, years	Rest	Exercise			
	1 MET	4 METs	6 METs	8 METs	10 METs
25	16.0	19.3	20.8	22.3	23.8
35	16.3	19.6	21.6	23.5	25.2
45	16.7	20.2	22.4	23.5	24.8
55	17.0	20.9	23.4	25.5	27.5

[a] 1 kPa = 7.5 torr.
Source: Based on data of S.M. Fox, personal communication.

Resting systolic and diastolic pressures (kPa) measured in home environment by Canada Fitness Survey (Fitness Canada, 1983)

Age	Men	Women	All subjects
20–29	16.0/10.7	14.5/9.9	15.3/10.3
30–39	16.7/10.4	15.6/9.7	16.1/10.1
40–49	17.1/10.9	15.7/10.3	16.4/10.6
50–59	17.6/10.9	17.2/10.7	17.4/10.8
60–69	18.9/11.5	17.7/10.9	18.3/11.2
70–79	19.1/10.9	18.0/10.8	18.5/10.9

optimum recommendation for the hypertensive patient is to continue moderate exercise to a pressure that is well tolerated by the heart.

Muscle-strengthening exercises may help in controlling hypertension, since the rise of blood pressure during exercise reflects difficulty in perfusing muscles that are contracting at an excessive fraction of their maximal voluntary force (46).

Failure of Blood Pressure to Rise.   Failure of the blood pressure to show the rise anticipated with an increase of work rate (Table 9) is an ominous sign of a failing circulation (36). It may reflect aortic valvular or vascular stenosis or simply failure of a weakened and ischemic myocardium to respond to the challenge of an increased afterload during vigorous exercise. Again, the prescribed intensity of effort should be held below a level where this sign appears.

Exercise-Induced Symptoms.   Significant symptoms are not common during routine stress testing. PVCs may be detected as "thumps," in the chest. Sometimes, on close questioning, a patient with an apparently silent myocardial ischemia may also admit to a little tightness in the chest, a sense of constriction in the throat, or a tingling sensation along the inner aspect of the left arm. If the patient learns to recognize and admit such symptoms, this may be helpful both in the monitoring of exercise sessions and in self-pacing of physical activity.

Evaluation of Symptoms

Sometimes it may be unclear whether a symptom is of cardiac origin or whether it originates in the musculoskeletal system. It is then useful to exercise the patient in the laboratory until the symptom is elicited. If there is pain in the chest or in the left arm but the ECG remains normal, it is unlikely that the symptom has a basis in myocardial ischemia.

Work Assessment

Work assessment is increasingly required as a condition of employee recruitment, promotion, and retention in jobs with a heavy physical demand. Although laboratory tests can form part of a work assessment, it is more common to use occupationally relevant field tasks—for example, in the case of police officers, scaling a 3-m fence, dragging a simulated casualty across a freeway, and handcuffing a strongly resisting dummy. Courts have a more ready understanding of such tests than of such alternatives as a direct treadmill measurement of maximal oxygen intake.

Effectiveness of Drugs and Rehabilitation

When drugs are administered to modify heart rate or blood pressure, it is very helpful to examine their effectiveness during exercise. For example, some hypotensive medications offer quite good control of resting blood pressures but are relatively ineffective during exercise (27).

Responses to rehabilitation and return to work are heavily influenced by psychosocial factors; it is therefore useful to obtain objective assessments of working capacity in the clinical laboratory.

Body Composition

"Ideal" Body Weight

Actuarial tables of "ideal weight" become harder to interpret in the case of older adults [Fig. 3 (76)]. The "ideal" figure, as assessed when an individual purchases life insurance in early adulthood, may not be relevant in middle age and later life. Mortality is lowest in those whose body mass has increased no more than 10% over the working span (4,6,18,29,45,62,89). The advantage persists after effects attributable to current smoking habits (4) and preexisting disease are eliminated, although it is less certain that data have been adjusted adequately for the effects of former smoking and clinically "silent" disease. Postmenopausal

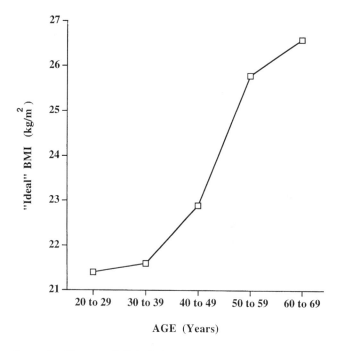

FIGURE 3   Changes of "ideal" body mass with age. (Based on data from Ref. 4.)

women synthesize significant amounts of estrogen in body fat, and possibly there are health disadvantages in maintaining the body mass of a young adult through a combination of a sedentary lifestyle and rigid dieting, which causes a loss of lean tissue.

Fat Distribution

As adults grow older, there is not only an increase in total body fat content (Table 10) but also an alteration in fat distribution. A "central," masculine pattern of accumulation over the abdomen is associated with an increased risk of ischemic heart disease (7,8,12). The proportion of deep to superficial fat also rises with age (5,16).

Assessment of Body Composition

Because of changes in the distribution of body fat, skinfold equations developed on young adults no longer predict either body density or body fat content accurately in older people. The loss of bone calcium also leads to a substantial decrease in the density of lean tissue, so that the standard assumption of hydrometry (a fat density of 0.9 g/ml and a lean tissue density of 1.1 g/ml) overestimates body fat content (22,23,52,74,83).

Body composition assessments based on the lean tissue compartment (body impedance, total body water, and total body potassium measurements, for example) can also be complicated by age-related changes in the water and potassium content of the tissues and the screening effect from superficial fat. Age-specific equations should thus be used to predict body composition (22,52,74,83).

TABLE 10   Changes in Excess Body Mass and Average Skinfold Thicknesses with Aging[a]

Age, years	Men		Women	
	Excess body mass, kg[b]	Skinfold, mm[c]	Excess body mass, kg[b]	Skinfold, mm[c]
20–29	1.7 ± 8.7	11.3 ± 5.3	8.3 ± 5.3	16.2 ± 3.8
30–39	6.4 ± 8.5	16.1 ± 10.6	1.4 ± 5.3	13.5 ± 5.2
40–49	9.3 ± 9.5	14.0 ± 5.8	6.8 ± 8.4	17.3 ± 5.4
50–59	8.8 ± 7.7	15.2 ± 6.7	4.9 ± 7.2	18.2 ± 5.1
60–69	5.1 ± 7.3	15.4 ± 2.7	4.5 ± 9.5	22.5 ± 7.9

[a]Mean ± SD of data for average Canadians living in metropolitan Toronto.
[b]Relative to actuarial "ideal" value for a person of equivalent height and average body build.
[c]Based upon the average of eight skinfold readings.

Methods of measuring bone density (dual photon absorptiometry, computed tomography, and whole-body calcium counts following neutron activation) are becoming more readily available (32,74,83,88) and should be considered in older adults who give a history of fractures with insignificant amounts of trauma.

Muscle Strength and Flexibility

Assessments of muscle strength in the older adult are hampered by a lack of representative normative data. The peak isometric force is affected substantially by small alterations in joint angle and harnessing, and isokinetic measurements are influenced by the allowances that are made for damping and gravitational forces. All scores also depend strongly on motivation and thus the persuasive powers of the observer.

Much of the available information relates to early measurements of hand-grip force (20) (Fig. 4), but even results for this simple test depend heavily upon the design of the dynamometer, the motivation of the subject, and opportunity for test practice. There is only a limited correlation between peak hand-grip force and the maximal strength of muscles about the knee joint or in the back. For example, a tennis player is likely to have preserved hand-grip force as he or she becomes older.

Studies of master's athletes who have maintained regular training into old age show little decrease of either strength or lean tissue mass through to the age of 65 years (42), but there is an accelerating loss of lean tissue during the retirement years, even in those who claim to be maintaining their volume and intensity of training.

The problem of a lack of generality also affects determinations of joint flexibility (82). The largest volume of normative data is for scores on the "sit and reach" test; values for this decrease substantially over the span of adult life.

PRESCRIBING PHYSICAL ACTIVITY

General Considerations

The objectives in recommending physical activity to an older adult are to suggest a safe ceiling intensity of effort, to motivate the individual to participate in various appropriate types of physical activity on a regular basis, and to sustain or restore the function that has been lost since early adulthood. A moderate increase in physical activity is beneficial to health, even if it is unsupervised, and care should be taken not to overmedicalize what should be perceived as normal behavior. Detailed advice and examination are required mainly by those who are proposing a return to rigorous competition (see Table 4).

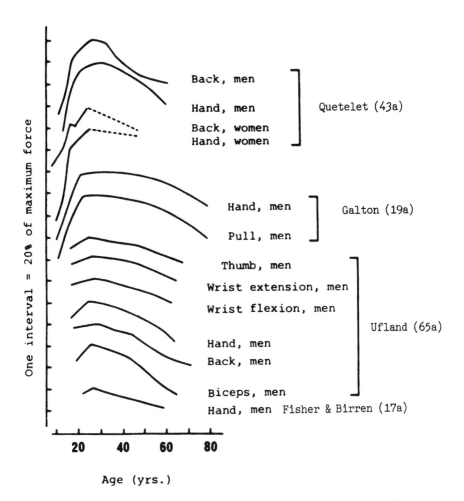

FIGURE 4   Age-related changes in maximal isometric force in selected muscle groups. (Based in part on data from Ref. 20.)

Safety

Moderate physical activity is a very safe undertaking for the older adult (98). Even in those who have already sustained a myocardial infarction, the average risk of a cardiac incident is only about 1 in 300,000 person-hours for an unsupervised program and 1 in 100,000 person-hours for a supervised program (33,81). Nevertheless, the immediate risk of a cardiac incident is 5 to 50 times higher during a bout of physical activity than when the same person is sedentary (39,

47,67,86,87,94,98). Moreover, although the absolute risk of physical activity is lower for middle age than for the retirement years, the relative risk is somewhat greater for the younger age groups (Table 11). One possible explanation of this paradox is that middle-aged men who have been sedentary for a number of years are sometimes reluctant to admit their poor physical condition and, when challenged, are tempted to embark on very demanding bouts of physical activity for which they are not prepared. In contrast, most elderly people adopt a very cautious approach to exercise.

The physician may encounter particular difficulty in regulating the activity patterns of a busy and overly competitive executive. Sometimes, such an individual will try to beat a superior opponent at squash or tennis even when he or she has become extremely fatigued; or one employee may seek to progress faster than a rival when both are enrolled in a sequential training plan. A hectic schedule may also encourage such individuals to exercise without an adequate warm-up [a common cause of cardiac problems (7)], and they may decide that if a 30-min session of exercise has been recommended, an even greater health benefit can be obtained from a continuous 2-h bout. Such people must be warned firmly against exceeding their exercise prescription.

Older individuals may have encountered previous problems with their backs or knees, and it is important to inquire about previous disabilities before recommending an activity program. City jogging and violent aerobic dance classes are particularly likely to exacerbate musculoskeletal problems. Repeated pounding on a hard surface such as a concrete sidewalk or a tiled concrete floor in a dance studio can also give rise to stress fractures, particularly of the metatarsal bones. A weakening of tendons and muscles combined with a slowing of reflexes can lead to a high incidence of musculotendinous tears and strains, particularly if an overly long weekly training distance is attempted (42,61).

TABLE 11   Relative Risks of Sudden Death During Nonstrenuous and Strenuous Exercises in Relation to Age

Age, years	Nonstrenuous exercise[a]		Strenuous exercise[a]	
	M	R	M	R
20–39	26.0	2.5	6.1	10.0
40–49	5.2	3.6	1.2	13.1
50–69	3.4	2.5	1.2	5.3

[a]Number of exercise sessions ($\times 10^6$) for a single death (M) and risk of sudden cardiovascular death in exercise relative to sedentary state (R).
Sources: Based on data from Refs. 98 and 99.

The tolerance of hot and cold conditions also decreases with age (Chapter 5). Thus, the middle-aged adult must be more cautious than a younger person if the climate is unfavorable for a particular type of competition or vigorous physical activity.

Recruitment and Compliance

Recruitment and motivation to continued compliance are major problems with most exercise programs for middle-aged adults. For instance, if a corporate fitness program is introduced at the worksite, only about one-third of eligible employees are likely to be recruited initially, and many of these are people who were previously active elsewhere (44). Moreover, some 50% of initial recruits are lost to the exercise program after 6 months, and a steady attrition continues thereafter, so that despite an influx of new employees, our 10-year experience has been that only 13% of employees remain significantly involved with the program (72). Moreover, many of these people are infrequent rather than frequent participants.

Minimizing Barriers to Exercise

The reason usually cited for dropping out of an exercise program (Table 12) is "lack of time" (21,75,91). At first inspection, this seems a feeble excuse. Most older adults have 3–4 h of free time per day, much of which is spent in watching television. However, there is a substantial "opportunity cost" if a large segment of the available time is spent not in the exercise itself but rather in travel to and from the exercise facility (Chapter 22) (69,70). Participants decide that the opportunity foregone is too great relative to the immediate benefits they may derive from the exercise session (Table 13).

The simplest way to change this unfavorable assessment is to lower the opportunity cost—particularly the unproductive travel component. Thus if the exercise facility is near the home or at the place of employment, the yield of physical activity per hour of time invested is much greater than for a distant (if well-appointed) fitness club. A similar advantage is gained if the activity is built into the normal day (the "active living" approach, Chapter 22).

Other barriers to participation can be very simple, such as the need to leave the worksite with other members of a car pool. Such difficulties can often be surmounted by developing flexible hours of work or of program operation. The cost of facility membership is rarely a significant barrier in the middle aged, but lack of child care and a need for expensive equipment, clothing, and footwear can discourage the participation of single parents.

Optimizing Rewards

A second approach to improved compliance is to augment the dividends from exercising. The physiological and biochemical rewards of enhanced function bear

TABLE 12   Obstacles to Exercise and Factors that Would Encourage Participation in Adults Aged 20–69 Years

Obstacles	Current participants, % of category	Nonparticipants, % of category
Obstacles to exercise		
Work pressures	56	39
Laziness	30	26
Lack of facilities	21	13
Lack of time	22	9
Cost	16	10
Injury or illness	17	39
Factors that would encourage personal participation		
More time	40	
Better facilities	27	
Partner	22	
Family interest	18	
Friend's interest	17	
Cheaper facilities	16	
Fitness classes	11	
Fitness test	9	
Organized sports	9	
Activities sponsored by union or employer	7	
Information on benefits	6	
Nothing	20	

Source: Based on data from Ref. 21.

a relatively fixed relationship to the energy expended, but external rewards (Table 14) can be increased by an upgrading of the fitness facility (a more pleasant decor, attractive incidental music, a better control of temperature and humidity, improved shower and locker facilities, greater opportunities for socializing), provision of positive feedback from the instructor (reporting of favorable test scores, presentation of award pins, T-shirts, and other symbols of achievement), and maximizing gains of mood state by optimizing the type, intensity, duration, and frequency of class sessions.

It is also helpful to reduce negative feedback. A person who is in poor physical condition and who has become obese may be embarrassed to exercise with those of the opposite sex, and the unrealistic demands of a fit instructor can also be discouraging. It is useful to arrange unisex classes for such individuals. At the other end of the spectrum, a person who has maintained an excellent level of physical condition may be disillusioned if an age-stratified exercise class offers

TABLE 13 Scores on an Intention-to-Exercise Scale in
Relation to Specific Beliefs About Exercise

Belief about exercise	Intention to exercise	
	Low	High
Control body mass	0.06	1.29[a]
Look younger	0.06	1.29[a]
Fill recreational time	−0.25	0.99[a]
Be healthy	1.94	2.50[b]
Be more energetic	1.38	2.07[b]
Improve appearance	0.63	1.56[b]
Live longer	1.25	1.10
Relieve tension	1.63	1.66
Be tired	1.69	0.90
Feel good	1.81	2.14
Meet people	0.44	0.91
Consume time	1.25	1.17
Improve thinking	0.69	1.11
Be physically fit	1.44	1.90

Note: All beliefs were scored on an arbitrary seven-point scale (-3
to $+3$).
[a]$p < 0.01$.
[b]$p < 0.05$.
Source: From Ref. 30.

TABLE 14 Possible Rewards That Can Provide Positive Feedback in an Exercise
Program

Rewards	
Symbolic	Badges; pins; T-shirts, awards, club membership
Material	Money, prizes, release time, assistance with dues
Psychological	Encouragement from instructor, recognition of achievements by group or family, attention, friendship
Punishment	
Symbolic	Exclusion from group
Material	Pain, injury, costs of tuition and clothing, loss of time, physical effort and fatigue
Psychological	Discouragement or ridicule (from instructor, group, or family), failure to achieve goals, family complaints about absence, psychological fatigue due to program

Source: Based on an analysis by R. Danielson and K. Danielson, in *Employee Fitness: the How To*
(L. Wanzel, ed.). Ministry of Tourism and Recreation, Toronto (1979).

so little physical challenge that it fails to improve physical fitness or to stimulate the desired release of endorphins.

Effectiveness

Considerations governing an appropriate and effective pattern of physical activity in the older person are much the same as those for a younger adult (Chapter 1), although in terms of avoiding musculoskeletal and cardiac problems, it is desirable to reduce the intensity of effort (commencing, for example, at 60% rather than 70 or 80% of maximal oxygen intake). The duration of training sessions can be extended to compensate for their lower intensity (2,96). Quite low intensities of exercise offer a satisfactory way of restoring cardiorespiratory condition provided that sessions are repeated regularly (17,85) (see Chapter 5, Fig. 3).

Muscle-strengthening exercises remain important in middle age, but it is important to avoid straining against a closed glottis, particularly if the muscles are initially weak.

In terms of controlling obesity, improving lipid profile, and extending calendar life span, an effective regimen calls for a substantial weekly energy expenditure (Fig. 5), but this can usually be achieved by such activities as rapid walking and vigorous stair climbing (54,55,58,59). Benefit commences with an added leisure energy expenditure of about 2.2 MJ/week (500 kcal/week); an optimal response is seen with an expenditure of 8.8 MJ/week (2000 kcal/week), the latter being equivalent to an hour or more of brisk walking on most days of the week.

Optimal Types of Physical Activity

Cardiorespiratory Conditioning

Any large-muscle activity (fast walking or jogging, cycling, vigorous swimming, rowing, canoeing, or cross-country skiing) is an effective means of developing cardiorespiratory condition. Such pursuits can be combined with daily commuting needs (the "active living" approach, Chapter 22), or they can be undertaken in beautiful areas of the countryside (increasing personal rewards and possibly relaxation). Unfortunately, some of the most effective types of endurance activity lack a social component (which is an important motivator for some people), and they do little to develop muscle strength.

Classes in gymnastics and aerobics or social dance maximize social rewards, but the intensity of activity may be too light to augment cardiorespiratory condition unless movements are performed at a fast tempo. The speed of movement can be increased by an appropriate choice of music, but there is a danger that fast twisting movements may provoke joint injuries.

Tennis and squash are very popular with middle-aged executives. Such

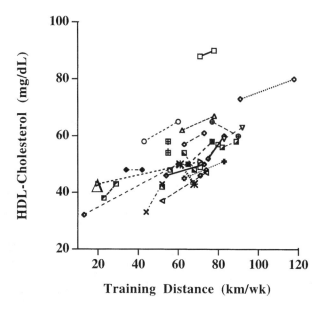

FIGURE 5   Influence of weekly jogging distance on plasma HDL concentration. Each line represents a pair of observations on individual patients who prepared themselves for marathon participation by an increase in their weekly jogging distance. The large triangle represents the average values for the less active members of this patient group. [Redrawn from Kavanagh, T., Shephard, R. J., Lindley, L. J., and Pieper, M., *Arteriosclerosis,* 3: 249–259 (1983); used with permission.]

games provide a substantial cardiorespiratory stimulus if they are played against a vigorous opponent, and their competitive nature can be an important motivator. However, competition leads to a substantial secretion of catecholamines for a given intensity of effort (9) (Fig. 6), with a corresponding increase in the risk of premature ventricular contractions (57) and fatal cardiac arrhythmias.

Team sports offer substantial camaraderie and appeal particularly to hourly workers. But as age advances, it becomes increasingly difficult to assemble a full team of players at an appropriately matched level of fitness and skill. Moreover, competition and excitement increase the catecholamine output for a given intensity of exercise, and the body contact inherent in many team sports becomes increasingly hazardous for weakened bones.

Building Muscle Strength

The most effective approach to muscle building is a circuit training program (for instance, lifting weights about each of the major joints in turn). At each station

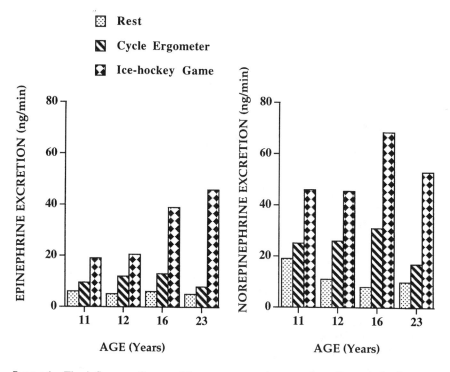

FIGURE 6   The influence of competitive sport upon the excretion of catecholamines at different ages. Urinary output of epinephrine and norepinephrine compared between rest, the period following a game of ice hockey, and following an equivalent intensity of cycle-ergometer exercise. (Redrawn from Ref. 9; used with permission).

on the circuit, a series of perhaps three sets of 10 repetitions is performed at 50–60% of the single-repetition maximum force for the movement in question. Some people find motivation from an improvement in performance at each of the various stations, but unfortunately such gains tend to plateau as training continues (35).

Other recreational activities that require the lifting of heavy weights can also develop muscle mass. In recommending such activities, it is important to emphasize the avoidance of straining and the resulting hypertension. Nevertheless, it is interesting that 3 of 14 participants in the Canada/USSR Polar Ski Trek carried a 40-kg back pack some 2000 km across the arctic ice cap in difficult winter and early spring conditions despite substantial resting and exercise-induced hypertension (79).

Some people seek to combine muscle building with aerobic exercise by carrying light weights while walking or jogging. Commonly purchased barbells add little to the energy cost of movement (50) and seem to represent an unnecessary expense. Simpler options are to swing the arms vigorously while walking with a briefcase or a bag of groceries or to mow the lawn briskly with a hand lawnmower.

Increasing Flexibility

Flexibility is developed and maintained by taking all of the major joints gently through their full ranges of motion on a regular basis. In this regard, rowing and swimming are more effective than other types of activity.

Preventing Osteoporosis

Any weight-bearing activity is effective in strengthening the bone at the prime sites of osteoporotic fracture (the hip and the neck of the femur). Some authors have suggested that the practice of vigorous swimming is associated with well-conserved bone density. This is a little surprising, since normal gravitational forces are countered by buoyancy while a person is in the water. If indeed there is such an association, it may reflect the pull of the active muscles on the bone, or it may simply be that patients who choose to swim also engage in other forms of physical activity that involve weight bearing.

Enhancing Mood State

If mood elevation is a major goal of a physical activity program, cerebral arousal can be increased through vigorous movement, but prolonged exercise is normally required in order to increase the secretion of endorphins.

If the patient's problems seem related to an overly hectic schedule, relaxation may be achieved most effectively by rhythmic, noncompetitive activity, performed alone or with a close friend, in a quiet, relaxing setting (78).

Spontaneous Choice

The spontaneous choice of the older adult concentrates increasingly upon walking and gardening as the preferred forms of physical activity (53,96) (see Fig. 7).

Slow walking (2–3 km/h) is unlikely to contribute more to health than a pleasant form of relaxation. However, if the patient is encouraged to walk rapidly (up to 7–8 km/h), the activity can become quite demanding—indeed, for most people, the energy demand is similar to running at an equivalent speed. Fast walking brings many older adults close to their maximal oxygen intake (68,77), particularly if they are climbing a moderate rise.

Walking has the advantage that the forces imposed on the knee and spine are only about one-third as great as in jogging. Moreover, since one foot is always

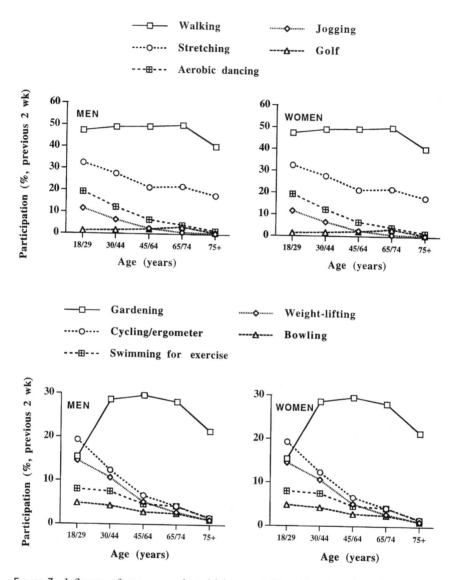

FIGURE 7 Influence of age upon selected leisure activities. (Based on data obtained by the U.S. National Health Interview Survey of 1991.)

in contact with the ground, there is less danger of slipping and falling. Walking can be performed as a social activity (with family or friends), and if the route is appropriately chosen, it can be combined with other motivating pursuits (for instance, the study of nature or urban architecture).

Gardening is an activity of very variable intensity. For some people, it amounts to no more than a stroll through the flower beds, sitting on a power mower, or holding the nozzle of a hose on a summer evening. However, planting and weeding give valuable exercise to the knees, hips, and back, and digging in heavy soil provides a substantial stimulus to both cardiovascular and muscular systems. The intensity of effort when digging depends on the texture and wetness of the soil, the size of the shovel, and the pace of shoveling. Demand can be reduced to meet the effects of aging by use of a smaller shovel at a slower pace and by taking longer rest pauses. In countries such as Canada and the United States, it is important to recognize that gardening is a seasonal activity. A few days should be allowed each spring so that muscles and joints can readapt to tasks that were readily accomplished at the end of the previous season.

As with snow shoveling, there is some danger that heavy digging may provoke a heart attack. There is also some risk from the pruning of larger trees by handsaw, since heavy muscular exercise must then be performed with the arms lifted above the head. Caution is necessary when using ladders, particularly if reflexes and/or the sense of balance have deteriorated. In addition to its physiological benefits, gardening can offer quiet, relaxation, and a sense that something of permanence is being created—an appreciable reward, particularly for an older person.

Although alternative modes of exercise can be considered, both walking and gardening have considerable potential as methods of meeting the activity needs of the older adult. It may thus be appropriate for governments—and others interested in the promotion of fitness—to recognize this trend and to encourage it. Policy options would include a diversion of funds from the construction of hockey arenas to the building of hiking trails as well as the development of garden plots that would enable older people could get both good exercise and sound nutrition by growing their own vegetables.

ACKNOWLEDGMENT

Dr. Shephard's studies are supported in part by a research grant from Canadian Tire Acceptance Ltd.

REFERENCES

1. American College of Sports Medicine, *Guidelines for Graded Exercise Testing and Prescription,* 1st ed. Lea & Febiger, Philadelphia (1975).

2. American College of Sports Medicine, *Guidelines for Graded Exercise Testing and Prescription,* 5th ed. Lea & Febiger, Philadelphia (1995).
3. Andersen, K.L., Shephard, R.J., Denolin, H., Varnauskas, E., and Masironi, R., *Fundamentals of Exercise Testing.* World Health Organization, Geneva (1971).
4. Andres, R., in *Exercise, Fitness and Health* (C. Bouchard, R.J. Shephard, T. Stephens, J. Sutton, and B. McPherson, eds.) Human Kinetics, Champaign, Illinois, pp. 133–136 (1990).
5. Ashwell, M., Cole, T.J., and Dixon, A.K., *Br. Med. J.,* 290: 1691–1694 (1985).
6. Avons, P. Ducimitière, P., and Rakatovao, R., *Lancet* 1: 1104 (letter) (1983).
7. Bjorntorp, P., *Exerc. Sports Sci. Rev.,* 11: 159–180 (1983).
8. Blair, S.N., Ludwig, D.A., and Goodyear, N.N., *Hum. Biol.,* 60: 111–122 (1988).
9. Blimkie, C.J., Cunningham, D.A., and Leung, F.Y., in *Frontiers of Activity and Child Health* (H. Lavallée and R.J. Shephard, eds.). Editions du Pélican, Québec City (1977).
10. Bonow, R.O., Kent, K.M., Rosing, D.R., Lau, K.K., Lakatos, E., Borer, J.S., Bacharach, S.L., Green, M.V., and Epstein, S.E., *N. Engl. J. Med.,* 311: 1339–1345 (1984).
11. Bosco, C., and Komi, P.V., *Eur. J. Appl. Physiol.* 43: 209–219 (1980).
12. Bouchard, C., in *Metabolic Complications of Human Obesities* (J. Vague et al., eds.). Elsevier, Amsterdam, pp. 87–96 (1985).
13. Buskirk, E.R., in *Exercise, Fitness and Health* (C. Bouchard, R.J. Shephard, T. Stephens, J. Sutton, and B. McPherson, eds.). Human Kinetics, Champaign, Illinois, pp. 687–697 (1990).
14. Chiang, B.N., Montoye, H.J., and Cunningham, D.A., *Am. J. Epidemiol.,* 91: 368–377 (1970).
15. Cooper, K.H., *J.A.M.A.,* 211: 1663–1667 (1970).
16. Durnin, J.V.G.A., and Womersley, J.A., *Br. J. Nutr.,* 32: 77–97 (1974).
17. Durnin, J.V.G.A., Brockway, J.M., Whitcher, H.N., *J. Appl. Physiol.,* 15: 161–165 (1960).
18. Dyer, A.R., Stamler, J., Berkson, D.M., and Lindberg, H.A., *J. Chronic Dis.,* 28: 109–123 (1975).
19. Fagard, R.H., and Tipton, C.M., in *Physical Activity, Fitness and Health* (C. Bouchard, R.J. Shephard, and T. Stephens, eds.), Human Kinetics, Champaign, Illinois, pp. 633–655 (1994).
20. Fisher, M.B., and Birren, J.E., *J. Appl. Psychol.,* 31: 490–497 (1949).
21. Fitness Canada, *Fitness and Lifestyle in Canada.* Fitness Canada, Ottawa (1983).
22. Forbes, G.B., *Human Body Composition: Growth, Aging, Nutrition and Activity.* Springer-Verlag, New York (1987).
23. Forsyth, R., Plyley, M.J., and Shephard, R.J., *Can. J. Appl. Sport Sci.,* 9: 5P (1984).
24. Fox, S., and Haskell, W.L., *South Carolina Med. J.,* Suppl. 1 (1996).
25. Franklin, B., and Kahn, J.K., *Sport Sci. Rev.,* 4: 85–105 (1995).
26. Franklin, B.A., Fink-Bennett, D., Savas, V., Pavlides, G., and Safian, R.D., in *Resource Manual for Guidelines for Exercise Testing and Prescription,* 2nd ed. (Durstine, L.J., King, A.C., Painter, P.L., Roitman, J.L., Zwiren, L.D., and Kenney, W.L. eds.). Lea & Febiger, Philadelphia, pp. 285–308 (1993).
27. Franz, I.W., *Can. J. Sport Sci.,* 16: 296–301, (1991).

28. Gardin, J.M., Henry, W.L., Savage, D.D., and Epstein, S.E. *Am. J. Cardiol.* 39: 277 (1977).
29. Garn, S.M., Hawthorne, V.M., Pilkington, J.J., and Pesick S.D., *Am. J. Clin. Nutr.* 38: 313–319 (1983).
30. Godin, G., and Shephard, R.J., in *International Perspectives on Adapted Physical Activity* (M. Berridge and G. Ward, eds.). Human Kinetics, Champaign, Illinois, pp. 243–249 (1986).
31. Goodman, J., *Sport Sci. Rev.,* 4: 14–30 (1995).
32. Harrison, J.E., McNeill, K.G., Hitchman, A.J., and Britt, B.A., *Invest. Radiol.,* 14: 27–34 (1979).
33. Haskell, W.L., *Circulation,* 57: 920–924 (1978).
34. Health Canada, *Canadian Standardized Test of Fitness, Operations Manual,* 4th ed. Health Canada, Ottawa (1997).
35. Hettinger, T., *Physiology of Strength.* Charles C Thomas, Springfield, Illinois (1961).
36. Ivanova, L.A., Mazur, N.A., Smirnova, T.M., Sumarokov, A.B., Svet, E.A., Nazarenko, V.A., and Kotlyarov, V.V., in *Sudden Cardiac Death* (B.A. Lown and A.M. Vihkert, eds.). NIH Publ. 81-2101. National Heart and Lung Institute, Washington, D.C. pp. 23–38 (1980).
37. Jennings, K., Reid, D.S., Hawkins, T., and Julian, D.J., *Br. Med. J.,* 288: 185–187 (1984).
38. Jetté, M., Landry, F., Sidney, K.H., and Blumchen, G., *J. Cardiopulm. Rehabil.,* 8: 171–177 (1988).
39. Kabisch, D., and Funk, S., *Dtsche. Z. Sportmed.,* 42: 464–470 (1991).
40. Kannel, W.B., and Brand, F.N., in *Principles of Geriatric Medicine* (R. Andres, E.L. Bierman, and W.R. Hazzard, eds.). McGraw-Hill, New York, pp. 104–119 (1985).
41. Kavanagh, T., and Shephard, R.J., *Ann. N.Y. Acad. Sci.,* 301: 656–670 (1977).
42. Kavanagh, T., Lindley, L.J., Shephard, R.J. and Campbell, R., *Ann. Sports Med.* 4: 55–64 (1988).
43. Kavanagh, T., Mertens, D.J., Matosevic, V., Shephard, R.J., and Evans, B., *Clin. Sports Med.,* 1: 72–88 (1989).
44. Leatt, P., Hattin, H., West, C., and Shephard, R.J., *Can. J. Publ. Health,* 79: 19–25 (1988).
45. Lew, E.A., and Garfinkel, L., *J. Chronic Dis.,* 32: 563–576 (1979).
46. Lind, A.R., and McNicol, G.W., *Can. Med. Assoc. J.,* 96: 706–712 (1967).
47. Löllgen, H., and Dirschedl, P., *Dtsche. Z. Sportmed.,* 40: 212–221 (1989).
48. Londeree, B., and Moeschberger, M.L., *J. Card Rehabil.,* 4: 44–49 (1984).
49. Madsen, E.B., and Gilpin, E., *J. Cardiopulm. Rehabil.,* 3: 481–488 (1983).
50. Makalous, S.L., *Phys. Sportsmed.,* 16(4): 139–148 (1988).
51. Maron, B.J. (Chair: Sudden Death Committee and Congenital Cardiac Defects Committee, Am. Heart Assoc.), *Med. Sci. Sports Exerc.,* 28: 1445–1452 (1996).
52. Mernagh, J.R., Harrison, J., Krondl, A., McNeill, K.G., and Shephard, R.J., *Nutr. Res.,* 6: 499–507 (1986).
53. Montoye, H.J., *Physical Activity and Health: An Epidemiological Study of an Entire Community.* Prentice Hall, Englewood Cliffs, New Jersey (1975).
54. Morris, J.N., Everitt, M.G., Pollard, R., Chave, S.P.W., and Semmence, A.M., *Lancet* 2: 1207–1210 (1980).

55. Morris, J.N., Clayton, D.G., Everitt, M.G., Semmence, A.M., and Burgess, E.H., *Br. Heart J.,* 63: 325–334 (1990).

56. Noakes, T.D., Opie, L.H., and Rose, A.G., in *Symposium on Sports Medicine, Clinics in Sports Medicine* (B.A. Franklin and M. Rubenfire, eds.), Saunders, Philadelphia, pp. 527–543 (1984).

57. Northcote, R.J., Flannigan, C., and Ballantyne, D., *Br. Heart J.,* 55: 198–203 (1986).

58. Paffenbarger, R.S., Hyde, R.T., Wing, A.L. and Hsieh, C.C., *N. Engl. J. Med.,* 314: 605–613 (1986).

59. Paffenbarger, R.S., Hyde, R.T., Wing, A.L., Lee, I-M., and Kampert, J.B., in *Physical Activity, Fitness and Health* (C. Bouchard, R.J. Shephard, and T. Stephens, eds.). Human Kinetics, Champaign, Illinois, pp. 119–133 (1994).

60. Pollock, M.L., Foster, C., Knapp, D., Rod, J., and Schmidt, D., *J. Appl. Physiol.,* 62: 725–731 (1987).

61. Pollock, M.L., Graves, J., Leggett, S., Braith, R., and Hagberg, J., *Med. Sci. Sports Exerc.,* 21: S88 (1989).

62. Rhoades, G.G., and Kagan, A., *Lancet,* 1: 492–495 (1983).

63. Sawada, S.G., Segar, D.S., Ryan, T., Brown, S.E., Dohan, A.M., Williams, R., Fineberg, N.S., Armstrong, W.F., and Feigenbaum, H., *Circulation,* 83: 1605–1614 (1991).

64. Scanlan, J.G., Gustafson, D.E., Chevalier, P.A., Robb, R.A., and Ritman, E.L., *Am. J. Cardiol.,* 46: 1263–1268 (1980).

65. Schelbert, H.R., Phelps, M.E., Hoffman, E., Huang, S.C., and Kuhl, D.E., *Am. J. Cardiol.,* 46: 1269–1277 (1980).

66. Seals, D., Hagberg, J., Hurley, B., Ehsani, A., and Holloszy, J.O., *J. Appl. Physiol.,* 57: 1024–1029 (1984).

67. Shephard, R.J., *Ischemic Heart Disease and Exercise.* Croom Helm, London (1981).

68. Shephard., R.J., *Br. J. Sports Med.,* 16: 220–229 (1982)

69. Shephard, R.J., *Fitness and Health in Industry.* Karger, Basel (1986).

70. Shephard, R.J., *Economic Benefits of Enhanced Fitness.* Human Kinetics, Champaign, Illinois (1986).

71. Shephard, R.J., *Sports Med.,* 5: 185–195 (1988).

72. Shephard, R.J., in *Parke-Davis/AFB/TCOM Conference on the Economic Impact of Employee Health Promotion* (B. Kaman, ed.). Texas College of Osteopathic Medicine, Fort Worth, Texas (1990).

73. Shephard, R.J., in *Textbook of Clinical Sports Medicine* (C.B. Rians, ed.). Human Kinetics, Champaign, Illinois (1991).

74. Shephard, R.J., *Body Composition in Biological Anthropometry.* Cambridge University Press, London (1991).

75. Shephard, R.J., in *Advances in Exercise Adherence* (R. Dishman, ed.). Human Kinetics, Champaign, Illinois, pp. 343–360 (1995).

76. Shephard, R.J., *Physical Activity, Aging and Health.* Human Kinetics, Champaign, Illinois (1997).

77. Shephard, R.J., in *Consensus Conference on Physical Activity and Health* (A. Leon, ed.), Human Kinetics, Champaign, Illinois pp. 76–87 (1977).

78. Shephard, R.J. *Sports Med.* 23:211–217 (1997).

79. Shephard, R.J., and Rode, A., *Observations on the Soviet/Canadian Transpolar Ski Trek.* Karger, Basel (1992).
80. Shephard, R.J., Allen, C., Benade, A.J.S., Davies, C.T.M., diPrampero, P.E., Hedman, R., Merriman, J.E., Myhre, K., and Simmons, R., *Bull. W.H.O.,* 38: 757–764 (1968).
81. Shephard, R.J., Kavanagh, T., Tuck, J., and Kennedy, J., *J. Cardiopulm. Rehabil.,* 3: 321–329 (1983).
82. Shephard, R.J., Montelpare, W., and Berridge, M., *Res. Q.,* 61: 326–330 (1990).
83. Shephard, R.J., Kofsky, P.R., Harrison, J.E., McNeill, K.G., and Krondl, A., *Hum. Biol.,* 57: 671–686 (1985).
84. Shephard, R.J., Thomas, S., and Weller, I., *Sports Med.,* 11: 358–366 (1991).
85. Sidney, K.H., and Shephard, R.J., *Med. Sci. Sports,* 10: 125–131 (1978).
86. Siscovick, D.S., in *Exercise, Fitness and Health* (C. Bouchard, R.J. Shephard, T. Stephens, J. Sutton, and B. McPherson, eds.), Human Kinetics, Champaign, Illinois pp. 707–713 (1990).
87. Siscovick, D.S., Laporte, R.E., and Newman, J.M., *Public Health Rep.,* 100: 180–188 (1985).
88. Smith, E., Reddan, W., and Smith, P., *Med. Sci. Sports Exerc.,* 13: 60–64 (1981).
89. Society of Actuaries, *Build Study, 1979.* Society of Actuaries, Chicago (1980).
90. Stack, R., and Kislo, J., *Am. J. Cardiol.,* 46: 1117–1124 (1980).
91. Stephens, T., and Craig, C., *The Well-Being of Canadians.* Canadian Fitness and Lifestyle Research Institute, Ottawa (1990).
92. Tanaka, H., Bassett, D.R., and Turner, M.J., *Am. J. Hypertens.,* 9: 1099–1103 (1996).
93. Thompson, P.D., in *Resource Manual for Guidelines for Exercise Testing and Prescription,* 2nd ed. (Durstine, J.L., King, A.C., Painter, P.L., Roitman, J.L., Zwiren, L.D., and Kenney, W.L., eds.). Lea & Febiger, Philadelphia, pp. 359–363 (1993).
94. Thompson, P.D., and Fahrenbach, M., in *Physical Activity, Fitness and Health* (C. Bouchard, R.J. Shephard, and T. Stephens, eds.). Human Kinetics, Champaign, Illinois, pp. 1019–1028 (1994).
95. Tipton, C.M., *Exerc. Sport Sci. Rev.,* 12: 245–306 (1984).
96. U.S. Surgeon General, *Physical Activity and Health.* U.S. Department of Health and Human Services, Washington, D.C. (1996).
97. Vedin, J.A., Wilhelmsson, C.D., Wilhelmsen, L., Bjure, J., and Ekstrom-Jodal, B., *Am. J. Cardiol.,* 30: 25–30 (1972).
98. Vuori, I., *Sport Sci. Rev.,* 4: 46–84 (1995).
99. Vuori, I., Suurnakki, L., and Suurnakki, T., *Med. Sci. Sports Exerc.,* 14: 114–115 (1982).

5

Exercise in the Old and Very Old

ROY J. SHEPHARD
University of Toronto
Toronto, Ontario, Canada

INTRODUCTION

In this chapter, we look specifically at patterns of exercise and physical activity that are appropriate for the old and the very old (65–85 years of age and older). Firstly, we must consider the definition of old age and make an appropriate classification of the elderly. We then examine particular problems of exercise testing and prescription, the likely benefits from encouraging an increase of physical activity, and safety precautions appropriate to this age group.

DEFINITION OF THE ELDERLY

Onset of Old Age

Influenced by considerations of safety and convenient access to subjects, many research articles supposedly dealing with exercise for the elderly have focused upon people in the latter half of their working careers (subjects ranging in age from 40 to 65 years). Such individuals are essentially late-middle-aged rather than elderly. Problems of exercise prescription peculiar to this group have already been discussed in Chapter 4.

One convenient milestone indicating passage into old age is normal retirement from work. This commonly occurs at the age of 65 years in Canada and the United States but is allowed a few years earlier in some European countries (157). Those who are suffering from chronic illness or are otherwise unfit for work often retire several years earlier than those who have maintained their working capacity (154,157). In North America, "equal opportunity" and "human rights" commissions are seeking to abolish a mandatory retirement age unless this is a bona fide occupational criterion (151), but at the same time automation and technological change are making it difficult for older people to continue in the labor force, and those who have accumulated adequate savings are retiring at what would previously have been regarded as late middle age.

Gradations of Aging

Even if the age of onset of old age is agreed, the elderly cannot be regarded as a homogenous group. Most people show a very substantial and progressive deterioration of physical abilities between their retirement and death at an age of 80 to 90 years.

One method of reducing interindividual differences is to subdivide the elderly on the basis of their calendar ages. Three subcategories may be distinguished: the young old (65–75 years), the middle old (75–85 years), and the very old (over 85 years). Demographers are concerned because advances in medical treatment are leading to a rapid increase in numbers of the very old in most countries.

A simple calendar classification ignores the existence of very substantial differences of biological and functional age between individuals who share an identical calendar age (31,65). This has been an important legal issue, exploited by those arguing against mandatory retirement. There has been corresponding interest in developing both general scales of biological age (using a variety of anthropometric, physiological and psychological markers) and functional indices closely related to job performance. Unfortunately, it has been far from clear how to combine data from widely disparate disciplines, obtained using very different techniques and differing scales of measurement. Too often, calculations of biological age have proven little more than a complicated way of determining calendar age (157).

Functional Classification

Neither calendar age nor biological age provides an entirely satisfactory basis for classification of the elderly. Nevertheless, differences between individuals are incontrovertible and obvious even to the lay person. There is thus much to commend the adoption of a simple functional classification, whether evaluating continued employability, recommending a physical activity program, or determining the need for institutional support.

The *young old* may then be considered as a group who can live independently, with few symptoms of chronic disease and little or no restriction upon their physical activity. The *middle old* have developed some physical disability, and as they grow older, they require progressively more assistance with their daily activities. The *very old* are those who have become almost totally disabled and require extensive support, often within an institution.

Prevalence of Disability

The Canada Health Survey (23) found that 26.5% of individuals over the age of 65 years had some major limitation of their habitual physical activity, and 8.9% of senior citizens were totally unable to undertake major activities. By the age of 80 years, a large proportion of subjects were limited by disturbances of either cardiac or mental function. Likewise, in the United States (93), 80% of older people had some type of chronic disability, arthritis (44%) and heart disease (27%) being the commonest problems.

Although they represent only 11% of the total population, the chronically disabled account for 30% of medical costs, 40% of acute hospital bed usage, and 90% of demand for home-care nursing. By the age of 60 years, the *active* life expectancy of the typical North American is only 60% of the remaining 16.5 years of life, and by age 85, the active life expectancy is only 40% of the remaining 7.3 years (73).

Although the totally disabled make up only a small fraction of the elderly population, they account for a large part of the growing medical and institutional costs that currently alarm health economists (146). On average, Canadian senior citizens live for 8–10 years in the category of the middle old and a final year in that of the very old (14,148). Moreover, women live 7–8 years longer than men, but they also have a much longer period of partial and total disability (14).

Distinguishing Disease from Aging

The onset of chronic disease is one important variable potentially limiting the physical activity of many old and very old people (148,157); 85.6% of Canadians over the age of 65 years are said to have some type of health problem (23), and in the Canada Fitness Survey (49), "illness" was perceived as the major impediment to physical activity among the elderly. On the other hand, many of the chronic conditions that afflict senior citizens are relative rather than absolute contraindications to physical activity, and many patients with such diseases are helped by an increase in their physical activity. Given a suitably adapted prescription, such individuals are capable of achieving substantial gains in physical condition.

There is often no clear dividing line between the effects of aging and those of disease. For example, it is generally held that the elderly have difficulty in sustaining cardiac stroke volume as maximum aerobic effort is approached, because the aging myocardium has difficulty in expelling blood against a heavy afterload (117). However, Lakatta and associates (88) argue that a decline of stroke volume at high work rates reflects undiagnosed cardiac disease. In their view (which is not unanimously accepted), if patients with silent myocardial ischemia are carefully excluded by electrocardiography, scintigraphy, and other advanced techniques, then those of the elderly with healthy hearts can compensate fully for the inevitable age-related decline in peak heart rate by application of the Frank-Starling mechanism; an increase of end-diastolic volume yields a compensatory *increase* of stroke volume, and peak cardiac output is maintained as in a young adult.

This chapter focuses mainly upon the outwardly healthy elderly, recognizing that as they age, they constitute a diminishing fraction of the total population, and that the dividing line between health and illness becomes progressively blurred. The operational definition of *healthy* we have adopted is the absence of any well-defined symptoms, regular medication, or gross medical condition that would restrict the ability of the individual to participate effectively in a program of progressive conditioning exercises.

SPECIFIC PROBLEMS OF EXERCISE TESTING IN THE OLD AND VERY OLD

General Considerations

It may be wise to begin by considering the need for exercise testing of the elderly. Some guidelines recommend a stress test as a part of preliminary screening if there is to be any substantial increase in physical activity (3). However, the results obtained in the elderly patient are often puzzling because of minor pathologies, and discovery of a seemingly dangerous but clinically silent condition may lead to a prohibition of exercise that the patient had previously enjoyed. Exercise testing is certainly desirable if very strenuous activity is contemplated (for example, preparation for a master's competition). It may also be helpful for personal motivation, to assess obscure symptoms, to help in diagnosis and prognosis, to assess programs and to evaluate the results of individual medical or surgical treatment, including cardiac rehabilitation (Chapter 4). However, a formal test is not necessary if only a moderate increase of daily activity such as light walking is envisaged. Indeed, insistence upon rigorous preliminary testing may be counterproductive, suggesting to the individual patient that such activity is a dangerous habit.

Exercise programs have traditionally focused on endurance activities, and—as in younger age groups—exercise testing has also centered on the measurement or the estimation of aerobic power. However, as age increases, the development of muscle strength and flexibility assumes increasing functional importance. A well-designed test protocol should provide information not only on aerobic power (with the electrocardiographic and blood pressure response to a graded treadmill or cycle ergometer test) but also on muscle function, flexibility, and body composition.

Maximal Oxygen Intake

Value of Test Data

Maximal oxygen intake determinations are helpful in exercise prescription, monitoring of occupational fatigue, and assessing the capacity for independent living.

Exercise Prescription. The determination of maximal oxygen intake is important in setting a safe upper limit for the person who wishes to begin a program of vigorous physical activity. The elderly individual should normally keep the intensity of effort below the ventilatory threshold, about 70% of maximal oxygen intake.

Regulation is best achieved in terms of a specified walking or jogging speed. Since heart rates are monitored during testing, it is also possible to specify an appropriate target pulse rate, although many older people have difficulty in counting this accurately. On average, the ventilatory threshold corresponds to a perception of ''somewhat hard'' activity (13 units on the original Borg scale), but individual perceptions have an unsatisfactory standard deviation of some 20% about this target (165). Finally, breathlessness should be kept below a level where conversation becomes difficult. However, heart rate, ratings of perceived exertion, and breathlessness are all best used simply to modulate a speed-based prescription in the face of adverse circumstances (such as a period of hot weather).

Occupational Monitoring. Determinations of maximal oxygen intake provide a useful guide to those who are monitoring occupational activity. Fatigue is likely to develop over an 8-h working day if the average energy consumption demands more than 40% of the individual's maximal oxygen intake (67,157).

Capacity for Independent Living. In the very old person, maximal oxygen intake scores may drop to such a low level that oxygen transport becomes the main factor limiting independent living. The critical level for functional independence is commonly a peak oxygen transport of $12-14$ ml·kg^{-1}min^{-1}, although in some patients with chronic cardiac disease apparent maxima as low as $7-10$ ml·kg^{-1}min^{-1} are observed (148,157).

Choice of Test Equipment

The young old can usually undertake the same laboratory tests of aerobic performance that are adopted for middle-aged individuals—uphill treadmill walking, cycle ergometry, and stair climbing. However, many even of the young old have not undertaken vigorous exercise recently. Relative to a young person, more time must thus be allowed for familiarization with both the laboratory and the test equipment. For example, when walking on a treadmill for the first time, an older person may adopt an awkward posture, taking small and hesitant steps, in part because of a fear of falling. However, a more normal gait is restored with a chance to practice the test. Likewise, the older person often makes rather clumsy initial attempts to operate a cycle ergometer.

The knee joints often become unstable with aging, and older people often welcome a light hand support, both for treadmill walking and for stepping. The use of such support necessarily alters the oxygen cost of the activity; therefore the oxygen consumption must be measured directly, rather than predicted from the supposed intensity of treadmill or stepping exercise (50,142). If a treadmill is not available, jogging in place has been suggested as a possible alternative method of testing for those who are reasonably fit (127). Again, measurement of oxygen consumption is essential for such an assessment to have any precision. A final alternative for those with very unstable knees or a history of back problems is the use of a cycle ergometer. With this approach, maximal effort may be limited by quadriceps weakness; it is also difficult to dismount in an emergency, and in some older men further difficulties arise from a varicocele or prostatic problems.

Direct Maximal Testing

As in a younger person, the most accurate method of determining maximal oxygen intake is a progressive exercise test, carried to voluntary exhaustion unless there are clinical indications to halt the test (3). If this is the case, data are reported as a "symptom-limited" peak oxygen intake.

A short bout of maximal effort is tolerated surprisingly well by the young old (33,168,182). The only changes of treadmill protocol that are needed relative to a younger person are a longer period of familiarization and warm-up, smaller increments of speed or slope per test stage, and a lower peak rate of working. If a stepping bench is chosen as the means of exercise, a step height of 0.35–0.40 m rather than 0.45 m may suffice to elicit maximal effort, and the use of a lower step is also desirable because the range of motion at the hip joint is reduced.

A traditional "plateau" of oxygen consumption can be demonstrated in as many as three-quarters of healthy elderly who undertake a maximal stress test on a treadmill (168). However, since the maximal oxygen intake decreases with age, the usually accepted definition of a plateau (an increment of <2 $ml \cdot kg^{-1}min^{-1}$ with an increase of power output) represents a larger fraction (7–10%) of total aerobic power than in a younger person. The proportion of subjects reaching a plateau has been much lower in some studies (for example, Ref. 182), but the observed peak values have nevertheless remained quite reproducible from one test day to another. Ancillary criteria of a good maximal effort (peak heart rate, blood lactate concentration, and respiratory gas-exchange ratio) all become more fallible in an old person, so that if a plateau reading cannot be elicited, the only option may be to report the peak voluntary effort (Table 1).

If maximal effort tests are conducted on a cycle ergometer, peak performance is commonly halted by complaints of local weakness and fatigue in the quadriceps muscle rather than by the intended central circulatory limitation (148, 157). Cycle ergometer values for directly measured or predicted peak oxygen intake thus show a steeper age-related decline than the corresponding treadmill or step-test data (7).

Submaximal Exercise Tests

Because of fears about test safety, some authors have attempted to predict the maximal performance of older individuals from data obtained during submaximal exercise. Unfortunately, such predictions (which are already imprecise in young adults) become progressively more unsatisfactory in the elderly (Table 2). The maximal heart rate (an essential element in most prediction formulae) shows a large and very variable decrease with aging (4,157). The coefficient of variation for heart rate-based predictions of maximal oxygen intake may be 15–25%, sometimes with a substantial superimposed systematic error (148,157). Attempts to estimate oxygen consumption from the rate of working are also unsatisfactory in the elderly. A short-paced, tentative pattern of treadmill walking is mechanically inefficient, and the energy cost of the activity is further modified relative to anticipated values if the subject clutches the hand rail while walking. Likewise, rapid stair climbing is often performed awkwardly, and stiff joints and lack of recent familiarity give a mechanical efficiency of cycling that is less than the "constant" value of 23% assumed in young subjects (157). A final important variable is medication. Old people consume a wide range of prescribed and non-prescribed drugs. Some agents, such as β-blockers, impair both the heart rate and the metabolic response to a given intensity of physical activity, precluding the use of submaximal tests based upon heart rate readings. Possible alternatives are to determine the ventilatory threshold (110,193) or to rate perceived exertion (17).

Alternative Approaches to Assessment

As age increases, physicians are increasingly reluctant to require even vigorous submaximal exercise testing, since a large proportion of older populations show electrocardiographic abnormalities that would contraindicate vigorous physical activity in a younger adult (169) (Fig. 1). During the Canada Fitness Survey, for example, 19% of subjects in the 60–69 age group saw themselves as unable to perform a simple submaximal step test, and a total of 55% of potential subjects

TABLE 1   Results of Exercise Testing[a]

	Oxygen intake plateau		Peak heart rate		Respiratory gas exchange ratio		Arterial lactate >8.8 mmol	Systolic BP >200 mmHg
	<2 ml·kg⁻¹min⁻¹	<1 ml·kg⁻¹min⁻¹	>160 beats per minute	>165 beats per minute	>1.00	>1.15		
Men								
Fair effort	42.8%	14.2%	42.8%	14.2%	85.7%	0%	25.0%	57.1%
Good effort	78.9	63.2	84.2	68.4	100.01	77.8	77.8	57.9
All men	69.2	50.0	73.1	53.8	96.2	68.2	68.2	57.7
Women								
Fair effort	44.4	33.3	44.4	22.2	55.6	0%	11.1	33.3
Good effort	75.0	55.0	60.0	35.0	80.0	20.0	50.0	35.0
All women	65.5	48.2	55.2	31.0	72.4	13.8	37.9	34.5

[a]Percentages of a sample of elderly subjects meeting selected criteria of maximal effort in relation to quality of effort as rated by observer; sample of 26 men and 29 women of average age 65 years performing progressive treadmill test.
Source: From R.J. Shephard, Physical Activity and Aging. Croom Helm, London (1978), based on data from Ref. 169.

Table 2 Errors in the Prediction of Maximal Oxygen Intake from Progressive Submaximal Test Data[a]

Test method	Number of patients	Aerobic power (L/min STPD)			Percent error
		Predicted	Measured	Discrepancy	
Cycle ergometer (4 min per load)	13 M	1.72 ± 0.36	2.27 ± 0.42	−0.56 ± 0.33	−24.7 ± 14.5
	17 F	1.37 ± 0.36	1.62 ± 0.17	−0.25 ± 0.26	−15.4 ± 16.0
Treadmill (3 min per load)	26 M	2.11 ± 0.38	2.27 ± 0.36	−0.16 ± 0.35	−7.0 ± 15.4
	29 F	1.83 ± 0.43	1.60 ± 0.22	0.23 ± 0.41	14.3 ± 25.6

[a]Findings for sample of 65-year-old individuals, using the Åstrand nomogram.
Source: From R.J. Shephard, Physical Activity and Aging. Croom Helm, London (1978), based on data from Ref. 169.
STPD: Standard temperature and pressure, dry gas.

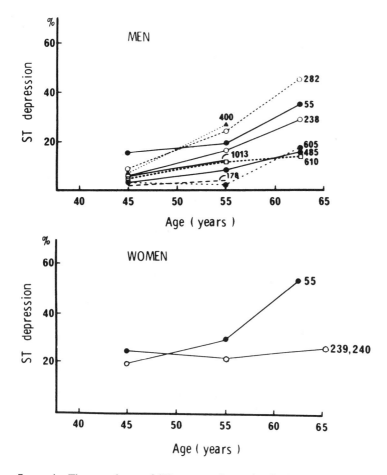

FIGURE 1 The prevalence of ST-segment depression in the electrocardiogram during or immediately following maximal exercise in relation to age. [From R.J. Shephard, *Physical Activity and Aging.* Croom Helm, London (1987), based on data from Ref. 169.]

in the same age category were "screened out" by the health professionals who were conducting the tests (49,147). Equally, if testing is conducted in a clinical laboratory, effort may soon be halted because of symptoms, signs, or electrocardiographic findings that appear dangerous to the patient or the supervising physician (3).

Possible alternatives to a laboratory physical assessment, which avoid the risk that testing may provoke a cardiac catastrophe, are (a) to observe the range of normal daily activities (92), (b) to measure the normal pace of walking (10,

22,35,36), or (c) to determine the heart rate that is developed at a moderate walking pace such as 1.3 m/s (11,36). The coefficient of correlation between walking speed and maximal oxygen intake is unfortunately too weak to give more than a general impression of an individual's fitness. For example, Cunningham et al. (36) reported a correlation of only 0.25 when walking speeds were compared with maximal oxygen intakes over a broad age range from 19 to 66 years. The correlation of walking speed with maximal oxygen intake was indeed only slightly greater than that between speed and age (-0.13). Bassey et al. (11) noted that walking speed was also influenced by the strength of the calf muscles. In subjects over the age of 65 years, correlations of 0.41 and 0.36 linked strength and walking speed in men and women respectively.

Very old individuals may be unable to stand. Smith and Gilligan (176) proposed a progressive "step test" that could be performed while sitting in a straight-backed chair; this test increased metabolism progressively from 2.3 to 3.9 METs (ratios to basal metabolic rate). Mechanical efficiency is inevitably very variable during seated exercise, being affected among other things by habitual posture and thigh length. Direct measurements of oxygen consumption are thus needed in order to draw useful conclusions from such a test. Unfortunately, limited dentition may hamper use of a mouthpiece, and hollowed cheeks also limit the effectiveness of gas collection by face mask. Nevertheless, the peak MET value reached in such simple activities gives some indication of both the potential to initiate an exercise program and the subsequent prognosis of the individual.

Another possible method of evaluating fitness in the very old is to assess their ability to perform specific activities of daily living (92). This approach lacks scientific precision, since the tasks that are accomplished depend greatly upon the living environment and the determination of the individual concerned. Nevertheless, an inventory of this sort may allow a ranking of aerobic fitness, providing some indication of the activities that an elderly person is able to undertake.

Electrocardiographic Changes

As age increases, an ever-increasing proportion of people (both sedentary and highly active) show premature ventricular contractions (PVCs) and other exercise-induced abnormalities of ECG rhythm and waveform (76,113,169) (Fig. 1). However, as in a younger person, questions remain about the reliability and validity of such information (141) and an appropriate clinical response.

It has been argued that because of an increased prevalence of clinically significant myocardial ischemia, the number of false-positive results should be lower in the elderly than in a younger person. At first inspection, Bayes' theorem supports such a hypothesis. However, other complicating factors are a high incidence of resting ECG abnormalities and an overall physical weakness that prevents many of the frail elderly from reaching a diagnostically adequate level of exercise. Many old people take diuretics on a regular basis, and the resulting potassium ion excretion influences both ECG appearances and vulnerability to an abnormal cardiac rhythm. Other medications, such as β-blockers and calcium channel antagonists, also influence the extent of ST-segment depression by altering exercise heart rate and/or modifying myocardial contractility. For these various reasons, a fair number of the apparently abnormal records seen in older people are still false-positive responses (169).

In general, an abnormal ECG is more likely to be a true-positive result if it is associated with other cardiac risk factors, abnormalities of heart rhythm, failure of the blood pressure to show the expected rise with exercise, chest pain of anginal type, or a low peak power output. False-positive tests can generally be clarified by further laboratory investigation, but at substantial cost to the patient or the insuring agency.

A proportion of exercise-induced ECG changes undoubtedly reflect the onset of significant myocardial ischemia, with implications of an adverse prognosis. Questions that then arise are (a) Is it safe for such individuals to undertake regular physical activity? (b) Should continuous electrocardiographic monitoring be provided during such exercise? and (c) Can the threshold for such abnormalities be used to set an appropriate ceiling of exercise intensity?

Safety

Appropriately prescribed exercise is very safe, even for patients with established cardiovascular disease. Our studies of some 5000 "postcoronary" patients, followed over a 20-year period, have shown a mortality of about 1 in 300,000 person-hours for supervised exercise programs and 1 in 100,000 person-hours for unsupervised activities (163). A survey of 167 supervised cardiac rehabilitation programs in the United States (186) provided data on 51,303 patients (not all of whom had sustained a myocardial infarction). They completed 2,351,916 person-hours of prescribed exercise. During this time, there were a total of 21 incidents of cardiac arrest and 8 myocardial infarctions. The incidence rates were 1 per 111,996 patient-hours of exercise for cardiac arrest, 1 per 293,990 hours for myocardial infarction, and 1 per 783,972 patient hours for a fatality (Table 3). The risks were apparently similar for large- and small-scale programs and were uninfluenced by the availability of continuous ECG monitoring.

We lack such large-scale statistics for elderly persons who have not yet sustained a myocardial infarction, but it seems unlikely that they are at greater risk than the postcoronary patients provided that they undertake a similar pattern of moderate, progressive physical activity appropriate to their initial physical condition. It is thus very safe to recommend an increase of physical activity to an older person. Indeed, Vuori (191) has suggested that because the elderly are

TABLE 3   The Incidence of Cardiovascular Complications During Cardiac Rehabilitation Programs in Relation to Program Size

Program size, PH[a]	Reports, number	Patients, number	Exposure, total PH	Cardiac arrests per 10⁶ PH	Fatalities per 10⁶ PH	Total MI per 10⁶ PH
<5000	51	8582	115,152	8.7	0	0
5000–24,999	94	30,335	1,135,157	8.8	0.9	4.4
>25,000	22	12,386	1,101,607	9.1	1.8	2.7
Total	167	51,303	2,351,916	8.9	1.3	34

[a]PH = patient-hours.
Source: Based on data from Ref. 186.

unlikely to undertake feats for which they are ill prepared, the relative risk of death from either "nonstrenuous" or "strenuous" exercise is lower in the 50- to 69-year-old group than in younger individuals (Table 4).

Moreover, if account is taken of the entire day, a modest increase of physical activity is generally less risky than prolonged sitting or bed rest (141,173, 174). Very vigorous activity may shorten life span slightly in the very old (97), but it would seem inappropriate to restrict the activity of the elderly simply on the basis of asymptomatic electrocardiographic abnormalities. Why persuade an 80-year-old man who enjoys a weekly game of golf that it would be "safer" to give up this habit? What social good would be served if the patient lived 5 years longer but spent 4 of those years paralyzed by a severe stroke, unable to recognize his golfing friends?

Need for Continuous ECG Monitoring

Given the safety of moderate physical activity, it seems counterproductive to suggest that such activity requires minute-by-minute electronic surveillance. Insistence on such monitoring (Gorden et al., 1983) discourages participation, implying that exercise is a dangerous habit rather than a normal feature of life.

Empirical data show that ambulatory ECG monitoring is an unnecessary luxury, even if there is a history of myocardial infarction. DeBusk et al. (40) arranged home exercise programs for cardiac patients up to the age of 70 years. The only communication with the physician was a twice-weekly transmission of ECG signal and heart-rate-monitor data. None of the patients assigned to this

TABLE 4 Influence of Age on the Relative Risk of Sudden Death During Exercise

| Type of activity | Subject age, years | | | | | |
| | 20–29 | | 40–49 | | 50–69 | |
	Deaths[a]	Rel. risk[b]	Deaths	Rel. risk	Deaths	Rel. risk
Walking			37.9	0.2	11.7	0.5
Jogging	14.3	9.3	4.5	4.7	6.7	0.7
Nordic skiing	10.0	9.3	1.3	9.0	0.6	6.1
Ballgames	11.9		3.8		6.2	
Nonstrenuous exercise	26.0	2.5	5.2	3.6	3.4	2.5
Strenuous exercise	6.1	10.0	1.2	13.1	1.2	5.3

[a]Deaths expressed per 10^6 exercise sessions.
[b]Relative risk expressed as observed deaths/expected deaths for resting subjects over the same time interval.
Source: Based on data from Ref. 191; by permission of author.

regimen developed any cardiovascular complications over a 26-week period of vigorous exercise, although it must be admitted some individuals with high-risk conditions such as congestive heart failure and unstable angina were excluded from the trial.

Prescription Ceiling

It seems prudent to set the ceiling of physical activity a little below the intensity that provokes adverse symptoms (angina, abnormalities of pulse rhythm), signs (such as a fall in systolic pressure), or major ECG abnormalities.

On the other hand, exercise-induced ECG abnormalities give only a statistical indication of cardiovascular risk, even when they are considered in conjunction with adverse symptoms and signs. The most commonly discussed finding (>0.2 mV, horizontal or downsloping depression of the ST segment) is associated with about a twofold increase in the risk of exercise-induced cardiac incidents (140,143).

The safe ceiling of energy expenditure is lower for activities that involve small muscles, an awkward posture, straining, or movements of the arms above the head, because in all of these situations the exercise-induced rise in blood pressure is augmented. Tolerance of exercise is also diminished by recent illness, emotional stress, and adverse environmental conditions (extremes of heat or cold, the excitement of intense competition).

Blood Pressure Responses

Exercise normally induces a progressive rise of systolic blood pressure in the body's attempt to sustain the perfusion of muscles that are contracting at a large fraction of their maximal force (77,96,136). The cardiovascular response is most obvious during isometric straining against a closed glottis. In such circumstances large increases of blood pressure can develop within a minute (96). However, a slower increase of systolic pressure also develops over 10–15 min of vigorous endurance activity. The resultant increase of cardiac afterload is one factor contributing to the commonly observed decrease of cardiac stroke volume when older people approach peak power output (Fig. 2).

The rise of blood pressure is commonly exacerbated in those who are at risk of hypertension (69). In contrast, if the myocardium is weakened by chronic fibrotic degeneration or left ventricular contractility is impaired by myocardial ischemia, there may be not only a decrease of stroke volume but also difficulty in sustaining blood pressure at high work rates. Failure of blood pressure to show the anticipated rise over a progressive exercise test is a warning that effort should be halted urgently (3). An abnormally low blood pressure response to exercise also indicates a poor prognosis following myocardial infarction (55).

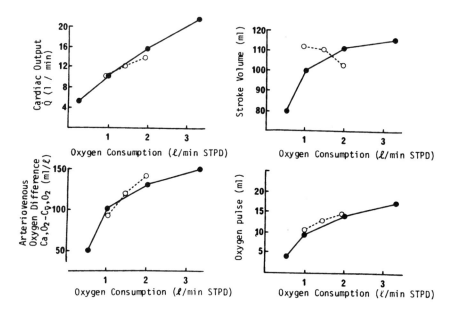

FIGURE 2   A comparison of exercise responses between young adults (solid line, average age 25 years) and elderly subjects (interrupted line, average age 65 years). (Graphs drawn from data of Ref. 117; first published in Ref. 141. Used with permission.)

Postural hypotension immediately following a vigorous bout of physical activity is a further problem (37,98). Possible contributing factors include poor general physical condition, bed rest, varicosities, a diuretic-induced reduction of blood volume, the administration of blood-pressure-lowering drugs, "drop" attacks from arthritic compression of a vertebral artery (122), a substantial rise of core temperature, prolonged swimming or aquabics, lack of an adequate cooldown, and standing in hot and humid shower areas (141). The fall in pressure may be sufficient to cause a loss of consciousness, with associated risks of physical injury and drowning. The resulting decrease of coronary perfusion may also precipitate cardiac arrhythmias and sudden death. The few reported fatalities in cardiac rehabilitation programs have tended to occur in shower areas following exercise (100,141).

In examining blood pressure responses in the frail elderly, it is important to obtain full details of any continuing medication, as many commonly prescribed drugs can lead to hypotension during and following exercise. If there is a history of frequent fainting, it may be worth undertaking a tilt-tolerance test. A person with good cardiovascular reflexes shows a small increase rather than a fall of systemic blood pressure on tilting rapidly to the upright position.

Muscle Function

Muscle function is important to the cardiovascular system for several reasons. If the muscles are weak, they must contract at a large fraction of peak force, increasing the cardiac afterload. Further, frailty progressively limits daily activities, to the point that the very old have difficulty in taking sufficient exercise to maintain cardiovascular condition.

Laboratory Tests

Standard laboratory approaches can be applied to the assessment of isometric, isokinetic, and isotonic muscle function, even in old and very old patients (48, 157). Until recently, observations on senior citizens were limited to measurements of peak isometric force on a few key muscle groups (157). Both isokinetic and isotonic data are now becoming available (48,55) (Table 5). The commonly used hand-grip dynamometer score, although important in a functional context, does not provide a good index of overall body strength. Moreover, the results for this are lower if overall weakness precludes measurement in a standing position (181).

It is important that testing be preceded by inquiry regarding musculoskeletal disorders affecting the joints under investigation. There must also be an adequate warm-up to avoid causing musculoskeletal injury and/or cardiac arrest during testing. Finally, prolonged straining against a closed glottis is to be avoided because of the associated rise in systemic blood pressure. Relative to young adults, longer periods of practice may be needed to reach stable scores, not only during the dynamometric or tensiometric assessment of maximal isometric force

TABLE 5   Isokinetic Torque About Knee Joint at Rotation Speeds of 180°/s and 240°/s (Data for Three Groups of Older Males)

Average age, years	Knee flexion torque		Knee extension torque	
	180°/s, nm	240°/s, nm	180°/s, nm	240°/s, nm
57.1	47.9	47.9	66.0	65.3
63.1	45.0	34.9	68.1	57.4
74.0	34.6	28.1	51.1	42.4

Source: Adapted from Ref. 55; used with permission.

TABLE 6   Force and Power Developed During Squatting Jump in Men of
Various Ages

Age, years	n	Body mass, kg	Average force, newtons	Average leg power W/kg
18–28	35	80	618	23
29–40	16	79	508	17
41–49	18	77	435	14
54–65	4	76	320	19
71–73	11	74	315	7

Source: Based on data of C. Bosco and P.V. Komi, *Eur. J. Appl. Physiol.,* 43: 209–219 (1980).

but also in determinations of isokinetic strength (using a device such as the Cybex
II or the Kin-Com isokinetic tester) and during measurements of isotonic strength
(using, for instance, an incremental dynamic lifting task).

Field Tests

Under field conditions, explosive strength could theoretically be evaluated by a
squatting jump (Table 6), a standing broad jump, or a jump-and-reach test, although in a frail elderly population, unstable knees, poor coordination, impaired
balance and a lack of recent practice of the skill frequently lead to scores that are
unrepresentatively low relative to actual muscle mass. A combination of muscle
strength and endurance can be assessed from such items as timed push-ups and
sit-ups (147), but such tests are hard upon an aging vertebral column and may
give rise to undesirably large rises of systemic blood pressure.

Functional abilities also provide some guide as to muscle function in the
middle old and very old (Table 7). The relationship of triceps surae strength to

TABLE 7   Percentage of U.S. Adults of Various
Ages Who Have Difficulty in Doing Heavy
Housework

Age, years	Men	Women
65–69	9.8%	21.8%
70–74	13.0	27.3
75–79	14.6	33.2
80–84	18.9	41.7
>85	33.3	54.2

Source: U.S. National Center for Health Statistics, *Advanced Data Report 133* (1987).

walking pace (11) has already been noted. One particularly important item in the context of physical activity is the ability to lift the body mass from a chair (157).

Issues of Motivation

The observed scores for most laboratory and field tests of strength depend heavily upon the motivation of the subject. More encouragement may be needed to elicit maximal effort in an old person than in someone who is younger. Pain may also limit effort about an arthritic joint. Rapid movements are probably unwise in those with a history of joint pain, and in the frail elderly with signs of osteoporosis such as the "dowager's hump," there is some risk that overvigorous muscular efforts could cause a fracture.

One method of avoiding problems of motivation is to estimate the lean body mass by computed tomography or hydrodensitometry. Our studies in master's athletes showed relatively constant values until the eighth decade of life, but values for athletes aged 70–79 years decreased even in those who reported that they were continuing training (76).

DeVries (41) suggested that problems of motivation and physical injury during testing could be avoided by relating the development of submaximal force to the corresponding level of electromyographic activity. A strong person can develop a large muscle force with less electromyographic activity than a weaker individual.

Body Composition

An excess of body fat is widely recognized as a risk factor for atherosclerotic heart disease, although it is less certain that the risk is independent of resulting increases in serum cholesterol and blood pressure. Obesity also decreases effective aerobic power, since the energy cost of most tasks is linked fairly closely to body mass.

The simple assessment is based on weight-for-height tables. Other approaches are to determine the thickness of various skinfolds, to measure waist and hip circumferences, or to carry out hydrostatic weighing. Finally, there are various more sophisticated methods of estimating lean tissue mass and bone density (152).

Weight for Height

Actuarial tables of weight-for-height and ratios of body mass to $(height)^2$ (the body mass index, or BMI) have some value as epidemiological tools in young adults, but there are several potential problems in applying such an approach to the evaluation of body composition in elderly patients:

1.   Special weighing devices are needed for patients who have difficulty in standing. Alternatively, body mass can be estimated from calf (C) and arm (A) circumferences, knee height (K), and subscapular skinfold thickness (SS), all measured in centimeters (28):

For men, $M = 0.98\ C + 1.16\ K + 1.73\ AC + 0.37\ SS - 81.69$

For women, $M = 1.27\ C + 0.87\ K + 0.98\ AC + 0.40\ SS - 62.35$

2.   The setting of an "ideal weight" is complicated by an age-related decrease of stature due to kyphosis and vertebral collapse. Stature may thus need to be estimated from knee height K:

For men, $H = 2.20\ K$ (cm) $- 0.04\ A$ (year) $+ 64.19$
For women, $H = 1.83\ K$ (cm) $- 0.24\ A$ (year) $+ 84.88$

3.   The "ideal weight" indicated in the actuarial tables applies to survival from the age when insurance was purchased, usually in young adulthood. However, there is growing evidence that the "ideal" value is larger in older adults (5).

4.   A substantial accumulation of body fat may be masked by loss of muscle protein and bone calcium, giving a normal weight for height.

Skinfold Measurements

Determination of the thickness of representative double folds of skin and superficial fat is a second simple way to examine body composition. Again, there are some specific problems in applying this method to the elderly. The patient may be reluctant to shed the necessary layers of clothing, and in any event undressing is time-consuming in this age group. Measurement errors may arise because the skin moves independently of subcutaneous fat. Moreover, the skin is thinner and more compressible than in a young adult, and the ratio of deep to superficial fat is often increased (152,175). A given skinfold reading thus implies a greater amount of body fat in an older person.

All of these issues point to the need for age-specific formulas if an attempt is to be made to predict body density or total body fat from skinfold readings (152). The alternative preferred by many investigators is to interpret the skinfold data in their own right—but again, age-specific norms are required (Table 8).

Particular attention has recently been directed to the relative amounts of fat over the chest and the hips. If the ratio is high (the so-called masculine pattern of fat distribution), there is an increased risk of ischemic heart disease and other chronic disorders (152).

Underwater Weighing

Underwater weighing is often regarded as providing the "gold standard" of body composition determinations (152). Body mass is partitioned into two arbitrary

TABLE 8   Age-Related Increase of Skinfold
Thicknesses at Selected Sites[a]

Body site	Percentage increase relative to young adult	
	Men	Women
Central sites		
Subscapular	31%	77%
Chest	49	106
Waist	62	101
Suprapubic	111	68
Suprailiac	8	59
Peripheral sites		
Chin	39%	67%
Triceps	12	26
Knee	37	90
Average (all sites)	25	51

[a]Data from seven surveys of elderly adults compared with
norms for young adults approximating the "ideal" body mass.
Values expressed as a percentage increase.
Source: From R.J Shephard, *Physical Activity and Aging*.
Croom Helm, London (1978).

components ("fat" and "fat-free" tissue), and the percentage of body fat is
estimated by assigning a fixed density to each compartment. Unfortunately, a
progressive loss of bone mineral greatly reduces the density of "lean" tissue in
the elderly, and a two-compartment model has limited validity unless lean tissue
is assigned an age-specific density (109,152).

Technically, it remains quite possible to undertake underwater weighing
in the young old, but there are practical difficulties when dealing with the middle
old and very old. Many old people are nervous about total immersion. There may
be a history of blackouts or hypotensive episodes on emerging from a pool, and
there is also a danger of slipping on wet decks, particularly if balance is impaired
(157).

Because chronic chest disease is common in old people, it is no longer
possible to assume the residual gas volume or to predict it from vital capacity,
as is sometimes done in younger individuals. Chronic chest disease also slows
expulsion of air from the lungs if a forced expiration is attempted while under
water, and a combination of uneven gas distribution and frank bronchospasm
may delay the equilibration of helium or oxygen when residual gas volume is
being estimated. Finally, the use of a closed-circuit breathing apparatus may be

complicated by mouthpiece leakage around poorly fitting dentures. One helpful possibility is to measure the residual gas volume with the head out of the water (43).

Determinations of Lean Tissue

Methods of lean tissue determination based upon body potassium measurements (109,152) require access to a whole-body counter, but have the important advantage that minimal cooperation is required from the patient. Difficulties of interpretation arise in senior citizens because the potassium (^{40}K) content of lean tissue is generally lower than in younger adults (152,190). Changes may arise because of the administration of diuretics, and the natural ^{40}K radiation emanating from the muscles may be screened from the scintillation counter by an increased thickness of subcutaneous fat.

Likewise, estimates of lean tissue mass that are based on the dilution of deuterated or tritiated water are complicated by assumptions about the water content of the tissues, which changes substantially with aging (152).

Other Techniques

A variety of other methods of determining body composition are now available (152). These include ultrasound, nuclear magnetic resonance imaging, computed tomography, dual-photon absorptiometry, whole body-impedance, and infra-red reactance. However, many of these procedures are too costly for routine use.

Whole-body impedance can be determined relatively simply, but if body fat is to be predicted from such measurements, major assumptions must be made regarding both the electrical conductivity of lean tissue and the geometry of body parts. These assumptions are often not valid for an older person because of differences in the amount and distribution of body water and the thickness of fascial sheaths (87,152,187).

Flexibility

Flexibility is usually only a minor part of fitness assessment in a young adult. However, it becomes an increasingly important determinant of function and the ability to maintain cardiorespiratory function as age increases.

One difficulty in assessing flexibility is that it is specific to a given articulation (164). There are general effects of aging upon collagen (61,157,189), but limitations on the range of movement become highly joint-specific in elderly people, as general changes and the impact of inherited local anatomical peculiarities are compounded by local arthritic change.

For those patients who can sit on the floor, the standard sit-and-reach test

TABLE 9   Scores for Sit-and-Reach Test of
Flexibility at Various Ages

Age, years	Men, meters	Women, meters
20–29	0.303	0.327
30–39	0.288	0.318
40–49	0.249	0.299
50–59	0.246	0.295
>60	0.221	0.276

Note: Measurements are made with the subject seated. However, a score of 0.250 m implies that the person tested has flexibility equivalent to an ability to touch the floor with the tips of the fingers when the knees are fully extended.
Source: From Ref. 49.

(50,52,194) provides a reproducible measure of spinal flexibility (Table 9). The range of movement at other joints can be assessed by a simple goniometer, although the observed range of motion depends largely on success in aligning the goniometer with the axis of rotation of the joint (164).

Balance

A progressive deterioration of balance can impose a substantial limitation upon function in the middle old and the very old. Laboratory determinations of balance can be based on stabilometer scores (142) or more precisely on movements of the center of gravity as observed when the subject is standing on a force platform. In the field, approximate data can be obtained by timing the ability to stand on one leg with and without the eyes closed.

Bone Density

A decrease in bone density leaves the very old vulnerable to "spontaneous" fractures. Determinations of bone density by whole-body calcium estimation or dual photon absorptiometry require referral to specialized centers (44,152). However, such referral may be warranted if fractures are occurring with little application of external force.

Prescription of Physical Activity for the Elderly

We now consider the principles of physical activity prescription for the elderly, discussing the issues of an appropriate intensity, frequency, and duration of activity and making optimum recommendations for several categories of older patients. Finally methods of sustaining motivation are considered.

Principles of Physical Activity Prescription

The majority of elderly people who wish to exercise are interested in moderate physical activity that is perceived as appropriate to their age group (121). They seek a prescription that will maintain physical condition, improving their general health and appearance. Some master's athletes still want to stress themselves to the limit of their potential (76,120,166), although even in this group many become interested in social interaction rather than unbridled competition.

Such needs were, until recently, at variance with perceptions of the exercise scientist, since it was assumed that physical activity had to be relatively intense to restore function and assure health benefit. However, this dogma of intensive exercise has come under increasing scrutiny (3,13,123), particularly with respect to the elderly. Physicians now realize that in a very sedentary senior, both functional capacity and health can be improved by quite modest increases of regular physical activity. Moreover, resulting gains of health and function may outstrip observed gains in maximal oxygen intake (107). However, maximization of the potential training response still depends on compliance with a regimen where intensity of effort is progressively increased.

As in younger individuals, a large part of the conditioning response is dissipated by 2–3 weeks of detraining or bed rest (32,112).

Intensity: Traditional Concept

The traditional concept was that, at all ages, endurance training required regular 30- to 60-min sessions of large-muscle exercise—such as jogging, cycling, or vigorous swimming—pursued on at least alternate days at an initial intensity of 60–70% of maximal oxygen intake (2). It was further assumed that in order to maximize gains in physical condition, there should be a progression of training intensity from 60–70% to 70–80% of maximal oxygen intake as soon as the condition of the patient permitted.

Possible Dangers of Intensive Activity.   There is little evidence that regular endurance exercise predisposes to osteoarthritis (90,126), but an overvigorous program can aggravate preexisting disease. The impact stress on the knee joint is three to six times greater during jogging than during rapid walking at an equivalent oxygen consumption (128).

The chances of an exercise-induced cardiac emergency [although low with all patterns of physical activity (141,155,191)] may be increased if training progresses to strenuous exercise (191).

However, the main argument against an intensive program is probably motivational; those who are initially unfit perceive it as beyond their capacity.

The Case for Low-Intensity Activity.   Recent data suggest that much of the health advantage is gained from quite light physical activity (185). This is particularly true in older people, since another important determinant of the training response is the initial fitness of the individual relative to the prescribed intensity of effort. Thomas et al. (182) suggested that intensity and frequency of physical activity together accounted for only 10% of the training-induced gains of performance in the elderly.

Sidney and Shephard (171) compared various self-selected patterns of training in a sample of young-old volunteers (Fig. 3). The largest and most rapid increase of aerobic power (a dramatic 33% over 7 weeks) was seen in subjects who averaged 3.3 training sessions per week at an intensity rising from 60–80% of their maximal oxygen intake. However, a useful 10% increment of aerobic power over 14 weeks was seen in subjects who exercised frequently but failed to progress beyond an intensity demanding 60% of maximal oxygen intake. The improvement of cardiovascular endurance in response to low-intensity training was subsequently confirmed by Badenhop et al. (6). They found equal gains of maximal oxygen intake with training at 30–45% and 60–75% of heart rate reserve. Likewise, Seals et al. (139) found some response to 6 months of training at 40% of heart rate reserve, although further gains were seen when the intensity of training was increased to 75–80% of heart rate reserve. Such observations

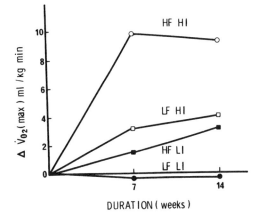

FIGURE 3   Influence of frequency (high versus low) and intensity of exercise (high versus low) on increasing the predicted aerobic power of 65-year-old adults participating in a 14-week training program. (From Ref. 171; used with permission.)

have considerable practical importance for the frail elderly, who initially may find great difficulty in exercising at more than 30–45% of their heart rate reserve.

Implications for "Postcoronary" Patients. Several recent reports have examined the influence of low-intensity training following myocardial infarction. In the first few months of rehabilitation, there seems little advantage to the adoption of a vigorous regimen (16,130,134). On the other hand, if training is continued for a year or more, intensive activity induces a continuing increase in peak stroke volume, whereas lighter exercise merely improves peripheral circulatory function (46,130).

Conclusions. Any special benefit of intensive training seems focused upon myocardial performance. In contrast, the consumption of body fat may be greater with prolonged bouts of moderate exercise than with shorter periods of intensive effort, since fat cannot be metabolized under anaerobic conditions (142). Thus, if an objective of an exercise regimen is to reduce the amount of body fat, a program calling for moderate physical activity may be more effective than an intensive training plan.

Frequency and Duration of Effort

The beneficial effects of exercise on calendar life span are most likely to be realized if a critical volume of training is undertaken every week. For example, in Harvard alumni, extended survival is associated with an added leisure energy expenditure; benefit begins at 2.2 MJ/wk (500 kcal/wk), and is maximized at 8.8 MJ/wk (2000 kcal/wk) (124). Little benefit is obtained from irregular or seasonal bursts of physical activity, and attempts to sustain activity at a level beyond current capacity may actually provoke a heart attack (141,155,191).

Cardiovascular Benefits. The cardiovascular benefits of regular physical activity seem less marked in senior citizens than in younger people (94), possibly in part because the more vulnerable individuals have already died (124,125,131). For example, the gain of longevity associated with a leisure energy expenditure of 8.8 MJ/wk decreases from about 2.5 years at age 35–39 years to only 0.4 years at age 75–79 years (124). The optimum training time for the elderly person has yet to be defined, but a greater total duration may be required to compensate for a low intensity of activity (3). Barry (9) suggested that the optimum session length was related to the prescribed intensity of effort in METs by the formula:

$$\text{Duration (min)} = 218/\text{MET} - 60$$

For example, if an intensity of 2 METs is selected, then the recommendation is to undertake a total of 49 min of exercise per day.

However, prolonged exercise sessions are impractical for the frail elderly. If they are to undertake any substantial volume of training, it must be broken into several sessions per day or at least several segments of moderate effort with alternating periods of rest and light activity. It appears that such a plan can be followed without a serious decrease in training response (3,185). Some authors have found a good response to a circuit training plan where 1- to 2-min periods of light activity are interspersed between 5-min bouts at five or six different tasks (196).

Metabolic Benefits. If optimization of the serum lipid profile is seen as an important component of training (106,197), data on middle-aged adults suggest the need for an energy expenditure equivalent to walking or jogging at least 18–20 km per week (45,75,195). In the elderly, the optimum tactic to sustain HDL cholesterol levels may be a combination of dietary restriction sufficient to reduce body mass by 4–5 kg coupled with 3–4 km of brisk walking on most days (180).

Recovery processes, such as the replenishment of glycogen stores, recovery of immune function (158), and repair of tissue microtrauma are likely to proceed more slowly in the elderly than in young adults, taking at least 2 days to complete. From the viewpoint of tissue metabolism, the optimal pattern of exercise for older people may thus be three formal sessions per week, with light walking on intervening days.

Other Benefits. Other benefits of training—such as the strengthening of muscles (3,48,60) or an increase of joint flexibility—may require relatively brief periods of definitive activity per session. Some objectives (such as an increase in social contacts) may be satisfied by program attendance, irrespective of the level of active participation.

Anticipated Response

It might be anticipated that training would be accomplished less easily in a frail elderly person than in a young adult. Functional adaptations to most types of stress are reduced with aging, and slower rates of protein synthesis could reduce the likelihood of morphological adaptations such as hypertrophy of cardiac or skeletal muscle. Nevertheless, Fiatarone et al. (48) found large gains of strength from resistance training in nonagenarians, and in at least some of her sample there were appreciable increases in muscle mass. Further, the physiological gap between the sedentary person and the active individual or the continuing athlete remains much as in a younger individual (157). The implication is that although the old person may move more slowly from a sedentary to a trained state, the ultimate potential of the conditioning response is unaltered by aging.

It is difficult to make formal comparisons of trainability between young and older individuals because the low initial fitness levels of many old people in themselves facilitate the training response (72,157). The ideal experiment would train people of different ages but at the same level of physical condition relative to their age-matched peers. If this is done, 65-year-old people seem to show at least the same percentage gains of fitness as younger individuals (171), although in the short term (14 weeks) their absolute response is generally less than in a younger sample. Certainly, training cannot restore tissue that has been destroyed by disease, but it can maximize residual function.

IDEAL PHYSICAL ACTIVITY PROGRAM

The ideal program of physical activity is tailored to the physical and medical condition of the individual, without circumscribing the pursuit of modest activities by a discouraging excess of tests and restrictions. The search is for a recommendation that is safe, effective in promoting health and function, and sufficiently motivating to offer a good chance of sustained compliance.

Effectiveness

An effective regimen checks the commonly observed age-related deterioration of cardiovascular function and muscle strength, maintains flexibility and balance, and counters osteoporosis while enhancing social interactions, mood-state, and overall quality of life.

Cardiovascular Function

Cardiovascular function is improved by any activity that involves a substantial fraction of the body musculature—for example, regular walking, cycling, cross-country skiing, rowing, or vigorous swimming. Unfortunately, loss of balance and difficulty in standing preclude some of these activities for the middle old and the very old. Nevertheless, a considerable cardiovascular stimulus can be developed using the muscles of the arms and shoulder girdle (150). For instance, several arm and wheelchair ergometers are now available (150), and McNamara et al. (102) have described chair exercises to mimic both cycling and rowing.

Many elderly people have undertaken almost no activity for many years, and in such individuals heart rates in the range 100–120 beats per minute initially provide some cardiovascular stimulus, although gains of condition quickly plateau unless the intensity of exercise is increased as fitness improves. Some patients have difficulty in palpating their heart rates accurately. Abnormalities of heart rhythm and the administration of drugs that modify the heart-rate response to exercise limit the possibility of using heart rate to regulate the intensity of effort. The simplest guideline is to undertake an intensity of effort that is a little more than attempted recently but leaves no more than pleasant tiredness a few hours later. Other practical guidelines suggest an intensity of effort that is perceived as "somewhat hard" and that induces some sweating but that permits conversation even though it induces some breathlessness.

Initially, exercise bouts may be limited to a duration of 10–15 min, but as condition improves, the patient should be encouraged to extend each session to 30–60 min.

Muscle Strength

Many early exercise prescriptions neglected to sustain muscular strength because of fears of provoking an excessive rise of blood pressure. However, an exclusive cardiovascular focus can weaken important muscle groups, particularly in the upper half of the body.

The fears of hypertension are now recognized as overstated. At any given fraction of maximal voluntary force, isometric exercise gives a similar rise of systemic blood pressure in young and older adults (136). Both cardiac patients and the young old can undertake the full range of isotonic, isometric, and circuit-training exercises that younger adults use to develop muscle function, provided that muscle contractions are held for no more than a few seconds and an adequate recovery interval is allowed between contractions (51,64,79). Fiatarone et al. (48) have demonstrated that even institutionalized nonagenarians can make large gains of strength in response to high-intensity isotonic contractions. For the middle-old or very old person who is bedridden, muscle condition can still be improved by tensing one muscle group against another, or pressing periodically against the bed board. It may also be possible to condition the leg muscles—for instance, by placing books on a short plank that is balanced across the ankles, and lifting this load in a rhythmic manner.

Flexibility and Balance

Era (47) has argued that exercise programs for the elderly should pay particular attention to the development of balance, coordination, agility, joint flexibility, and reaction speed. The normal leisure activities of the elderly are unlikely to take all major joints through their full range of motion, and the patient should thus be encouraged to exercise all major joints on a regular basis. The mobility of most joints can be improved by a combination of flexibility exercises and dance-type movements (95).

Weight-supported activities in a heated swimming pool provide a useful component of training if individual joints have become painful or unstable (84,91,144). If movements are becoming restricted, it may also be helpful to engage in gentle stretching at the extremes of motion, using either body weight or a partner as the driving force for such stretching. However, sudden, jerky movements could cause injury and are to be avoided.

Countering Osteoporosis

The precise pattern of exercise needed to reduce the risk of osteoporosis is still debated (44,137). The loss of bone mineral during actual and simulated space missions suggests that normal gravitational acceleration is one important factor conserving bone density. Walking provides a good stimulus to the bones of the legs, hips, and spine, but weights must be held in the hands or lifted if the arm bones are to receive adequate stimulation. There have been suggestions that the muscle forces associated with resistance exercise can also stimulate bone development (27). Smith et al. (170,171) have even claimed that 80-year-old subjects derive some protection from chair exercises at an intensity of 1.5–3.0 METs. However, moderate swimming and water-supported gymnastics seem unlikely to provide an adequate stimulus to strengthen the bones.

Mood Elevation

In younger adults, an elevation of mood may arise from the secretion of endorphins, other hormones, and cytokines, together with alterations in tryptophan metabolism (24,39,63), but elderly subjects are unlikely to engage in the prolonged and intensive activity needed to induce such responses. Mood state can also be enhanced by an increase of cerebral arousal. The intensity of physical activity needed for this response is much more likely to be achieved by seniors; indeed, some proprioceptive stimulation can be realized even while sitting in bed.

Nevertheless, the main factors enhancing mood in the elderly are probably an increase in social contacts, the development of new interests, an enhancement of self-image, development of a sense of self-efficacy, and even the pleasant esthetic experience of, for example, a walk in the country or a city park.

Irrespective of mechanisms, the end result is a lessening of anxiety and depression (89,114,118).

Overall Recommendation

An appropriate program for the senior citizen will include a fairly lengthy warmup, endurance work involving a variety of the major muscle groups, weight-bearing activity (if possible), some strengthening of the major muscles by resistance activity, and an extended cool-down period (10–15 min following a bout of vigorous endurance exercise).

Motivation

Perhaps the most difficult part of an exercise program at any age is to ensure continued motivation of the participants. Even in young adults, the 6-month dropout rate is commonly a discouraging 50% of those initially recruited (145). In old people, poor memory and inevitable interruptions of training by lack of transportation, severe weather, and intercurrent illness give even poorer compliance.

Unfortunately, gains of fitness cannot be stored (32,112), and benefits to health and functional status are realized only if the recommended physical activity is repeated on a regular basis several times per week.

Factors encouraging a retention of initial enthusiasm include a careful matching of the regimen to the goals, aptitudes, interests, and skills of the individual and an avoidance of injuries.

Goals

The primary goals of an older exerciser are an improvement of health and function and (particularly in women) an increase of social contacts (170). The search for activities that involve speed, danger, and demanding competition is diminished even in continuing master's athletes (76).

The instructor should thus emphasize linkages between the recommended activities, health, function, and continued independence, preferably within the framework of a comprehensive health-promotional "package." Feedback should be provided to participants in terms of gains in health-related fitness: an increase in cardiovascular endurance, a reduction in body fat, a faster walking speed, and a reduction of fatigue during everyday activities.

Care should also be taken to allow adequate time for social interaction within the structure of formal exercise classes, without compromising the underlying training objectives.

Aptitudes

Habit has a strong influence upon exercise behavior (57,58). Thus it can be helpful to build an exercise prescription around the past aptitudes and experiences of the patient, using sporting equipment that may be hidden in the corner of an attic and skills sequestered in a forgotten area of the brain. However, much depends on the personality of the individual. In some instances, the patient's poor current performance of a previously mastered skill can have a negative impact on his or her motivation, and attempts to match performances achieved at an earlier time can occasionally have fatal consequences.

Interests

It is vital that the recommended activities be matched with the interests of the patient—a solitary jogging program is unlikely to be accepted if the person concerned hates jogging and is looking for new social contacts. For such a person, pool or gymnasium exercise, social dancing, and folk games will be a much more appropriate regimen (188). On the other hand, an introverted person may react negatively to the somewhat artificial jollity of an exercise class (104) while showing a positive response to a graded walking program.

Skill and Fitness Levels

The person who drops out of an exercise program is typically obese and a heavy smoker (104,170). This reflects in part the lesser interest of such individuals in all aspects of health, but a further factor may be that the gap between the skill and fitness levels of such participants and the expectations of the instructor is too wide. Attempts to meet program demands are thus unsuccessful, with a negative impact upon both body image and motivation to continued participation (170).

It is sometimes helpful if exercise classes are taught by an older instructor, since such individuals are likely to have more empathy for the problems of the elderly. Specific classes for the obese and for those with low skill levels are further tactics that reduce embarrassment and encourage the setting of goals that the patient perceives as attainable.

Other Motivational Tools

Regular positive feedback is important to motivation. The form of feedback may be physiological (demonstration of an improvement in exercise test scores), psychological (words of encouragement), or symbolic (provision of T-shirts or pins for specific achievements within the capacity of the participants). It may also be helpful to have the patient draw up a decision balance sheet or to contract for the attainment of specific fitness goals (42).

Obstacles to participation should be minimized. As in younger age groups, "lack of time" is a frequently stated reason for failure to achieve the recommended quantity of exercise. Opportunity costs should thus be minimized (Chapter 22) by incorporating as much as possible of the regimen into the normal activities of daily living. For example, the patient should be encouraged to walk rather than drive to the store when buying a newspaper, and to use hand rather than power tools around the home and garden. Failing memory can be countered by telephone reminders and/or provision of specific transport to activity classes, and limited socioeconomic resources should be recognized by minimum-cost programs that avoid demands for the purchase of expensive clothing and equipment.

BENEFITS OF REGULAR PHYSICAL ACTIVITY

Many of the accepted benefits of an active lifestyle apparently have a differing impact as a person ages. For example, regular exercise controls obesity in a younger adult. However, the "ideal" body mass increases with age (5). The cross-sectional data of Hammond and Garfinkel (62) suggest that the actuarial risk associated with a 20% excess of body mass drops from 225% of the standard value in men aged 40–49 years to 119% of standard at an age of 70–79 years. This may reflect not only an approach to the "square" part of the mortality curve, where death becomes inevitable (54) but also an increased influence of lean tissue loss on total body mass and thus "ideal" weight.

The same cross-sectional data suggest an increasingly adverse effect of physical inactivity (from 180% of standard mortality in sedentary men aged 40–49 years and 131% in men aged 50–59 years to 285% in men aged 70–79 years).

However, cross-sectional comparisons can be misleading. For example, those who report that they are still taking heavy exercise at the age of 70–79 years are presumably both a health-conscious and a healthy subsegment of the elderly population, and some of those who are very sedentary may be incapacitated by terminal illnesses. Longitudinal studies (124,131) suggest that regular physical activity has progressively less influence on longevity as a person ages. The survival curves for active and sedentary individuals come together around the age of 80 years (131); in those who are still older, vigorous physical activity may actually shorten life expectancy (97). In this age group, a healthy lifestyle (regular exercise, avoidance of smoking, and a low consumption of saturated fat) has relatively little effect, since many of those with inherited susceptibilities to the various cardiac risk factors have already died.

Particular benefits of exercise in the elderly include (a) the maintenance of function, independence, and life quality; (b) the halting of osteoporotic changes; (c) improvements in metabolic health; (d) social gains; and (e) the relief of depression and anxiety.

Independence and Quality of Life

Not all of the factors that lead to institutionalization are amenable to an increase in habitual physical activity, but an active lifestyle nevertheless has a positive impact on several causes of loss of independence (160,199), including a lack of the aerobic power, muscle strength, and flexibility needed to perform the activities of daily living and the age-related deterioration in cerebral function.

Aerobic Power

Aging is associated with a progressive loss of aerobic power, amounting to 0.4–0.5 ml·kg^{-1}min^{-1} per year. In a sedentary individual, maximal oxygen intake drops below the threshold needed to sustain independent living (12–14 ml·kg^{-1}min^{-1}) soon after the age of 80 years (Fig. 4). In those with an active lifestyle, the handicap of an increase in body mass may be avoided. The rate of loss of maximal oxygen intake is only marginally less than in a sedentary person

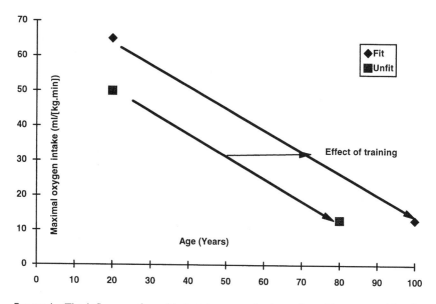

FIGURE 4   The influence of aerobic training upon the loss of aerobic power with aging. In a sedentary subject, the maximal oxygen intake drops by some 0.4–0.5 ml·kg^{-1}min^{-1} each year, dropping below the threshold for independent living (12–14 ml·kg^{-1}min^{-1} soon after the age of 80 years. The rate of aging is only marginally less in an endurance athlete, but because such an individual begins with a much larger reserve, it takes 10–20 years longer for aerobic power to drop below the independence threshold. Involvement in an endurance training program increases the aerobic power of a sedentary person toward the level of the endurance athlete over the course of 2–3 months, so that the trained individual also takes 10–20 years longer to drop below the independence threshold. In effect, training has reduced this aspect of biological age by 10–20 years. (From Shephard, R.J., *Exercise Physiology* B.C. Decker, Burlington, Ontario, and Philadelphia, 1987.)

(149), but because an active person begins with a much larger reserve, it takes 10–20 years longer for aerobic power to drop below the threshold for independence.

An optimal training regimen can increase the maximal oxygen intake of a sedentary 65-year-old by as much as 10 ml·kg^{-1}min^{-1} (171), moving the individual concerned from the sedentary aging line to that for active individuals and giving the equivalent of a 20-year gain in what has been termed "functional aerobic age" (21,73). Moreover, the renewal of physical activity has delayed the crossing of the independence threshold by a similar margin.

Muscle Strength

Independence can also be threatened by a loss of muscle strength. For example, a senior may be unable to lift his or her body mass from a chair or toilet seat unaided. In middle age, continued involvement in training for master's competition does seem to preserve lean mass; but in the oldest competitors, there is a loss of lean tissue despite continued training (76).

Nevertheless, appropriate resistance training can lead to large gains in muscle strength, even in nonagenarians (38,48,157). Part of the response is due to better coordination and a more effective recruitment of motor units, but if the training is continued, some increase in lean tissue also occurs (48).

The active person thus follows a different aging curve than the sedentary individual, and at any given calendar age the active individual remains much further from the limiting values of muscle strength and power needed to sustain independence (103).

Flexibility

A third problem of advancing years is loss of movement at key joints. Flexibility becomes insufficient to allow such daily activities as climbing into a bath or dressing unaided. Exercise does not reverse the aging of collagen, but if the main articulations are taken regularly through their full range of motion, the critical level of function for independent living may be conserved to a much greater age.

Again, exercise cannot restore damaged articular surfaces, but a reduction of obesity and a strengthening of the major muscles around an arthritic hip, knee, or ankle can substantially improve the stability of these joints, enabling continued performance of the vital activities of everyday living.

Cerebral Function

A final important cause of loss of independence is a progressive deterioration of cognition. There is some evidence that mental ability can be conserved by regular physical activity (18,133,159). Possible mechanisms include an increase of cerebral perfusion, alterations in the secretion of cytokines, and alterations in tryptophan metabolism (24,39).

Halting of Osteoporotic Changes

Senescence is associated with a progressive loss of both mineral content and matrix from the bones (25,44,135,178). There is now increasing evidence that manual labor (68) or regular weight-bearing activity during leisure hours can check this process (1,20,27,44,86,172,178), particularly if care is taken to ensure an adequate intake of calcium and vitamins (184). The need to supplement such exercise and good nutrition by hormone replacement therapy in postmenopausal women (44) remains more controversial.

Improvements in Metabolic Health

Regular exercise makes an important contribution to the prevention (26,53,82) and control (8) of obesity, avoiding the loss of lean tissue that characterizes rigorous dieting. The decrease in body mass reduces the load on arthritic joints and increases the effective aerobic and muscular power per kilogram of body mass.

The control of blood glucose is also improved, reducing the susceptibility of the individual to maturity-onset diabetes and its various complications (66).

Finally, the active individual has a lower risk of various cancers, particularly tumors of the descending colon (56,153,185).

Social Gains

For a variety of reasons—including a deterioration of the special senses, the death of friends and relations, and increasing poverty—the social world of the middle old and the very old becomes increasingly circumscribed (159). An exercise class provides a valuable occasion for friendly contact with other people and can thus be helpful in reversing the process of social disengagement.

Relief of Depression and Anxiety

Depression is a common accompaniment of aging. There are obvious physical, social, and economic reasons why the life of a senior citizen can be hard.

Like younger adults, many seniors claim that ''exercise makes them feel better.'' Experimental demonstration of the enhanced mood state is more difficult, although some reports show a lessening of anxiety and a relief of depression, particularly where patients were initially anxious or depressed (89,114,118). Possible mechanisms include not only greater cerebral arousal but also the development of new interests and social contacts, an improved body image, and a greater feeling of self-efficacy.

SAFETY OF EXERCISE

A discussion of the safety of exercise for the elderly inevitably raises potential dangers of physical injury, an adverse response to environmental hazards, and susceptibility to infection and death, all of which must be weighed against the gains in calendar and quality-adjusted life expectancy discussed above.

Most old people are cautious about exercising. With a few exceptions, they err by engaging in too little physical activity. The usual role of the physician is thus to encourage physical activity rather than to beset it with many rigid precautions and constraints. Although there is a transient increase in the risk of a cardiac catastrophe while exercise is being undertaken, an increase in physical activity is clinically justified, since the overall risk for a 24-h period is substantially lower for an active than for an inactive person (141,155,173,183).

Because they are inherently cautious, exercise for the elderly is usually very safe. The main emphasis of any prescription must be to do just a little more than was accomplished safely in the preceding week. If the enhanced program can be accomplished without symptoms, then there is no need for detailed and costly clinical surveillance.

Nevertheless, a few simple precautions should be observed. The recommended intensity of physical activity should normally leave the patient with no more than pleasant tiredness a few hours later. The intensity of activity should be held below a level provoking deep ST-segment depression, frequent premature ventricular contractions, or a decline in systolic blood pressure. Moderation of the prescription is advisable during extremes of hot or cold weather; in both situations, the optimal arrangement is to shift the activity to an air-conditioned facility such as a gymnasium, swimming pool, or indoor shopping mall. An excessive exercise-induced rise of blood pressure should be avoided by prohibiting the prolonged lifting of heavy weights and straining against a closed glottis. Where necessary, the impact stress on the knees and the vertebral column should be reduced by substituting walking and pool exercises for jogging. Violent twisting movements of the spine should also be avoided, as should situations predisposing to a fall (particularly in the frail elderly with disturbances of balance and a history of "drop attacks").

Injury

Well-conceived epidemiological surveys of the injuries sustained in various types of sport and physical activity are infrequent (85,115,129). There is no great difficulty in accumulating sport-specific injury totals, but much less is known about the number of participants and the average period for which they were active.

The participation of office workers in the average North American worksite exercise class has little influence on orthopedic expenditures (162), but in Europe many forms of sport and adventurous activities bring a substantial toll of preventable injuries (115,157).

Leg, ankle, and back injuries apparently occur with some frequency among older individuals who engage in strenuous exercise. Koplan et al. (83) noted that as many as one-third of participants in a 10-km race had been injured in the previous year, and we also found that about a half of master's competitors were injured in a typical year (76); one participant in six had to stop training for 4 weeks or longer. One study of older individuals attending an outpatient sports medicine clinic suggested that the majority of problems were due to overuse (Table 10). Recovery usually occurred with conservative treatment, and surgery was required in only 4% of consultations (105).

Violent muscular efforts and sudden twisting movements seem particularly undesirable: straight-leg lifts, traditional knee bends, and hyperextension of the back have all been criticized as increasing the likelihood of injury (99). Old people generally recognize their limitations; relative to younger people, they are less likely to engage in excessive competition or dangerous pastimes. Nevertheless, safety can be increased further by age-specific athletic leagues, simple modifications of the rules, and skillful "officiating," which slows the pace of a team sport when necessary.

With activities such as jogging, the incidence of stress injuries rises sharply once a certain weekly distance—perhaps 40–50 km—is exceeded (132). The influence of calendar or biological age on this injury threshold is unknown, but

TABLE 10   Types of Injuries Incurred by Older (Mean Age, 57 Years) and Younger (Mean Age, 30 Years) Patients Attending an Outpatient Sports Injury Clinic

	Percentage of sample	
Diagnosis	Older patients	Younger patients
Tendinitis	25.3%	26.2%
Patellofemoral pain	10.9	22.6
Ligament sprain	7.9	12.6
Muscle sprain	7.0	9.0
Metatarsalgia	6.9	2.8
Osteoarthritis	6.6	1.7
Plantar fasciitis	6.6	2.5
Meniscal injury	5.4	1.4
Degenerative disk disease	4.8	1.5
Stress fracture	4.2	11.2
Morton's neuroma	3.2	0.5
Inflammatory arthritis	2.6	1.1
Vascular compartment	1.5	0.3
Bursitis	1.0	2.2
Multiple diagnoses	2.3	1.3
Unknown	3.8	3.1
Total	100.0	100.0

Source: From Ref. 105.

it seems likely that the tolerated distance will decrease with aging. On the other hand, most older people have less inclination to indulge in excessive and obsessional amounts of physical activity, and for this reason the proportion who sustain injury may decrease with age (105).

A number of factors predispose to mechanical injury in an older person. Poor vision, disturbed balance (29), unstable knee and hip joints, reduced foot lift, postural hypotension, and "drop attacks" all increase the likelihood of slips and falls (122). Moreover, osteoporosis increases the likelihood of a fracture if a fall is sustained (15,34,108). Care must thus be taken to provide nonslip flooring, free of obstacles that could trip up the unwary. When an older person is playing competitive games, a reduction in the field of vision plus some impairment of hearing increase the risk of collision with an opponent and/or moving or stationary obstacles (157). Good design of an exercise facility can minimize such risks, although as age increases it may be wise to avoid competitive activities where there is a substantial risk of colliding with an opponent, a racquet, or a ball. Impairments of balance, attacks of unconsciousness, and hypotension on leaving the water all increase the risks of swimming and other forms of aquatic exercise; hand rails and nonslip flooring reduce accidents on the deck, but elderly subjects should avoid swimming alone. Pursuits such as cycling and downhill skiing may also become inappropriate if balance is disturbed.

Environmental Hazards

Aging is associated with increased difficulty in adapting to all forms of stress, including extremes of both heat and cold.

Heat

In hot environments, problems of a low general level of fitness and poor cardiovascular function (111,179) are compounded by a greater rate of body heat production (because mechanical efficiency is reduced, a larger fraction of the total energy expenditure appears as heat and less as usable work). There is also a decreased secretion of sweat at any given intensity of effort (80), and accumulated heat is less readily eliminated because of an increased thickness of subcutaneous fat and poorer vascular regulation (81).

Even moderate physical activity can cause fatalities in the frail elderly who are exposed to extremes of continental heat (119,138). Methods of combating heat and other environmental hazards are discussed in Chapter 1.

Cold

The elderly have an increased vulnerability to the various general, local cutaneous, and local respiratory problems of a cold environment, including hypothermia, chilblains, frostbite, and exercise-induced bronchospasm.

Because of their poor general condition, they cannot work hard enough to avoid hypothermia under cold conditions. An excessive drop in core temperature also reflects difficulty in regulating the distribution of blood flow. Limited intramuscular stores of glycogen and an impaired shivering response further restrict the maximum rate of heat production. There may also be an impaired function of the cutaneous thermoreceptors, an inappropriate setting of the hypothalamic thermostat (30), a lesser capacity for cutaneous vasoconstriction (192), treatment with vasodilator drugs that increase the rate of heat loss (12), and in some instances lack of money to purchase adequate protective clothing and footwear.

One important factor predisposing the elderly to the peripheral effects of cold is a poor circulation (for instance, from peripheral atherosclerosis). Loss of cutaneous sensitivity and a lack of adequate clothing may also contribute to the development of lesions.

Other Environmental Hazards

The frail elderly have an increased vulnerability to the other environmental hazards discussed in Chapter 1. They are unwise to engage in underwater exploration, as even a brief loss of consciousness under water is likely to prove fatal. Care is needed to avoid hypotensive episodes following normal swimming or pool exercises (144).

The moderate hypoxia of mountain resorts (3000–4000 m altitude) may be sufficient to provoke an attack of myocardial ischemia, although the elderly are remarkably tolerant of reduced ambient pressures (198).

Finally, the very old are particularly vulnerable if they attempt to exercise outdoors during episodes of severe air pollution.

Susceptibility to Infection

Strenuous bouts of physical activity impair the function of the immune system, at least briefly (19,78,116). Potential mechanisms include immune responses to tissue microtrauma and a depletion of plasma amino acids. The elderly are unlikely to undertake the volume of exercise associated with immunosuppression in young adults, but because their resting immune function is impaired and they are more susceptible to tissue injury (161), their immune function may be suppressed by a much smaller volume of physical activity.

On the other hand, moderate aerobic training helps to maintain the immune function of older adults (167), and by augmenting the resting activity of natural killer cells, it may protect against both viral infections and the development of neoplasms (101,158).

A combination of incipient diabetes mellitus, a poor blood supply to the skin, poor venous drainage, and a slow rate of healing increases the risk of ulcers, and abrasions, and serious staphylococcal infections of the skin. An older person must thus be very careful to avoid superficial injuries, to ensure cleaning and drying of the skin after exercising, and to monitor the healing of any minor skin injuries that may be incurred.

Risk of Death and Quality-Adjusted Life Expectancy

When a middle-old or very old patient asks a physician for advice about exercising, the common reply is ''Be careful.'' However, such advice largely ignores both the limited life expectancy of the old person and the likely impact of ''being careful'' upon the quality of the remaining years of life.

If there are no close relatives and the prognosis for the ultracareful individual is 9 years of partial dependency, followed by a year of total dependency with a painful death from cancer, then there is much to commend a more carefree attitude to life. Such a philosophy would recognize that, on occasion, vigorous physical activity can not only provoke sudden death (141,155,191) but also increase overall survival prospects. It would also note that an increase in the range of physical pursuits commonly enhances the quality of life, in part by maintaining the physical condition essential to independent living. Above all, it would place more emphasis on the quality than the total length of life (70,156).

It is perhaps dangerous to draw conclusions from cross-sectional data, since the results may be influenced by cohort effects. Nevertheless, the figures of Vuori (191) suggest that the relative risk of provoking sudden death by physical activity is actually lower in a person aged 50–69 years than in a younger individual.

Certainly, the dangers of exercise for the elderly have been greatly overstated, and it may well be the chair- or bed-bound senior citizen who needs regular medical surveillance rather than the person who is prepared to increase his or her physical activity. A moderate, progressive exercise regimen is a safe and desirable recommendation, even for persons of advanced age.

REFERENCES

1. Aloia, J.F., Cohn, S.H., Ostuni, J.A., Cane, R., and Ellis,K., *Ann. Intern. Med.,* 89: 356–358 (1978).
2. American College of Sports Medicine, *Guidelines for Graded Exercise Testing and Exercise Prescription.* Lea & Febiger, Philadelphia, 1975.
3. American College of Sports Medicine, *Guidelines for Graded Exercise Testing and Exercise Prescription,* 5th Ed. Lea & Febiger, Philadelphia, 1995.
4. Andersen, K.L., Shephard, R.J., Denolin, H., Varnauskas, E., and Masironi, R., *Fundamentals of Exercise Testing.* World Health Organization, Geneva (1971).
5. Andres, R., in *Exercise, Fitness and Health* (C. Bouchard, R.J. Shephard, T. Ste-

phens, J. Sutton, and R.J. Shephard, eds.). Human Kinetics, Champaign, Illinois, pp. 133–136 (1990).

6. Badenhop, D.J., Cleary, P.A., Schaal, S.F., Fox, E.L., and Bartels, R.L., *Med. Sci. Sports Exerc.*, 15: 496–502 (1983).

7. Bailey, D.A., Shephard, R.J., and Mirwald, R., *Can. J. Appl. Sport Sci.*, 1: 67–78 (1976).

8. Ballor, D.L., and Keesey, R.E., *Int. J. Obesity*, 15: 717–726 (1991).

9. Barry, H.C., *Geriatrics*, 34: 155–162 (1986).

10. Bassey, E.J., Fentem, P.H., MacDonald, I.C., and Scriven, P.M., *Clin. Sci. Mol. Med.*, 51: 609–612 (1976).

11. Bassey, E.J., Bendall, M.J., and Pearson, M., *Clin. Sci.*, 74: 85–89 (1988).

12. Besdine, R.W., and Harris, T.B., in *Principles of Geriatric Medicine* (R. Andres, E.L. Bierman, and W.R. Hazzard, eds.). McGraw-Hill, New York, pp. 209–217 (1985).

13. Blair, S.N., in *Physical Activity, Fitness and Health* (C. Bouchard, R.J. Shephard, and T. Stephens, eds.). Champaign, Illinois, Human Kinetics, pp. 579–590 (1994).

14. Blanchet, M., in *Exercise, Fitness and Health* (C. Bouchard, R.J. Shephard, T. Stephens, J. Sutton, and B. McPherson, eds.), Human Kinetics, Champaign, Illinois, pp. 127–132 (1990).

15. Block, J.E., and Genant, H.K., in *Physical Activity, Aging and Sports* (R. Harris and S. Harris, eds.). Center for Studies of Aging, Albany, New York, pp. 295–299 (1989).

16. Blumenthal, J.A., Rejeski, W.J., Walsh-Riddle, M., Emery, C.F., Miller, H., Roark, S., Ribisl, P.M., Morris, P.B., Brubacker, P., and Williams, R.S., *Am. J. Cardiol.*, 61: 26–30 (1988).

17. Borg, G., in *Frontiers of Fitness* (R.J. Shephard, ed.). Charles C Thomas, Springfield, Illinois, pp. 280–294 (1971).

18. Bortz, W.M., *J.A.M.A.*, 248: 1203–1208 (1982).

19. Brenner, I.K.M., Shek, P.N., and Shephard, R.J., *Sports Med.* 17: 86–107 (1994).

20. Brewer, V., Meyer, B.M., Keele, M.S., Upton, S.J., and Hagan, R.D., *Med. Sci. Sports Exerc.*, 15: 445–449 (1983).

21. Bruce, R.A., in *Principles of Geriatric Medicine* (R. Andres, E.L. Bierman, and W.R. Hazzard, eds.), McGraw-Hill, New York, pp. 87–105 (1985).

22. Butland, R.J.A., Pang, J., Gross, E.R., Woodcock, A.A., and Geddes, D.M., *Br. Med. J.*, 284: 1607–1608 (1982).

23. Canada Health Survey, *Health and Welfare, Canada*. Ottawa, 1982.

24. Chaouloff, F., *Med. Sci. Sports Exerc.*, 29: 58–62 (1997).

25. Chestnut, C.H., in *Principles of Geriatric Medicine* (R. Andres, E.L. Bierman, and W.R. Hazzard, eds.). McGraw-Hill, New York, pp. 801–812 (1985).

26. Ching, P.L.Y.H., Willett, W.C., Rimm, E.B., Coldlitz, G.A., Gortmaker, S.L., and Stampfer, M.J., *Am. J. Publ. Health*, 86: 25–30 (1996).

27. Chow, R.K., Harrison, J., and Notarius, C., *Br. Med. J.*, 295: 1441–1444 (1987).

28. Chumlea, W.C., Roche, A., and Mukherjee, D., *Nutritional Assessment of the Elderly through Anthropometry*. Ross Laboratories, Columbus, Ohio (1987).

29. Claussen, C-F., and Claussen, E., in *Physical Activity, Aging and Sports* (R. Harris and S. Harris, eds.). Center for Study of Aging, Albany, New York, pp. 123–132 (1989).
30. Collins, K.K., Dore C., Exton-Smith, A.N., Fox, R.H., MacDonald, I.C., and Woodward, P.M., *Br. Med. J.* (i): 353–356 (1977).
31. Comfort, A., *Lancet,* 2: 411–414 (1969).
32. Convertino, V., Hung, J., Goldwater, D., et al., *Circulation,* 65: 134–140 (1982).
33. Cumming, G.R., and Borysyk, L.M., *Med. Sci. Sports,* 4: 18–22 (1972).
34. Cummings, S.R., Nevitt, M.C., Browner, W.S., Stone, K., Fox, K.M., Ensrud, K.E. et al., *N. Engl. J. Med.,* 332: 767–773 (1995).
35. Cunningham, D.A., Rechnitzer, P.A., Pearce, M.E., and Donner, A.P., *J. Gerontol.,* 37: 560–564 (1982).
36. Cunningham, D.A., Rechnitzer, P.A., and Donner, A.P., *Can. J. Aging,* 5: 19–26 (1986).
37. Dambrink, J.H.A., and Wieling, W., *Clin. Sci.,* 72: 335–341 (1987).
38. Davies, C.T.M., and White, M.J., *Gerontology,* 29: 19–25 (1983).
39. Davis, J.M., and Bailey, S.P., *Med. Sci. Sports Exerc.,* 29: 45–57 (1997).
40. DeBusk, R.F., Houston, N., Haskell, W.L., Fry, G., and Parker, M., *Am. J. Cardiol.,* 44: 1223–1229 (1979).
41. DeVries, H., *J. Gerontol.,* 25: 325–336 (1970).
42. Dishman, R., *Exercise Adherence: Its Impact on Public Health,* 2nd ed. Human Kinetics, Champaign, Illinois (1995).
43. Donnelly, J.E., and Sintek, S.S., in *Perspectives in Kinathropometry* (J.A.P. Day, ed.). Human Kinetics, Champaign, Illinois (1986).
44. Drinkwater, B., in *Physical Activity, Fitness and Health* (C. Bouchard, R.J. Shephard, and T. Stephens, eds.). Human Kinetics, Champaign, Illinois, pp. 724–736 (1994).
45. Drygas, W., Jegler, A., and Kunski, H., *Int. J. Sports Med.* 9: 275–278 (1988).
46. Ehsani, A.A., Martin, W.H., Heath, G.W., and Coyle, E.F., *Am. J. Cardiol.,* 50: 246–254 (1982).
47. Era, P., *Scand. J. Soc. Med.,* 39(Suppl.): 1–77 (1987).
48. Fiatarone, M., O'Neill, E.F., Doyle Ryan, N., Clements, K.M., Solares, G.R., Nelson, M.E., Roberts, S.B., Kehayias, J.J., Lipsitz, L.A., and Evans, W.J., *N. Engl. J. Med.,* 330: 1769–1775 (1994).
49. Fitness Canada, *Fitness and Lifestyle in Canada.* Fitness Canada, Ottawa, 1983.
50. Fitness Canada. *Canadian Standardized Test of Fitness,* 4th ed. Fitness Canada, Ottawa (1997).
51. Franklin, B.A., Hellerstein, H.K., Gordon, S., and Timmis, G.C., *J. Cardiopulm. Rehabil.* 6: 62–79 (1986).
52. Frekany, G., and Leslie, D., *Gerontologist,* 15: 182–183 (1975).
53. French, S.A., Jeffery, R.W., Forster, J.L., McGovern, P.G., Kelder, S.H., and Baxter, J.E., *Int. J. Obesity,* 18: 145–154 (1994).
54. Fries, J.F., *N. Engl. J. Med.,* 303: 130–135 (1980).
55. Gandee, R., Hollering, B., Kikukawa, N., Rogers, S., Narraway, A., Newman, I. and Haude, R., in *Physical Activity, Aging and Sports* (R. Harris and S. Harris, eds.). Center for Study of Aging, Albany, New York, pp. 369–373 (1989).

56. Giovannucci, E., Ascherio, A., Rimm, E.B., Coldlitz, G.A., Stampfer, M.J., and Willett, W.C., *Ann. Intern. Med.,* 122: 327–334 (1995).
57. Godin, G., and Shephard, R.J., *Sports Med.,* 10: 103–121 (1990).
58. Godin, G., Valois, P., Shephard, R.J., and Desharnais, R., *J. Behav. Med.,* 10: 145–158 (1987).
59. Gorden, N.F., Levinrad, R.I., Faitelson, H.L. et al., *South Afr. Med. J.,* 64: 169–172 (1983).
60. Grimby, G., Aniansson, A., Danneskold-Samsoe, B., and Saltin, B., *Med. Sci. Sports,* 12: 95 (1980).
61. Hall, D.A. in *Textbook of Geriatric Medicine and Gerontology,* 2nd Ed. (J.C. Brocklehurst, ed.). Churchill Livingstone, Edinburgh, pp. 18–36 (1978).
62. Hammond, E.C., and Garfinkel, L., *Arch. Environ. Health,* 19: 167–182 (1969).
63. Harber, V.J., and Sutton, J., *Sports Med.,* 1: 154–171 (1984).
64. Haslam, D.R.S., McCartney, N., McElvie, R.S., and McDougall, J.D., *J. Cardio-pulm. Rehabil.,* 8: 213–225 (1988).
65. Heikkinen, E., in *Recent Advances in Gerontology* (H. Orimo, K. Shimada, M. Iriki, and D. Maeda, eds.). Excerpta Medica, Amsterdam, pp. 501–503 (1979).
66. Helmrich, S.P., Ragland, D.R., Leung, R.W., and Paffenbarger, R.S., *N. Engl. J. Med.,* 325: 147–152 (1991).
67. Hughes, A.L., and Goldman, R.F., *J. Appl. Physiol.* 29: 153–159 (1970).
68. Jaglal, S.B., Kreiger, N., and Darlington, G.A., *Ann. Epidemiol.,* 5: 321–324 (1995).
69. Jetté, M., Landry, F., Sidney, K.H., and Blümchen, G., *J. Cardiopulm. Rehabil.,* 8: 171–177 (1988).
70. Kaplan, R., in *Behavioral Epidemiology and Disease Prevention* (R. Kaplan and M.H. Criqui, eds.), Plenum Press, New York, pp. 31–56 (1985).
71. Kasch, F., and Kulberg, J., *Scand. J. Sports Sci.,* 3: 59–62 (1981).
72. Kasch, F., Wallace, J.P., and Van Camp, S.P., *J. Cardiopulm. Rehabil.,* 5: 308–312 (1985).
73. Kasch, F.W., Boyer, J.L., Van Camp, S.P., Verity, L.S., and Wallace, J.P., *Age Ageing,* 22: 5–10 (1993).
74. Katz, S., Branch, L.G., Branson, M.H., et al., *N. Engl. J. Med.,* 309: 1218–1224 (1983).
75. Kavanagh, T., Shephard, R.J., Lindley, L.T., and Pieper, M., *Arteriosclerosis,* 3: 249–259 (1983).
76. Kavanagh, T., Lindley, L.J., Shephard, R.J. and Campbell, R., *Ann. Sports Med.,* 4: 55–64 (1988).
77. Kay, C., and Shephard, R.J., *Int. Z. Angew. Physiol.,* 27: 311–328 (1969).
78. Keast, D., Cameron, K., and Morton, A.R., *Sports Med.,* 5: 248–267 (1988).
79. Keber, R.E., Miller, R.A., and Najjar, S.M., *Chest,* 67: 388–394 (1975).
80. Kenney, W.J., and Fowler, S.R., *J. Appl. Physiol.,* 65: 1082–1086 (1988).
81. Kenney, W.L., and Hodgson, J.L., *Sports Med.,* 4: 446–456 (1987).
82. Klesges, R.C., Klesges, L.M., Haddock, C.K., and Eck, L.H., *Am. J. Clin. Nutr.,* 55: 818–822 (1992).

83. Koplan, J.P., Powell, K.E., Sikes, R.K., Shirley, R.W., and Campbell, C.C., *J.A.M.A.*, 248: 3118–3121 (1982).
84. Koszuta, L.E., *Phys. Sportsmed.*, 17(4): 203–206 (1989).
85. Kraus, J.F., and Conroy, C., *Annu. Rev. Public Health*, 5: 163–192 (1984).
86. Krølner, J.P., Toft, B., Nielsen, S.P., and Tondevold, E., *Clin. Sci.*, 64: 541–546 (1983).
87. Kushner, R.F., and Schoeller, D.A., *Am. J. Clin. Nutr.*, 44: 417–424 (1986).
88. Lakatta, E.G., *Physiol. Rev.*, 73: 413–467 (1993).
89. Landers, D.M., and Petruzzello, S.J., in *Physical Activity, Fitness and Health* (C. Bouchard, R.J. Shephard, and T. Stephens, eds.), Human Kinetics, Champaign, Illinois, pp. 868–882 (1994).
90. Lane, N.E., *Bull. Rheum. Dis.*, 41: 5–7 (1992).
91. Lawrence, G., *Aquafitness for Women*. Personal Library, Toronto (1981).
92. Lee, T.H., Shammash, J.B., Ribeiro, J.P., Hartley, L.H., Sherwood, J., and Goldman, L., *Am. Heart J.*, 115: 203–204 (1988).
93. Lenfant, C., and Wittenberg, C.K., *Physical Activity, Aging and Sports* (R. Harris and S. Harris, eds). Center for Study of Aging, Albany, New York, pp. 7–16 (1989).
94. Leon, A., *Med. Clin. North Am.*, 69: 3–20 (1985).
95. Levarlet-Joye, H., and Simon, M., *J. Sports Med. Phys. Fitness*, 23: 8–13 (1983).
96. Lind, A., and McNicol, J.W., *Can. Med. Assoc. J.*, 96: 706–712 (1967).
97. Linsted, K.D., Tonstad, S., and Kuzma, J.W., *J. Clin. Epidemiol.*, 44: 355–364 (1991).
98. Lipsitz, L.A., Wei, J.Y., and Rowe, J.W., *Quart. J. Med.*, 55: 45–54 (1985).
99. MacCallum, M., in *The Coming of Age of Aging* (R.C. Goode and D.J. Payne, eds.). Ontario Heart Foundation, Toronto, pp. 83–111 (1980).
100. McDonough, J., and Bruce, R.A., *J. South Carolina Med. Assoc.*, 65 (Suppl. 1): 26–33 (1969).
101. Mackinnon, L.T., *Sports Med.*, 7: 141–149 (1989).
102. McNamara, P.S., Otto, R.M., and Smith, T.K., *Med. Sci. Sports Exerc.*, 17: 266 (Abstr.) (1985).
103. Makrides, L., Heigenhauser, G.J., McCartney, N., and Jones, N.L., *Clin. Sci.*, 69: 197–205 (1985).
104. Massie, J., and Shephard, R.J., *Med. Sci. Sports*, 3: 110–117 (1971).
105. Matheson, G.O., MacIntyre, J.G., Taunton, J.E., Clements, J.E., Clement, D.B., and Lloyd-Smith, R., *Med. Sci. Sports Exerc.*, 21: 379–385 (1989).
106. Matter, S., Stanford, B.A., and Weltman, A., *J. Gerontol.*, 35: 332–336 (1980).
107. Mazzeo, R.S., Brooks, G.A., and Horvath, S.M., *J. Appl. Physiol*, 57: 1369–1374 (1984).
108. Melton, L.J., in *Biological and Behavioral Aspects of Falls in the Elderly*. National Institute of Aging, Bethesda, Maryland, pp. 17–18 (1984).
109. Mernagh, J.R., Harrison, J.E., Krondl, A., McNeill, K.G., and Shephard, R.J., *Nutr. Res.*, 6: 499–507 (1986).
110. Mertens, D.J., Kavanagh T., Baigrie R.S., Shephard R.J., *Sports Med. Training Rehabil.*, 3: 37–48 (1991).
111. Minson, C.T., and Kenney, W.L., *Med. Sci. Sports Exerc.*, 29: 75–81 (1997).

112. Miyashita, M., Haga, S., and Mizuta, T., *J. Sports Med. Phys. Fitness,* 18: 131–137 (1978).

113. Montoye, H.J., *Physical Activity and Health: An Epidemiological Study of an Entire Community.* Prentice-Hall, Englewood Cliffs, N.J. (1975).

114. Morgan, W.P., in *Physical Activity, Fitness and Health* (C. Bouchard, R.J. Shephard, and T. Stephens, eds.). Human Kinetics, Champaign, Illinois, pp. 851–867 (1994).

115. Nicholl, J.P., Coleman, P., and Williams, C.T., *Injuries in Sport and Exercise.* British Sports Council, London (1993).

116. Nieman, D.C., Johanssen, L.M., Lee, J.W., and Arabatzis, K., *J. Sports Med. Phys. Fitness,* 30: 316–328 (1990).

117. Niinimaa, V., and Shephard, R.J., *J. Gerontol.,* 33: 362–367 (1978).

118. North, T.C., McCullagh, P., and Tran, Z.V., *Exerc. Sport Sci. Rev.,* 18: 379–415 (1990).

119. Oeschli, F.W., and Buechley, R.W., *Environ. Res.,* 3: 277–284 (1970).

120. Oja, P., Kukkonen-Harjula, R., Nieminen, R., Vuori, I., and Passanen, M., *Int. J. Sports Med.,* 9: 45–51 (1988).

121. Ostrow, A.C., and Dzewaltowski, D.A., *Res. Q.,* 57: 167–169 (1986).

122. Overstall, P.W., in *Principles and Practice of Geriatric Medicine,* 2nd Ed. (M.S.J. Pathy, ed.). Wiley, Chichester, England, pp. 1231–1240 (1991).

123. Paffenbarger, R.S., and Lee, I.M., *Res. Q.,* 67 (Suppl. 3): S11–S28 (1996).

124. Paffenbarger, R.S., Hyde, R.T., Wing, A.L., Lee, I-M., and Kampert, J.B., in *Physical Activity, Fitness and Health* Human Kinetics, Champaign, Illinois, pp. 119–133 (1994).

125. Palmore, E.D., in *Physical Activity, Aging and Sports* (R. Harris and S. Harris, eds.). Center for Study of Aging, Albany, New York, pp. 151–156 (1989).

126. Panush, R.S., in *Physical Activity, Fitness and Health* (C. Bouchard, R.J. Shephard, and T. Stephens, eds.). Human Kinetics, Champaign, Illinois, pp. 712–723 (1994).

127. Papazoglou, N.M., Kolokouri-Dervou, E.S., Viaros, P.A., Vassilou, S.V., and Korkodilos, G.A., *Am. J. Cardiol.,* 61: 1146–1147 (1988).

128. Pascale, M., and Grana, W.A., *Phys. Sportsmed.,* 17(3): 157–166 (1989).

129. Pate, R.R., and Macera, C.A., in *Physical Activity, Fitness and Health* (C. Bouchard, R.J. Shephard, and T. Stephens, eds.). Human Kinetics, Champaign, Illinois, pp. 1008–1018 (1994).

130. Paterson, D.H., Shephard, R.J., Cunningham, D., Jones, N.L., and Andrew, G., *J. Appl. Physiol.,* 47: 482–489 (1979).

131. Pekkanen, J., Marti, B., Nissinen, A., Tuomilehto, J., Punsar, S., and Karvonen. M.J., *Lancet,* 1: 1473–1477 (1987).

132. Pollock, M.L., Gettman, L.R., Milesis, C.A., Bahn, D., Durstine, L., and Johnson, R.B., *Med. Sci. Sports,* 9: 31–36 (1977).

133. Powell, R.R., *J. Gerontol.,* 29: 157–161 (1974).

134. Quaglietti, S., and Frolicher, V.F., in *Physical Activity, Fitness and Health* (C. Bouchard, R.J. Shephard, and T. Stephens, eds.). Human Kinetics, Champaign, Illinois, pp. 591–608 (1994).

135. Raab, D.M., and Smith, E.L., *Topics Geriatr. Med.,* 1: 31–39 (1985).

136. Sagiv, M., and Grodjinovsky, A., in *Physical Activity, Aging and Sports* (R. Harris

and S. Harris, eds.). Center for Study of Aging, Albany, New York, pp. 51–55 (1989).

137. Schoutens, A., Laurent, E., and Poortmans, J.R., *Sports Med.,* 7: 71–81 (1989).

138. Schuman, S.H., *Environ. Res.,* 5: 59–75 (1972).

139. Seals, D.R., Hagberg, J.M., Hurley, B.F. et al., *J. Appl. Physiol.,* 57: 1024–1029 (1984).

140. Shephard, R.J., *Eur. J. Cardiol.,* 11: 147–157 (1980).

141. Shephard, R.J., *Ischemic Heart Disease and Exercise,* Croom Helm, London (1981).

142. Shephard, R.J., *Physiology and Biochemistry of Exercise,* Praeger, New York (1982).

143. Shephard, R.J., *J. Cardiovasc. Pulm. Med.,* 12: 29–32 (1984).

144. Shephard, R.J., *CAHPER J.,* 50(6): 2–5, 20 (1985).

145. Shephard, R.J., *Sports Med.,* 2: 348–366 (1985).

146. Shephard, R.J., *Economic Benefits of Enhanced Fitness.* Human Kinetics, Champaign, Illinois (1986).

147. Shephard, R.J., *Fitness of a Nation. Lessons from the Canada Fitness Survey.* Karger, Basel (1986).

148. Shephard, R.J., in *International Perspectives on Adapted Physical Activity* (M. Berridge and G. Ward, eds.). Human Kinetics, Champaign, Illinois, pp. 235–242 (1987).

149. Shephard, R.J., in *Physical Activity and Aging: The Academy Papers* (W.W. Spirduso and H.M. Eckert, eds.). Human Kinetics, Champaign, Illinois, pp. 175–185 (1988).

150. Shephard, R.J., *Fitness in Special Populations.* Human Kinetics, Champaign, Illinois (1990).

151. Shephard, R.J., *Sports Med.* 12: 94–109 (1991).

152. Shephard, R.J., *Body Composition in Biological Anthropology.* Cambridge University Press, London (1991).

153. Shephard, R.J., *Sports Med.,* 15: 258–280 (1993).

154. Shephard, R.J., *Ergonomics,* 38: 617–636 (1995).

155. Shephard, R.J., *Sport Sci. Rev.,* 4: 1–13 (1995).

156. Shephard, R.J., *Quest,* 48: 354–365 (1996).

157. Shephard, R.J., *Physical Activity, Aging and Health.* Human Kinetics, Champaign, Illinois, 1997.

158. Shephard, R.J., *Physical Activity, Immune Function and Health.* Cooper Publications, Carmel, Indiana (1997).

159. Shephard, R.J., and Leith, L. in *Cognitive Change and Aging* (M.L. Howe, ed.). Springer-Verlag, New York, pp. 153–180 (1989).

160. Shephard, R.J., and Montelpare, W.M., *J. Gerontol.,* 43: M86–M90 (1988).

161. Shephard, R.J., and Shek, P.N., *Int. J. Sports Med.,* 16: 1–6 (1995).

162. Shephard, R.J., Corey, P., Renzland, P., and Cox, M., *Can. J. Publ. Health,* 73: 259–263 (1982).

163. Shephard, R.J., Kavanagh, T., Tuck, J., and Kennedy, J., *J. Cardiac Rehabil.,* 3: 321–329 (1983).

164. Shephard, R.J., Berridge, M., and Montelpare, W., *Res. Q.* 61: 326–330 (1990).

165.   Shephard, R.J., Vandewalle, H., Gil, V., Bouhlel, E., and Monod, H., *Med. Sci. Sports Exerc.,* 24: 556–567 (1992).
166.   Shephard, R.J., Kavanagh, T., and Mertens, D.J., *Br. J. Sports Med.* 29: 35–40 (1995).
167.   Shinkai, S., Kohno, H., Kimura, K., Komura, T., Asai, H., Inai, R., Oka, K., Kurokawa, Y., and Shephard, R.J., *Med. Sci. Sports Exerc.,* 27: 1516–1526 (1995).
168.   Sidney, K.H., and Shephard, R.J., *J. Appl. Physiol.,* 43: 280–287 (1977).
169.   Sidney, K.H., and Shephard, R.J., *Br. Heart J.,* 39: 1114–1120 (1977).
170.   Sidney, K.H., and Shephard, R.J., *Med. Sci. Sports,* 8: 246–252 (1977).
171.   Sidney, K.H., and Shephard, R.J., *Med. Sci. Sports,* 10: 125–131 (1978).
172.   Sidney, K.H., Shephard, R.J., and Harrison, J., *Am. J. Clin. Nutr.,* 30: 326–333 (1977).
173.   Siscovick, D., in *Exercise, Fitness and Health* (C. Bouchard, R.J. Shephard, T. Stephens, J. Sutton, and B. McPherson, eds.). Human Kinetics, Springfield, Illinois, pp. 707–713 (1990).
174.   Siscovick, D., Laporte, R.E., and Newman, J.M., *Public Health Rep.,* 100: 180–188 (1985).
175.   Skerlj, B., Brozek, J., and Hunt, F.E., *Am. J. Phys. Anthropol.,* 11: 577–600 (1953).
176.   Smith, E.L., and Gilligan, C., *Phys. Sportsmed.,* 11(8): 91–101 (1983).
177.   Smith, E.L., Reddan, W., and Smith, P.E., *Med. Sci. Sports Exerc.,* 13: 60–64 (1981).
178.   Smith, E.L., Smith, K.A., Gilligan, C., in *Exercise, Fitness and Health* (C. Bouchard, R.J. Shephard, T. Stephens, J. Sutton, and B. McPherson, eds.). Human Kinetics, Champaign, Illinois, pp. 517–528 (1990).
179.   Soltysiak, J., Golec, L., and Soklowski, E., *Acta Physiol. Pol.,* 22: 639–648 (1971).
180.   Stefanick, M.L., and Wood, P.D., in *Physical Activity, Fitness and Health* (C. Bouchard, R.J. Shephard, and T. Stephens, eds.)., Human Kinetics, Champaign, Illinois, pp. 417–431 (1994).
181.   Teraoka, T., *Kobe Med. J.,* 25: 1–17 (1979).
182.   Thomas, S., Cunningham, D.A., Rechnitzer, P.A., Donner, A.P., and Howard, J.H., *Can. J. Sport Sci,* 12: 144–151 (1987).
183.   Thompson, P.D., and Fahrenbach, M.C. in *Physical Activity, Fitness and Health* (C. Bouchard, R.J. Shephard, and T. Stephens, eds.). Human Kinetics, Champaign, Illinois, pp. 1019–1028 (1994).
184.   Tiidus, P., Shephard, R.J., and Montelpare, W.M., *Can. J. Sport Sci.,* 14: 173–177 (1989).
185.   U.S. Surgeon General, *Physical Activity and Health.* U.S. Department of Health and Human Services, Washington, D.C. (1996).
186.   Van Camp, S.P., and Peterson, R.A., *J.A.M.A.,* 256: 1160–1163 (1986).
187.   Van Loan, M., and Mayclin, P., *Hum. Biol.,* 59: 299–309 (1986).
188.   Van Rensel, B., Renson, R., and deMeyer, H., *Int. Rev. Sports Sociol.,* 18: 103–114 (1983).
189.   Viidik, A., *Biomed. Eng.,* 2: 64–67 (1967).
190.   Von Kriegel, W., and Airsherl, W., *Acta Endocrinol.,* 46: 47–64 (1964).
191.   Vuori, I., *Sport Sci. Rev.,* 4(2): 46–84 (1995).

192. Wagner, J.A., Robinson, S., and Marino, R.P., *J. Appl. Physiol.,* 37: 562–565 (1974).
193. Wasserman, K., Beaver, W.L., and Whipp, B.J., *Med. Sci. Sports Exerc.,* 18: 344–352 (1986).
194. Wells, K.F., and Dillon, E.K., *Res. Q.,* 23: 115–118 (1952).
195. Williams, P.T., Wood, P.D., Haskell, W.L., and Vranizan, K., *J.A.M.A.,* 247: 2672–2679 (1982).
196. Wolfel, E.E., and Hossack, K.F., *J. Cardiopulm. Rehabil.,* 9: 40–45 (1989).
197. Yano, K., Reed, D.M., Curb, J.D., Hankin, J.H., and Albers, J.J., *Arteriosclerosis,* 6: 422–433 (1986).
198. Yaron, M., Hultgren, H.N., and Alexander, J.K., *Wilderness Environ. Med.,* 6: 20–28 (1995).
199. Young, D.R., Masaki, K.H., and Curb, J.D., *J. Am. Geriatr. Soc.,* 43: 845–854 (1995).

6

Exercise, Hypertrophy, and Cardiomyopathy in Young and Older Athletes

ROY J. SHEPHARD
University of Toronto
Toronto, Ontario, Canada

THE CONCEPT OF ATHLETE'S HEART

The large hearts of endurance athletes (particularly of rowers, cyclists, and distance runners) (22,57,63) have been recognized from the early days of sports medicine. Many physicians regarded such hypertrophy as a healthy response to prolonged exercise, but others drew a parallel to the large hearts observed in various cardiac pathologies, worrying that the enlargement was a risk factor for sudden death on the sports field "because it indicates undue strain or because of the danger of eventual degeneration" (28).

Recognition of the prevalence of cardiac hypertrophy became more widespread as examination of cardiac radiographs began to supplement such simple clinical approaches as thoracic percussion (20) and detection of a prominent, displaced apical impulse and/or a right ventricular lift (59). Investigators quickly found that the cardiothoracic ratios of many athletes exceeded the supposed normal limit of 0.50 (20,28,66,72). Addition of a lateral radiograph (69) allowed a crude estimation of cardiac volume—values averaged about 700 ml in sedentary young men—but in endurance athletes figures rose to 1000—1100 ml (Fig. 1). Later, radiographic information was supplemented by electrocardiography (ECG) (3) (Fig. 2). Left ventricular hypertrophy was diagnosed if the sum of SV_1 and RV_5 exceeded 35 mm (3.5 mV), and right ventricular hypertrophy if the sum of

223

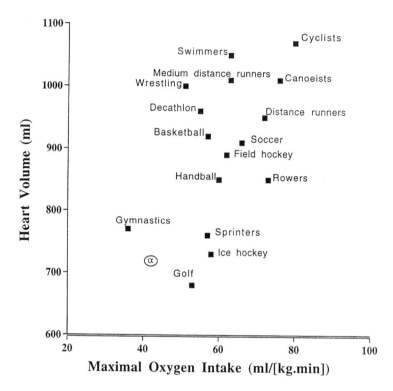

FIGURE 1 Relationship of radiographic estimate of heart volume to maximal oxygen intake. [Based on data of R. Rost, *Athletics and the Heart.* Year Book, Chicago (1987).]

V_1 and V_5 exceeded 10.5 mm (1.05 mV) (88,89). Such criteria suggested that 14 to 85% of athletes had developed left ventricular hypertrophy (24). Other investigators developed more complicated evaluations of the ECG (73,79), but correlations of the ECG findings with radiography, echocardiography, or ultimate postmortem evaluation remained poor (18), in part because hypertrophy of the chest muscles (typical of rowers and other prime candidates for ventricular hypertrophy) attenuated ECG voltages (59).

It remained difficult to distinguish physiological from pathological hypertrophy using chest radiographs and ECG records. One might anticipate a distinction between the firm, rounded radiographic contours of a heart with physiological hypertrophy; the sagging, distended form of a failing myocardium (82); and the irregular contours of a heart with what is generally an asymmetrical hypertrophic cardiomyopathy (30,40). However, in practice, the two ventricles and the atria make varying contributions to the cardiac sihouette, and it is not easy to

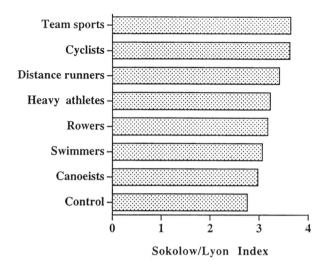

FIGURE 2   Sokolow/Lyon Index for selected categories of athlete. Based on data of R. Rost, Athletics and the Heart. Year Book Publishers, Chicago (1987).

distinguish the left ventricle from the other chambers of the heart. Perhaps the most important distinction is functional. Rheumatic valvular disease and hypertrophic cardiomyopathy each lead to a poor cardiac ejection fraction and a limited effort tolerance. In contrast, the cardiac hypertrophy of the endurance athlete is associated with a large ejection fraction and an outstanding peak power output.

ECHOCARDIOGRAPHIC AND MAGNETIC RESONANCE IMAGING DATA

The introduction of wide-angle, two-dimensional echocardiography (10,39,54) and magnetic resonance imaging (15,52) led to new interest in cardiac enlargement as a possible cause of sudden, exercise-related death. Rost and Hollmann (75) recognized the overdiagnosis of abnormalities and described hypertrophic myocardiopathy as an ''ultrasound-specific'' disease. However, warnings against the dangers of ''athlete's heart'' have continued until quite recently (2,4,38, 55,77).

   The new techniques allowed the cardiologist to make relatively accurate measurements of both wall thicknesses and chamber dimensions (39). Differences were noted between the heart of the endurance athlete, where the thicker ventricular walls seemed an adaptation to volume loading of the heart, and the heart of the resistance athlete, where thickened septal and free walls were not accompanied by any increase in left ventricular end-diastolic diameter (18,54, 87,95,102). The new methods also held the potential to distinguish such forms of hypertrophy from both the distended heart of cardiac failure and the irregularly hypertrophied cardiomyopathic heart. Nevertheless, the limits of resolution for echocardiography, approximately 2 mm for an individual measurement (64), are of a similar order to many of the differences between athletes and sedentary individuals and between those with "healthy" hearts versus those with pathological enlargement of the heart.

As many as 60% of endurance athletes have posterior wall diastolic thicknesses in excess of the originally specified ceiling of 11 mm (25,60,66,72). In consequence, normal limits for diastolic wall thickness have been revised upward to 16 mm (80,92,100), 18 mm (96), or even 19 mm (67). The new standards leave little margin between physiological hypertrophy and the 17- to 18-mm wall thickness typical of the pathological hypertrophy associated with pressure (aortic stenosis, hypertension) or volume (aortic or mitral regurgitation) overload (18). Hypertrophic cardiomyopathy commonly leads to a wall thickness of 20 mm or more, but some patients with this condition also have readings in the range 13–15 mm (44). Nevertheless, as recently as 1991, Pellicia et al. (63) wrote that the distinction between physiological and pathological hypertrophy "depends largely on the judgment whether the magnitude of the left ventricular wall thickness exceeds that expected as a result of athletic training alone." Some 7% of rowers, canoeists, and cyclists in their series had a wall thickness greater than 13 mm. All of these individuals also had enlarged left ventricular end-diastolic dimensions in the range 55 to 63 mm, a useful point of contrast with pathological hypertrophy (where the cavity is usually either normal or smaller than normal) (40).

The large heart of the athlete arises in part because many categories of competitors, such as rowers, have a large body size. If cardiac weight is expressed per unit of lean body mass, the values for resistance athletes become "normal" (32,87,96,102), and in endurance competitors only the septal thickness is greater than in control subjects (21). A further point of distinction between physiological and pathological hypertrophy is that the data of the endurance athlete quickly regress toward "normal" over several weeks or months of reduced training (14).

RATIO OF SEPTAL THICKNESS TO VENTRICULAR CAVITY DIMENSIONS

Some cardiologists have expressed concern if the ratio of interventricular septum to left posterior ventricular wall thickness exceeds 1.3:1 (24). Septal/wall thickness ratios can rise as high as 2.0 in athletes, much higher than in patients with pathological pressure or volume overload (49,72,80), but it has yet to be demonstrated that such ratios are in themselves either dangerous or pathological (24). Some 60% of basketball players (72) and 83% of child swimmers (1) have septal thicknesses that exceed accepted norms for the sedentary population. Oakley and Oakley (56) instanced an athlete who had a ratio of 1.5. Four years after ceasing training, both the ECG and the echocardiogram had returned to ''normal'' limits.

Other cardiologists have argued that the ratio of septal thickness to left ventricular end-systolic or end-diastolic diameter is the most useful diagnostic measurement (8,9,49,61,95). The upper limit of normality for the septal thickness/end-systolic diameter ratio has been set at 0.48 (3 SD above normal values) (24). A discrepancy between cardiac dimensions and ergometric performance (95) and associated abnormalities of cardiac rhythm are other helpful indicators that enlargement is pathological.

HYPERTROPHY AND MYOCARDIAL ISCHEMIA

A propensity for sudden death might arise if hypertrophy led to an altered pathway for conduction of electrical signals within the heart, subvalvular hypertrophy restricted ventricular ejection (thus increasing cardiac work rate), hypertrophy predisposed to myocardial ischemia by increasing the diffusion distance from the coronary vessels to myocardial mitochondria, or abnormalities of ventricular structure limited diastolic filling. Such problems arise mainly if not exclusively in a small group of individuals with congenital myocardial dystrophy (74,76, 90,93,99). This condition is prone to cause a disturbance of the electrical pathway (43,65), mitral regurgitation (80), limited ventricular compliance, poor diastolic filling (10), and/or hypotension (37,48).

However, an increase in heart size *per se* does not predispose the healthy athlete to myocardial ischemia. When the heart hypertrophies, there is a parallel development of the myocardial capillaries, as in hypertrophied skeletal muscle, so that the myocardial blood supply remains at least as good as in a hypotrophic heart. Moreover, determinants of myocardial hypoxia include (a) the relation of myocardial work rate to myocardial oxygen supply, (b) the tension developed in the ventricular wall, and (c) the relative duration of the systolic phase of the cardiac cycle.

The Relation of Myocardial Work Rate to Oxygen Supply

The myocardial work rate is approximated by the product of heart rate and systolic blood pressure. Because of myocardial hypertrophy, the endurance athlete can sustain a larger stroke volume than a less well trained person during vigorous exercise. A given external task can thus be performed at a lower heart rate and a lower cardiac work rate than in a sedentary individual (although during competition, an athlete reaches a much higher work rate than a sedentary person is likely to develop). The athlete's myocardial oxygen consumption is correspondingly reduced at a given external work rate; and during ordinary daily life, the risk of myocardial ischemia is much less than in a sedentary person.

Ventricular Wall Tension

According to the law of LaPlace (as modified for a thick-walled structure), the total tension exerted by the ventricular wall is approximately proportional to the product of intraventricular pressure and the average ventricular radius (83). The large average radius of the hypertrophied ventricle may cause some increase of tension for a given arterial pressure, but because the wall is also much thicker in the athlete than in a sedentary person, the force exerted per unit of wall cross-section at any given intraventricular pressure is lower in the athlete than in the untrained person (83).

Relative Duration of the Systolic Phase

The tension in the ventricular wall is high during systole, irrespective of a person's training status. Myocardial perfusion thus occurs mainly during diastole, giving an advantage to the athlete with a slow heart rate and a longer diastolic phase to the cardiac cycle.

EXERCISE AND SUDDEN DEATH

Fear of cardiac hypertrophy has arisen mainly because of occasional exercise-related deaths in young endurance athletes (2,31,76). Cardiac hypertrophy is often invoked to explain such deaths, and sometimes it is inferred that the condition should have been detected at preparticipation examination (2,11,53,86,98), despite growing evidence that such screening is not cost-effective (15) and indeed rarely succeeds in diagnosing the abnormality.

Exercise-related deaths in young athletes have many causes (2,7,19,74, 94,101). A proportion are due to injury or heat stress. Sometimes there is rupture of a congenital aneurysm in the circle of Willis. Sometimes there is an acute myocarditis due to recent influenza or some other viral infection (12,16,47), possibly associated with overtraining (5,26,29). Sometimes there is evidence of a fatal myocardial ischemia, but this is traced to a previously undetected congenital anomaly such as an abnormal origin of the coronary vessels (6,50,71,74). But where no other obvious pathology is seen, blame is frequently attached to myocardial hypertrophy; it is alleged that this is pathological in extent and has caused myocardial ischemia or led to a fatal arrhythmia. Others maintain that there is little relation between ventricular hypertrophy and sudden death in the absence of an inherited dystrophy with disarray of the myocardial fibers (48); the problem then becomes one of distinguishing a congenital, dystrophic hypertrophy from a physiological hypertrophy.

Hypertrophic cardiomyopathy is often diagnosed on the postmortem finding of an interventricular septal thickness that is "excessive" relative to arbitrary normal standards. However, the dice are then heavily loaded in favor of "proving" that septal hypertrophy is to blame for exercise-induced deaths, since training thickens both the ventricular wall and the interventricular septum, and postmortem examinations are being performed on individuals who have died on the sports field.

In order to establish that septal thickening had pathological significance, it would be necessary to make either a prospective comparison of outcomes between athletes with supposedly normal septa and those with thickened septa, or, alternatively, to carry out a blinded postmortem comparison between athletes who died on the sports field and others at a similar level of training who were killed in traffic accidents. Such a trial is unlikely to take place, since sudden death on the sports field is a rare event and no one group of investigators could accumulate sufficient cases for either type of study. Moreover, although details of athletic involvement would be readily available for a person dying on the sports field, it would be difficult to obtain comparable sports histories for those involved in traffic accidents or indeed to match other aspects of personal lifestyle between the two groups of data.

HYPERTROPHIC CARDIOMYOPATHY AND SUDDEN DEATH

Despite the diagnostic problems noted above, there are frequent claims that hypertrophic cardiomyopathy is the "commonest cause of death" in young athletes (2,4,38,55,91,96). Such statements must be viewed in the context of the overall number of exercise-related deaths in young athletes, which is extremely low. Winget et al. (101) set the total at around a hundred incidents per year in the United States, and Vuori (97) found one death per 11 million h of exercise in Finnish men aged 20–39 years. A recent study of 215, 413 marathon runners disclosed only four exercise-related deaths; three of the four fatalities were in runners aged 32–58 years, and all of these had evidence of coronary atherosclerotic disease. The one young person in this series was aged 19 years, and he had an anomalous coronary artery (45).

An early computerized search of the U.S. literature (7) covering a 50-year period revealed only *four* cardiac incidents that were considered as likely cases of hypertrophic cardiomyopathy! The view that hypertrophic cardiomyopathy is a ''common'' cause of exercise-related death can probably be traced to an early paper by Maron and associates (38). These authors collected case histories on 29 U.S. athletes between the ages of 13 and 30 who had died over a period of several years; 19 of the 29 were said to have hypertrophic cardiomyopathy, although only in 8 of the 19 did the septal/free wall ratio meet the minimum diagnostic criterion of 1.3/1.0. The whole hypothesis was thus founded on some two *possible* cases per year across the United States; plainly, in the absence of a documented family history and histopathology, even these two cases could have been a physiological rather than a pathological hypertrophy. Spirito et al. (91) pointed out that almost all reports concerning hypertrophic cardiomyopathy had come from two reference laboratories. The view that the condition is widely prevalent had arisen, at least in part, from a repeated description of the supposed 19 cases of Maron et al. (38) in a minimum of 25 independent publications, and the suggested prevalence (1 in 500 athletes) (2) seems a gross overestimate.

In one recent report, Maron et al. (46) accumulated 158 sudden exercise-related deaths in athletes under 35 years of age over a period of 10 years; 134 of these incidents apparently had a cardiovascular origin, with the nonendurance sports of basketball and football accounting for 92 of the 134 episodes (68%). One-third of the group were said to represent probable or definite cases of hypertrophic cardiomyopathy, although the diagnostic criteria were relatively weak: a hypertrophied and nondilated ventricle and one other supporting clinical or morphological feature. Even accepting that all of these diagnoses were correct, hypertrophic cardiomopathy would have caused only four to five exercise-related deaths per year in the United States.

Other authors have used even less satisfactory diagnostic criteria, classifying as ''probable hypertrophic cardiomyopathy'' all deaths where the cardiac mass exceeded 400 g in the absence of other systemic, valvular, or cardiac disorders (96). But despite this simplistic approach, the total incidence across the United States was apparently only about five cases per year.

This is not to deny the possibility that an individual who dies while exercising *may* be affected by a variety of extremely rare inherited malformations based on molecular abnormalities in the genes encoding protein molecules of the ventricular sarcomere (30,33,70), with resulting abnormalities of ventricular wall structure. However, even in such individuals the liability to premature death is very variable (34), and the establishment of such a diagnosis requires a clear family history, reinforced by evidence such as cardiac symptoms on exertion, abnormal patterns of left ventricular filling (41), and failure of the cardiac enlargement to regress out of season (42), preferably with demonstration of a characteristic abnormal gene-structure (70) and carefully blinded histopathology in the case of a postmortem diagnosis. In the familial hypertrophic form of cardiomyopathy, ventricular function may be normal or even supranormal (35,36); the dilated form of myopathy is lethal at an earlier age, and there is no particular reason why this form of myopathy should affect endurance athletes; indeed, because of the myocardial dysfunction, an exceptional athletic performance seems unlikely.

BENEFITS OF CARDIAC HYPERTROPHY

Any possible dangers of exercise for the person with ventricular hypertrophy must be weighed carefully against known benefits. The cardiac hypertrophy seen in the endurance athlete is associated with a large stroke volume and thus a large maximal cardiac output and peak oxygen transport. In consequence, any given physical task can be undertaken at a smaller fraction of maximal oxygen intake. Many aspects of exercise-related strain, from the increase of blood pressure to the sense of personal fatigue, are thus less for the person who has developed a large heart and a large maximal oxygen intake.

If cardiac hypertrophy is advantageous for a young person, it becomes even more important in an older individual. Maximal oxygen intake decreases progressively with each year of survival beyond early adult life. In a sedentary person, the loss averages about 500 $\mu l \cdot kg^{-1} min^{-1}$ per year (84). By the age of 75–80 years, a sedentary person often lacks sufficient aerobic power to climb even a slight slope without becoming excessively breathless. Soon, even the minor chores of daily life become very fatiguing, and the last 10 years of life are spent in growing institutional dependency.

It is difficult to determine the true rate of aging of cardiorespiratory function in an endurance athlete because competitors tend to reduce their volume of training as they grow older. Nevertheless, tests on those who have maintained their training programs suggest that the absolute rate of functional loss is a little slower in athletes than in sedentary subjects (27). Given a much higher initial aerobic power and possibly a slightly slower rate of aging, endurance athletes have a large advantage of maximal oxygen intake at any given age, equivalent to a 10- to 20-year reduction in biological age (84). Thus, endurance athletes have the functional capacity to live independently through 90 or even 100 years of age rather than needing institutional support around the age of 80 years. Given that regular exercise has only a minor influence on survival prospects in old age (58, 62), they are also likely to die of acute intercurrent disease before their physical condition has deteriorated to the point that institutional support is required.

IMPLICATIONS FOR HEALTH POLICY

Epidemiological data provide further evidence that cardiac hypertrophy in itself has little importance in terms of health policy. Although endurance athletes on average have larger hearts than sedentary individuals, their life expectancy compares favorably with that of the general population.

Sarna and associates (78) looked at 2613 athletes who had represented Finland in either the Olympic Games or the World or the European championships between 1920 and 1965. The analysis was not flawless, since there are likely to have been differences of personal lifestyle, particularly cigarette consumption, between the endurance athletes and the general population. Moreover, it is uncertain how far either endurance athletes or the participants in power sports continued their exercise involvement in the long interval between competition and the average age at death. Nevertheless, the endurance athletes survived to an average age of 75.6 years, compared with 69.9 years in a sample of 1712 sedentary adults, and 71.5 years for those who had been Finish champions in power sports. There was thus no evidence that endurance competition had shortened life span; rather, survival appeared to be enhanced by such activity.

Independence during old age is a further important argument in favor of developing and maintaining a large heart. Physicians have worried too long about the one in 10 million chance that athletic participation might cause sudden death while neglecting the major public health problem presented by the millions of sedentary senior citizens who require full-time geriatric care. Health policy must be assessed not simply in terms of survival but also in terms of quality-adjusted life expectancy (85). And in such terms, a large, hypertrophied heart offers an important advantage to the active individual.

It is plain that the risk of death during exercise is extremely small. Although we cannot design an entirely satisfactory experiment to see whether cardiac hypertrophy makes any significant contribution to the phenomenon, current evidence suggests that physical activity reduces rather than increases the risk of sudden death.

The recent position statement of the American Heart Association (2) seems ambivalent about the need for mass echocardiography. Although pointing to problems of high cost and false-positive conclusions, it still states that ''This viewpoint, however, is not intended to actively discourage all efforts at population screening.'' Nevertheless, the best practical advice for the young athlete seems to avoid any preparticipation cardiac screening beyond a standard clinical examination, whether the ventricle appears normal or increased in its dimensions. The routine performance of echocardiography and other sophisticated laboratory examinations is likely to do little more than precipitate a chain of costly invasive procedures, with attendant cardiac phobias, unnecessary medical costs, premature cessation of sport involvement, and loss of life insurance coverage (17). Maron et al. (46) found that most of the young athletes who died while exercising had been screened, but cardiovascular disease had been diagnosed in only 5% of those examined, and the diagnosis had been correct in less than 1% of the sample!

Specifically, only 1 of 48 suspected cases of hypertrophic cardiomyopathy had been diagnosed prior to death!

CONCLUSIONS

Although ventricular hypertrophy is sometimes suggested as the commonest cause of sudden, exercise-related death in the young adult, the total number of exercise induced deaths is very small, and their relation to either ventricular hypertrophy in general or cardiomyopathy in particular is far from established. There is a rare inherited form of myocardial dystrophy that predisposes to sudden death, but this is not peculiar to athletes; indeed, because of a low work capacity, those affected are unlikely to have become involved in sport. Detailed preparticipation studies of an athlete's heart are unwarranted unless there is a strong family history of early cardiac death. In general, the ''athlete's heart'' should be viewed as a beneficial adaptation to training, enhancing work capacity and reducing the likelihood of dependency in old age.

SUMMARY

Development of the concept of ''athlete's heart'' is traced through early clinical and radiographic studies to modern echocardiography and magnetic resonance imaging. The lower limits of criteria for the diagnosis of a ''pathological'' enlargement of the heart have repeatedly been revised in an upward direction, as the prevalence of large hearts has been recognized among healthy competitors in both endurance and power sports. Belief that hypertrophic cardiomyopathy is the commonest cause of sport-related death is traced to acceptance of weak diagnostic criteria and frequent republication of details obtained on a very small group of cases. The existence of a congenital myocardial dystrophy is well established, but the condition is extremely rare and has no particular predilection for athletes. Genetically based screening tests may become available in the future, but the exclusion of young adults from sport participation on echocardiographic evidence of cardiac hypertrophy appears costly, ineffective, and inappropriate. For most people, the development of a large heart is not a pathological sign; rather, it is a desirable outcome that will enhance performance on the sports field and allow longer independence in old age. The screening of participants in school and university sports programs should thus be limited to a competent history and physical examination.

ACKNOWLEDGMENT

Dr. Shephard currently receives funding as the Canadian Tire Acceptance Limited Resident Scholar in Health Studies at Brock University.

REFERENCES

1. Allen, H.D., Goldberg, S.J., Sahn, D., Schy, N., and Wojcik, R., *Circulation,* 55: 142–155 (1976).
2. American Heart Association, *Med. Sci. Sports Exerc.,* 28: 1445–1452 (1996).
3. Bramwell, C., and Ellis, R., *Q. J. Med.,* 24: 329–346 (1931).
4. Brandenburg, R.O., *J. Am. Coll. Cardiol.,* 15: 962–964 (1990).
5. Cabinian, A.E., Kiel, R.J., Smith, F., Ho, H.K.L., Khatib, R., and Reyes, M.P., *J. Lab. Clin. Med.,* 115: 454–462 (1990).
6. Cheitlin, M., DeCastro, C., and McAllister, H., *Circulation,* 50: 780–787, 1974.
7. Chillag, S., Bates, M., Voltin, R., and Jones, D., *Phys. Sports Med.,* 18 (3): 89–94 (1980).
8. Colan, S.D., Sanders, S.P., and Borow, K.M., *J. Am. Coll. Cardiol.,* 9: 776–783 (1987).
9. Dickhuth, H.H., Röcker, K., Hipp, A., Heitkamp, H.C., and Keul, J., in *Kardiologie im Sport* (R. Rost and F. Webering, eds.). Deutscher Arzte Verlag, Cologne, pp. 132–145 (1987).
10. Dickhuth, H.H., Jakob, E., Staiger, L., and Keul, J., *Int. J. Sports Med.,* 4: 21–26 (1983).
11. Dickhuth, H.H., Röcker, K., Hipp, A., Heitkamp, H.C., and Keul, J., *Int. J. Sports Med.,* 15: 273–277 (1994).
12. Drory, Y., Kramer, M.R., and Lev, B. *Med. Sci. Sports Exerc.* 23: 147–151 (1991).
13. Durand, J.B., Bachinski, L.L., Beiling, L. et al., *Circulation,* 92: 3387–3389 (1995).
14. Ehsani, A.A., Hagberg, J.M., and Hickson, R.C., Am. J. *Cardiol.,* 42: 52–56 (1978).
15. Fleck, S.J., Henke, C., and Wilson, W., *Int. J. Sports Med.,* 10: 329–333 (1989).
16. Francis, G.S., *Phys. Sportsmed.,* 23 (7): 63–83 (1995).
17. Franklin, B., and Kahn, J.K., *Sports Sci. Rev.,* 4: 85–105 (1995).
18. George, K.P, Wolfe, L.A., and Burggraf, G.W., *Sports Med.,* 11: 300–331 (1991).
19. Goodman, J.M., *Sports Sci. Rev.,* 4: 14–30 (1995).
20. Gott, P.H., Roselle, H.A., and Crampton, R.S., *Arch. Int. Med.,* 122: 340–344 (1968).
21. Hagan, R.D., Laird, W.P., and Gettman, L.R., *J. Cardiopulm. Rehabil.,* 5: 554–560 (1985).
22. Henschen, S., *Skilanglauf und Skiwettlauf: Eine medizinische Sport Studie* Jena: Mitt. med. Klin. Uppsala, 1899 (cited by Rost and Hollmann, Ref. 75).
23. Hillis, W.S., McIntyre, P.D., Maclean, J., Goodwin, J.F., and McKenna, W.J., *Br. Med. J.,* 309: 657–660 (1994).
24. Huston, T.P., Puffer, J.C., and Rodney, W.M., *N. Engl. J. Med.,* 313: 24–32 (1985).
25. Ikäheimo, M.J., Palatsi, I.J., and Takkunen, J.T., *Am. J. Cardiol.,* 44: 24–30 (1979).

26. Ilbäck, N.G., Fohlman, J., and Friman, G., *Am. Heart J.,* 117: 1298–1302 (1989).
27. Kavanagh, T., Mertens, D.J., Metosevic, V., Shephard, R.J., and Evans, B., *Clin. J. Sports Med.,* 1: 72–88 (1989).
28. Keys, A., and Friedell, H.L., *Science,* 88: 456–458 (1938).
29. Kiel, R.J., Smith, F.E., Chason, J., Khatib, R., and Reyes M.D., *Eur. J. Epidemiol.,* 5: 348–350 (1989).
30. Klues, H.G., Schiffers, A., and Maron, B.J., *J. Am. Coll. Cardiol.,* 26: 1699–1708 (1995).
31. Kohl, H.W., and Powell, K.E., *Sports Med.,* 17: 209–212 (1994).
32. Longhurst, J.C., Kelly, A.R., Gonyea, W.J., and Mitchell, J.H., *J. Appl. Physiol.,* 48: 154–162 (1980).
33. Marian, A.J., Kelly, D., Mares, A., Fitzgibbons, J., Caira, T., Qun-Tao, Hill, R., Perryman, B.J., and Roberts, R., *J. Sports Med. Phys. Fitness,* 34: 1–10 (1994).
34. Marian, A.J., Mares, A., Kelly, D.P. et al., *Eur. Heart J.,* 16: 368–376 (1995).
35. Marian, A.J., and Roberts, R., *Circulation,* 92: 1336–1347 (1995).
36. Marian A.J., and Roberts, R., *Annu. Rev. Med.,* 46: 213–222 (1995).
37. Maron, B.J., *Phys. Sportsmed.,* 21 (9): 83–91, 1993.
38. Maron, B.J., Roberts, W.C., McAllister, H.A., Rosing, D.R., and Epstein, S.E., *Circulation,* 62: 218–229 (1980).
39. Maron, B.J., Gottdiener, J., Bonow, R.O., and Epstein, S.E., *Circulation,* 63: 409–418 (1981).
40. Maron, B.J., Bonow, R.O., Cannon, R.O., Leon, M.B., and Epstein, S.E., *N. Engl. J. Med.,* 316: 780–789, 1987.
41. Maron, B.J., Spirito, P., Green, K.J., Wesley, Y.E., Bonow, R.O., and Arce, J., *J. Am. Coll. Cardiol.,* 10: 733–742 (1987).
42. Maron, B.J., Pellicia, A., Spataro, A., and Granata, M., *Br. Heart J.,* 69: 125–128, 1993.
43. Maron, B.J., Isner, J.M., and McKenna, W.J., *Med. Sci. Sports Exerc.,* 26: S261–S267 (1994).
44. Maron, B.J., Pellicia, A., and Spirito, P., *Circulation,* 91: 1596–1601 (1995).
45. Maron, B.J., Poliac, L.C., and Roberts, W.C., *J. Am. Coll. Cardiol.,* 28: 428–431 (1996).
46. Maron, B.J., Shirani, J., Poliac, L.C., Mathenge, R., Roberts, W.C., and Mueller, F.C., *J.A.M.A.,* 276: 199–204, 1996.
47. McCaffrey, F.M., Braden, D.S., and Strong, W.B., *Am. J. Dis. Child.,* 145: 177–183, 1991.
48. McKenna, W.J., and Camm, A.J., *Circulation,* 80: 1489–1492 (1989).
49. Menapace, F.J., Hammer, W.J., Ritzer, T.F., Kessler, K.M., Warner, H.F., Spann, J.F., and Bove, A.A., *Med. Sci. Sports Exerc.,* 14: 72–75 (1982).
50. Menke, D., Waller, B., and Pless, J., *Chest,* 88: 299–301 (1985).
51. Michels, V.V., Moll, P.P., Miller, F.A. et al., *N. Engl. J. Med.,* 326: 77–82 (1992).
52. Milliken, M.C., Stray-Gundersen, J., Pesjock, R.M., Katz, J., and Mitchell, J.H., *Am. J. Cardiol.,* 62: 301–305 (1988).
53. Mitten, M.J., and Maron, B.J., *Med. Sci. Sports Exerc.,* 26: S238–S241 (1994).
54. Morganroth, J., Maron, B.J., Henry, W.L., and Epstein, S.E., *Ann. Intern. Med.,* 82: 521–524 (1975).

55. Nienhaber, C.A., Hiller, S., Spielmann, R.P., Geiger, M., and Kuck, H., *J. Am. Coll. Cardiol.,* 15: 948–955 (1990).
56. Oakley, D.G., and Oakley, C.M., *Am. J. Cardiol.,* 50: 985–989 (1982).
57. Osler, W., *The Principles and Practice of Medicine.* New York: Appleton, p. 635 (1892).
58. Paffenbarger, R.S., Hyde, R.T., Wing, A.L., Lee, I-M., and Kampert, J.B., in *Physical Activity, Fitness and Health* (C. Bouchard, R.J. Shephard, and T. Stephens, eds.). Human Kinetics, Champaign, Illinois, pp. 119–133 (1994).
59. Park, R.C., and Crawford, M.H., *Curr. Probl. Cardiol.,* 10: 1–73 (1985).
60. Parker, B.M., Londeree, B.R., Cupp, G.V., and Dubiel, J.P., *Chest,* 73: 376–381 (1978).
61. Pearson, A.C., Schiff, M., Mrosek, D., Labovitz, A.J., and Williams, G.A., *Am. J. Cardiol.,* 58: 1254–1259 (1986).
62. Pekkanen, J., Marti, B., Nissinen, A., Tuomilehto, J., Punsar, S., and Karvonen, M.J., *Lancet,* 1: 1473–1477 (1987).
63. Pellicia, A., Maron, B.J., Spataro, A., Proschan, M.A., and Spirito, P., *N. Engl. J. Med.,* 324: 295–301 (1991).
64. Perreault, H., and Turcotte, R.A., *Sports Med.,* 17: 288–308 (1994).
65. Pye, M.P., and Cobbe. S.M., *Cardiovasc Res.,* 26: 740–750, 1992.
66. Raskoff, W.J., Goldman, S., and Cohn, K., *JAMA,* 236: 158–162 (1976).
67. Reguero, J.J.R., Cubero, G.I., de la Iglesia, J.L., Terrados, N., Gonzalez, V., Cortina, R., and Cortina, A., *Eur. J. Appl. Physiol.,* 70: 375–378 (1995).
68. Reichek, N., and Devereux, R.B., *Circulation,* 63: 1391–1398 (1981).
69. Reindell, H., König, K., and Roskamm, H., *Functionsdiagnostik des gesunden und kranken Herzens.* Stuttgart: Thieme, 1966.
70. Roberts, R., *Sports Med,* 23: 1–10 (1997).
71. Roberts, W., Siegel, R., and Zipes, D., *Am. J. Cardiol.,* 49: 863–868, 1982.
72. Roeske, W.R., O'Rourke, R.A., Klein, H., Leopold, G., and Karliner, J.S., *Circulation,* 53: 286–292 (1976).
73. Romhilt, D.W., and Estes, E.H., *Am. Heart J.,* 75: 752–758 (1968).
74. Rosenzweig, A., Watkins, H., Hwang, D-S., Miri, M., McKenna, W., Traill, T.A., Seidman, J.G., and Seidman, C.E., *N. Engl. J. Med.,* 325: 1753–1760 (1991).
75. Rost, R., and Hollmann, W. in *Endurance in Sport* (R.J. Shephard, and P.O. Åstrand, eds.). Blackwell, Oxford, pp. 438–451 (1992).
76. Sadaniantz, A., and Thompson, P.D., *Sports Med.,* 9: 199–204 (1990).
77. Sandric, S., in *Sports Cardiology* (T. Lubich and A. Venerando, eds.). Aulo Gaggi, Bologna, pp. 707–716 (1980).
78. Sarna, S., Sahi, T., Koskwenvuo, M., and Kaprio, J., *Med. Sci. Sports Exerc.,* 25: 237–244 (1993).
79. Scott, R.C., *Cardiovasc. Clin.,* 5: 219–254 (1973).
80. Shapiro, L.M., *Br. Heart J.,* 52: 130–135 (1984).
81. Shapiro, L.M., *Sports Med.,* 4: 239–244 (1987).
82. Shephard, R.J., *Endurance Fitness.* University of Toronto Press, Toronto (1969).
83. Shephard R.J., *Physiology and Biochemistry of Exercise.* Praeger, New York (1982).
84. Shephard, R.J., *Physical Activity and Aging,* 2nd Ed. Croom Helm, London (1987).

85. Shephard, R.J., *Quest,* 48: 354–365 (1996).
86. Smith, D.M., *Sports Med.,* 18: 293–300 (1994).
87. Snoeckx, L.H.E.H., Abeling, H.F.M., Lambregts, J.A.C., Schmitz, J.J.F., Verstappen, F.T.J., and Reneman, R.S., *Med. Sci. Sports Exerc.,* 14: 428–434 (1982).
88. Sokolow, M., and Lyon, T.P., *Am. Heart J.,* 37: 161–186 (1949).
89. Sokolow, M., and Lyon, T.P., *Am. Heart J.,* 38: 273–294 (1949).
90. Solomon, S.D., Jarcho, J.A., McKenna, W., Geisterfer-Lowrance, A., Germain, R., Salerni, R., Seidman, J.G., and Seidman, C.E., *J. Clin. Invest.,* 86: 993–999 (1990).
91. Spirito, P., Chiarella, F., Carratino, L., Berisso, M.Z., Bellotti, P., and Vecchio, C., *N. Engl. J. Med.,* 320: 749–755 (1989).
92. Spirito, P., Pelliccia, A., Proschan, M.A., Granata, M., Spataro, A., Bellone, P., Caselli, G., Biffi, A., Vecchio, C., and Maron, B.J., *Am. J. Cardiol.,* 1994; 74: 802–806.
93. Thierfelder, L., Watkins, H., MacRae, C., Lamas, R., McKenna, W., Vosberg, H-P., Seidman, J.G., and Seidman, C.E., *Cell,* 77: 701–712 (1994).
94. Torg, J. in *Current Therapy in Sports Medicine 3* (J. Torg and R.J. Shephard, eds). Mosby–Year book, Philadelphia, pp. 8–10 (1995).
95. Urhausen, A., and Kindermann, W., *Sports Med.,* 13: 270–284 (1992).
96. Van Camp, S.P., Bloor, C.M., Mueller, F.O., Cantu, R., and Olson, H.G., *Med. Sci. Sports Exerc.,* 27: 641–647 (1995).
97. Vuori, I., *Sport Sci. Rev.,* 4: 46–84, 1995.
99. Weidenbener, E.J., Krauss, M.D., Waller, B.F., and Talierco, C.P., *Clin. J. Sports Med.,* 5: 86–89 (1995).
99. Wigle, E.D., Sasson, Z., Henderson, M.A., Ruddy, T.D., Fulop, J., Rakowski, H., and Williams, W.G., *Progr. Cardiovasc. Dis.,* 28: 1–83 (1985).
100. Williams, C.C., and Bernhardt, D.T., *Sports Med.,* 19: 223–234 (1995).
101. Winget, J.P., Capeless, M.A., and Ades, P.A., *Sports Med.,* 18: 375–383 (1994).
102. Zeppilli, S., Sandric, S., Cecchiti, F., Spataro, A., and Fanelli, R., in *Sports Cardiology* (T. Lubich and A. Venerando, eds.). Aulo Gaggi, Bologna, pp. 723–734 (1980).

7

Exercise and the Female Cardiac Patient

JACK M. GOODMAN and LORI D. KIRWAN
University of Toronto
Toronto, Ontario, Canada

INTRODUCTION

Cardiovascular disease is no longer considered a chronic disease unique to men. Among the older female population, it is *the* leading cause of death. In fact, cardiovascular diseases of all types have killed more women than men on an annual basis for more than 15 years, and annually such diseases account for more than twice as many fatalities as all cancers combined. Nevertheless, most women do not consider coronary artery disease (CAD) a major health risk, particularly in later life. In spite of a significant reduction in CAD mortality in men since 1975, the mortality rates for women remains stubbornly high, having declined only 50% as much as that of men. The delay in clinical manifestation of CAD until later life complicates treatment strategies. Male-female ratios for death rates remain between 3.4 and 4.3 for those aged 45–64 years but drop to less than 2.0 in some countries after the age of 65 years (1). Those aged 35–64 years still experience a low non-fatal infarction rate (0.2% per year), but by the age of 70, CAD is manifest in 15–20% of all women (2).

Aside from gender differences in the presentation of symptoms, manifestation of the disease, and treatment, there is a paucity of information to guide the practitioner regarding the roles of primary and secondary prevention of CAD for the female patient. This is particularly true with respect to exercise interventions. Only recently have studies explored possible gender differences in cardiovascular responses to acute and chronic exercise. A growing literature suggests that women and men may have similar physiological responses to training yet differ significantly in psychosocial needs during the rehabilitation process. To date, in excess of 5200 patients have been included in reviews and meta-analyses of cardiac rehabilitation intervention trials, yet women represent less than 3% of the total sample (3). This gender bias is not confined to cardiac rehabilitation. It remains a critical factor in the clinical assessment and treatment of CAD in general. For example, there appears to be a significant gender bias in referral to tertiary-care hospitals (4) and in enrollment patterns of cardiac rehabilitation programs (500 sampled) in the United States (3). More disturbing is the lack of information regarding women who have participated in a cardiac rehabilitation program.

This chapter highlights key issues relating to the female cardiac patient, from the challenges involved in CAD diagnosis to the application of exercise as a key intervention in primary and secondary prevention.

CLINICAL ASSESSMENT AND TREATMENT: GENDER DIFFERENCES

Clinical Presentation

Women with CAD present with different characteristics than men. In general, women have more comorbidity, a worse prognosis, and higher death rates after myocardial infarction (5). In addition, they are more likely to present with angina pectoris as their initial symptom of CAD (65 versus 35% of men), and fewer women than men (29 versus 43%) develop a myocardial infarction (MI) as their first manifestation of ischemic heart disease (6). Women appear to be more likely than men to sustain an unrecognized MI, which is typically diagnosed during a subsequent routine medical examination (6). The tendency of women to delay seeking medical attention following a coronary event (e.g., MI) may contribute to their higher fatality rate (7). They show an adverse experience for cardiac sudden death (36% of women die of sudden cardiac death) (6), death within 60 days of MI, and death within 1 year following an event (39 versus 31%) (8). Age is another factor that distinguishes the genders in CAD. Women are typically 7–10 years older than men when an MI occurs, and this may contribute to a more extensive lesion (7). Collectively, these factors complicate strategies for both diagnosis and treatment in female patients.

Assessment and Treatment

There are considerable gender differences in the tactics used to assess CAD; consequently less aggressive treatment is afforded to the female patient. This tendency has been termed the "Yentl phenomenon" (9), named after the nineteenth-century tale in which a woman named Yentl could gain acceptance for talmudic study only by disguising herself as a man. Do women receive different diagnostic tests solely on the basis of gender? It appears so. Women are more likely to receive noninvasive rather than invasive assessment for CAD, and even if a positive result is obtained, women are scheduled for further testing 20% less often than men (10). Despite greater relative CAD morbidity and mortality in women, they are referred for revascularization procedures less often than men (11), possibly owing in part to the higher operative mortality and excess of peri-procedural complications in female patients. It is more probable, however, that diagnostic criteria currently used to evaluate clinical status and suitability for surgery are either inappropriate for women or are applied less aggressively than in the treatment of men. This is also true of routine procedures such as coronary angiography, which are performed much less often in women (11–13). Even when age and severity of disease are controlled for, women receive fewer procedures, including bypass surgery and coronary angiography, than do men. Of great concern is the finding that even when data are controlled for disease severity, women still die from CAD in hospital more often than men (14). Complicating the issue and relieving the burden of treatment bias to some extent is the finding that although angiography is positive in over 80% of men with angina, only 50% of women with similar symptoms demonstrate diseased vessels (15,16). The triad of angina pectoris, a positive exercise electrocardiogram, and angiographically patent coronary arteries is widely referred to as *syndrome X* (17).

The presence of ischemia without angiographic evidence of disease implies that coronary angiography may not be the ideal method of diagnosing CAD, especially in women. In addition, the cost and risks associated with coronary angiography have led to greater interest in noninvasive methods for the diagnosis and screening of women with suspected CAD (11). However, noninvasive methods of assessment [e.g., electrocardiography (ECG)] have less predictive value in women than men (18); there is a high rate of false positive tests when exercise ECG tests are compared with coronary angiograms in women. Given that women are more likely to have microvessel atherosclerotic lesions that would not be detected by angiography, use of the angiogram as a "gold standard" for comparison may not be appropriate. It is also likely that the standard reporting of scores for angina and other symptoms has not been adequately validated for women, limiting the usefulness of such scores in diagnosis.

Changes in left ventricular function during exercise have been used for noninvasive detection of CAD; however, these may also be of limited value. Like the exercise ECG, the exercise ejection fraction (EF) may have a poor specificity for women (19,20), thus limiting the clinician's ability to assess and treat this condition. Although the sensitivity and specificity of exercise ECGs can increase when the information is combined with the results of thallium-201 scintigraphy, the procedure remains less accurate in women than in men, largely because of

TABLE I   Factors Influencing Diagnosis and Treatment in Women with Coronary Artery Disease

Primary factor	Implications
Age	Advanced disease, with more complications
Onset of coronary artery disease seen later in life	
Delayed presentation to primary care physician	
Comorbidity	Treatment and follow-up more complex
Greater likelihood of diabetes mellitus, hypertension	
Manifestation of symptoms	Inadvertent denial of treatment
Different symptomatology from men	Less aggressive treatment
Denial of symptoms	
Absence of symptoms despite positive findings	
Sensitivity/specificity tests	May require ancillary testing (imaging) to enhance accuracy of diagnosis
Lower for noninvasive testing	
Presence of "syndrome X"	
Surgical/diagnostic outcomes	May reflect selection bias and/or increased comorbidity
Increased complications	
Increased hospital death rates	Limited clinical information to guide treatment

the greater attenuation of myocardial radioactivity (and hence image quality) by breast tissue. Soft tissue attenuation often produces apparent nonuniform anterior and septal distributions of perfusion (11).

In summary, women display several characteristics that make the diagnosis and treatment of CAD more difficult (Table 1). They are more likely to present with acute MI and less likely to be referred for an angiogram and revascularization procedures. Diagnostic testing in women is difficult because of the lack of sensitivity and specificity of current techniques.

RISK FACTORS FOR CORONARY ARTERY DISEASE IN WOMEN

The impact of various CAD risk factors differs between women and men, some risk factors being unique to women (15). In men, the primary CAD risk factors include physical inactivity, hypertension, an atherogenic cholesterol profile, and cigarette smoking. Secondary risk factors include a family history of heart disease, race, advanced age, high plasma triglyceride levels, and diabetes mellitus (21). However, in women, the relative importance of the primary risk factors is unclear, possibly owing to differences in their prevalence. Obesity, diabetes, and high blood lipids appear to play a larger role in the development of CAD in women than in men (21).

Complicating the analysis of risk factors and CAD incidence is the well-described postmenopausal increase in risk factors (22,23). The so-called pre-menopausal protective factor is linked to normal ovarian function, since pre-menopausal oophorectomy leads to a high risk for MI (24). Estrogen deficiency has been identified as a CAD risk factor in postmenopausal women, and estrogen replacement therapy (ERT) has now emerged as a significant deterrent of CAD in older women (25–27).

ESTROGEN DEFICIENCY AND CAD IN WOMEN: AN EMERGING THERAPY?

There are likely several mechanisms by which estrogens reduce CAD risk (Table 2). Still, the effect of ERT on cardiovascular morbidity and mortality has not been completely clarified, and no consensus has been reached regarding its use. Benefits for the heart and bone tissue must be set against an increased risk of cancer. The wide variation in experimental designs and in the size and characteristics of study populations—together with intertrial differences in hormone formulations, treatment regimens, and duration of estrogen administration—have produced conflicting recommendations. It is clear that benefits exist (risk reduction), but individual clinical status dictates treatment—not a clinically accepted protocol. Most epidemiological studies (meta-analyses) indicate as much as a 60% reduction in risk for CAD in estrogen-treated women (25–27). The addition of progestin does not appear to attenuate the cardioprotective effects of postmenopausal estrogen therapy.

The strongest effects relate to the favorable effect of unopposed estrogen on lipoprotein metabolism (Fig. 1); this increases levels of high-density lipoprotein cholesterol (HDL-C) and decreases those of low-density lipoprotein cholesterol (LDL-C) (23,28,29).

Estrogen replacement therapy may have its greatest effect directly on the atherosclerotic process in the arterial wall, acting independently of changes in plasma lipoprotein levels (30). However, estrogen also decreases the accumulation of LDL-C in to the arterial wall (30), and protection against oxidation damage due to LDL remains an important contributing factor. The decrease in LDL-C is partially due to an estrogen-enhanced hepatic clearance of atherogenic LDL particles by upregulated LDL receptors (31). Estrogen increases HDL levels, thus removing lipoprotein from the blood. The improvement in HDL-C levels is due

TABLE 2 Acute and Chronic Effects of estrogen Replacement Therapy

Organ/system	Acute effect	Chronic effect
Lipoprotein plasma levels	—	↑HDL; ↓LDL; ↓athero-genic remnants (34)
Blood vessel wall	—	↓LDL oxidation (39) ↓LDL accumulation in arterial wall (30)
Coagulation	Remote risk of ↑coronary artery thrombosis (depending on dose and clinical presentation of woman) (71) No consensus	Not known
Glucose metabolism		↓Insulin resistance (72)
Cardiac	↑Coronary blood flow (73) ↓Inotropic (nonconclusive) (74)	Not known
Peripheral vascular	↑Vasodilation (endothelium-dependent and -independent (75)	Not known
Reproductive tissue (endometrium, breast)	—	↑Risk of endometrial hyperplasia (76) ↑Risk of endometrial cancer (77) ↑Risk of breast cancer (77)

Note: Effects vary with (a) route of administration (oral versus transdermal), (b) presence of progesterone, (c) in vivo versus in vitro assessment.
↑ = increase; ↓ = decrease.

to an estrogen-induced decrease in the activity of hepatic lipase, the enzyme that promotes the hepatic uptake of cholesterol from HDL particles (32). Estrogen also improves postprandial lipid metabolism—an important observation, because humans are in the postprandial state at most times (32). In the postprandial state, the intestine produces chylomicron particles, which contain triacylglycerols and cholesterol. In the postprandial state, these "intestinal lipoproteins" compete with hepatic lipoproteins for removal from the circulation, and this can lead to the accumulation of remnant particles in the bloodstream. The remnants are atherogenic (33) and can be taken up by both the arterial wall and macrophages. The atherogenicity of these remnants is further increased through a transfer of cholesterol from HDL to the remnants, thus decreasing the concentration of

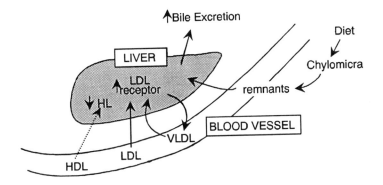

FIGURE I   Effects of estrogen on lipoprotein metabolism. A high rate of traffic is shown by broad lines, a low rate of traffic by dashed lines. Estrogen increases removal of chylomicron remnants and LDL from the blood and decreases the removal of HDL. HL-hepatic triglyceride lipase, which changes inversely with HDL concentrations.

HDL-C. Estrogens reduce the blood level of chylomicron remnants (there is an increased rate of removal of chylomicron remnants by the liver (34); as a result, the transfer of cholesterol from HDL to remnant particles is decreased, sparing HDL-C (32,35–37). Estrogen's ability to increase hepatic synthesis of HDL particles may also contribute to its beneficial effects (34). Estrogen causes an increased secretion of very low density lipoprotein (VLDL) from the liver but also an increased hepatic uptake of VLDL remnants (34). Even the secretion of bile acid is increased, providing a further mechanism for increased removal of cholesterol from the body (34,38). Transdermal or percutaneous administration of estrogen induces less alteration of hepatic metabolism than oral administration, because the drug then bypasses the portal circulation.

The effects of added progestin are related to the dose used and the androgenic potency of the hormone relative to the concomitant dose of estrogen. Generally, progestins inhibit the rate of metabolism at steps in lipoprotein transport associated with both the delivery of cholesterol to the tissues and its removal (34).

Antioxidant properties have been observed for antiestrogens (i.e., tamoxifen and raloxifene), and the dietary phytoestrogens found predominantly in soy products (39). Both endothelium-dependent and endothelium-independent vasodilation have been observed following estrogen treatment in vitro and in vivo, the former confirmed by observations that estrogen withdrawal produces an increased sensitivity of the endothelium to vasoconstrictor stimuli.

The different formulations, doses, and routes of administration of the hormones prescribed for postmenopausal women make interpretation and comparison of studies extremely difficult, yet the potential benefits of such therapy should be considered carefully (Table 2).

EXERCISE AND THE PRIMARY PREVENTION OF CAD IN WOMEN

The American Heart Association has recognized physical inactivity as a primary risk factor for CAD (40). However, the inverse relationship that has been demonstrated between CAD incidence and habitual physical activity is based primarily on male-dominated cohorts (41–44). Few epidemiological studies on physical activity and CAD incidence have included women or have separated men and women in their analyses (41,42). It is only recently that a large prospective study of 2260 post-menopausal women demonstrated a graded, inverse association between physical activity and all-cause mortality after a 7-year follow-up (45). Interpretation and comparison of studies is difficult, in part because of the challenge of defining physical activity and physical fitness. Most studies rely on personal inventories, and each defines activity status differently. More importantly, the assessment of activity status is based primarily on questionnaires validated on male subjects; the reliability and validity of such instruments for heterogeneous groups of women has not been established (21). In fact, low cardiovascular fitness may be a stronger predictor of risk in women than in men, and even a modest increase in physical activity can substantially reduce risk independent of blood pressure, smoking habits, serum cholesterol, or family history of cardiac disease (46).

An exercise training program at least 12 weeks in duration, which results in an increase in $\dot{V}_{O_2 max}$ will increase HDL levels (47). Early work in this area was based largely on male subjects, but a similar dose response has now been confirmed for females; this suggests that an energy expenditure in excess of 8 MJ/week can significantly reduce the risk of CAD (48,49).

EXERCISE AND CARDIOVASCULAR FUNCTION

There are significant differences in oxygen transport between women and men. Women have a lower blood volume, a lower haematocrit and a 10% lower hemoglobin concentration. Consequently, their submaximal response to exercise is characterized by a higher cardiac output and a lower arteriovenous oxygen difference. Peak exercise values are proportionately lower, although a smaller body surface area and cardiac mass also contribute to their lower peak cardiac output and lower peak oxygen consumption.

Clinical gender differences in the acute response to exercise arise in part from a limited specificity of the techniques used (e.g., ventriculography). The LV ejection fraction increases approximately 24% with exercise in men (20), but there is a limited increase in women (19). This may be related to the different mechanisms by which women and men increase their cardiac output during exercise. Several supine exercise studies have demonstrated that women increase cardiac output primarily by increasing end-diastolic volume without significantly increasing ejection fraction; in contrast, men tend to decrease end-systolic volume and raise ejection fraction (19,20,50). It is possible that women exhaust their end-diastolic reserve with increasing age, thereby limiting its use as an adaptive mechanism during training. Unfortunately, there is little information about cardiac function and training in females with CAD. In healthy males, the improvement in $\dot{V}_{O_2max}$ with endurance training reflects both central and peripheral adaptations (51–54). However in women with CAD, central adaptations have yet to be demonstrated (55–57). Healthy older women may not have the capacity to improve central function following training, whereas more than 60% of the improvement seen $\dot{V}_{O_2max}$ seen in normal individuals may be dependent on changes in cardiac function (58). The gender-specific adaptive response may relate to inherent ventricular compliance characteristics. Training-induced cardiac adaptations in older males are achieved from changes in LV compliance and not from improvements in inotropic function. This response is not seen in women; therefore changes in $\dot{V}_{O_2max}$ of women depend largely on peripheral adaptations (59).

PHYSIOLOGICAL ADAPTATIONS IN CARDIAC REHABILITATION

Older women can substantially improve risk-factor profiles and physiological function following training; the extent of such adaptation is comparable with that in men (61,63–68). Those who enter with the lowest fitness generally demonstrate the largest gains in aerobic power (69). Changes in lipid profile, body mass index (BMI), anaerobic threshold, and body composition have also been observed, in addition to an enhanced utilization of fat during exercise (70). Despite limited data from prospective studies that have focused on women, there is no reason to assume that their physiological outcomes will be inferior to those in males. It remains to be seen whether cardiac adaptations can be demonstrated or if improvements in diastolic function are possible. In addition, there is as yet no information on the potential role of estrogen in the adaptation process. Preliminary data from our laboratory suggest that training responses are similar, whether estrogen replacement therapy is given or not. Improvements in peak $\dot{V}_{O_2}$ are substantial, but more than 16 weeks may be needed before they become statistically significant. Changes seem secondary to changes in peripheral function. Improvements in peak $\dot{V}_{O_2}$ anaerobic threshold, and blood pressure responses are important to submaximal performance and quality of life. Given that the female cardiac patient is typically older and more deconditioned, even small increments in aerobic power may make it possible for light activities such as walking and gardening to be undertaken without precipitating early fatigue, dyspnea, or angina.

THE EFFECTS OF CARDIAC REHABILITATION ON QUALITY OF LIFE

Quality of life (QQL) and behavioral characteristics (anxiety, depression, somatization, and hostility) are generally similar between genders (63), but women tend to have lower scores for energy, function, and total QOL than men. After cardiac rehabilitation and exercise training, these indices are generally improved, although depression, hostility, and mental health appear less affected in women. Gender-related differences in these factors may reflect differing perceptions and needs among women, together with differing social responsibilities, family roles, and expectations.

BARRIERS TO PARTICIPATION OF WOMEN IN CARDIAC REHABILITATION PROGRAMS

There are significant differences between male and female cardiac rehabilitation participants with respect to psychosocial needs and clinical status, and these differences may limit compliance and physiological outcomes in women. Regardless of their clinical evaluation, women are less likely than men to enroll in cardiac rehabilitation programs following MI or coronary artery bypass graft surgery, particularly if they are older than 65 years of age. Cardiac risk-factor profiles are also worse in women than men upon entry to rehabilitation programs, and this in itself may be a perceived barrier to participation. Women are more likely to be hypertensive and/or diabetic and to have high cholesterol levels (3,60). Older women report higher levels of perceived exertion than men at the same relative work rates, and given that they also have a lower exercise capacity, the greater perception of effort may lead to poor compliance if the recommended intensity of exercise is estimated using conventional formulas. In addition, females participants in exercise rehabilitation programs are more likely to manifest symptoms such as angina (61), further discouraging compliance. Because of their greater age, female participants are likely to have more severe musculoskeletal limitations of effort. In addition to these factors, fewer women are referred to rehabilitation programs in the first instance (62), particularly in older age groups (61). Perhaps the most important factor that explains the negative experience of women in cardiac rehabilitation programs is the failure to address women's needs, which differ considerably from those of men. Women differ in their perceptions and expectations of rehabilitation and exercise, and the models that most rehabilitation programs adopt may not be applicable to them (60). Unfortunately, data are lacking to establish a model explaining exercise participation for women, but a number of determinants have recently been identified, including the need for group interaction, flexibility and convenience of programs, and emotional support (62).

CONCLUSIONS

Exercise training is a key intervention for primary and secondary prevention in the female cardiac patient. If compliance can be maintained, there is every reason to expect that women of any age will benefit significantly from participating in an exercise training program. Early detection and aggressive treatment are critical, given the increased likelihood of comorbidy and the advanced nature of CAD. Furthermore, efforts to optimize compliance are needed to facilitate long-term exercise participation and resulting benefits in this rapidly growing segment of the population.

REFERENCES

1. Thom, T., *Total Mortality and Mortality from Heart Disease Cancer and Stroke from 1956 to 1987 in 27 Countries: Highlights of Trends and Their Interrelationships Amongst Causes of Death.* National Institutes of Health, National Heart, Lung, and Blood Institute, Bethesda Maryland (1992).
2. Newnham, H., *Lancet,* 346: 13–16 (1997).
3. Thomas, R.J., Houston Miller, N., Lamendola, C., Berra, K., Hedback, B., Durstine, J.L., and Haskell, W., *J. Cardiopulm. Rehab.* 16: 401–412 (1996).
4. Blackburn, G.G., Sprecher, D.L., and Apperson-Hansen, C., *Circulation,* 94: I-582 (1996).
5. Wenger, N.K., Speroff, L., and Packard, B., *N. Engl. J. Med.,* 329: 247–256 (1993).
6. Lerner, D.J., and Kannel, WB., *Am. Heart J.,* 111: 383–390 (1986).
7. Greenland, P., Reicher-Reiss, H., and Goodhourt, U., *Circulation,* 83: 484–491 (1991).
8. American Heart Association, Silent epidemic: American Heart Association, Dallas, Texas (1989).
9. Healy, B., *N. Engl. J. Med.,* 60: 274–276 (1991).
10. Jaglal, S.B., Goel, V., and Naylor, C.D., *Can. J. Cardiol.,* 10: 239–244 (1994).
11. Heller, L.I., disease. *Cardiology,* 86: 318–323 (1995).
12. Ayanian, J.Z., and Epstein, A.M., *N. Engl. J. Med.,* 325: 221–225 (1991).

13. Steingart, R.M., Packer, M., and Hamm, P., *N. Engl. J. Med.,* 325: 226–230 (1991).
14. Iezzoni, I., Ash, A.S., Shwartz, M., and MacKiernay, D. *Med. Care,* 35: 158–171 (1997).
15. Schenck-Gustafsson, K., *Eur. Heart J.,* 17: SD2–8 (1996).
16. Wenger, N.O., *Ann. Intern. Med.,* 112: 557–558 (1990).
17. Rosano, G.M.C., Peters, N.S., Lefroy, D., Lindsay, D.C., Sarrel, P.M., Collins, P., and Poole-Wilson, P.A., with syndrome X. *J. Am. Coll. Cardiol.,* 28: 1500–1505 (1996).
18. Steingart, R.M., Forman, S., Coglianese, M., Bittner, V., Mueller, H., Frishman, W., Handberg, E., Gambino, A., Knatterud, G., and Conti, R., *Clin. Cardiol.,* 19: 614–618 (1996).
19. Hanley, P., Zinsmeister, A.R., Clements, I.P., Bove, A.A., Brown, M.L., and Gibbons, R.J., *J. Am. Coll. Cardiol.,* 13: 624–629 (1989).
20. Higginbotham, M.B., Morris, K.G., and Coleman, R.E., *Circulation,* 70: 357 (1984).
21. Shoenhair, C.L., and Wells, C.L., *Med. Exerc. Nutr. Health,* 4: 200–216 (1995).
22. Lobo, R.A., and Speroff, L., *Fertil. Steril.,* 62(Suppl. 2): 176S–179S (1994).
23. The Postmenopausal Estrogen/Progestin Interventions (PEPI) Trial, *J.A.M.A.,* 273: 199–208 (1995).
24. Barrett-Connor, E., and Bush, T.L., *J.A.M.A.,* 265: 1861–1867 (1991).
25. Gorodeski, G.I., and Utian, W.H., in *Treatment of the Postmenopausal Women* (R.A. Labo, ed.). Raven Press, New York, pp. 199–221 (1994).
26. Stampfer, M.J., and Colditz, G., *Prev. Med.,* 20: 47–63 (1991).
27. Bush, T.L., Barrett-Connor, E., and Cowan, L.D., *Circulation* 75: 1102–1109 (1987).
28. Applebaum-Bowden, D., McLean, P., Steinmetz, A., Fontana, A., Matthys, C., Warnick, G.R., Cheung, M., Albers, J.J., and Hazzard, W.R., *J. Lipid Res.,* 30: 1895–1906 (1989).
29. Walsh, B.W., Schiff, I., Rosner, B., Greenberg, L., Ravnikar, V., and Sacks, F.M., *N. Engl. J. Med.* 325: 1196–1204 (1991).
30. Wagner, J.D., Clarkson, T.B., St. Clair, R.W., Schwenke, D.C., Shively, C.A., and Adams, M., *J. Clini. Invest.,* 88: 1995–2002 (1991).
31. Angelin, B., Olivecrona, H., Reihner, E., Ruding, M., Stahlberg, M., Eriksson, M., Ewerth, S., Hendriksoon, P., and Einarsson, K., *Gastroenterology,* 103: 1657–1663 (1992).
32. Westerveld, H.T., Meyer, E., de Bruin, W.A., and Erkelens, D.W., *Biochem. Soc. Trans.,* 25: 45–49 (1997).
33. Slyper, A.H., *Lancet.* 340: 8814, 289–291 (1992).
34. Knopp, R.H., Zhu, X., and Bonet, B., *Atherosclerosis,* 110: S83–S91 (1994).
35. Demacker, P.N.M., Mol, M.J.T.M., and Stalenhoef, A.F.M., *Biochem. J.,* 272: 419–429 (1990).
36. Jackle, S., Rinninger, F., Greeve, J., Greten, H., and Windler, E., *Lipid Res.,* 33: 419–429 (1992).
37. Cohn, J.S., McNamara, J.R., Cohn, S.D., Ordovas, J.M., and Schaefer, E.J., *J. Lipid Res.,* 29: 469–474 (1988).
38. Wild, R.A., *J. Obst. Gynecol.,* 87: 27S–35S (1996).
39. Wiseman, H., and O'Reilly, J., *Biochem. Soc. Trans.,* 25(1): 50–54 (1997).

40. American Heart Association, *Statement on Exercise: Benefits and Recommendations for Physical Activity Programs for All Americans.* American Heart Association, Dallas, Texas (1992).
41. Berlin, J.A., and Colditz, G.A., *Am. J. Epidemiol.,* 132: 612–628 (1990).
42. Powell, K.E., Thompson, P.D., Caspersen, C.J., and Kendrick, J.S., *Annu. Rev. Public Health,* 8: 253–287 (1987).
43. Morris, J.N., Clayton, D.G., Everitt, M.G., and Semmence, A.M., *Br. Heart J.,* 63: 325–334 (1990).
44. Paffenbarger, R.S., Hyde, R.T., Wing, A.L., and Steinmetz, C.H., *J.A.M.A.,* 252: 491–495 (1984).
45. Kushi, L.H., Fee, R.M., Folsom, A.R., Mink, P.J., Anderson, K.E., and Sellers, T.A., *J.A.M.A.,* 277: 1287–1292 (1997).
46. Blair, S.N., Kohl, H.W., Paffenbarger, R.S., Clark, D.G., Cooper, K.H., and Gibbons, L.W., *J.A.M.A.,* 262: 2395–2401 (1989).
47. Rohm Young, D., and Steinhardt, M.A., *Sports Med.,* 19: 303–310 (1995).
48. Jette, M., Sidney, K., Quenneville, J., and Landry, F., *Can. Med. Assoc. J.,* 146: 1353–1360 (1992).
49. Owens, J.F., Matthews, K.A., Wing, R.A., and Kuller, L.H., *Prev. Med.,* 19: 147–157 (1990).
50. Younis, L.T., Melin, J.A., Robert, A.R., and Detry, J.M.R., *Eur. Heart J.,* 11: 916–924 (1990).
51. Clausen, J.P., *Physiol. Rev.,* 57: 779–815 (1977).
52. Ehsani, A.A., Biello, D.R., Schultz, J., Sobel, B.E., and Hollozy, J.O., *Circulation,* 74(2): 350–358 (1986).
53. Hagberg, J.M., Eshani, A.A., and Holloszy, J.O., *Circulation,* 67(6): 1194–1199 (1983).
54. Stromme, S.B., and Ingier, F., *Scand. J. Med.,* 29: 37–45 (1982).
55. Higginbotham, M.B., Morris, K.G., Williams, R.S., McHale, P.A., Coleman, R.E., and Cobb, F.R., *Circ. Res.,* 58: 281–291 (1986).
56. Cobb, F.R., Williams, R.S., McEwan, P., Jones, R.H., Coleman, R.E., and Wallace, A.G., *Circulation,* 66: 100–108 (1982).
57. Blumenthal, J.A., Rejeski, W., Walsh-Riddle, M., Emery, E., Miller, H., Roark, S., Ribisl, P.M., Morris, P.B., Brubaker, P., and Williams, R.S., *Am. J. Cardiol.,* 61: 26–30 (1988).
58. Spina, R.J., Ogawa, T., Miller, T.R., Kohrt, W.M., and Ehsani, A.A., *Am. J. Cardiol.* 71: 99–104 (1993).
59. Spina, R.J., Miller, T.R., Bogenhagen, W.H., Schechtman, K.B., and Ehsani, A.A., *J Gerontol.,* 51A: B232–B237 (1996).
60. Cannistra, L.B., Balady, G.J., O'Malley, C.J., Weiner, D.A., and Ryan, T.J., *Am. J. Cardiol.,* 69: 1274–1279 (1992).
61. Ades, P.A., Waldmann, M.L., Polk, D.M., and Coflesky, J.T., *Am. J. Cardiol.,* 69: 1422–1425 (1992).
62. Moore, S.M., *J. Cardiopulm. Rehabi.,* 16: 123–129 (1989).
63. Lavie, C.J., and Milani, R.V., *Am. J. Cardiol.,* 75: 340–343 (1995).
64. Kavanagh, T., Mertens, D., and Kennedy, J., *Circulation,* 94: 2445 (1996).
65. Lavie, C.J., and Milani, R.V., *Am. J. Cardiol.,* 79: 664–666 (1997).

66. Lavie, C.J., and Milani, R.V., *Am. J. Cardiol.,* 79: 397–401 (1997).

67. Lavie, C.J., Milani, R.V., *Am. J. Cardiol.,* 76: 177–179 (1995).

68. Ades, P.A., Waldmann, M.L., and Gillespie, C., *J. Gerontol.,* 50A: M7–M11 (1995).

69. Shiran, A., Kornfeld, S., Zur, S., Laor, A., Karelitz, Y., Militaianu, A., Merdler, A., and Lewis, B.S., *Cardiology* 88: 207–213 (1997).

70. Ades, P.A., Waldmann, M.L., Poehlman, E.T., Gray, P., Horton, E.D., Horton, E.S., and LeWinter, M.M., *Circulation,* 88: 572–577 (1993).

71. Notelovitz, M., in *Treatment of the Postmenopausal Woman: Basic and Clinical Aspects* (R.A. Lobo, ed.). Raven Press, New York pp. 271–279 (1994).

72. Skouby, S.O., in *Treatment of the Postmenopausal Woman: Basic and Clinical Aspects* (R.A. Lobo, ed.). Raven Press, New York (1994).

73. Rosano, G., Sarrel, P., Poole-Wilson, P., and Collins, P., *Lancet,* 342: 133–136 (1993).

74. Scheuer, J., Malhortra, A., Schaible, T., and Capasso, J., *Circ. Res.,* 61: 12–19 (1987).

75. White, M., Zamudio, S., Stevens, T., Tyler, R., Lindenfeld, J., Kimberly, L., and Moore, L., *Endocr. Revi.,* 16: 739–751 (1995).

76. Gambrell, R.D., in *Treatment of the Postmenopausal Woman: Basic and Clinical Aspects* (R.A. Lobo, ed.). Raven Press, New York (1994).

77. Ross, R.K., and Bernstein, L., in *Treatment of the Postmenopausal Woman: Basic and Clinical Aspects* (R.A. Lobo, ed.). Raven Press, New York (1994).

8
Exercise Programs for Middle-Aged and Older Women

Roy J. Shephard
University of Toronto
Toronto, Ontario, Canada

INTRODUCTION

Women make up more than half of the adult population, and their participation in both the labor force and athletic competitions is growing rapidly. Moreover, some 15% of the patients who attend the Toronto Rehabilitation Centre for cardiac rehabilitation following myocardial infarction are women (2), and in 1988 the annual economic burden due to heart disease in U.S. women was estimated at $20 billion (3). Nevertheless, there remains a dearth of information on how women respond to exercise, physical conditioning, and cardiac rehabilitation programs.

Inferences are too often based simply on the reactions that have been observed in male patients. This approach can be quite fallacious, since women have different physiological and psychological reactions to both acute and chronic exercise, and they usually develop manifestations of ischemic heart disease at a much later age than men. Moreover, they are likely to present at a physician's office with symptoms of angina pectoris rather than myocardial infarction, and there are many gender-specific features of diagnosis and treatment in atherosclerotic heart disease.

This chapter thus reviews issues concerning the prescription of exercise for middle-aged and older women, looking at normal female responses to exercise and conditioning programs. We adopt the clinical terminology of primary and secondary prevention of cardiac disease, nothing that epidemiologists (1) have sometimes classified these two types of exercise programs as "secondary prevention" and "tertiary prevention." Among specific issues to be discussed, we may note gender-related differences in:

1. Acute responses to exercise in healthy adults
2. Physiological and psychological responses of healthy adults to aerobic training ("primary prevention")
3. Acute responses to exercise after myocardial infarction
4. Physiological and psychological responses to aerobic training following myocardial infarction ("secondary prevention")
5. Hormonal status and the response to a secondary preventive regimen
6. Indicators of prognosis after myocardial infarction

A final section considers the implications of current knowledge for management of the female patient.

GENDER-RELATED DIFFERENCES IN ACUTE RESPONSES TO EXERCISE

Current data suggest substantial gender differences in functional capacity electrocardiographic (ECG) responses, tolerance of environmental stress, biomechanics, and metabolic function between women and men, but it is less clear how far these differences are biological in nature and how far they are caused by the sociocultural environment of growing children.

Functional Capacity

The average adult woman has a poorer score than her male counterpart on many current tests of exercise performance, but a fit, well-trained female can outperform most men of similar age, particularly in terms of aerobic power, balance, and flexibility. Functional capacity thus overlaps widely between female and male populations.

There is some value in attempting to distinguish gender differences that have a biological basis (what are sometimes described as "sex-linked" characteristics) from features of the exercise response that are largely or entirely determined by such aspects of the sociocultural environment as gender-related barriers to vigorous physical activity during the developmental years.

Small gender-related differences in average functional capacity can be detected from an early age, but these first assume practical significance at puberty. Relative to young men, women of similar age (4,5) are 4–8% shorter in height, with a 20–30% lower body mass, a 30% greater body fat content, a 30–40%

lower lean tissue mass (gender-related differences of muscle development being particularly marked in the upper limbs), and a 10% lower hemoglobin concentration. The heart of the average woman also has a smaller volume than that of a man, even when an appropriate adjustment is made for gender differences in body size or body mass (6). But, given the potential for heavy aerobic training to induce ventricular hypertrophy, differences in relative cardiac volume could have a sociocultural rather than a biological basis.

The shorter height of the typical woman is indisputably biological in origin. Shorter limb length inevitably reduces the leverage of arm and leg muscles. In consequence, a woman has more difficulty than a man in making rapid, repetitive movements, but she finds the performance of fine, highly coordinated motor tasks easier than her male counterparts. The lower hemoglobin level also has a strong biological component, reflecting the combined influences of monthly menstrual blood loss and low levels of circulating androgens. There is a biological basis to at least a part of gender differences in body fat content, muscle development and bone strength, but much of the currently observed differences in body composition is undoubtedly attributable to gender stereotypes (7,8), which have held that girls should have physically less active roles than boys throughout their developmental years.

It is difficult to design conclusive experiments that will identify the relative contributions of biological and sociocultural factors to current physique. However, the progressive diminution of gender-related differences in aerobic and muscular fitness is most easily explained as a consequence of the progressive elimination of barriers to female participation in vigorous physical activity.

Both sex-linked and socioculturally determined factors thus contribute to gender differences in functional responses to an acute bout of exercise. Because they have a lower hemoglobin level, women who are making a peak effort generally carry less oxygen carriage per liter of cardiac output than men. Other factors remaining equal, they thus have a smaller maximal oxygen transport. Because body fat content is greater than in a typical man, a woman's oxygen transport per unit of body mass is further reduced relative to that of her male counterpart, and unfortunately relative aerobic power is the critical variable that determines a person's ability to undertake most aerobic tasks. Weak skeletal muscles limit the average woman's tolerance of activities that demand great strength and if a woman with weaker muscles attempts to match the muscle force developed by a male peer, she will show a larger and more rapid rise of systemic blood pressure, a higher heart rate, a heavier afterloading of the left ventricle, and a greater increase of cardiac work rate. Several authors have noted that the increase of ejection fraction during a progressive, maximal exercise test is smaller in older women than in men of similar age (6,9–11), although it remains unclear how far this is attributable to a greater afterloading of the left ventricle.

ECG Responses

The proportion of otherwise healthy individuals who report exercise-induced chest pain and/or show "ischemic" electrocardiograms is substantially higher in women than in men (12–14). Cumming et al.(12) found that as many as 25% of women aged 20–39, 50% of women aged 40–59, and 66% of those over the age of 60 years had exercise ECGs that (on male criteria) would have been suggestive of myocardial ischemia. However, the specificity of exercise-induced ST depression as an indicator of myocardial ischemia is poor in women (59 to 66%) (14), with many false-positive test results. Whereas 18% of men with such an ECG will develop overt cardiac disease within 5 years, only 4.6% of women show such a progression (15). The checking of apparently ischemic ECGs by such techniques as thallium scintigraphy may also be difficult in women, since signals are attenuated by the substantial fat content of overlying breast tissue (3).

In many female patients, the explanation of an apparently abnormal ECG remains unclear. The great majority of women with positive ECGs show no angiographic evidence of coronary vascular narrowing, although in some instances a poor ejection fraction suggests that a relative myocardial ischemia may have developed during exercise (12), perhaps due to small vessel disease, which is not readily detected by techniques such as angiography.

Part of the diagnostic problem in those women who are finally shown to be free of disease is Bayesian: because the prevalence of coronary disease is low in women, a high proportion of apparently ischaemic records are inevitably false-positive results, and the ability of the exercise ECG to detect clinically significant coronary vascular disease is correspondingly poor. Another factor is the small average heart size (above); the cross-sectional thickness of the ventricular wall is substantially less in a woman than in a man. Since blood pressures are at least as high in women as in men, women must develop a greater tension per unit cross-section of ventricular wall during a given bout of vigorous exercise, and the intramural tension may rise to a level that occludes the penetrating coronary vessels.

Application of the law of LaPlace indicates that at any given intraventricular pressure, the wall tension is proportional to the average ventricular diameter. Thus, the situation of the typical female exerciser is exacerbated by a lesser catecholamine-mediated increase of ventricular contractility than would occur in a male patient (16). During exercise, there is a greater increase of ventricular dimensions and in consequence a higher wall tension than in a man (13). Other possible disadvantages of a female test candidate include a poor physical condition relative to her potential, evaluation by exercise test protocols that include work rates which are appropriate for men and therefore too stressful for smaller women, a heavy afterloading of the left ventricle because blood flow through the working limbs is impeded by skeletal muscle weakness, and a depression of myocardial contractility by a digitalis-like action of estrogens (17).

Tolerance of Environmental Stress

Women tend to have a larger ratio of body surface area to mass than men (18); in consequence, they react less favorably to both cold and hot environments.

The peak rate of heat production is lower in women than in men (19), and they also have a lesser ability to generate heat by nonshivering thermogenesis (20). Despite a thicker layer of subcutaneous fat, they thus tend to lose heat faster than men when they are exposed to a cold environment.

They also gain heat more rapidly than a typical man when exercising under hot and dry conditions (21). There have been suggestions that women sweat less readily than men (22), although, since the rate of sweating at any given body temperature is influenced by the individual's training status, investigators making such comparisons have had difficulty in deciding whether female and male subjects were appropriately matched for initial physical condition.

Biomechanics

Because women have a lower center of gravity, greater joint flexibility, different angles of limb carriage and different patterns of habitual physical activity than men, there are gender-related differences in motor coordination and the oxygen cost of many everyday tasks.

Published tables of oxygen costs have generally been determined on male subjects, and such information has limited value when prescribing exercise in females, even if the results are standardized per unit of body mass [as when MET (metabolic equivalent) units are used, or the prescribed activity involves mainly the displacement of body weight; for example, in jogging at a fixed speed].

In contrast, prescriptions that are based on exercise heart rate or a rating of perceived exertion generally impose a similar relative stress on women and men of comparable age.

Metabolic Function

There is some evidence that exercise mobilizes body fat less readily in women than in men. When a woman undertakes prolonged physical activity, she thus imposes heavier demands on alternative sources of energy, particularly muscle glycogen reserves.

The greater stability of depot fat in the female may reflect a woman's biological need to conserve food energy for pregnancy and lactation (23–26). On the other hand, at any given level of habitual daily physical activity, women have higher HDL cholesterol levels than men (27). Indeed, the HDL cholesterol level found in a sedentary woman commonly matches the values anticipated in male endurance athletes.

At any given age, the bones are both lighter and less densely calcified in a woman than in a man. This imposes a greater risk of fracture from collision with external objects, although currently the overall prognosis of the active female patient remains good; because as yet fewer women engage in contact sports, patterns of play are based on skill rather than physical aggression, and the risk of mechanical injury during falls is offset by a lighter body mass.

GENDER-RELATED DIFFERENCES IN RESPONSE TO TRAINING

Pattern of Change

When women undertake aerobic training, they show an overall change in physiological responses similar to those anticipated in men. Resting data commonly show a decrease of resting blood pressure in both normotensive and hypertensive subjects of 5–10 mmHg (28). Insulin responsiveness is also increased, although probably without normalizing the response to a glucose challenge (29,30).

In both sexes, training-induced decreases in exercise blood pressure and heart rate reduce the cardiac work rate and thus the oxygen demand of the myocardium at any given power output. The bradycardia allows a lengthening of the diastolic phase of the cardiac cycle; this improves left ventricular perfusion, particularly in the critical subendocardial zone, since most of the blood flow to the heart wall occurs during diastole.

Over 2–3 months of participation in a progressive exercise regimen, both sexes show an increase of peak power output, associated with gains of maximal oxygen intake and peak respiratory minute volume. Moreover, at any given intensity of submaximal exercise, there are decreases in both heart rate and respiratory minute volume.

Magnitude of Change

It is unclear whether the intrinsic magnitude of the aerobic training response is equal for women and for men because of difficulties in matching initial levels of fitness between the sexes.

Studies at West Point Military Academy found larger gains of maximal oxygen intake in female cadets than in their male counterparts, but this was thought to be because the women were initially in poorer physical condition than the male recruits (31). Kavanagh (2) maintained that the gain in aerobic power he observed during a secondary preventive program for patients seen 2–3 months after myocardial infarction was similar in women and in men; in his studies, both sexes began training from little more than bed rest.

Because of the low concentrations of circulating androgens, women who engage in resistance exercise programs are unable to induce the massive muscle hypertrophy that is seen in men (32,33). Nevertheless, weight-lifting programs can produce considerable gains of strength in women, probably through such mechanisms as improved neuromuscular coordination.

Training also reduces the percentage of body fat less readily in women than in men, probably because the hormone prolactin helps female subjects to conserve depot fat against the needs of pregnancy and lactation. However, if an adequate weekly amount of exercise is pursued for sufficient time, the body fat content of a woman does decrease, and blood lipid profiles are optimized. In particular, the HDL_2 component and the A-2 apoprotein are increased (34–36). There is even a danger that some younger women who have a distorted body image may develop not only a high level of habitual physical activity but also an inadequate food intake, progressing to manifestations of anorexia nervosa.

Reasons for Exercising

The perceived reasons for engaging in primary and secondary programs of preventive exercise are generally similar for men and women, but there are nevertheless some important differences.

Responses to open ended questions regarding reasons for participation in a university preretirement class of primary preventive exercise revealed four main determinants in men: a wish to improve fitness or health, availability of the program and athletic facility, a desire to ''assist science'' through the experimental phase of the study, and recreational or hedonistic reasons (37). In women, there were six main determinants. A wish to improve health or fitness and the availability of programs and facilities adapted to the needs of their age group were the two commonest citations, but other responses included a search for psychological well-being, a desire to assist science, recreational/hedonistic objectives, and a desire to socialize or make friends (37,38).

Women commonly place more value on detailed exercise programming than do men. The latter are attracted rather by the convenience and quality of the facility and by respect for the personnel who are offering the program (39). Women commonly perceive exercise as a means of losing weight and improving health, but men place more value on the relief of tension and ''feeling better'' (40). Women often begin an exercise program with a lesser sense of self-efficacy than their male peers (41). Perhaps because some female participants emphasize the social aspects of an exercise program at the expense of physical effort, their regular involvement has only a limited impact on other forms of health behavior.

Over the first year of one worksite fitness program, male participants showed a substantial reduction in several types of risk-taking behavior, with a 2.4-year decrease in their biological age (as assessed by the Canadian Health Hazard Appraisal schema). In contrast, female participants in the same program showed only a 0.1 year reduction of biological age (42).

One study of healthy individuals noted a similar overall program compliance in men and women (43). However, a second study involving postcoronary patients found a 19% dropout rate in women compared with 8% in men (44). It is unclear how far any gender-related differences in compliance reflect the physiological and psychological problems that women encounter if they are directed to exercise programs that have been uniquely tailored to the desires, needs, and abilities of male participants (3). Currently identified characteristics of female dropouts do not seem strongly related to program content; they include high anger scores on the Profile of Mood States and poor flexibility on the sit-and-reach test (43).

Health Benefits of Participation

The health benefits of regular exercise have been examined much less frequently in women than in men (45,46). In terms of cardiac disease, one meta-analysis found that data on female subjects had been reported in only 4 of 43 studies (47). Two epidemiological studies of women found that questionnaire reports of regular physical activity had little association with protection against cardiac disease (48,49). However, this may merely reflect the fact that current physical activity questionnaires have been designed for men, and therefore they fail to detect forms of physical activity that provide a significant training stimulus for many traditional women (for example, the care of children or of the elderly). Other studies, using different (and sometimes simpler) activity questionnaires (50–52) or initial fitness scores (53) have shown that women can indeed decrease their risks of cardiac disease by adopting an active lifestyle.

ACUTE RESPONSES OF WOMEN TO EXERCISE AFTER MYOCARDIAL INFARCTION

The various gender-related influences (physiological and psychological) that limit the physical performance of healthy women during a bout of vigorous exercise assume even greater significance following myocardial infarction.

Acute Response to Exercise

Because of the small overall dimensions of the heart, a given-sized infarct is likely to destroy a larger fraction of the total ventricular muscle in a woman than in a man. A given infarction-related decrease in aerobic power also has greater functional significance in a woman than in a man, because the average woman has a smaller reserve of functional capacity prior to infarction.

Loss of lean tissue during the acute phase of hospital stay (whether for infarction or for cardiac surgery) exacerbates the problems associated with muscles that are initially weak. A rapid return to heavy physical activity is thus more likely to provoke acute ischemia and related disturbances of myocardial function (54,55) in a woman than in a man. Only about one-half of the women who report typical angina and less than one-fifth of those with atypical chest pain show significant coronary vascular obstruction at angiography (3). However, such observations are usually made at rest and without exposure to cigarettes; it seems likely that a higher proportion of abnormalities would be detected if observations were made under conditions that were representative of the patient's normal daily habits.

The likelihood that exercise will cause a decrease of ejection fraction in those who develop chest pain is three times greater in women than in men (55), suggesting that exercise temporarily compromises either myocardial oxygen supply or contractile function through some combination of vascular spasm, microvascular narrowing, weak skeletal muscles, a large increase of heart rate and blood pressure, and a high cardiac work rate.

Risk of Exercising

The average female coronary patient is quite elderly. Typically, the first symptoms of coronary heart disease appear 10 years later than in a man, and even at this stage a woman is much less likely to be referred for angiography and subsequent coronary vascular surgery (56–58). Indeed, the incidence of diagnosed coronary heart disease does not peak in women until around 75 years of age. The full picture of myocardial infarction commonly develops 20 years later than in a man (3); even prior to the critical ischemic episode, many female patients have become frail and dependent, with a very low level of habitual physical activity. It might thus be anticipated that the risks of exercising after myocardial infarction would be greater in women than in men.

Attempts to implement a program of secondary preventive exercise for women are hampered not only by chest pain and frailty but also by the common concomitants of advanced aging: rheumatoid and/or osteoarthritis, poor pulmonary function, deterioration of vision, neurological problems, nutritional deficiencies, and a distorted perception of exertion that leads them to curtails physical activity voluntarily before an adequate training stimulus has developed (59).

Although chest pain is a difficult symptom to diagnose, a high proportion of elderly women report an exercise-induced pain that is anginal in type. Some also have a tendency to develop congestive failure secondary to undiagnosed myocardial infarction (60). In the first few weeks after myocardial infarction, death is twice as common in women as in men, and 39% of women (as compared with 31% of men) are likely to die during the first year of rehabilitation (61).

However, because women usually pursue exercise in a less aggressive manner than men, the proportion of deaths that are induced by exercise is actually smaller in women than in men (62).

Exercise and Coronary Bypass Surgery

There are theoretical reasons why the response to exercise after coronary bypass surgery might be poorer in women than in men (see prognosis below), but in practice the gains from rehabilitation seem essentially similar in both sexes (63), possibly because any initial gender-related impairments of left ventricular function in the women are corrected during hospital treatment.

GENDER-RELATED DIFFERENCES IN RESPONSE TO SECONDARY PREVENTIVE PROGRAMS

Investigators have had difficulty in demonstrating the precise impact of exercise rehabilitation upon cardiac function, myocardial perfusion and survival, even in the large pool of male postcoronary patients that is available in most urban centers. It is thus hardly surprising that no definitive randomized controlled experiments have been conducted on the much smaller and older pool of female patients. Although Kavanagh claimed that the effectiveness of secondary prevention was unaffected by gender (2), a majority of authors now seem agreed that women show a less favorable immediate clinical response to the usual patterns of treatment following myocardial infarction.

Differences in Morbidity and Mortality

Mortality statistics show that women have a higher age-adjusted in-hospital mortality rate for myocardial infarction (17% versus 12% in the study of Walling et al., Ref. 64), with an increased incidence of postinfarct complications, comorbid events that limit exercise participation, and a higher mortality over the next 1–4 years (65,66).

An older age at infarction and a greater prevalence of hypertension (65) are obvious factors contributing to a poor prognosis, but it is difficult to attribute all of the female disadvantage to such features. A number of other, more subtle influences, both biological and cultural, contribute to a poor outcome. Sometimes, the health of the myocardium has been compromised by previous, undetected infarctions (60). A given size of lesion also has a greater functional impact in a woman because her heart is smaller than a man's. It can be difficult for the patient to implement an effective program of exercise-based rehabilitation if she is already frail and elderly before infarction occurs. A high proportion of women experience angina and other types of chest pain, and this makes participation in a program of vigorous exercise an uncomfortable experience.

Whereas the majority of male patients are quite willing to take an initial 3–4 weeks of graded rest following myocardial infarction, women have been socialized to feel guilty if they are not personally attending to household chores (67). They do not understand the oxygen requirements of domestic tasks, and do not regard such activities as demanding exercise. They thus have a tendency to return to quite heavy housework, including lifting and reaching above their heads, as soon as they leave hospital. In consequence, they become physically fatigued—sometimes developing acute congestive failure—and this discourages them from subsequent participation in a structured exercise program that may be appropriate to their needs.

Cardiac rehabilitation programs commonly require thrice-weekly attendance at a facility which may be quite distant from the participant's home. Often, older female patients lack the personal transportation needed to reach the rehabilitation facility, and the domestic duties they have resumed also preclude attendance at the typical postcoronary exercise class at 6 to 7 P.M. Assuming that these practical obstacles can be overcome, compliance with a formal exercise program is still strongly influenced by the individual's mood state, and, as in the general population, it is well documented that women with myocardial infarction more frequently suffer from feelings of depression, anxiety, and guilt than do their male peers (68–70). The end result is that women are less likely than men to be recruited to a formal exercise program, and those who are recruited show a poorer compliance with their exercise prescription (66,67). The practical corollary is that personnel responsible for cardiac rehabilitation programs must devote more time to recruiting female patients and to encouraging their continued participation in exercise classes (71).

Functional Response

Although the typical woman faces a considerable gender handicap when she attempts to participate in a secondary preventive program, the poor initial fitness level of the elderly woman gives the successful participant greater scope to develop a gain in functional capacity; one report has claimed that women who are persuaded to exercise show a similar increase in functional capacity to men, despite their poorer program compliance (72).

The value of estrogen replacement therapy as a component of a secondary preventive regimen is discussed below. No randomized controlled trials have examined the contribution of smoking cessation programs, the aggressive treatment of hyperlipidemia, or the rigorous control of hypertension to the success of exercise-centered rehabilitation programs. However, the information that is available from less rigorous types of experiment suggests a similar pattern of response to that observed in men. After a myocardial infarction, prognosis is improved most by smoking cessation. In Toronto, the percentage of heavy smokers dropped from 80 to 35% during the acute phase of hospital treatment. Subsequent involvement in phase II and III exercise rehabilitation programs apparently did no more that prevent recidivism, although this in itself can be an important dividend of an exercise program in a woman who has been strongly addicted to cigarettes.

Return to Paid Employment

Women typically have a longer period of poor health than men following myocardial infarction, and fewer women ultimately return to the paid labor force (68, 73).

In men, an early return to work is often associated with denial of disease and type A behavior (74,75); both of these behavioral characteristics are less prevalent among female patients. Depression is a negative factor, inhibiting return to work, and, as noted above, this symptom is more prevalent in women than in men following myocardial infarction. If employment makes heavy physical demands, the low initial functional capacity of a woman is also more easily pushed below the minimum job requirement by a period of illness or hospitalization (76).

Motivation to return to paid employment often differs between the sexes. Women in traditional marriages have fewer incentives than their male peers to return to paid work. Outside employment may provide them with no more than a source of discretionary income. When paid work is attempted, this must frequently be combined with all of the responsibilities of a homemaker (68). In contrast, single women are strongly motivated to work because they have only limited financial resources; they account for the majority of female patients who make a successful return to work following myocardial infarction (68).

HORMONAL STATUS AND CORONARY VASCULAR DISEASE

There have been suggestions that women develop coronary atheromas just as rapidly as men, but they seem either to escape or at least to retard the fatal consequences of the disease process for many more years than their male counterparts (77). Such assertions are difficult to evaluate, given the differential access to medical services already noted here (56,57,58) and in the accompanying chapter by Goodman and Kirwan. Nevertheless, the fact that in women angina pectoris often antedates infarction supports the view that atherosclerotic disease exists but that for some reason it does not cause death.

Possibly, gender-related differences in the hormonal milieu and mineral reserves make the female myocardium less vulnerable to a given extent of cardiovascular disease (78). Certainly, the risk of developing myocardial infarction seems to rise quite steeply following the menopause (79–81). However, other factors—both constitutional and cultural—may keep middle-aged women from making sudden competitive physical efforts and engaging in the aggressive, hostile forms of behavior that convert "silent" atheromas to overt heart attacks in male patients.

Administration of estrogen as a contraceptive agent increases rather than decreases the risk of a cardiovascular incident. However, after menopause or oophorectomy, the therapeutic administration of estrogen substantially reduces the risk of cardiovascular death, both in those who are free of clinical coronary vascular disease (82) and in those with mild to moderate coronary stenosis (83, 84). One potential mechanism of benefit in the postmenopausal patient is that estrogens increase HDL cholesterol levels, although the effects on lipid profile do not seem sufficient to account for all of the protection that is gained from hormone replacement therapy.

PROGNOSTIC INDICES IN WOMEN

There are several important gender-related differences in cardiac risk factors between men and women. Both biological and sociocultural factors contribute to these differences.

Estrogens

Particularly in young women, myocardial infarction is strongly related to the use of estrogens, whether these are administered as contraceptive agents (relative risk about 15) or as a treatment for other medical conditions (relative risk about 9). However, the cardiovascular risk drops rapidly once the use of oral contraceptives is stopped (84).

Cigarette Smoking

Cigarette smoking in itself carries a risk ratio of 5 (85–87), and this risk continues after myocardial infarction if the patient does not succeed in stopping smoking (88–92). The risk of premenopausal estrogen therapy is also exacerbated if the patient is a cigarette smoker.

The nature of the functional problems associated with cigarette smoking seem much as in men—tachycardia (with a resultant increase in cardiac work rate), coronary vascular spasm, poor left ventricular function, and a reduced efficacy of antianginal drugs (93–96). These various side effects of smoking exacerbate myocardial ischaemia, and favor a recurrence of clinical disease.

Cardiovascular Factors

Runs of ventricular premature beats are not an independent risk factor in women (97). Women are more vulnerable to hypertension than men, and hypertension is a significant cardiac risk factor for them (87). Perhaps because of the prevalence of hypertension, women are more vulnerable to congestive failure after myocardial infarction (70), even though they commonly have a better left ventricular ejection fraction than men when they are discharged from hospital (67).

Angina is apparently a less significant risk factor for women than for men (98,99), and a substantial proportion of women who complain of chest pain remain free of clinically diagnosed myocardial infarction for many years. Nevertheless, it is difficult to dissociate this difference from (a) a greater prevalence of pain without angiographic evidence of coronary artery narrowing in women (3,100) and (b) differential patterns of diagnosis and treatment, as discussed by Goodman and Kirwan.

Lipid Profile and Metabolic Factors

An adverse lipid profile is a cardiac risk factor for women (101), although when assessing the extent of risk, due account must be taken of gender differences in normal values. When eating a traditional "western" diet that is rich in saturated animal fats, even quite sedentary women often have a much higher HDL to total cholesterol ratio than physically active men. Triglycerides also seem to be an independent cardiac risk factor in women (49,102).

Perhaps because of gender differences in the distribution of body fat, obesity does not appear to be a direct risk factor in women (87). Nevertheless, an excessive accumulation of body fat limits the functional capacity of a woman with a weakened heart, and it can also predispose to maturity-onset diabetes mellitus. Women with diabetes mellitus have about twice the risk of dying of a heart attack as do men, and their risk of death from a cerebrovascular accident is also higher than in their male peers (88,103,104). A combination of diabetes mellitus and hypertension in women is apparently associated with an increased risk of sudden death (105), perhaps because the cardiac work-rate is increased in such individuals.

Access to Treatment

The outcome of an acute cardiac incident depends on speedy treatment. Somewhat at variance with the hypotheses of Goodman and Kirwan, men seem more likely than women to die outside of hospital (106). In part, this paradox arises because of their younger age; thus, men are more likely to develop a cardiac incident when they are working or playing in circumstances where prompt emergency treatment is lacking.

There may also be gender-related differences in symptom denial, self-medication, willingness to call a physician or emergency services, and the nature of the service rendered, all of which should be considered in planning secondary preventive treatment.

Risk Factors After Myocardial Infarction and Coronary Vascular Surgery

The progression of atherosclerosis after coronary bypass surgery is essentially similar in women and in men (107).

Relatively few studies have examined the influence of cardiac risk factors on the prognosis of women after recovery from myocardial infarction. One of the more insistent exponents of the need for such research (108) examined a sample of 96 women following myocardial infarction (88), but practical problems in recruiting adequate subject numbers were underlined by the limited number of female cardiovascular deaths available for analysis (only 16). In this study, the only useful predictors of increased risk were continued cigarette smoking and a personal history of diabetes mellitus (88).

Demonstration of exercise-induced chest pain or ST-segment depression does not seem to be associated with an adverse prognosis after infarction, at least if arteriography shows a normal or near normal coronary vascular supply to the functional myocardium (9,109). However, persistent congestive failure has an adverse impact upon prospects for long-term survival. The incidence of congestive failure following infarction is about twice as great in women as in men (70).

The Timolol Trial suggested a slight trend for this particular β-blocking agent to improve prognosis after myocardial infarction, although any benefit was smaller in women than in men; in the case of women, the difference in recurrence rate was not statistically significant (110,111). Low-dose aspirin (112,113) and streptokinase (113,114) are also useful adjuvants to an exercise rehabilitation program.

There is a greater short-term risk of bradycardia, hypotension and coronary dissection in women than in men following percutaneous transluminal coronary angioplasty, and account should be taken of such potential complications in planning postoperative exercise programs. In a longer-term perspective, the risk of restenosis seems to be lower in women than in men (115). Coronary artery bypass grafts have a higher perioperative mortality in women, possibly because the coronary vessels are smaller than in men (70), but possibly also related to the other factors that contribute to a poor early prognosis after myocardial infarction (above). The operation less frequently relieves chest pain in women, complicating attempts at exercise rehabilitation programs following such surgery (3,116).

IMPLICATIONS FOR PATIENT MANAGEMENT

The objectives of patient management following either myocardial infarction or coronary vascular surgery include the relief of any immediate symptoms, a reduction of morbidity and early mortality, and an optimization of the overall quality of the remaining years of life. It is important to functional objectives, and probably also to survival, that women be encouraged to persist with an exercise rehabilitation program, and the supervising physician should recognize that many of them will find compliance difficult.

The exercise prescription should take full account of gender-related differences in acute and chronic responses to physical activity. Programs should be arranged in a format and at a time that encourages the attendance and active participation of women (based on female aptitudes and motives for exercising, as discussed above). Because feelings of depression, anxiety and guilt are more prevalent in women than in men (70), female class members may have a greater need than men for associated sessions of psychotherapy. They should be taught the normality of a depressed mood state following myocardial infarction and, perhaps more importantly, a parallel program should be instituted to educate their spouses regarding both the physical and the emotional problems of life during the recovery process. If vigorous physical activity is still limited by anginal-type pain, appropriate medication should be provided, and an interval training regimen should be considered as a substitute for continuous aerobic exercise.

Because of the high incidence of coronary vascular spasm, nitrites and calcium-channel blocking drugs may be particularly effective in helping women to begin an effective exercise program. However, nonspecific β-blocking drugs should be given with care, since the vulnerability to peripheral vascular spasm under cold conditions is greater in women than in men.

Obesity is not in itself a major cardiac risk factor for women. Nevertheless, correction of obesity will increase the patient's relative aerobic power and relative strength, thus increasing her functional capacity and improving her quality of life. The need to strengthen skeletal muscles, now gaining recognition in male patients, is even greater in women, given their lower initial levels of strength. Given that most women either cannot or will not abandon their traditional roles as homemakers, it is finally important that they be taught techniques that will reduce the energy costs of household work, thus extending the range of activities that they can undertake in the face of limited cardiovascular function (71).

Continuing risk factors should be corrected where possible, with a particular focus on cigarette smoking, oral contraceptives (in premenopausal women), diabetes, and hypertension. Regular monitoring and periodic repetition of counseling is important to success. One study found that treatment of hypertension was adequate in only 27% of women following myocardial infarction (117), and others have noted a strong tendency for the recidivism of smokers after they have recovered from a myocardial infarction (2,118).

Estrogen replacement has not been formally evaluated as an adjuvant to an exercise rehabilitation program, although there is some evidence of benefit when it is administered to postmenopausal patients. If given alone to premenopausal women, there would be an offsetting increase in the risk of uterine and breast cancers (119), and it is still unclear how far the coronary protection would be attenuated if it were given in combination with progesterone.

Exercise may offer some help in encouraging smoking withdrawal, but the moderate levels of socially focused activity popular with many women have less impact in discouraging smoking than would a demanding aerobic-type endurance training program.

Finally, attempts should be made to reduce the intake of saturated fats. However, women have a less favorable response than men on switching to a diet of unsaturated fat. In particular, they show a fall of HDL cholesterol, so that the LDL/HDL ratio rises to male levels (120). Women with the APO E 3/2 phenotype are at a particular disadvantage in this respect.

CONCLUSIONS

There are many important gender-related differences in responses to acute bouts of exercise and to training programs. The interaction of these differences with cardiac risk factors must be given careful consideration in designing programs of exercise and cardiac rehabilitation for women. However, given a program that has been designed to meet the needs of women and strong encouragement of the individual participant, there is good reason to anticipate that female patients will derive substantial therapeutic benefit from programs of both primary and secondary prevention.

ACKNOWLEDGMENT

Dr. Shephard's studies are supported in part by research grants from the Toronto Rehabilitation Centre and Canadian Tire Acceptance Limited.

REFERENCES

1. Mausner J.S., and Bahn A.K., *Epidemiology: An Introductory Text.* Saunders, Philadelphia (1974).
2. Kavanagh, T., *The Healthy Heart Programme.* Van Nostrand, Toronto (1985).
3. Packard, B., in *Rehabilitation of the Coronary Patient.,* 3rd Ed. (N.K. Wenger and H.K. Hellerstein, eds). Churchill Livingstone, New York, pp. 217–230 (1992).
4. Klafs, C.E., and Lyon, M.J., *The Female Athlete: A Coach's Guide to Conditioning and Training.* Mosby, St. Louis (1978).
5. Wells, C.L., *Women, Sport and Performance.* Human Kinetics, Champaign, Illinois (1985).
6. Hanley, P.C., Zinsmeister, A.R., Clements, I.P., Bove, A.A., Brown, M.L., and Gibbons, R.J., *J. Am. Coll. Cardiol.,* 13: 624–629 (1989).
7. Hall, M.A., in *Canadian Sport: Sociological Perspectives.* (R.G. Gruneau and J.G. Albinson, eds.). London: Addison-Wesley, London, pp. 170–199 (1976).
8. Loy J.W., McPherson B.D., and Kenyon, G., *Sport and Social Systems.* Addison-Wesley, London (1978).
9. Houghton, J.L., Price, C., Chatterjee, B., and Adams, K.F., *J. Cardiopulm. Rehabil.,* 10: 58–64 (1990).
10. Franquiz, J.M., Alvarez, A., Fernandez, R., and Maltas, A.M., *J. Cardiopulm. Rehabil.,* 12: 183–187 (1992).
11. Higginbotham, M.B., Morris, K.G., Coleman, E., and Cobb, F.R., *Circulation,* 70: 357–366 (1984).
12. Cumming, G.R., Dufresne C., and Samm, J., *Can. Med. Assoc. J.,* 109: 108–111 (1973).
13. Sidney, K.H., Shephard, R.J., *Br. Heart J.,* 39: 1114–1120 (1977).
14. Chaitman, B.R., Bourassa, M.G., and Lam, J., *Coronary Heart Disease in Women.* (E.D. Eaker, B. Packard, N.K., Wenger, et al., eds.). Haymarket Doyma, New York, p. 222 (1987).
15. Manca, C, Dei Cas, L., Albertini, D., Baldi, G., and Visioli, O., *Cardiology* 63: 312–319 (1978).
16. Jones, R.H., McEwan, P., Newman, G.E., Port, S., Rerych, S.K., Scholz, P.M., Upton, M.T., Peter, C.A., Austin, E.H., Leong, K.-H., Gibbons, R.J., Cobb, F.R., Coleman R.E., and Sabiston, D.C., *Circulation,* 64: 586–601 (1981).
17. Glazer, M.D., and Hurst, J.W., *Am. J. Noninvas. Cardiol.,* 1: 61 (1987).
18. Kollias. J., Bartlett, L., Bergsteinova, V., Skinner, J.S., Buskirk, E.R., and Nicholas, W.C., *J. Appl. Physiol.,* 36: 577–580 (1974).
19. Graham, T.E., *Hum. Biol.,* 55: 463–476 (1983).
20. Shephard, R.J., *Sports Med.,* 16: 266–289 (1993).
21. Drinkwater, B., *Ex. Sport Sci. Rev.,* 12: 21–51 (1984).
22. Frye, A.J., and Kamon, E., *J. Appl. Physiol.,* 50: 65–70 (1981).
23. Murray, S.J., Shephard, R.J., Greaves, S., Allen, C., and Radomski, M., *Eur. J. Appl. Physiol.,* 55: 610–618 (1986).
24. Brownell, K.D., Bachorik, P.S., Ayerle, R.S., *Circulation,* 65: 477–484 (1982).
25. Goldberg, L., and Elliot, D.L., *Sports Med.,* 4: 307–321 (1987).

26. Després, J.P., Bouchard, C., Savard, R., et al., *Eur. J. Appl. Physiol.*, 53: 25–30 (1984).
27. Rifkind, B.M., Tamir, I., Heiss, G., Wallace, R.B., and Tyroler, H.A., *Lipids*, 14: 105–112 (1979).
28. Tipton, C.M., *Ex. Sport Sci. Rev.*, 19: 447–506 (1991).
29. King, D.S., Galsky, G.P., Staten, M.A., et al., *J. Appl. Physiol.*, 63: 2247–2252 (1987)
30. Holloszy, J.O., Schultz, J., Kusni, J., Hagberg, J.M., and Ehsani, A.A., *Acta Med. Scand. Suppl.*, 711: 55–65 (1986).
31. Daniels, W.L., Kowal, D.M., Vogel, J.A., and Stauffer, R.M., *Aviat. Space Environ. Med.*, 50: 562–566 (1979).
32. Brown, C.H., and Wilmore, J.H., *Med. Sci. Sports Exerc.*, 6: 174–177 (1974).
33. Oyster, N., *J. Sports Med. Phys. Fitness*, 19: 79–83 (1979.)
34. Durstine, J.L., Pate, R.R., Sparling, P.B., et al., *Int. J. Sports Med.*, 8 (Suppl.): 119–123 (1978).
35. Rotkis, T., Boyden, T.W., Pamenter, R.W., Stanforth, P., and Wilmore, J., *Metabolism* 30: 994–995 (1981).
36. Hardman, A.E., Hudson, A., Jones, P.R., and Norgan, N.G., *Br. Med. J.*, 299: 1204–1205 (1989).
37. Sidney, K.H., and Shephard, R.J., *Med. Sci. Sports*, 8: 246–252 (1977).
38. Sidney, K.H., Niinimaa, V., and Shephard, R.J., *J. Sports Sci.*, 1: 195–210 (1983).
39. Morgan, P.P., Shephard, R.J., Finucane, R., Schimmelfing, L., and Jazmaji, V., *Can. J. Appl Sport Sci.*, 9: 87–93 (1984).
40. Godin, G., and Shephard, R.J., *Can. J. Appl. Sport Sci.*, 10: 36–43 (1985).
41. Godin, G., and Shephard, R.J., *Percept. Motor Skills*, 60: 599–602 (1985).
42. Shephard, R.J., Corey, P. and Cox, M.H., *Can. J. Public Health*, 73: 183–187 (1982).
43. Ward, A., and Morgan, W.P., *J. Cardiac Rehabil.*, 4: 143–152 (1984).
44. Oldridge, N.B., LaSalle, D., and Jones, N.L., *Am. Heart J.*, 100: 755–757 (1980).
45. Healy, B., *N. Engl. J. Med.*, 325: 274–276 (1991).
46. Gurwitz, J.H., Col., N.F., and Vaorn, J., *J.A.M.A.*, 268: 1417–1422 (1992).
47. Powell, K.F., Thompson, P.D., Caspersen, C.J., and Kendrick, J.S., *Annu. Rev. Public Health*, 8: 253–287 (1987).
48. Kannel, W.B., and Sorlie, P., *Arch. Intern. Med.*, 139: 857–861 (1979).
49. Lapidus, L., and Bengtsson, C., *Br. Heart J.*, 55: 295–301 (1986).
50. Magnus, K., Matroos, A., and Strackee, J., *Am. J. Epidemiol.*, 110: 724–733 (1979).
51. Scragg, R., Stewart, A., Jackson, R., and Beaglehole, R., *Am. J. Epidemiol.*, 126: 77–85 (1987).
52. O'Connor, G.T., Buring, J.E., Goldhaber, S.Z., et al., *Am. J. Epidemiol.*, 126: 741–742 (abstr.) (1987).
53. Blair, S.N., Kohl, H.W., Paffenbarger, R.S., Clark, D.G., Cooper, K.H., and Gibbons, L.W., *J.A.M.A.*, 262: 2395–2401 (1989).
54. Berger, H.J., Sands, M.J., and Davies, R.J., *Ann. Intern. Med.*, 94: 186–191 (1981).
55. Gibbons, R.J., Lee, K.L., Cobb, F., and Jones, R.H., *Circulation*, 64: 952–957 (1981).

56. Ayanian, J.Z., and Epstein, A.M., *N. Engl. J. Med.,* 325: 221–225 (1991).
57. Steingart, R.M., Packer, M., Hamm, P., Coglianese, M.E., Gersh, B., Geltman, E.M., et al., *N. Engl. J. Med.,* 325: 226–230 (1991).
58. Petticrew, M., McKee, M., and Jones, J., *Br. Med. J.,* 306: 1164–1166 (1993).
59. Shephard, R.J. *J. Cardiopulm. Rehabil.,* 9: 17–23 (1989).
60. Lerner, D.J., and Kannel, W.B., *Am. Heart J.,* 111: 383–390 (1986).
61. Kannel, W.B., and Abbott, R.D., in *Coronary Heart Disease in Women,* (E.D. Eaker, B. Packard, N.K., Wenger et al., eds.). Haymarket Doyma, New York, p. 208 (1987).
62. Romo M. Factors relating to sudden death in acute ischaemic heart disease. A community study in Helsinki. *Acta Med. Scand.,* Suppl. 547. (1972).
63. Hanson, P., Stevens, R., Berkoff, H., Chopra, P., Kroncke, G., Myerowitz, D., Albrecht, A., Christopherson, M.S., Eyherabide, A., and Bruskewitz, E., *J. Cardiopulm. Rehabil.,* 5: 389–397 (1985).
64. Walling, A., Tremblay, G.J.L., Jobin, J., Charest, J., Delage, F., LeBlanc, M-H., Tessier Y., and Villa, A., *J. Cardiopulm. Rehabil.,* 8: 99–106 (1988).
65. Puletti, M., Sunseri, L., Curione, M., Erba, S.M., and Borgia, C., *Am. Heart J.,* 108: 63–66 (1984).
66. Tofler, G.H., Stone, P.H., Muller, J.E., Willich, S.N., Davis, V.G., Poole, K.W., Strauss, H.W., Willerson, J.T., Jaffe, A.S., Robertson, T., Passamani, E., Braunwald, E., and the MILIS Study Group, *J. Am. Coll. Cardiol.,* 9: 473–482.
67. Boogaard, M.A.K., and Briody, M.E., *J. Cardiopulm. Rehabil.,* 5: 379–388.
68. Chiricos, T.N., and Nickel, J.L., *Women Health,* 9: 55–74 (1984).
69. Wenger, N.K., *Annu. Rev. Med.,* 36: 285–294 (1985).
70. Fisher, L.D., Kennedy, J.W., Davis, K.B., Maynard, C., Fritz, J.K., Kaiser, G., Myers, W.O., and participating CASS clinics, *J. Thorac. Cardiovasc. Surg.,* 84: 334–341 (1982).
71. Wenger, N.K., in *Rehabilitation of the Coronary Patient* (NK Wenger and HK Hellerstein, eds.). Churchill-Livingstone, New York, p. 415. (1992).
72. O'Callaghan, W.G., Teo, K.K., O'Riordan, J., Webb, H., Dolphin, T., and Horgan, J.H., *Eur. Heart J.,* 8: 649–651 (1984).
73. Maeland, J.G., and Havik, O.E., *Scand. J. Soc. Med.* 14: 183–195 (1986).
74. Burgess, A.W., Lerner, D.J., D'Agostino, R.B., Vokonas, P.S., Hartman, C.R., and Gaccione P., *Soc. Sci. Med.,* 24: 359–370 (1987).
75. Degré-Coustry, C., and Grevisse, M., *Adv. Cardiol.,* 29: 126–131 (1982).
76. Smith, G.R., and O'Rourke, D.F., *J.A.M.A.,* 259: 1673–1677 (1988).
77. Kannel, W.B., and Brand, F.N., in *Principles of Geriatric Medicine.* (R. Andres, E.L., Bierman, and W.R. Hazzard, eds). McGraw Hill, New York, pp. 104–119 (1985).
78. Anderson, T.W., *Lancet,* 2: 1084–1085 (1973).
79. Szadjerman, M., and Oliver, M.P., *Lancet,* 1: 962–965 (1963).
80. Rosenberg, L., Hennekens, C.H., Rosner, B., Belanger, C. Rothman, K.J., and Speizer, F.C., *Am. J. Obstetr. Gynecol.,* 139: 47–51 (1981).
81. Gordon, T., Kannel, W.B., Hjortland, M.C. and McNamara, P.M., *Ann. Intern. Med.,* 89: 157–161 (1978).

82. Bush, T.L., Barrett-Connor, E., Cowan, L.D., Criqui, M.H., Wallace, R.B., Such-indran C.M., Tyroler, H.A., and Rifkind, B.M., *Circulation*, 75: 1102–1109 (1987).

83. Sullivan, J.M., Vander Zwaag, R., Hughes, J.P., Maddock, V., Kroetz, F.W., Rama-nathan, K.B., and Mirvis, D.M., *Arch. Intern Med.*, 150: 2557–2562 (1990).

84. Royal College of General Practitioners, *Oral Contraceptives and Health*. Pitman, London (1974).

85. Mann, J.I., Vessey, M.P., Thorogood, M., et al., *Br. Med. J.*, 2: 241–245 (1975).

86. Jick, H., Dinan, B, Herman, R., and Rothman, K.J., *J.A.M.A.*, 240: 2548–2552, (1978).

87. Rosenberg, L., Miller, D.R., Kaufman, D.W., Helmrich, S.P., van de Carr, S., Stol-ley, P.D., and Shapiro, S., *J.A.M.A.*, 250: 2801–2806 (1983).

88. Khaw, K.-T., and Barrett-Connor, E., *J. Cardiopulm. Rehabil.*, 6: 474–480 (1986).

89. Johansson, S., Bergstrand. R., Pennert, K., Ulvenstam, G., Vedin, A., Wedel, H., Wilhelmsson, C., Wilhelmsson, L. and Aberg, A., *Am. J. Epidemiol.*, 121: 823–831 (1985).

90. Perkins. J., and Dick, T.B., *Postgrad. Med. J.*, 61: 295–300 (1985).

91. Salonen, J.T., *Br. Heart J.*, 43: 463–469 (1980).

92. Mulcahy. R., *Br. Heart J.*, 49: 410–415 (1983).

93. Rode, A., Ross, R., and Shephard, R.J., *AMA Arch. Environ. Health*, 24: 27–36 (1972).

94. Winniford, M.D., Jansen, D.E., Reynolds, G.A., Apprill, P., Black, W.H., and Hillis, L.D., *Am. J. Cardiol.*, 59: 203–207 (1987).

95. Deanfield, J.E., Shea, M.J., Wilson, R.A., Horlock, P., de Landsheere, C.M., and Selwyn, A.P., *Am. J. Cardiol.*, 57: 1005–1009 (1986).

96. Mauoad, J., Fernandez, F., Hebert, J.L., Zamani, K., Barrillon, A., and Gay, J., *Cathet. Cardiovasc. Diagn.*, 12: 366–375 (1986).

97. Moss, A.J., Carleen, E., and Multicenter Postinfarction Research Group, in *Coronary Heart Disease in Women* (E.D. Eaker, B, Packard, and N.K. Wenger, eds.). Haymarket Doyma, New York, p. 204 (1987).

98. Elveback, L.R., and Connolly, D.C., *Mayo Clin. Proc.*, 60: 305–311 (1985).

99. Lerner, D.J., and Kannel, W.B., *Am. Heart J.*, 111: 383–390 (1986).

96. Harris, T., Cook, E.F., Kannel, W.B., and Goldman, L., *J. Am. Geriatr. Soc.*, 36: 1023–1028 (1988).

101. Kannel, W.B., and Feinleib, M., *Am. J. Cardiol.*, 29: 154–163 (1972).

102. Johansson, S., Bondjers, G., Fager, G., Wedel, H., Tsipsgianni, A., Olofsson, S.O., Vedin, A., Wiklund, O., and Wilhelmsson, C., *Arteriosclerosis*, 8: 742–749 (1988).

103. Westlund, K., *Mortality of diabetics*. Universitetsforlaget, Oslo (1969).

104. Tansey, M.J.B., Opie, L.H., and Kennelly, B.M., *Br. Med. J.*, 1: 1624–1629 (1977).

105. Kannel, W.B., Sorlie, P., Castelli, W.P., and McGee, D., *Am. J. Cardiol.*, 45: 326–330 (1980).

106. Gillum, R.F., *Circulation*, 79: 756–765 (1989).

107. Campeau, L., Enjalbert, M., Lesperance, J., Bourassa, M.G., Kwiterovich, P., Wac-holder, S., and Sniderman, A., *N. Engl. J. Med.*, 311: 1329–1332 (1984).

108. Khaw, K.T., *Br. Med. J.,* 306: 1145–1146 (1993).
109. Kemp, H.C., Kronmal, R.A., Vliestra, R.E., and Frye, R.L., *J. Am. Coll. Cardiol.,* 7: 479–483 (1986).
110. Pedersen, T.R., *N. Engl. J. Med.,* 313: 1055–1058 (1985).
111. Beta-blocker Heart Attack Trial Research Group, *J.A.M.A.,* 247: 1707–1717 (1982).
112. Shekelle, R.B., Gale, M., and Norusis, M., *Am. J. Cardiol.,* 56: 221–225 (1985).
113. ISIS-2 (Second International Study of Infarct Survival) Collaborative Group, *Lancet* 2: 349–353 (1988).
114. Italian Group for the Study of Streptokinase in Myocardial Infarction (GISSI), *Lancet,* 1: 397–401 (1986).
115. Cowley, M.J., Mullin, S.M., Kelsey, S.F., Kent, K.M., Gruentzig, A.R., Detre, K.M., and Passamani, E.R., *Circulation,* 71: 90–97 (1985).
116. Stanton, B.A., Zyzanski, S.J., Jenkins, C.D., et al., *Psychopathological and Neurological Dysfunctions Following Open-Heart Surgery* (R. Becker ed.). Heidelberg: Springer-Verlag, p. 217 (1982).
117. Connolly, D.C., Elveback, L.R., and Oxman, H.A., *Mayo Clin. Proc.,* 58: 249–254 (1983).
118. Young, D.T., Kottke, T.E., McCall, M.M., and Blume, D., *J. Cardiac Rehabil.,* 2: 32–36 (1982).
119. American Medical Association, Council on Scientific Affairs (N.M. Kaplan, Chair). *J.A.M.A.,* 249: 359–367 (1983).
120. Cobb, M.M., Teitlebaum, H., Risch, N., Jekel, J., and Ostfeld, A., *Circulation,* 86: 849–857 (1992).

9

General Principles of Exercise Testing and Training in a Cardiac Population

HENRY S. MILLER, JR., and JASON L. FOX
Wake Forest University
 School of Medicine
Winston-Salem, North Carolina

PETER H. BRUBAKER
Wake Forest University
Winston-Salem, North Carolina

INTRODUCTION

The principles of exercise testing and training outlined in this chapter apply to the population of patients with valvular disease, cardiomyopathy, and coronary artery disease in addition to those who are at high risk for coronary atherosclerosis. Exercise prescription and training specific for patients with coronary disease, congestive failure, and others may be outlined in more detail in the chapters related to these problems.

Prompt use of thrombolytic therapy at the onset of myocardial infarction, percutaneous transluminal coronary angioplasty, atherectomy, stenting, and coronary artery bypass graft surgery improve myocardial blood flow. The use of angiotensin converting enzyme inhibitors, angiotensin-II blockers, beta blockers, and other drugs significantly improve the clinical and functional status of patients with heart failure and other complications of coronary heart disease. Repair of valvular and congenital heart abnormalities now restores exercise capacity. Medications and cardiac transplantation have improved survival and functional capacity of the patients with cardiomyopathy. Transvenous application of antitachycardia/defibrillation devices, pacemakers, and ablation of arrhythmia-generating sites have dramatically reduced the morbidity and mortality related to rhythm disturbances. These therapies and procedures have markedly increased the number of patients surviving a wide range of cardiovascular problems. All these individuals can benefit from exercise conditioning and improved fitness.

It is important to note that the general principles of cardiac exercise testing and training are essentially the same regardless of the patient population. Since the exercise prescription establishes a safe and effective individual exercise program specifically defining intensity, duration, frequency, and mode of activity, these parameters are specifically adjusted to meet the individual patient needs.

EXERCISE TESTING

Although there have been many advances in the technology related to the diagnosis and treatment of cardiovascular disease (CAD), as previously noted, the exercise test remains an indispensable tool for assessing cardiorespiratory function. The properly performed exercise test yields valuable diagnostic, prognostic, functional, and therapeutic information at a relatively low cost and with minimal risk to the patient. Data from several studies indicate that exercise testing is very safe, even in high-risk patients, with one or fewer deaths, four or fewer myocardial infarctions, and approximately five hospital admissions per 10,000 exercise tests (1). To minimize the risk to the patient while achieving the objectives of the exercise test, it is important that recommended guidelines from professional organizations including the American College of Sports Medicine (ACSM), the American Association of Cardiovascular and Pulmonary Rehabilitation (AACVPR), and the American Heart Association (AHA) are closely followed (2–4). This section describes such guidelines and address the many important issues to consider in the administration of exercise tests to individuals with cardiovascular disease or at high risk for its development.

Pretest Considerations

Prior to the exercise test, information from a medical history and physical examination should be reviewed for all patients with known or suspected CAD to identify contraindications for exercise testing (2). The medical history should include any remote or recent medical problems, symptoms, medications, and findings from previous examinations and tests. Physical activity patterns, vocational requirements, and family history of cardiopulmonary and metabolic disorders should also be assessed. Identification of absolute contraindications (Table 1) should result in cancellation of the test and referral of the patient to the cardiologist or primary physician for further medical management. Patients with relative contraindications may be tested only after careful evaluation of the risk/benefit ratio. The identification of major CAD risk factors and signs and symptoms suggestive of cardiopulmonary disease is important to determine the need for extra caution during the test and in stratifying the patient for risk (2). The ACSM and other guidelines include pertinent information for all of these procedures.

Detailed verbal and written instructions, provided to the patient in advance,

TABLE 1   Contraindications to Exercise Testing

Absolute contraindications
1. A recent significant change in the resting ECG suggesting infarction or other acute cardiac event.
2. Recent complicated myocardial infarction (unless patient is stable and pain-free).
3. Unstable angina.
4. Uncontrolled ventricular arrhythmia.
5. Uncontrolled atrial arrhythmias that compromises cardiac function.
6. Third degree AV heart block without pacemaker.
7. Acute congestive heart failure.
8. Severe aortic stenosis.
9. Suspected or known dissecting aneurysm.
10. Active or suspected myocarditis or pericarditis.
11. Thrombophlebitis or intracardiac thrombi.
12. Recent systemic or pulmonary embolus.
13. Acute infections.
14. Significant emotional distress (psychosis).
Relative contraindications:
1. Resting diastolic blood pressure >115 mm Hg or resting systolic blood pressure >200 mm Hg.
2. Moderate valvular heart disease.
3. Known electrolyte abnormalities (hypokalemia, hypomagnesemia).
4. Fixed-rate pacemaker (rarely used).
5. Frequent or complex ventricular ectopy.
6. Ventricular aneurysm.
7. Uncontrolled metabolic disease (e.g., diabetes, thyrotoxicosis, or myxedema).
8. Chronic infectious disease (e.g., mononucleosis, hepatitis, AIDS).
9. Neuromuscular, musculoskeletal, or rheumatoid disorders that are exacerbated by exercise.
10. Advanced or complicated pregnancy.

Source: From Ref. 2.

should include information about refraining from the ingestion of food, alcohol, caffeine, or use of tobacco products within 3 hrs prior to testing. It is best if the patient is well rested before the exercise test and has not been vigorously active on the day of the test. Patients should be instructed to continue their prescribed medications unless instructed otherwise. Tapering beta blockers or discontinuing antianginal medications for several days prior to testing may increase the sensitivity of a diagnostic test; but because of the effect on symptoms, blood pressure and pulse rate, they should be continued in the patients with known disease who will be taking these medications while exercising. Clothing should be comfortable and provide freedom of movement and easy access for electrode and the placement of a blood pressure cuff. Well-fitting walking shoes with rubber soles should be worn to ensure good traction, particularly if a treadmill is the mode of testing.

A thorough explanation of the potential risks and discomforts associated with exercise testing as well as a demonstration concerning how to get on and off the testing apparatus is required prior to testing. Enhanced test results may be obtained if steps are taken to reduce pretest anxiety, answer questions, and describe expectations such as reporting symptoms, level of test endpoints, and required exertion. An informed consent, as is noted by the ACSM's *Guidelines for Exercise Testing and Prescription* (2), has important ethical and legal implications and ensures that the patient knows and understands the purpose and risks associated with the exercise test when properly reviewed and explained.

Exercise Test Selection

The purpose of the test, the health and fitness of the patient, the exercise modality, and the exercise protocol are fundamental considerations in testing. In many exercise testing laboratories, these issues may be dictated by the equipment available, but each of these factors can have a profound effect on the response to the exercise test.

Modes

An ideal exercise mode increases total body and myocardial oxygen demand at safe increments and within a reasonable time period. This requires a dynamic exercise device that uses major muscle groups, permitting large increases in cardiac output, oxygen delivery, and gas exchange. Many modalities have been used for diagnostic testing, including cycle ergometers, treadmills, arm ergometers, steps, and, recently, chemical stressors.

The bicycle ergometer and the treadmill are the most commonly used dynamic exercise devices. The bicycle is generally less expensive and occupies less space. Upper body motion is decreased, making blood pressure and electrocardiographic (ECG) recordings easier. The work rate administered by simple, mechanically braked cycle ergometers is not always accurate, as it is dependent upon pedaling speed. Though more expensive, the electronically braked bicycle ergometers maintain the work rate at a specified level over a wide range of pedaling speeds. The cycle ergometer workload is usually expressed in kilogram-meters per minute (kgm/min) or watts and is related to body weight.

The treadmill is used most often for exercise testing in North America (5). Researchers comparing treadmill and bicycle ergometer exercise tests have reported maximal oxygen uptake to be 10–20% higher (range, 6–25%) and maximal heart rate has been reported to be 5–20% higher on the treadmill (6–8). ST-segment changes are reported and angina is elicited more frequently during treadmill testing compared with the cycle ergometer (7–9). Exercise-induced myocardial ischemia by thallium scintigraphy was recently reported to be greater after treadmill testing than after cycle ergometry (8).

Protocols

As discussed, exercise testing may be performed for diagnostic purposes, for functional assessment, and/or for risk stratification. The purpose of the test and the individual influence the selection of a protocol. For example, a maximal, symptom-limited test on a relatively demanding protocol would not be appropriate (or very informative) for a severely limited patient. Likewise, a very gradual protocol might not be used for an apparently healthy, active individual. Utilization of submaximal testing, gas exchange techniques, the presence of a physician, and exercise modes are dictated by the individual and goals of the test.

Submaximal exercise testing is most appropriate clinically for predischarge, post–myocardial infarction evaluations. It has been shown to be important in stratifying these patients for risk (10), for making appropriate activity recommendations, and for recognition of the need for modification of the medical regimen or the need for vascular interventions. Submaximal testing is also appropriate for patients with a high probability of serious arrhythmias. A submaximal predischarge test appears to be as predictive for future events as a symptom-limited test when performed less than 1 month post-MI. The testing endpoints for submaximal testing have traditionally been arbitrary but should always be based on clinical judgment. A heart rate limit of 140 beats per minute and a metabolic equivalent (MET) level of 7 are often used for patients younger than 40 years of age and limits of 130 beats per minute and a MET level of 5 are often used for patients over age 40. For those on beta blockers, a Borg perceived exertion level in the range of 7 to 8 (1 to 10 scale) or 15 to 16 (6 to 20 scale) is a conservative endpoint. Maximal testing is probably more appropriate for those more than 1 month post-MI but has been used safely earlier for risk stratification.

A 1980 survey suggests that roughly two-thirds of practitioners in North American employ the Bruce protocol for exercise testing (5). Since then, however, an appreciation for more gradual, individualized protocols has occurred (6,7,11–15). Large and unequal work increments have been shown to result in less accurate estimates of exercised capacity, particularly for patients with CAD. Recent investigations (15) demonstrate that work-rate increments that are too large or rapid result in a falsely increased estimate of exercise capacity, less reliability for studying the effects of therapy, and a reduction in test accuracy for detecting CAD.

Individualizing the protocol appears to offer several advantages for cardiopulmonary assessment. Protocols should include a low-intensity warm-up phase followed by progressive, continuous exercise in which the demand is elevated to a patient's maximal level within a total duration of 8–12 min. It is important to report exercise capacity in METs and not treadmill time, so that exercise capacity can be compared uniformly between protocols. Modifications of the Balke Ware protocol are often used with a constant treadmill speed between 2 and 3.3 mph and equal increments in grade (2.5 or 5.0%) every 2 min.

The ramp test can overcome some of the limitations of incremental protocols. The ramp protocol employs a constant and continuous increase in metabolic demand that replaces the "staging" used in conventional exercise tests. The uniform increase in work allows for a steady rise in cardiopulmonary responses and permits a more accurate estimation of oxygen uptake (7,10). Investigators in one laboratory have developed a Bruce ramp protocol to reduce the problems encountered with large increments of work (16).

A key issue emphasized in recent studies is the individualization of the exercise protocol. Individualizing the test appears to optimize the information yield, and permits targeting the test duration to the recommended duration of 8–12 min. This duration has been justified not only on the basis of convenience but also in terms of evaluating the responses and limits of the cardiorespiratory system and predicting exercise capacity from work rate attained.

Monitoring Techniques

Electrocardiography

Although echocardiographic, nuclear, and invasive techniques add valuable diagnostic information to the exercise test, the ECG remains an integral part of the cardiopulmonary assessment of patients at high risk or with documented disease. Patient safety mandates a quality exercise ECG under all testing conditions. Critical to obtaining a high-quality ECG tracing is proper skin preparation and precise electrode placement.

The complete ECG should be recorded in the position of rest (supine or sitting) and exercise (standing or sitting) to note ECG changes that may occur in change in position.

In clinical settings, the Mason-Likar placement (Fig. 1) is generally employed, since this configuration provides a 12-lead ECG with less artifact and less restriction of movement than the standard limb placement. However, the Mason-Likar placement can result in differences in amplitude and axis when compared with the ECG with standard limb placement (17). Because these shifts may be misinterpreted as diagnostic changes, it may be advisable to do a resting supine ECG using the standard limb-lead placement prior to the test if the changes are of concern. The majority (probably exceeding 90%) of ST-segment changes will occur in the lateral precordial leads (18). Miranda and associates (18) recently studied 178 men who had undergone both exercise testing and coronary angiography to evaluate the diagnostic value of ST-segment depression in the inferior leads. Lead V_5 had better sensitivity and specificity than lead II, and this study suggested that ST-segment depression, isolated in the inferior leads, is frequently a false-positive response. During the exercise test, at least three ECG leads, representing the lateral, inferior, and anterior regions of the heart, should be continuously monitored to identify changes in rhythm, conduction, and evidence of myocardial ischemia. ECG tracings of the full 12 leads should be recorded at least once in the latter part of each stage, every 2 min during a ramp protocol, or more often if abnormalities or symptoms are observed.

The occurrence of "serious" arrhythmias during exercise, although rare, is an indication to terminate the exercise test. Serious arrhythmias may be overt, such as ventricular tachycardia, or more subtle, such as unifocal premature ventricular contractions or (PVCs) increasing in frequency or an episode of nonsustained supraventricular tachycardia. Arrhythmias for which the test should be stopped include second- or third-degree heart block, sustained supraventricular tachycardia, and ventricular tachycardia of any duration. When there is doubt as to the nature or origin of the arrhythmia, the test should be stopped. Isolated PVCs, even when they occur frequently, are not as ominous as previously thought. Recent studies have demonstrated that the occurrence of PVCs during an exercise test have minimal prognostic impact (19). PVCs should be interpreted in the context of "the company they keep," such that the decision to terminate the test should be made based on the patient's history and whether the patient remains hemodynamically stable and/or the arrhythmias are accompanied by symptoms.

A variety of medications taken by patients referred for exercise testing can have profound effects on the heart-rate response to exercise. The most common include beta blockers and certain calcium channel–blocking agents, which attenuate heart rate at rest and during exercise, and nitrates, which can increase heart rate (see Ref. 2). Because of the effects of medications on heart rate, age-predicted maximal heart rate should not be used as an endpoint during functional testing.

Blood Pressure

Assessment of systolic and diastolic blood pressure at rest and during the exercise test is important for patient safety and can provide important diagnostic and prognostic information. Property trained personnel can obtain accurate and reliable blood pressures by using noninvasive auscultatory techniques (20) and following recommended procedures (21). Blood pressure should be measured at rest prior to the exercise test in the supine and standing positions to diagnose postural hypotension. Blood pressure prior to an exercise test may be elevated compared with normal "resting" conditions owing to pretest anxiety. Persistent pretest hypertension is a relative contraindication to exercise testing (2). However, if blood pressure is elevated because of anxiety, it is common to observe a slight drop in blood pressure in the initial stages of an exercise test. Systolic and diastolic blood pressure should be assessed during the last minute of each exercise stage, every 2 min of a ramp test, and more frequently if hypo- or hypertensive responses are observed. Normally, systolic blood pressure increases in parallel with an increased in work rate and commonly exceeds 200 mmHg in healthy individuals. In general, a value above 260 mmHg is an indication to terminate the exercise test (2). Diastolic pressure normally stays the same or increases slightly during exercise. The fifth Korotkov sound, however, can frequently be heard all the way to zero in a young, healthy individual. A diastolic blood pressure exceeding 115 mmHg is an indication to terminate the exercise test (2). A drop in systolic blood pressure with increasing workloads should be immediately remeasured and the test terminated if it continues to decrease or is accompanied by symptoms. A drop in systolic blood pressure below baseline during exercise is a poor prognostic sign (22).

Expired-Gas Analysis

The measurement of gas exchange and ventilatory variables provides a valuable addition to the exercise test and increases knowledge of the patients cardiopulmonary function. Maximal oxygen consumption is the most common and generally the most useful measurement derived from gas-exchange data during an exercise test. This measurement defines the upper limits of the cardiorespiratory system and is dependent on the ability to increase heart rate, augment stroke volume, and/or increase extraction of oxygen by the active muscles.

The clinical importance of an objective and accurate measurement of exercise capacity is underscored by studies on the prognosis in patients with heart disease. In a recent review, exercise capacity was chosen more frequently than any other variable (including clinical history, markers of ischemia, or other exercise test variables) as a significant determinant of survival (23). In patients with congestive heart failure, peak oxygen consumption has been identified as one of the best predictors of survival and is widely used to determine the timing of cardiac transplantation. In one study (24), patients awaiting cardiac transplantation with a peak oxygen uptake of ≥ 14 ml/kg^{-1}·min^{-1} had a 1 year survival of 94%, whereas patients with a peak value of < 14 ml/kg^{-1}·min^{-1} decreased the 1 year survival rate to 45%.

Although peak oxygen consumption is most accurately determined from direct measurement of expired gases, this technology is not always available in clinical facilities. Consequently there have been numerous attempts to estimate the peak oxygen consumption from the exercise test time or workload. The ACSM's *Guidelines For Exercise Testing and Prescription* (2) describes equations to predict peak oxygen consumption for walking, running, arm and leg ergometry, and stair-stepping. These equations were developed primarily on young healthy subjects, and their use in other populations may result in significant errors in predicting peak oxygen consumption. A number of factors including age, functional capacity, disease status, medications, and the use of hand-rail support are known to affect the accuracy of these prediction equations. Other, recently published equations have been shown to improve the prediction of peak oxygen consumption in clinical populations (25,26) (Table 2).

Symptoms, deconditioning, and/or unwillingness to tolerate fatigue prevent many patients from attaining a true maximal level. When possible, ventilatory and gas-exchange variables should be monitored continuously during exercise, since they will be useful in determining the patient's maximum level of exertion and the subsequent endpoints of the test. Although most commercially available metabolic systems allow breath-by-breath measurement of oxygen consumption and other gas-exchange parameters, reported peak exercise values should be based on data averaged over the last 30 s of a maximum level of exercise attained or at a specific submaximal level, if that is the purpose of the test (15).

Subjective Assessments

Assessment of symptoms and perception of effort during the exercise test are important to maximize safety and may yield valuable diagnostic information. Angina and dyspnea are the most common cardiopulmonary symptoms elicited during exercise testing, and each is typically evaluated with a four-point scale (2). These scales should be shown and explained to patients prior to the exercise test. Patients should be encouraged to report any and all symptoms during the exercise test.

It is important to distinguish between typical and atypical angina, since they yield different diagnostic information. Exercise-induced discomfort in the

TABLE 2 · Prediction Equations or Estimating Maximal $\dot{V}_{O_2}$

ACSM (walking): $\dot{V}_{O_2}$ (ml/kg/min^{-1}) = 3.5 (ml/kg/min^{-1}) + 0.1 $\times$ speed (m/min^{-1}) + grade (frac) $\times$ speed (m/min^{-1}) $\times$ 1.8

FAST (walking): $\dot{V}_{O_2}$ (ml/kg/min^{-1}) = 0.0698 $\times$ speed (m/min^{-1}) + 0.8147 $\times$ grade(frac) $\times$ speed (m/min^{-1}) + 7.533 (ml/kg/min^{-1})

FOSTER (with hand-rail support): $\dot{V}_{O_2}$(ml/kg/min^{-1}) = 0.694 $\times$ (ACSM) + 3.33

chest, upper extremities, neck, and jaw that is reproducible with effort and relieved with nitroglycerin is characteristic of angina and is associated with the
presence of coronary artery disease more than any other test response. A patient
exhibiting the combination of typical angina and an abnormal ST response has
a 98% probability of having significant coronary artery disease. An important
indication to stop the exercise test is moderately severe angina (grade III) or
pain that would normally cause the patient to stop daily activities and/or take
nitroglycerin (27).

Dyspnea may be the predominant symptom in some patients with CAD,
but it is more often associated with reduced left ventricular function or chronic
obstructive pulmonary disease (COPD). In the former, it is usually accompanied
by a poor exercise capacity and can occur with impaired systolic blood pressure
responses to exercise. Dyspnea is appropriately quantified using a four-point scale
(2).

Levels of perceived exertion, when properly assessed during the exercise
test, can be used to help determine the endpoint of the test by identifying maximal
effort. The Borg perceived exertion scales have been shown to provide reproducible measures of effort within a wide range of human subjects. They are generally
not affected by cardiovascular medications such as beta blockers (19). The presence of cardiopulmonary symptoms such as angina and dyspnea and a rating of
perceived exertion should be obtained from the patient at a minimum of once
per stage. Signs and symptoms can be obtained while measuring expired gases
through the use of hand signals and/or pointing to charts.

Test Termination

The overall goal of the exercised test in patients with known or suspected disease
is to obtain a near maximal level of exertion to evaluate the response of a number
of cardiopulmonary variables. A symptom-limited maximal test is generally more
useful when assessing the cardiorespiratory responses of patients with known or
suspected disease. Patients should be instructed to exercise to the point which
they can no longer continue because of fatigue, dyspnea, or other symptoms and
be assured that the test will be terminated if abnormal responses (2) are observed.
Patients should be ''encouraged'' to exercise as long as possible, but they should
not be pushed beyond their capacity, and any request to stop the test should be
honored. Inability to fully monitor the patients' responses due to technical difficulties should result in immediate termination of the test.

Posttest Considerations

Some debate exists as to whether the postexercise recovery period should be an
active or passive process; selection of a method is dependent on the purpose of

performing the exercise test. If the test is performed for diagnostic purposes, it appears to be of value to place the patient in the supine position immediately after stopping exercise. The increase in venous return to the heart observed in the supine position results in increases in ventricular volume, wall stress, and, consequently, myocardial oxygen consumption. Several studies have show that ST-segment abnormalities are enhanced in the supine position and that an active recovery may attenuate the magnitude of these changes (28). ST-segment depression that may worsen or occur 3–4 mins into recovery correlates very closely with the presence of coronary insufficiency. Patients with symptom-limiting angina or dyspnea may become more uncomfortable in the supine position and should recover in a seated upright or semirecumbent position. If the test is performed for nondiagnostic purposes, an active recovery, at very low workloads, may be more comfortable. An active recovery decreases the risk of hypotension and minimizes the risk of dysrhythmias secondary to elevated catecholamines in the postexercise period. A passive, standing recovery should be avoided due to potential complications associated with venous pooling. Regardless of the method of recovery, patients should be monitored for at least 6–8 min into the postexercise period. The recovery period should be extended to resolve symptoms or abnormal hemodynamic and/or ECG responses. Blood pressure, ECG, and symptoms should be monitored and recorded at 2-min intervals for the duration of the recovery period and the patient observed for symptoms and signs of blood pressure change, angina, or undue fatigue while moving about the lab before leaving the area.

After completion of the observation, the patient should be given posttest instructions that include information about avoiding long hot showers or baths immediately following exercise. Furthermore, the patients should be told that they may experience fatigue and muscle soreness and to avoid any heavy exertion the remainder of the day. Any undue or suspicious discomfort during the posttest day should be reported to the physician immediately.

Data Interpretation

Except in a cardiac rehabilitation setting, the most common reason that individuals undergo exercise testing is to diagnose CAD. The majority of these patients are referred for testing for the evaluation of chest pain. In this role, the test serves the very important purpose of screening those who should or should not undergo further testing. How accurately the exercise test distinguishes individuals with disease from those without disease depends upon the population tested, the definition of disease, and the criteria used for an abnormal test.

The most common terms used to describe test accuracy are *sensitivity* and *specificity.* Sensitivity is the percentage of time a test correctly identifies those with CAD. Specificity is the percentage of time a test correctly identifies those without cardiovascular disease. Sensitivity and specificity are inversely related and are affected by both the population tested and the choice of discriminant value for test abnormality.

Prognosis

The exercise test has been shown to be of value for estimating prognosis in patients with a wide range of cardiovascular disease severity (29). There are several reasons why accurately establishing prognosis is important, and the exercise test plays a significant role in each. An estimate of prognosis may be useful to patients in planning their vocations, recreational activities, and for financial planning. Second, an estimated prognosis helps identify patients for whom interventions might improve outcome. Combining clinical and exercise test information has been shown to accurately estimate risk among men and women undergoing exercise testing (10).

Supplementary Diagnostic Tests

Radionuclide imaging techniques are a valuable complement to the exercise ECG for the evaluation of patients with known or suspected CAD. They are particularly helpful in patients with equivocal exercise ECGs, those likely to exhibit false-positive or false-negative responses, to clarify abnormal ST-segment responses in asymptomatic individuals, and to identify those in whom the cause of chest discomfort remains uncertain. Patients exhibiting both a positive exercise ECGs and positive radionuclide scans have been shown to have a 2.6-fold increased risk for subsequent coronary events (30).

Radionuclide and perfusion imaging techniques of the coronary anatomy have been shown to be somewhat more sensitive and specific than the exercise ECG for detecting CAD. An extensive review of the literature suggested that the sensitivity and specificity of exercise thallium scintigraphy for detecting coronary disease were in the order of 84 and 87% respectively (30). This modality also permits the localization of ischemia, which is not possible with ST-segment depression on the ECG. In addition, perfusion imaging permits the differentiation between fixed defects that reflect an area of myocardial infarction, versus reversible defects, which represent an area of ischemia. In addition to thallium, magnetic resonance imaging (MRI) with and without pharmacological stress is a very valuable method of noninvasive imaging to determine the presence or absence of coronary insufficiency as evidenced by myocardial perfusion.

Echocardiographic imaging of the heart is being increasingly utilized during exercise and pharmacological stress testing. Like that of standard exercise testing and radionuclide techniques, the diagnostic accuracy of echocardiography depends primarily on specific methodology used, the experience and technical ability of the personnel, and the pretest probability of coronary disease in the subjects tested. A summary of studies published since the advent of exercise echocardiography in the early 1980s suggests that the sensitivity and specificity of this technique for detecting coronary disease are both approximately 85% (31).

EXERCISE PRESCRIPTION

In order for exercise to be both safe and effective, each patient should be given an individualized exercise prescription based on his or her symptom-limited end-point from the graded exercise test, clinical status, activity history, noncardiac medical limitations, and individuals goals. It is very helpful for the physician or exercise physiologist prescribing exercise to follow guidelines established by several professional organizations, including the American College of Sports Medicine (2) and the American Association for Cardiovascular and Pulmonary Rehabilitation (3). This section includes information from these guidelines and offers some suggestions on how to optimize training in individuals with CAD. The ACSM has clearly defined the benefits of inpatient cardiac rehabilitation (Table 3).

In general, each exercise prescription should clearly articulate the following variables: type of activity, intensity, frequency, duration, rate of progression, warm-up, and cool down.

Type of Activity

The type of activity should be left to the discretion of the patient as long as it is aerobic in nature and available. Aerobic activity is defined as an activity for which the oxygen demands of the exercise can be met by the body's mechanisms for metabolizing substrates with oxygen. The activity should involve large muscle groups and entail rhythmic continuous movement, such as walking, jogging, cycling, swimming, rowing, hiking, endurance team activities. In general, walking,

TABLE 3 Benefits of Inpatient Rehabilitation

Offset the deleterious psychological and physiological effects of bed rest.

Provide additional medical surveillance of patients.

Identify patients with significant cardiovascular, physical, or cognitive impairments that may influence safety

Enable patients to return to activities of daily living within the limits imposed by their disease.

Prepare the patient and the support system at home to optimize recovery following hospital discharge.

Source: From Ref. 2.

the activity that provides the most aerobic benefit, is readily available, enjoyable, carries the least risk of causing orthopedic impairment.

Circuit weight training may have limited aerobic training benefit in that it is difficult to maintain heart rates at a consistent level to maximize cardiovascular improvement. However, resistance training that targets multiple muscle groups will help to develop strength, maintain functional capacity, maintain fat-free weight, and increase bone mineral density (32). Readers looking for more information on the rationale and guidelines for resistance training should refer to several recent publications (33,34). Research has shown that swimming may not be a good alternative for subjects whose main goals are weight loss but is a very useful modality for those patients with rheumatological and orthopedic limitations (35). Finally, it is important to consider obstacles for each type of activity— such as availability, cost, and degree of skill involved—if compliance and adherence are to be maximized.

Intensity

The exercise intensity for most cardiac patients is based on their symptom-limited maximum heart rate (HR) and HR range determined by the exercise test. To determine the patient's HR at the upper limit of his or her range, the following formula is used:

$$HR = 0.85 \times (\text{symptom-limited maximum HR} - \text{resting HR})$$

The lower limit of the HR range is determined by multiplying the difference between these two HRs by 0.5. If the patient exercises at a pace at which the HR is maintained between this upper and lower limit, they can feel confident that they are not exercising at a level that will cause cardiovascular problems. Moreover, by staying within the HR range, they will achieve aerobic training benefits. Research has shown that training benefits are not improved in normals or patients with coronary disease by exercising at a HR higher than the 85% range. Levels below 60% in subjects that have been inactive can be used for initial stages of the exercise program. Allow the subject to begin exercising at a comfortable level and then gradually increase the intensity. In cardiac patients who have not been exercising or who have recently had an MI, bypass surgery, or interventional therapy for unstable angina, an initial (1–2 months) prescription of 40–50% may be more appropriate. In patients with nonischemic forms of cardiac disease, the intensities used should be dependent on the exercise capacity and specific needs of the patients. Modifications related to special cardiac populations are discussed further on.

Frequency

As a general rule, patients should exercise three to five times per week depending, on their fitness levels, goals, and time constraints. Frequency will vary with changes in intensity and duration. Patients with low functional capacities benefit from multiple short daily exercise sessions; two to three sessions per day are appropriate for patients with three to five MET functional capacities; sessions 4 to 5 days per week are appropriate for patients with functional capacities greater than five METs (2).

Duration

The aerobic portion of the exercise should be maintained for 30–40 min per exercise session to achieve a good training effect. Many cardiac patients are not able to sustain activity for this length of time, but they should be encouraged to work toward this goal. Intermittent short periods of activity of 5–10 min alternating with rest periods can be very beneficial. In this way, the patient can gradually increase the length of activity periods and shorten rest periods, working toward the goals of exercise for 30–40 min 10–15 min two to three times per day at a higher intensity. Both methods will improve conditioning.

Rate of Progression

As patients increase their exercise capacity and tolerance with improved conditioning, either the frequency, intensity, or duration of activity must be increased. A four to six week progression (see Table 4) can be used as a general guideline.

TABLE 4   Example of Exercise Progression Using Intermittent Exercise[a]

Wk	% FC	Total Min at % FC	Min Exercise	Min Rest	Reps
A. Functional capacity (FC) >3 METs					
1	50–60	15–20	3–5	3–5	3–4
2	50–60	15–20	7–10	2–3	3
3	60–70	20–30	10–15	Optional	2
4	60–70	30–40	15–20	Optional	2
B. FC < 3 METs					
1	40–50	10–15	3–5	3–5	3–4
2	40–50	12–20	5–7	3–5	3
3	50–60	15–25	7–10	3–5	3
4	50–60	20–30	10–15	2–3	2
5	60–70	25–40	12–20	2	2

[a]Continue with two reps of continuous exercise, with one rest period, or progress to a single continuous bout.
Source: From Ref. 2.

However, each patient may adapt at a different level and the progression should be individualized.

Warm-Up

Each training bout should be started with a 5- to 10-min warm-up consisting of low-level range-of-motion exercises followed by low-level aerobic activity in the mode in which the patients will be exercising. This will allow the musculoskeletal and cardiovascular systems to adapt and prepare for higher levels of activity and will reduce the likelihood of injury.

Cool-Down

At the end of each exercise session, patients should spend 10 min cooling down, initially decreasing the intensity of the activity in which they are exercising, followed by range-of-motion exercises, games, or other types of low-level aerobic activities. This allows the cardiovascular system to slowly return to the resting level and avoid postural hypotension and minimize muscle cramping. Range-of-motion activities during these sessions will tend to increase flexibility.

Modifications of Exercise Prescription in Patients with Heart Failure, Cardiomyopathy, Valvular, and Congenital Disease

The modification of exercise prescriptions in heart failure are discussed in a chapter related to this problem. In general, patients who demonstrate poor myocardial function, as with ischemic and non-ischemic cardiomyopathy, exercise intensity and duration will need to be reduced. It may need to be started at a low level, approximately 20–40% capacity for 5–10 min, with activities interspersed with rest periods. Careful attention to dehydration and hypovolemia, particularly when the environmental humidity and temperatures are high, is very important in this group of patients to minimize the potential for syncopal episodes. Patients with coexistent ischemic heart disease requiring nitroglycerin for angina may develop syncope with light-headedness due to a drop in blood pressure and decreased preload coupled with the limited cardiac output. Arrhythmias are also commonly associated with cardiomyopathy and valvular disease and may worsen with exercise, causing a fall in blood pressure. Be sure the symptoms and signs are maximally controlled medically prior to beginning an exercise program.

Even in patients with severe congestive failure, including those who are pre- and post–cardiac transplant in a stable medical condition, significant benefits can be gained with physical training. The benefits will be related to peripheral adaptation primarily, but even minimal improvement in functional capacity is extremely beneficial to this population. More recently, studies have looked at both systolic and diastolic dysfunction and the benefits of exercise using a combination of weight-bearing and non-weight-bearing exercise (walking, bike ergometry). Results from the most recent study have not been reported, but preliminary information shows that there has been improvement in functional capacities in both categories of ventricular dysfunction.

EXERCISE TRAINING

Supervision of Training

Several risk-stratification models have been developed to give the clinician the opportunity to safely deliver cardiac rehabilitation services in an individualized and cost-effective manner (3,36,37). By applying these risk-stratification models, the clinician can classify patients based on the risk of untoward events as well as determining the level of exercise supervision, including ECG monitoring, the duration of the rehabilitation program, and the amount of reimbursement. In general, patients with depressed left ventricular function, complex ventricular arrhythmias, exertional hypotension, exercise-induced hypotension, a history of cardiac arrest, or a recent MI are considered at high risk and therefore require a higher level of supervision.

Patients at low risk may need only minimal supervision and may benefit from a home-based program, especially when barriers exist that interfere with their participation in a center-based program. DeBusk et al. (38) exercise-trained 66 patients after an uncomplicated myocardial infarction. The home-based exercise training was conducted three times per week for 26 weeks at 70–85% of the peak heart rate from a graded exercise test. No exercise-related cardiovascular complications were observed and all patients completed the study without harm.

SAFETY OF EXERCISE TRAINING PROGRAMS IN A CARDIAC POPULATION

Other chapters address specific concerns of patient populations with cardiovascular and associated disease, but the risk of death and other events in a well-monitored exercise test even in a disease and high risk population has been shown to be extremely low. Similarly, the risk is extremely low during exercise in cardiac rehabilitation programs in which all patients have coronary or other cardiovascular diseases. Documentation of the safety of testing and exercise in the cardiac population has been reported by Haskell (39) and VanCamp and Peterson (40); they surveyed cardiac rehabilitation programs in the late 1970s and later in the mid to late 1980s. The latter study noted 20 cardiac arrests in 52,300 patients exercising over 2,352,000 h. Eighteen of these were resuscitated, with only 8 sustaining a myocardial infarction. This event rate is equal to 1 arrest per 112,000 patient-hours, 1 infarction per 294,000 h, and a fatal occurrence every 784,000 patient-hours. The risk did not seem to differ whether the patients attended small or large programs or had ECG monitoring. Considering the fact that all the patients in these two survey studies had cardiovascular problems, the risk of problems in a cardiac rehabilitation program is extremely low.

In a separate study, Hossack and Hartwig evaluated their participants in the multiple exercise centers of the CAPRI Program (cardiopulmonary rehabilitation) in Seattle in which 2464 patients participated (41). Cardiac arrests occurred in 25 patients, all of whom were resuscitated. It was noted that most of these patients had been exercising above the exercise tolerance achieved during the exercise tests and were usually exercising above their prescribed heart rates. This finding has been observed in other studies. Patients should be watched closely and kept from exercising beyond those levels proven to be safe by exercise test.

As Thompson (42) noted, even though extremely low, the incidence of cardiac events was higher during the time the patients were exercising than when they were not. However, the overall mortality of patients who did exercise was significantly lower than that of those who were inactive. Thus, we should not be alarmed in having events in patient populations who have known coronary disease during exercise testing and training. As is well documented, the benefits of exercise far outweighs the risk, and careful attention to details during testing, prescribing, and administering exercise will improve the safety and benefit.

SUMMARY

This section provides an overview of methods and applications of exercise testing and exercise prescription for patients who have cardiovascular disease or have a high risk for the development of cardiovascular disease. The exercise test continues to occupy a critical place in the evaluation and management of patients with known or suspected coronary artery disease. In addition to being an inexpensive primary "gatekeeper" to more costly and invasive procedures, it is the most accessible tool to evaluate medical therapy, quantify exercise tolerance, help determine prognosis, and provide guidelines for exercise prescription. The exercise test has been shown to be extremely safe and yields an abundance of functional, diagnostic, and prognostic information. Optimizing the information yield from the test requires attention to proper methodology and an understanding of issues related to the basic physiology of exercise, safety, interpretation of ECG and hemodynamic responses, and, finally, a familiarity with various professional guidelines. The general information needed to develop an individual exercise prescription for each patient is required. Making the exercise safe, effective, and pleasurable with minimum discomfort and maximum compliance is the goal of each exercise prescription.

References

1. Thompson, P., In: *Guidelines for Exercise Testing and Prescription.* 2d ed. Lea & Febiger, Philadelphia, 359–363 (1993).
2. American College of Sports Medicine, *Guidelines for Exercise Testing and Exercise Prescription,* 5th ed. Williams & Williams, Baltimore, (1995).
3. American Association of Cardiovascular and Pulmonary Rehabilitation, *Guidelines for Cardiac Rehabilitation Programs.* 2d ed. Human Kinetics, Champaign, Illinois: (1995).
4. Fletcher, G.F., Froelicher, V.F., Hartley, L.H., Haskell, W.L., and Pollock, M.L., 91: 580–615 (1995).
5. Stuart, R.J., and Ellestad, M.H., *Chest,* 77: 94–97 (1980).
6. Buchfuhrer, M.J., Hansen, J.E., Robinson, T.E., Sue, D.Y., Wasserman, K., and Whipp, B.J., *J. Appl. Physiol.,* 55: 1558–1564 (1983).
7. Myers, J., Buchanan, N., Walsh, D., Kraemer, M., McAuley, P., Hamilton-Wessler, M., and Froelicher, V.F., *J. Am. Coll. Cardiol.,* 17: 1334–1342 (1991).
8. Hambrecht, R., Schuler, G.C., Muth, T., Grunze, M.F., Marfinger, C.T., Niebaur, J., Methfessel, S.M., and Kubler, W., *Am. J. Cardiol.,* 70: 141–146 (1992).
9. Wicks, J.R., Sutton, J.R., Oldridge, N.B., and Jones, N.L., *Circulation,* 57: 1066–1069 (1978).
10. Froelicher, V.F., *Manual of Exercise Testing.* Mosby, St. Louis, (1994).
11. Haskell, W., Savin, W., Oldrige, N., and DeBusk, R., *Am. J. Cardiol.,* 50: 299–304 (1982).
12. Webster, M.W.I., and Sharpe, D.N., *Am. Heart. J.,* 117: 505–508 (1989).
13. Tamesis, B., Stelken, A., Byers, S., Shaw, L., Younis, L., Miller, D., and Chaitman, B., *Am. J. Cardiol.,* 72: 715–720 (1993).
14. Panza, J., Quyyumi, A.A., Diodati, J.G., Callaham, T.S., and Epstein, S.E., *J. Am. Coll. Cardiol.,* 17: 657–663 (1991).
15. Myers, J., *Essentials of Cardiopulmonary Exercise Testing,* Human Kinetics, Champaign, Illinois, (1996).
16. Kaminsky, L.A., Roeker, M.S., Whaley, M.H., and Dwyer, G.B., *J. Cardio. Pulm. Rehab.* (in press).
17. Gamble, P., McManus, H., Jensen, D., and Froelicher, V.F., *Chest,* 85: 616–622 (1984).
18. Miranda, C.P., Liu. J., Kadar, A., Janosi, A., Froning, J., Lehman, K.G., and Froelicher, V.F., *Am. J. Cardiol.,* 69: 303–307 (1992).
19. Yang, J.C., Wesley, R.C., and Froelicher, V.F., *Arch. Intern, Med.,* 151: 349–353, (1991).
20. Bailey, R.H., and Bauer J.H., *Arch. Intern, Med.,* 153: 2741–2748 (1993).
21. Iyriboz, Y., and Hearon, C.M., *J. Cardiopulm. Rehabil.,* 12: 277–287 (1992).

22. Mazzotta, G., Scopinaro, G., Falcidieno, M., Claudiani, F., Decaro, E., Bonow, R.O., and Vecchio, C., *Am. J. Cardiol.,* 59: 1256–1260 (1987).

23. Morris, C.K., Ueshima, K., Kawaguchi,T., Hideg. A., and Froelicher, V.F., *Am. Heart J.,* 122: 1423–1431 (1991).

24. Mancini, D.M., Eisen, H., Kussmaul, W., Mull,R., Edmunds, L.H., and Wilson, J.R., *Circulation,* 83: 778–786 (1991).

25. Berry, M.J., Brubaker, P.H., O'Toole, M.L., Rejeski, W.J., Soberman, J., Ribisl, P.M., Miller, H.S., Afable, R.F., Applegate, W., and Ettinger, W.H., *Med. Sci. Sports. Exerc.,* 28: 808–814 (1996).

26. Foster, C., Crowe, A.J., Daines, E., Dumit, M., Green, M.A., Lettau, S., Thompson, N.N., and Weymier, J., *Med. Sci. Sports Exerc.,* 28:752–756 (1996).

27. Myers, J.N., *Med. Sci. Sports Exerc.,* 26:1082–1086 (1994).

28. Lachterman, B., Lehmann, K.G., Abrahamson, D., and Froelicher,V.F., *Ann. Intern. Med.,* 112: 11–16 (1990).

29. Chang, J.A., and Froelicher, V.F., of *Curr Probl. Cardiol.,* 19: 533–588 (1994).

30. Kotler, T.S., and Diamond, G.A., Exercise thallium-201 scintigraphy in the diagnosis and prognosis of coronary artery disease. *Ann. Intern. Med.,* 113: 684–702 (1990).

31. Greco, C.A., Alessandro S., Seccareccia, F., Ciavatti, M., Biferali, F., Valtorta, C., Guzzardi, G., Falcone M., and Palamara, A., *J. Am. Coll. Cardiol.,* 29: 267–271 (1997).

32. Braith, R.W., Mills, R.M., Welsch, M.A., Keller, J., and Pollock, M.L., *J. Am. Coll. Cardiol.,* 28: 1471–1477 (1996).

33. Feigenbaum, M.S., and Pollock, M.L., *Phys. Sports Med.,* 25: 2–10 (1997).

34. American College of Sports Medicine *Guidelines for Exercise Testing and Exercise Prescription,* 6th ed. Williams & Wilkins. Baltimore, In press.

35. Gwinup, G., *Am. J. Sports Med.,* 15: 275–279 (1987).

36. American College of Physicians, *Ann. Intern. Med.,* 15:671–673 (1988).

37. Fletcher, G.F., Froelicher, V.F., Hartley, L.H., Haskell, W.L., and Pollock, M.L., *Circulation,* 82: 2286–2322 (1990).

38. DeBusk, R.F., Haskell, W.L., Miller, N.H., et al., *Am. J. Cardiol.,* 55: 251–255 (1985).

39. Haskell, W.L., *Circulation,* 57: 920–924 (1978).

40. Van Camp, S.P., Cardiovascular complications of outpatient cardiac rehabilitation programs. *J.A.M.A.,* 256: 1160–1163 (1986).

41. Hossack, K.F., and Hartwig, R., *J. Cardiol. Rehab.,* 2: 402–408 (1982).

42. Thompson, P.D., *J.A.M.A.,* 259: 1537–1540 (1988).

10

The Prevention and Treatment of Coronary Disease: The Case for Exercise

HENRY S. MILLER, JR.
Wake Forest University School of Medicine
Winston-Salem, North Carolina

RALPH S. PAFFENBARGER, JR.
Stanford University School of Medicine
Stanford, California

INTRODUCTION

In the United States and throughout most of the world prior to the 1940s, workers were primarily employed in occupations requiring moderate to high levels of physical activity. With automation and industrialization, the level of physical activity has been gradually reduced even in those jobs that were considered manual labor. Labor-saving machines and robotics have gradually and progressively eliminated any significant physical activity related to most of the occupations in today's industrialized world. Therefore, to be physically active, one must add sports, games, or other leisure-time activities to obtain the amount of exercise that our ancestors attained through their gainful employment.

WORK AND LEISURE AND RISK OF CARDIOVASCULAR DISEASE

Few articles were written about the relationship of physical activity and the development of cardiovascular disease prior to 1950. But in 1953, Morris and his coworkers (1) pointed out that there was a relationship between physical activity and coronary disease in studies of London busmen. They compared the physical activity of the drivers with that of the "conductors," who repeatedly traversed the stairs between the upper and lower deck of the London bus, and they found the incidence of coronary disease incidence to be less in the more active conductors. Later they studied the health records of almost 18,000 British civil servants (2,3) with sedentary desk jobs. Again, they showed that those who had been vigorous in performing their yard work, hiking, running, and playing games had a coronary heart disease incidence one-half that of the workers who were less active. Paffenbarger and his coworkers (4,5) evaluated and followed over 6000 San Francisco longshoremen for over 22 years (early 1950s to early 1970s). The heavy physical activity of the cargo handlers, having an average energy expenditure of 8500 kcal or more per week, significantly lower their risk of fatal coronary heart disease, as compared with the men who had less physically demanding jobs, such as hoist operators, foremen, and clerks. In a 7-year follow-up of participants in the Multiple Risk Factor Intervention Trial (MRFIT), Leon et al. (6), having divided the subjects into tertiles according to their level of leisure time physical activity calculated in kilocalories per day, observed a decrease in the relative risk of coronary heart disease as the degree of physical activity increased. The lowest group was approximately half as active as the middle group and the high group more than twice as active as the middle group. Paffenbarger et al. (7,8) assessed the physical activity index in kilocalories per week based on habitual walking, stair climbing, leisure-time sports play, and similar activities in approximately 17,000 Harvard alumni over 10–16 years. In the 40% that had an index of 2000 kcal or more per week, the relative risk of developing coronary heart disease during the year follow-up was approximately 39% lower than the same risk in men who had an index of less than 2000 kcal. Additionally, in a longitudinal study of 14,786 subjects in 1988 (age 45–87 in 1977) of whom 3100 had chronic disease, there were 2343 deaths occurring in the population between 1977 and 1988. Again, the risk of premature death from all causes, versus increased longevity, was significantly related to energy expenditures expressed by high or low levels of the physical activity index, participation or nonparticipation in moderately vigorous recreational activities, absence or presence of cigarette smoking, absence of presence of hypertension, and other chronic diseases (15). This correlates closely with those subjects studied between 1962 or 1966 and 1977.

In review of these and similar studies, several interesting facts are noted. First, in contrast to the Harvard Alumni Studies, the MRFIT Study showed little or no benefit in mortality from exercise beyond a moderate level, even though there was significant benefit of moderate exercise compared to low of exercise. However, the MRFIT population differed in that the subjects were middle-aged men with a presumed high risk for coronary disease whose overall participation in vigorous physical activity was far less than that noted among the Harvard alumni. Secondly, in contrast to other groups, the cardiovascular disease risk was lower in the London Civil Servants Survey by Morris et al. (2) only when the physical activity included vigorous sports play in contrast to all leisure time moderate-level activities.

The differences in the findings between these studies may be related to the personal characteristics of the study population, the classification of exercise activities, and perhaps even the diagnostic criteria used for determining the presence or absence of cardiovascular disease. However, in these and some 30 studies reviewed, moderate to high levels of physical activity are related to decreased mortality and prolonged cardiovascular health.

PHYSICAL FITNESS AND RISK OF CARDIOVASCULAR DISEASE

More recent studies have looked at levels of physical fitness and the risk of subsequent cardiovascular and all-cause mortality by measuring cardiovascular fitness parameters during exercise testing. This method of population study, based on a single test measurement of fitness as it relates to mortality, is more direct than assessing leisure and work activity by various mechanisms, and the information seems to provide a valid comparison, as noted in the following studies. The evaluation of subjects in the MRFIT Study (6) show that treadmill times and percentage of subjects achieving target heart rates were significantly higher when their leisure-time activity assessment was greater. More importantly, coronary heart disease risk was less in those individuals as compared to those with the least exercise tolerance on treadmill testing. Lie and coworkers (9) evaluated the fitness by submaximal ergometer testing and followed approximately 2000 middle-aged male industrial government workers in Oslo for 7 years. They noted that the more fit participants had lower resting heart rates, blood pressure, and serum lipids; higher maximum heart rates and blood pressure during exercise; smoked less than the less fit individuals; and had approximately one-fifth the incidence of fatal coronary heart disease. Ekelund et al. (10) evaluated the 4276 middle-aged men in the Lipid Research Clinic Study by the heart rate determined at the second stage of a submaximal test and maximum time on the treadmill test. The subjects were divided into four groups and followed over an average of 8.5 years. The coronary heart disease mortality in the least fit quartile was six times greater than that in the most fit. Slatterly and coworkers (11) evaluated 2400 railway workers by recording the exercise heart rates at various stages of a treadmill fitness test. It was noted that the group with the slowest heart rate at each level had approximately one-third the number of deaths due to coronary heart disease as did those with the fastest heart rate response. Even when these studies were adjusted for age and in the Lipid Research Clinic Study for cigarette smoking, blood pressure levels, lipoprotein profiles, etc., the physical fitness levels proved to be an independent predictor.

Additionally, in 1989, Blair and associates divided 10,250 middle-aged men into five levels of fitness based on maximum treadmill performance during evaluation at the Cooper Clinic (12). They were followed for 8 years for all-cause mortality, with the death rate in the most fit group being 70% less than that in the least fit group. An increasing mortality gradient was noted from the most to least fit, with the middle group showing 45% less mortality than the lowest risk group. These trends persisted even when factoring out cigarette smoking, elevated blood pressure, elevated cholesterol, elevated glucose, and family history of high blood pressure. More recently, Blair et al. having reanalyzed the data and added subjects, again demonstrated a gradient in the reduction of mortality related to the increased fitness. Follow-up of 9777 men in this population showed that those who continued to be fit plus those that became fit between the first and second tests had a significant decrease in cardiovascular and all-cause mortality (16). This correlates with previous studies noting that even low to moderate exercise is significant as to its effect on mortality. All these studies suggest that significant protection against heart disease may be attained at a moderate level of physical fitness and exercise, with the highest levels of fitness and more aggressive training techniques allowing one to be more competitive but perhaps not increasing life expectancy or reducing the frequency of coronary events (17). From these and many other studies, one can surmise that being physically active and maintaining a good level of physical fitness lessens the mortality due to coronary disease.

EXERCISE AND MORTALITY AND REINFARCTION IN POST-MYOCARDIAL INFARCTION PATIENTS

For the patient with known cardiovascular disease who participates in an exercise program for rehabilitation and secondary prevention, the evidence of mortality reduction from any one study is encouraging but not statistically significant. However, two publications have performed meta-analyses of the available publications in which data on therapeutic physical activity training programs in patients with known heart disease could be compared with data on a controlled population. The individual studies differed in the length of time the subjects were in the training programs and the time in which they joined the exercise program following the cardiac event. However, all studies compared the patients in the exercise program with controls as to improvement in physical performance, the influence on risk factors, and, more importantly, the influence on all-cause and cardiovascular mortality and recurrence of myocardial infarction. In the first review, Oldridge and colleagues (13) surveyed a number of Scandinavian and European studies and one study from the United States. They found a significant reduction in all-cause and cardiovascular disease mortality in those subjects who were in the exercise training programs. Of interest, there were no significant group differences in the recurrence of myocardial infarction, but the mortality associated with the subsequent infarction was dramatically reduced in those patients in the physical exercise programs. Subsequently, O'Connor et al. (14) published a review some of the same studies reviewed by Oldridge (13) and added others based on slightly different inclusion criteria. Importantly, they reported the influence of the physical activity programs on mortality at 1, 2, and 3 years regardless of the patients' duration in an exercise program. They noted that the greatest reduction in all-cause and cardiovascular mortality and sudden death occurred in the first year. But even after 3 years, there was approximately a 20% decrease in these three parameters. Again, there was little effect on recurrence of myocardial infarction, but mortality from the recurrent myocardial infarction was quite low in the exercise group. In only one study was smoking control assessed; no other risk factors were addressed, as these studies were designed specifically to evaluate the influence of exercise on mortality and myocardial infarction recurrence rate following a cardiac event. As noted, because of the number of subjects in each study; the influence of exercise on mortality was not statistically significant; but by combining the number of subjects in each study, 2250 subjects and controls were analyzed, and this made the statistical difference significant. There are many skeptics who find it difficult to accept this, but whether analyzed individually or collectively, all studies follow the same trend, noting that the exercise group had a reduction in mortality.

To better examine the question of recurrent myocardial infarction, O'Connor et al. (18) evaluated 340 patients (266 men and 74 women) who survived an initial myocardial infarction between January 1, 1982, and December 31, 1983. These were matched by age, sex, and geographic area with 340 controls. The relative risk of subsequent myocardial infarction in those in the highest quartile of physical activity compared to the lowest was about 0.5 in men but 1 in women. When the subjects were further categorized by levels of energy expenditure and moderate to vigorous sports activities alone, men in the most active category had 0.39 times the risk of those in the least active category, and women had 0.43 times the risk. Adjustment for blood lipids, body mass, smoking, diet, alcohol intake, family history, and personality types did not substantially change these results. This strongly suggests that physical activity is inversely related to recurrent myocardial infarction risk independently of other coronary heart disease risk factors, even though the meta-analysis studies did not show this.

With the decrease in cardiovascular mortality, all-cause mortality, and decrease in recurrence of myocardial infarction related to increased fitness and conditioning, one must assume that longevity should be increased. As Lee et al.(19)

noted in a review of the major studies that have addressed physical activity, fitness, and all-cause mortality, physical activity is effective in delaying mortality and enhancing longevity.

Morris wrote "Exercise in the Prevention of Coronary Heart Disease: Today's Best Buy" (20). After review of many studies and proposing questions that should be addressed in regard to what is vigorous exercise for an individual, effect of coronary thrombosis, and need for rationalized study in a high risk population, he felt that in regard to the public need, physical activity could be today's "best buy" in public health in the western countries.

As the evidence builds supporting the premise that serum lipid reduction can decrease atherosclerotic plaque progression and, at times, may be related to minimal regression of the plaque size, one has to conclude that a well-designed multidisciplinary cardiac rehabilitation program of physical activity and risk-factor control should be extremely beneficial to the patient who has had a major coronary event in regard to mortality, morbidity, and quality of life.

SUMMARY

This very brief review of the relation of physical activity and fitness levels to mortality in the healthy and cardiovascular disease population is an introduction to the chapters that follow. It will be noted that patients with coronary artery disease treated medically for symptomatic and asymptomatic disease, and/or by interventional therapy—i.e., coronary artery bypass graft surgery, balloon angioplasty, etc.,—can benefit from exercise therapy. The more critically ill patients with congestive heart failure and those treated by cardiac transplant can also benefit from the effectiveness and safety of a rehabilitation program. Patients with congenital and valvular heart disease can also be functionally improved. Exercise is the base around which rehabilitation and prevention programs can be developed to positively return the patient to an as near normal a lifestyle as possible in a safe and effective way. It also creates an environment in which all other risk factors for coronary disease can be evaluated, treated, and hopefully controlled.

REFERENCES

1. Morris, J.N., Heady, J.A., Raffle, P.A.B., Roberts, C.G., and Parks, J.W., *Lancet,* 2: 1053–1057, 1111–1120 (1953).
2. Morris, J.N., Kagan, A., Pattison, D.C., Gardner, M., and Raffle, P.A.B., *Lancet,* 2: 552–559 (1966).

3. Morris, J.N., *Uses of Epidemiology,* 3rd Ed. Churchill Livingstone, Edinburgh, pp. 159–186 (1975).
4. Paffenbarger, R.S., Jr., Laughlin, M.E., Gima, A.S., and Black, R.A., *N. Engl. J. Med.,* 282: 1109–1114 (1970).
5. Paffenbarger, R.S., Jr., and Hale, W.E., *N. Engl. J. Med.,* 292: 545–550 (1975).
6. Leon, A.S., Connett, J., Jacobs, D.R., Jr., and Rauramaa, R., *J.A.M.A.,* 258: 2388–2395 (1987).
7. Paffenbarger, R.S., Jr., Wing, A.L., and Hyde, R.T., ''Am J. Epidemiol., 108: 161–175 (1978).
8. Paffenbarger, R.S., Jr., Hyde, R.T., Wing, A.L., and Hsieh, C.-C., *N. Engl. J. Med.,* 314: 605–613, 315: 399–401 (1986).
9. Lie, H., Mundal, R., and Erikssen, J., *Eur. Heart J.,* 6: 147–157 (1985).
10. Ekelund, L.G., Haskell, W.L., Johnson, J.L., Whaley, F.S., Criqui, M.H., and Sheps, D.S., *N. Engl. J. Med.,* 319: 1379–1384 (1988).
11. Slatterly, M.L., Jacobs, D.R., Jr., and Nichaman, M.Z., *Circulation,* 79: 304–311 (1989).
12. Blair, S.N., Kohl., H.W., Paffenbarger, R.S., Clark, D.G., Cooper, K.H., and Gibbons, L.W., J.A.M.A., 262: 2395–2401 (1989).
13. Oldridge, N.B., Guyatt, G.H., Fischer, M.E., and Rimm, A.A., *J.A.M.A.,* 260: 945–950 (1988).
14. O'Connor, G.T., Buring, J.E., Yusuf, S., Goldhaber, S.Z., Olmstead, E.M., Paffenbarger, R.S., Jr., and Hennekens, C.H., *Circulation,* 80: 234–244 (1989).
15. Paffenbarger, R.S., Kampert, J.B., Lee, I., Hyde, R.T., Leung, R.W., and Wing, A.L., *Med. Sci. Sports Exerc.,* 857–865 (1993).
16. Blair, S.N., Kohl, H.W., Barlow, C.E., Paffenbarger, R.S., Gibbons, L.W., and Macera, C.A., *J.A.M.A.,* 273: 1093–1098 (1995).
17. Blair, S.N., Kampert, J.B., Kohl, H.W., Barlow, C.E., Macera, C.A., Paffenbarger, R.S., and Gibbons, L.W., *J.A.M.A.,* 276: 205–210 (1996).
18. O'Connor, G.T., Hennekens, C.H., Willett, W.C., Gfoldhaber, S.Z., Paffenbarger, R.S., Breslow, J.L., Lee, I., and Buring, J.E., *Am J Epidemiol.,* 142: 1147–1156 (1995).
19. Lee, I.M., Paffenbarger, R.S. Jr. Hennekens, C.H., *Aging,* 9 (1–2): 2–11 (1997).
20. Morris, J.N., *Med. Sci. Sports Med.,* 26; 807–814 (1994).

11
Sudden Cardiac Death and Exercise in Healthy Adults

JACK M. GOODMAN
University of Toronto
Toronto, Ontario, Canada

Legend has it that in 492 B.C. Pheidippides ran over 100 mi from the plains of Marathon to Athens to announce the victory of the Athenians over the Persians and that he then died suddenly. This is likely the first widely reported case of exercise-related sudden death. Some 2000 years later, it was suggested that marathon running provided immunity against coronary heart disease (1). The so-called Bassler hypothesis has since been dismissed, as it is now widely accepted that atherosclerosis can develop in long-distance runners and that it is indeed a major culprit in cases of exercise-related sudden death, even among veteran marathon runners and those with a long history of physical activity.

Although exercise-related sudden cardiac death (SCD) occurs infrequently in the general population, sudden death remains the first symptom in 30–50% of those with coronary heart disease (2). To date, there have been over 600 reported cases of exercise-related sudden deaths occurring either during or immediately after participation in a wide range of sports. This chapter summarizes the etiology of sudden death in healthy adults and young athletes and also outlines the theoretical triggers for exercise-related SCD.

ETIOLOGY OF CARDIAC SUDDEN DEATH

Significance of Age and Gender

Analysis of autopsy data from numerous studies has established that the vast majority of SCD cases in those above the age of 30–35 years are secondary to acute complications of atherosclerosis (3). However, SCD in those below 30–35 years of age is most often ascribed to disorders of myocardial structure and/or conduction (3,4) secondary to various congenital conditions, the most common being hypertrophic cardiomyopathy. In both types of cases (Fig. 1), the immediate mechanism of death is likely fatal left ventricular arrhythmia (5). Women represent only a small fraction of SCD cases (approximately 10% of reported incidents). It is likely that men dominate the leading cause of sudden deaths (atherosclerosis) by a factor of 7–10.

Various pathological conditions become manifest as either myocardial ischemia or structural/mechanical factors that are directly attributed to SCD (Table 1). Conduction abnormalities acting independently of these conditions are rare, as are viral pathologies (myocarditis) and environmental factors that can lead to general circulatory collapse (e.g., heat stroke). Nevertheless, the last two types of conditions may precipitate cardiac sudden death if the appropriate pathophysiology is present (see "Potential triggers," below).

Morphological abnormalities of the cardiovascular system account for the vast majority of exercise-related SCD in conditioned athletes. Waller (3) has classified these abnormalities as coronary arterial, myocardial, valvular, and aortic in nature (Table 2). The first two are the most commonly seen in SCD.

ATHEROSCLEROTIC CORONARY ARTERY DISEASE IN SUDDEN DEATH

Atherosclerosis accounts for over 80% of exercise-related SCD in those over 35 years of age and over 95% in those above age 40. By definition, at least one major coronary artery must have at least 75% obstruction at autopsy if death is to be attributed to coronary artery disease (CAD) (6). Autopsy findings generally indicate prior or acute myocardial infarction or coronary thrombosis (6). The atherosclerotic lesions are typically well advanced, with close to half of autopsy-proven cases demonstrating three-vessel disease (6). Unlike anomalous origin of the coronary artery, occlusive disease is accompanied by prodromal symptoms and electrocardiographic (ECG) evidence in as many as 50% of victims prior to SCD (7). Contrary to the assertions of Bassler (1), there are a number of reports of advanced coronary disease in marathon runners (8), proving that SCD can

---

FIGURE 1   Etiologies of exercise-related sudden cardiac deaths in those above and below the age of 35 years. AVD = acquired valve disease; CAD = coronary artery disease; HCM = hypertrophic cardiomyopathy; LVH = left ventricular hypertrophy; MVP = mitral valve prolapse. (Adapted from Ref. 13.)

Exercise-Related Sudden Cardiac Death
Age < 35 yr

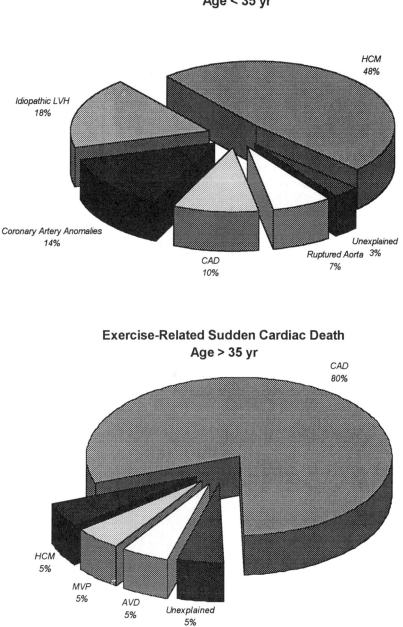

Exercise-Related Sudden Cardiac Death
Age > 35 yr

TABLE 1   Causes of Sudden Cardiac Death

Ischemia-related causes	Structural and mechanical causes
Atherosclerotic disease	Obstructive and nonobstructive hypertro-phic cardiomyopathy
Hypoplastic arteries	Mitral valve prolapse
Anomolous coronary arteries	Ruptured aorta/cystic medial necrosis
Tunneled coronary arteries	Aortic stenosis
Coronary spasm	Other myopathies

occur as a result of occlusive atherosclerotic disease despite a high commitment to endurance training (Fig. 2). Although this evidence led to categoric rejection of Bassler's hypothesis (1977), the incidence of SCD in endurance athletes is very low. Early reports estimated the risk to be at 1–2 per 18,000–25,000 marathon runners per year (8). More recent reports indicate that the risk may be even lower—0.002% or 1 in 50,000 race finishers (9). In fact, based upon a study of

TABLE 2   Pathophysiology of Exercise-Related Cardiac Sudden Death

Primary location	Potential pathophysiology
Coronary tree	Atherosclerosis
	Congenital anomalies
	Tunneled epicardial arteries
	High-takeoff coronary ostia
	Coronary trauma
	Coronary spasm
Myocardium	Hypertrophic cardiomyopathy
	Myocarditis
	Idiopathic concentric LV hypertrophy
	Right ventricular cardiomyopathy
	Marfan's syndrome
	Other congenital cardiac defects
Valves	Mitral valve prolapse
	Aortic stenosis
Aorta	Aortic rupture (Marfan's syndrome)
	Cystic medial necrosis
Conduction system	Nodal abnormalities (ischemic)
	Wolfe-Parkinson-White syndrome
	Paroxysmal tachycardias

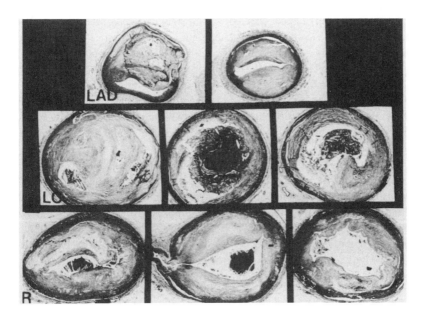

FIGURE 2   Evidence of atherosclerosis in a runner who had previously completed a number of marathons and had been averaging 80 km of running per week for more than 5 years. The right (R) left anterior descending (LAD) and left circumflex arteries (LC) were all more than 75% obstructed, with the latter obstructed completely by a thrombus. [From Virmani, R., Robinowitz, M., McAllister, H.A. Jr., *Pathology Annual, Part 2,* (Sommers, S.C., Rosen, P.P. and Fechner, R.E. eds.). Appleton-Century Crofts, Norwalk, Connecticut, p. 452 (1985), by permission.]

over 200,000 runners, Maron et al. (9) calculated that the overall risk of anyone dying in a given year (including all causes of mortality) was more than 100 times greater than that by running *one* marathon race.

The mechanism of thrombosis during exercise is unclear. Plaque hemorrhage and fissuring from mechanical trauma in the presence of advanced atherosclerotic lesions has been reported (10), yet advanced atherosclerosis is rare at a young age. Although this mechanism of luminal obstruction is not uncommon in older individuals, the cause is usually hemodynamic rather than mechanical per se. Fissuring of a previously fragile but nonocclusive plaque with thrombus formation leading to total occlusion is thought to account for most deaths with postmortem evidence of acute myocardial infarction. However, a fresh occlusive thrombus is found in only a small percentage of cases (11). In the absence of myocardial damage, transient myocardial ischemia is another possible mechanism of death; fissuring of a plaque may partially occlude a major coronary vessel, the lesion being sufficient to induce ischemia and/or vasospasm that evolves to malignant arrhythmias. In nonexercise cases of SCD, acute rupture or partial thrombosis evolving from a plaque is responsible for over 90% of the cases, occlusions often occurring at what had previously been thought to be noncritical lesions (7,12). This may explain why some individuals have previously been symptom-free or have failed to demonstrate ECG changes during a stress test; there is an acute progression in the disease state in the moments immediately preceding death (13).

In patients with CAD and moderate ischemia, the pathophysiological substrate of sudden death has been ascribed to a slowing in conduction of the electrical impulse (14). Other conduction-related arrhythmias may arise in conditions of mild ischemia, particularly if the ischemia is combined with increased circulating levels of catecholamines. Thrombus formation may also be enhanced by endothelial damage or magnesium deficiency (see below), increases in catecholamines and thrombolytic agents (15), coronary vasospasm, or paradoxical vasoconstriction secondary to CAD-induced endothelial dysfunction (16).

Pathology of the Coronary Tree

Congenital Coronary Artery Abnormalities

Abnormalities of the coronary arteries (Table 2) are observed in only 1% of those undergoing angiography and approximately 0.3% of those autopsied (17). However, such conditions are reported to be either the leading (3) or second most common (18) causes of death in athletes less than 35 years of age.

Anomalous origin of the major arteries from the sinuses of Valsalva is a common cause of SCD in athletes (7), accounting for approximately 30% of exercise-related SCD cases. It is rarely a primary cause of death in those under 30 years of age, although the older athlete who has significant atherosclerotic development in concert with this condition is at a considerably increased risk of SCD. A number of anomalies capable of causing sudden death have been reported, with close to 50% of such deaths occurring during or immediately after exercise (19). The conditions are generally asymptomatic, and they can be visualized only by techniques such as transthoracic or transesophageal echocardiography (20).

Various types of anomalous coronary artery origins have been described. The most common is an anomalous origin of the left coronary artery from the right sinus of Valsalva (7,18). The abnormal anatomy necessitates passage of the left main coronary artery between the aorta and the pulmonary trunk. This is in contrast to an anomalous origin of the right coronary artery, which may arise from the left sinus of Valsalva, passing between the aorta and pulmonary trunk (21).

The mechanism by which SCD occurs in these conditions is unclear, but it is possible that an obtuse angle of departure from the sinus may narrow the ostium of the involved artery, particularly when the stroke volume and minute ventilation are increased during exercise. The oblique takeoff from the aorta may cause a slit-like orifice in the aortic wall, which predisposes it for collapse upon diastole, particularly when the aortic root is distended during moderate to intense levels of exercise (19). Although impossible to demonstrate, the response is acute ischemia, leading to a lethal arrythmia (19,22,23).

Single coronary artery anomaly is rare, but when coupled with atherosclerosis and myocardial hypertrophy, can cause exercise-induced SCD. In such cases, the single vessel adapts and enlarges, typically evolving with other myocardial pathologies such as hypertrophic cardiomyopathy (24). Less common anomalies include *tunneled coronary arteries,* also known as myocardial bridges or intramyocardial arteries (25,26). *Hypoplasia of the coronary arteries* is a condition where the right or left circumflex artery extends beyond the lateral borders of the ventricle. Sustained ventricular tachycardia in the presence of these conditions can lead to myocardial ischemia during heavy exertion (4,19).

Coronary spasm (in the absence of CAD) is thought to cause some cases of SCD during exercise in both young athletes and older adults (3), but this is impossible to prove at autopsy. Spasm is a plausible mechanism, since it can cause local ischemia and the damaging effects of myocardial reperfusion (27). There have been reports of young athletes developing "cardiac fatigue" (depressed left ventricular function) following prolonged endurance events, with idiopathic coronary vasospasm mediated through endothelial damage as the postulated cause (15).

Marfan's Syndrome and Sudden Death

In cases of exercise-related SCD involving aortic or valvular lesions, Marfan's syndrome is usually present. Marfan's syndrome (MS) is an inherited disorder of connective tissue that involves the skeletal and ocular systems, in addition to the heart and aorta. Cardiac abnormalities include aortic dilatation secondary to cystic medial necrosis and mitral valve prolapse. Virtually all cases of SCD among individuals with MS occur through a combination of severe aortic insufficiency and ruptured aortic aneurysm or aortic dissection (28,29).

Aortic rupture is often but not necessarily secondary to MS; it has also been reported in cases of exercise-related SCD that did not show MS (18). In most cases, mediastinal hemorrhage, pericardial tamponade, and rapid congestive failure are the immediate causes of death. Even if MS is not diagnosed, aortic ruptures are often associated with classical evidence of cystic medial necrosis, reflecting an aorta that is less compliant than normal (3). Valvular pathologies independent of other pathologies (e.g., MS) are not common causes of sudden death in athletes. Despite their relatively high prevalence in the population (approximately 5%), they account for substantially less than 5% of exercise-induced deaths. Of valvular pathologies, mitral valve prolapse is most often the cause of death (4); typically, there are associated abnormal histological findings of the adjacent papillary muscles and myocardium (30) or an increased ventricular mass (e.g., hypertrophic cardiomyopathy). The mechanism of death in mitral valve prolapse is unclear, but it could involve the formation of emboli or ventricular tachycardia due to valve friction and a dislodged leaflet plaque. The leading risk indicators for exercise-induced SCD in those with mitral valve prolapse include (a) a history of syncope, (b) chest pain, (c) complex ventricular arrhythmias, (d) significant mitral regurgitation, (e) a prolonged QT interval, and (f) family history of MS (31).

Myocardial Tissue

Hypertrophic Cardiomyopathy is the most common cause of exercise-related sudden death in those under the age of 35 (18). Although this condition is rare in the general population (0.1% in young adults), 40% of HCM-related sudden deaths are associated with exertion of some type (32,33). The hallmark feature of HCM is left ventricular hypertrophy (>15 mm) without cavity dilation (Fig. 3A). The primary morphological abnormality lies in the septum, which exceeds the diameter of the free ventricular wall by a factor of 1.4 or more (4,34). Definitive diagnosis requires an abnormal histology of more than 5% of the total cardiac muscle mass (6). Although healthy endurance athletes may have modest wall thickening (13–14 mm), they usually demonstrate proportionally enlarged ventricular cavities. Associated pathologies that increase the risk of sudden death include left ventricular outflow tract obstruction, endocardial mural plaques, mitral valve disease, atrial dilation, abnormal intramural coronary arteries, and a disorganization of myocardial fibers in the septum.

The most striking feature of HCM is a focal disarray of the myocardial fibers down to the level of the myofilament (Figure 3B); this feature is seen in 90% of those with HCM (10). The morphological characteristics result in left ventricular functional impairment, including a distinct slowing of ventricular relaxation, particularly during the slow filling phase of diastole. Because of the non-physiological nature of the hypertrophy, systolic function is often diminished. The relatively small ventricular cavity size leads to a dysfunctional contraction, with supra-normal intracavitary pressure gradients (primarily due to mitral valve displacement against the enlarged septum). Outflow tract obstruction is often associated with sudden death in HCM, but it occurs in only 25% of reported cases (35).

The exact mechanism of exercise-related SCD in those with HCM is unclear (Table 3). The most likely pathology is arrhythmogenic (4,32,33). The action potential is lengthened in hypertrophied myocytes, and some experimental data suggest an ionic basis for this abnormality (36). Accessory conduction pathways, a mechanical stretching of myocytes (which can increase ectopic beat frequency) are other possible bases for the arrhythmias.

Exercise-related SCD in HCM may also arise from exertional hypotension; this is precipitated by impaired diastolic filling and a resulting low cardiac output (35). Malignant arrhythmias may arise, secondary to hypoperfusion and local ventricular ischemia; this chain of events is thought to be more common in older athletic victims, as opposed to the non-ischemic arrhythmogenic triggers found at younger ages.

Left ventricular hypertrophy secondary to hypertension is a strong risk factor in the general population (37); however, the hypertensive patient does not seem vulnerable to malignant dysrhythmias during exercise (38). Despite the known association between ventricular arrhythmias and an increase in ventricular mass, abnormal rhythms are more likely in HCM because of architectural pathologies in the left ventricular septum. Notwithstanding, hypertensive patients with left ventricular hypertrophy are at greater risk of ischemia and long-term myocardial necrosis, and these factors may be involved in the exercise-related deaths usually attributed to atherosclerosis in older individuals.

Ventricular Dysplasia

Arrhythmogenic right ventricular dysplasia (ARVD) usually affects the right ventricle but can also involve the septal region. It is a recognized cause of ventricular arrhythmias (39). However, this condition accounts for fewer than 1% of reported cases of exercise-induced CSD (39,40).

Conduction Abnormalities

Myocardial conduction abnormalities occurring independently of HCM and other congenital abnormalities are rarely the primary cause of exercise-related SCD (4). Nevertheless, a number of syndromes are associated with the sudden death of athletes, including the Wolff-Parkinson-White syndrome (41) and Lown-Ganong-Levine syndrome (42). Isolated conduction abnormalities may be a "concealed" cause of death in young athletes with normal histology because the conduction systems are rarely examined thoroughly (30). Atrioventricular and nodoventricular accessory pathways have been suggested as culprits in some

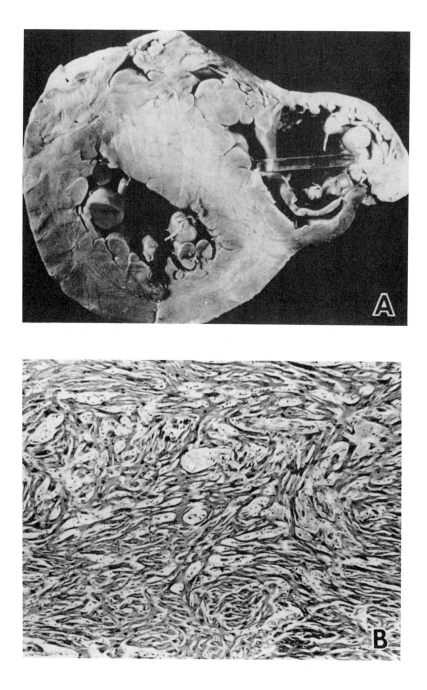

TABLE 3   Potential Mechanisms of Exercise-Related Death in Hypertrophic
Cardiomyopathy

Mechanism	Physiological cause/effect
Arrhythmogenic	
Ventricular tachy- and brady-arrhythmias	Prolonged action potential leads to increased chance of rapid depolarization and instability
Supraventricular arrhythmias with or without accessory atrioventricular pathway	Possibly due to altered ion content, abnormal electrical pathways, atrial stretching, latent ischemia and premature ventricular beats; leads to unresolved tachycardia
Other conduction abnormalities	Slowed conduction and increased chance of reentry of the electrical signal leading to ventricular tachycardia
Hemodynamic	
Hypotensive cardiac insufficiency	Arrhythmia-induced tachycardia leading to hypoperfusion, myocardial ischemia, and arrest

cases of exercise-related SCD (30). However, the lack of prior ECG evidence of such disorders in many of the athletes who die makes such speculations difficult to prove or disprove. In addition, various arrhythmias (e.g., paroxysmal supraventricular tachycardia, nonsustained ventricular tachycardia) are frequently reported in athletes but are rarely lethal.

Types of Physical Activity and Sudden Death

The distribution of sudden deaths in various sports shows a predominance of squash relative to other types of active leisure pursuits. However, this may simply

FIGURE 3   Hypertrophic cardiomyopathy (HCM) is characterized by asymmetrical and excessive hypertrophy of the ventricular septum, exceeding the normal septal to ventricular free-wall ratio of at least 1.3 (panel A). Areas of myopathic fiber disarray (panel B) are found upon histological examination; usually, they account for more than 5% of the total ventricular muscle mass. [From Virmani, R., Robinowitz, M., McAllister, H.A. Jr., *Pathology Annual, Part 2,* (Sommers, S.C., Rosen, P.P. and Fechner, R.E. eds.). Appleton-Century Crofts, Norwalk, Connecticut, p. 452 (1985), by permission.]

reflect the popularity of the sport (43). The explosive nature of squash, with sudden bursts of isometric activity, provides an ideal environment for the development of SCD if the individual has a severe cardiac pathology, yet the overall pressor response to this sport is very similar to that seen in moderate-intensity cycle ergometry (44). Unlike participants in other regular competitive sports or long-distance running, many recreational squash players engage in their chosen activity only infrequently and, being older (11), are therefore more likely to have advanced CAD. The substantial number of runners who also die suddenly (7) again reflects participation patterns in the general population, particularly in the coronary-prone age group.

Potential Triggers

In establishing a de facto *cause* of exercise-induced SCD, one must first identify a stimulus or "trigger" that must be coincident with a susceptible pathological state or underlying "environment" (*pathophysiological milieu*), typically multifactoral in nature (13). Various physiological triggers have been identified, each contributing to a general model describing the events that lead to SCD (Fig. 4).

Humoral and other blood borne triggers act to precipitate SCD in individuals who are *free* of CAD. The abnormalities identified include magnesium ion deficiency (15,45), hyperlipidemia, and hyperglycemia (46). Magnesium ion (Mg) deficiency often develops after prolonged effort and may persist for more than 12 weeks following competition. Because Mg deficiency usually elicits vasoconstriction (46), it has been proposed as triggering vasospasm-induced SCD (15) and even pronounced silent ischemia in a world-class marathon runner (47). Theoretically, Mg deficiency can also precipitate complex arrhythmias (45) that may progress to ventricular fibrillation in HCM.

Plasma catecholamine concentrations increase with both exercise intensity and duration and could elicit lethal arrhythmias. The myocardium that has unstable conduction pathways may be exposed to low-grade ischemia during exercise, perhaps owing to catecholamine-induced vasospasm. The catecholamines may also evoke electrical instability, producing nonhomogeneous electrical conduction and depolarization.

In cases of SCD where atherosclerosis is the primary pathology, shear stress on the coronary vessels may precipitate vasospasm and/or plaque fissuring (15, 48). An increased release of thromboxane A_2 (a coronary vasoconstrictor) would further enhance the likelihood of an arrhythmia (13,15,27).

Other triggers of SCD have been identified. Steroid use remains widespread in athletics, and the abuse of such drugs has been linked to both cardiomyopathy and increased thrombolytic activity (49). Cocaine derivatives are also known to stimulate arrhythmias, and cocaine abuse could be a strong stimulus for SCD if combined with HCM.

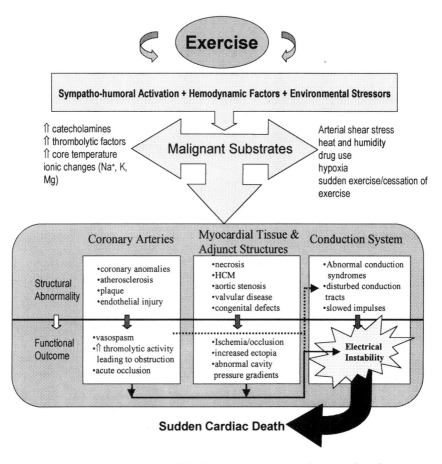

FIGURE 4   Model describing the possible factors and sequence of events triggering exercise-related cardiac sudden death. Physiological responses to exercise begin a cascade of actions that can interact with a pathological milieu to produce fatal results. These actions affect the coronary arteries, myocardial tissue, and conduction systems and can ultimately result in a malignant arrhythmia and/or thrombosis, leading to obstruction.

Sudden exercise and/or abrupt cessation of exercise may precipitate SCD in vulnerable individuals, including those with abnormal ECGs and ventricular dysfunction (50,51). Risk may be further exacerbated under adverse environmental conditions, as heat stroke has been associated with subendocardial necrosis (52). Prolonged endurance running in itself is an unlikely but possible long-term trigger for SCD (15). Prolonged effort may increase the risk of SCD via increases in core temperature, dehydration, and Mg depletion (45). Impaired diastolic and systolic performance (referred to as "cardiac fatigue") has been reported following prolonged effort (53) and may reflect subclinical myocardial damage (54). It may well increase risk, particularly in those individuals with underlying CAD.

CONCLUSIONS

The vast majority of exercise-related sudden deaths in individuals over the age of 30–35 are secondary to events caused by advanced atherosclerosis. In such cases, various malignant substrates interact and precipitate a fatal arrhythmia. In most cases, exercise-induced plaque rupture leads to thrombus formation, partial occlusion, and resultant myocardial ischemia. In rare instances, a complete obstruction is responsible for death. Malignant arrhythmias often evolve without evidence of plaque rupture. More importantly, in more than 50% of reported cases, prodromal symptoms have been reported, and thus the episode of SCD might have been avoided. For the younger population (less than 35 years of age), the common primary pathology is HCM, followed by anomolous coronary artery syndrome.

Sudden cardiac death during exercise remains extremely rare and is due to significant underlying ventricular pathology in over 95% of reported cases. Although the low incidence in the entire population does not justify mass screening procedures, efforts should be made to educate the participant to identify symptoms and the physician to identify risk factors within the general population, since there is typically an underlying pathology.

REFERENCES

1. Bassler, T.J., *Ann. N.Y. Acad. Sci.,* 301: 579–592 (1977).
2. Kannel, W.B., and Thomas, H.E. Jr. *Ann. N.Y. Acad. Sci.,* 382: 3–21 (1982).
3. Waller, B.F., in *Exercise and the Heart,* 2nd Ed. (N.K. Wenger, ed.). Davis, Philadelphia (1985).
4. Maron, B.J., Epstein, S.E., and Roberts, W.C., *J. Am. Coll. Cardiol.,* 7: 204–214 (1986).
5. Amsterdam, E.A., *Cardiology,* 77: 411–417 (1990).
6. Burke, A.P., Farb, A., and Virmani, R. *Cardiol. Clin.,* 303–317 (1992).
7. Thompson, P.D., *Med. Sci. Sports Exerc.,* 25: 981–984 (1993).
8. Noakes, T., *Med. Sci. Sports Exerc.,* 19: 187–194 (1987).
9. Maron, B.J., Poliac, L.C., and Roberts, W.O., *J. Am. Coll. Cardiol.,* 28: 428–431 (1996).
10. Maron, B.J., Anan, T.J., and Roberts, W.C., *Circulation,* 63: 882–894 (1981).

11. Northcote, R.J., Flannigan, C., and Ballantyne, D., *Br. Heart J.,* 55: 198–203 (1986).
12. Davies, M.J., and Thomas, A.C., *Br. Heart J.,* 53: 363–373 (1985).
13. Kohl, H.W., Powell, K.E., Gordon, N.F., Blair, S.N., and Paffenbarger, R.S., *Epidemiol. Rev.,* 14: 37–58 (1992).
14. Hurwitz, J.L., and Josephson, M.E., *Circulation,* 85 (suppl 1): 43–49 (1992).
15. Rowe, W.J., *Sports Med.* 16: 73–79 (1993).
16. Ciampricotti, R., el Gamal, M., and Relik, T., *Am. Heart J.,* 120: 1267–1278 (1990).
17. Baltaxe, H.A., and Wixson, D., *Radiology,* 122: 47–52 (1977).
18. Maron, B.J., Roberts, W.C., McAllister, H.A., Rosing, D.R., and Epstein, S.E., *Circulation,* 62: 218–229 (1980).
19. Taylor, A.J., Rogan, K.M., and Virmani, R., *J. Am. Coll. Cardiol.,* 20: 640–647 (1992).
20. Daliento, L., Fasoli, G., and Mazzucco, A. *Int. J. Cardiol.,* 38: 89–91 (1993).
21. Roberts, W.C., Siegel, R.J., and Zipes, D.P., *Am. J. Cardiol.,* 49: 863–868 (1982).
22. Barth, C.W., Bray, M., and Roberts, W.C., *Am. J. Cardiol.,* 57: 365–366 (1986).
23. Cheitlin, M.D., DeCastro, C.M., and McAllister, H.A., *Circulation,* 50: 780–787 (1974).
24. Van Camp, S.P., and Choi, J.H. *Phys. Sports Med.,* 16: 49–52 (1988).
25. Jokl, E., McClella, J.T., and Ross, G.D., Congenital anomaly of left coronary artery in young athlete. *J.A.M.A.,* 182: 572 (1962).
26. Morales, A.R., Romanelli, R., and Boucek, R.J., *Circulation,* 62: 230–237 (1980).
27. Myerburg, R.J., Kessler, K.M., and Castellanos, A., *Circulation,* 85 (Suppl. I): 2–10 (1992).
28. Van Camp, S.P., *Phys. Sports Med.,* 16: 92–112 (1988).
29. Van Camp, S.P., *Phys. Sports Med.,* 16: 47–55 (1988).
30. Corrado, D., Thiene, G., Nava, A., and Rossi, L., *Am. J. Med.,* 89: 588–595 (1990).
31. Jeresaty, R.M., *J. Am. Coll. Cardiol.,* 7: 231–236 (1986).
32. Maron, B.J., *Circulation* 85 (Suppl 1): 57–63 (1985).
33. Maron, B.J., and Fananapazir, L., *Circulation,* 85: I57–I63 (1992).
34. Goodwin, J.F., and Roberts, W.C., K, in *The Heart, Arteries and Veins* (J.W. Hurst ed.).McGraw-Hill, New York, pp. 1299–1362 (1982).
35. Maron, B.J., *Phys. Sports Med.,* 21: 83–91 (1993).
36. Pye, M.P., and Cobbe, S.M., *Cardiovasc. Res.,* 26: 740–750 (1992).
37. Messerli, F.H., and Grodzicki, T., *Eur. Heart J.,* 13: 66–69 (1992).
38. Dunn, F.G., and Pringle, S.D., *J. Hypertens.,* 11:1003–1010 (1993).
39. Fernando, E.S., Havenith, M., Burgada, P., Atie, J., Cheriex, E.C., et al., *Am. J. Cardiovasc. Pathol.,* 3: 329–332 (1990).
40. Maron, B., *N. Engl. J. Med.,* 318: 178–180 (1988).
41. Cantwell, J.D., and Watson, A., *Phys. Sports Med.,* 20: 115–129 (1992).
42. Sadaniantz, A., and Thompson, P.D., *Sports Med.,* 9: 199–204 (1990).
43. Northcote, R.J., and Ballantyne, D., *Int. J. Cardiol.,* 8: 3–12 (1985).
44. Brigdgen, G.S., Hughes, L.O., Broadhurst, P., and Raftery, E.B., *Eur. Heart J.,* 13: 1084–1087 (1992).
45. Eisenberg, M.J., *Am. Heart J.,* 124: 544–548 (1992).
46. Stendig-Lindberg, G., *J. Basic Clin. Physiol. Pharmacol.,* 3: 153–164 (1992).

47. Rowe, W.J., *Chest,* 99: 1306–1308 (1991).
48. Willich, S.N., Maclure, M., Mittleman, M., Arntz, H.R., and Muller, J.E., *Circulation,* 87: 1442–1450 (1993).
49. Ferenchick, G.S., Kirlin, P., and Potts, R., *Phys. Sports Med.,* 19: 107–110 (1991).
50. Foster, C., Anholm, J.D., Hellman, C.K., Carpenter, J., Pollock, M.L., et al., *Circulation.,* 63: 592–596 (1991).
51. Barnard, R.J., MacAlpin, R., Kattus, A.A., and Buckberg, G.D., *Circulation,* 48: 936–942 (1973).
52. O'Donnell, T.F. Jr., Clowes, G.M.A. Jr., *N. Engl. J. Med.,* 287: 734–737 (1972).
53. Ketelhut, R., Losem, C.J., and Messerli, F.H., *Int. J. Sports Med.,* 13: 293–297 (1992).
54. Laslett, L., Eisenbud, E., and Lind, R., Evidence of myocardial injury during prolonged strenuous exercise. *Am. J. Cardiol.,* 78: 488–491 (1996).

12

Exercise Therapy in Patients with Ischemic Heart Disease

GARY J. BALADY and DEBRA L. SHERMAN
Boston University Medical Center
Boston, Massachusetts

INTRODUCTION

Ischemic heart disease, most commonly a result of atherosclerotic coronary artery disease, remains a formidable problem in contemporary society. It is estimated that over 11 million persons in the United States are afflicted with this condition, and its broad-based impact has important consequences even among those without coronary disease. Nearly half of all deaths in the United States are a result of atherosclerotic heart disease. Affected individuals are subject to a wide range of personal limitations leading to restricted activity in domestic, occupational, and recreational spheres. Such disability and ensuing health expenditures translate to major socioeconomic problems with annual costs estimated to be in billions of dollars (1).

Underlying coronary artery disease is most often expressed in episodes of ischemia. Angina is the major clinical manifestation of this disease. Clinical decisions and management strategies in the past were often based on the presence or absence of angina. However extensive coronary artery disease may, in fact, be painless or silent.

A keen understanding of the pathophysiology of ischemia is necessary to affect its occurrence. A comprehensive familiarization with our current technologies to detect ischemia is essential to disclose the targets toward which our treatments are aimed. Contemporary therapeutic modalities continue to expand in every area. Revascularization techniques range from coronary artery bypass surgery, coronary angioplasty, and coronary stenting to the experimental (transmyocardial laser revascularization). Pharmacological agents encompass an ever-widening variety of drugs that affect β-adrenergic receptors, calcium channels, platelets, and numerous other receptors sites. Exercise is now considered an important part of the treatment strategy in the management of these patients (2).

An ever-increasing body of literature has yielded information regarding exercise and its effects on patients with atherosclerotic coronary artery disease. It is the purpose of this chapter to examine the role of exercise therapy among patients with ischemia, realizing that manifestations of coronary artery disease can be both painful or completely silent.

ISCHEMIC HEART DISEASE

Pathophysiology

Myocardial ischemia occurs when the supply of oxygen to the myocardial cells is inadequate to meet demands. This delicate balance of supply and demand for oxygenated blood can be affected by many factors. The variation in either supply, demand, or both is an area of great interest. Myocardial oxygen demand is related to heart rate, blood pressure, left ventricular contractility, and left ventricular wall stress (3). Left ventricular pressure, wall thickness, and cavity size will affect wall stress. Alterations in any of these factors—many of which are interdependent—can affect the myocardial need for oxygenated blood. Of these, the heart rate and blood pressure are the easiest parameters to measure and monitor. The product of the heart rate and systolic blood pressure, termed the *rate-pressure product,* has been found to be a very reliable index of myocardial oxygen demand (4) and therefore is the most widely used clinically.

Much data have accumulated to demonstrate that ischemia does not occur solely due to an increase in myocardial oxygen demand. This is supported by observations that during ambulatory or intensive care unit monitoring, ischemia can occur with little changes in the heart rate or systolic blood pressure (5). Therefore, transient reductions in coronary flow affecting regional myocardial oxygen supply must also be occurring. Nademanee (6) has found that exercise-induced ischemic parameters have a variability of 15–28% within any subject when compared with the variability of 44–64% as measured during ambulatory Holter monitoring. This suggests that there is a fixed threshold for myocardial oxygen demand but a wide variation in oxygen supply (coronary flow). Most commonly, coronary flow is compromised as a result of an atherosclerotic plaque within the lumen of the coronary artery. Such a plaque may cause minimal stenosis or complete occlusion of the artery. Factors that influence the significance of a given luminal stenosis include the degree of luminal obstruction, the length of the obstruction, the number and size of functioning collateral vessels, the magnitude of the supplied muscle mass, the shape and dynamic properties of the stenosis, and the autoregulatory capacity of the vascular bed (7).

Resistance flow across a given stenosis is dependent upon the residual lumen area (relative to normal) and the length of the stenosis. Resistance increases as flow increases owing to local turbulence. Therefore, the transtenotic pressure gradient will increase with increased flow. However, a considerable degree of stenosis is necessary to impair flow. A 50–70% reduction in luminal diameter will impair peak reactive hyperemia, whereas a stenosis of ≥75% will reduce resting flow (8).

Some 90% of vascular resistance resides at the level of the arterioles, which can dilate fourfold. The pressure remaining to perfuse myocardium distal to a stenosis is inversely related to flow and directly proportional to both the lumen area at the stenosis and resistance in the distal vessel (5). The amount of smooth muscle within a given plaque may lead to variability in the affected lumen diameter. Local changes in vasomotor tone can influence the supply of oxygenated blood to the myocardium, thus affecting the ischemic threshold. This variable flow reserve is subject to the dynamic nature of coronary stenoses. Changes in coronary vasomotor tone may be due to neuromodulation as well as endothelial control. Additionally, local thrombosis may occur and be accompanied by changes in vasomotor tone, further reducing or completely obstructing flow (8).

Endothelial Function and Dysfunction

The endothelium is now recognized as an important and complex structure that releases various vasoactive substances and mediates the interaction between blood components and vascular smooth muscle. Its normal function is crucial in the maintenance of vascular patency. One of the most important and widely studied of these substances is endothelium-derived relaxing factor (EDRF), which was discovered in 1980 by Furchgott and Zawadzki when they noted that rabbit aorta dilated when exposed to acetylcholine. However, if the endothelium was removed, acetylcholine caused either no change in vessel diameter or vasoconstriction (9). Since that time, EDRF has been identified as nitric oxide (NO) or a closely related molecule (10,11). Nitric oxide is produced from L-arginine by endothelial cell nitric oxide synthase (ecNOS) (12). It then diffuses from the endothelial cell and activates guanylyl cyclase to produce cyclic guanosine 3′, 5′ monophosphate (cGMP) in smooth muscle cells and platelets (13). This results in relaxation of vascular smooth muscle to maintain basal vasomotor tone (14) in response to a variety of stimuli, including platelet aggregation, serotonin, thrombin, acetylcholine, substance P, α_2 adrenergic stimulation, bradykinin, and shear stress (15,16). Other functions include inhibition of intimal growth, platelet adhesion, and leukocyte adhesion.

Endothelium produces many other substances that are important for the maintenance of vasomotor tone. Prostaglandins are fatty acid derivatives synthesized from arachidonic acid by the enzyme cyclooxygenase. Two powerful prostaglandins having opposite actions play an important role in the regulation of vasomotor tone and platelet function. *Prostacyclin* is formed by endothelial cells and stimulates smooth muscle cells and platelets to produce cyclic adenosine 3′, 5′ monophosphate (cAMP). This leads to vasodilation, decreased platelet aggregation and secretion, and inhibition of smooth muscle cell growth. *Thromboxane A_2* is produced by platelets and, in contrast to its endothelial counterpart, causes vasoconstriction and platelet activation (17). Endothelin-1 is the most potent vasoconstrictor known. It is produced by activated endothelial and smooth muscle cells and is important for the maintenance of vascular tone. Endothelin also causes adhesion and aggregation of neutrophils and stimulates smooth muscle growth. Various stimuli—including angiotensin II, catecholamines, growth factors, hypoxia, insulin, shear stress, and thrombin—cause rapid production and release of endothelin-1, resulting in vasoconstriction by binding to receptors on smooth muscle cells (18). In addition to EDRF, an endothelium-derived hyperpolarizing factor (EDHF) may also play a role in the vasodilation of smooth muscle. The release of EDHF is stimulated by acetylcholine, which causes transient hyperpolarization. EDHF may exert its effects by activating ATP-sensitive potassium channels, smooth muscle sodium-potassium ATPase, or both (19).

The endothelium produces several factors that maintain the balance between thrombosis and fibrinolysis. These factors are important at many levels of coagulation, including platelet and thrombin activation as well as fibrinolysis. The fibrinolytic system regulates the formation and removal of thrombi. The endothelium produces two important enzymes that regulate fibrinolysis and include tissue-type plasminogen activator (t-PA) and plasminogen activator inhibitor type 1 (PAI-1). t-PA is a serine protease that binds to fibrin and converts plasminogen to plasmin, the active form of the enzyme that produces clot lysis. Stimuli for t-PA release include shear stress, venous thrombosis, thrombin, histamine, and several cytokines (8). In contrast, PAI-1 binds and inactivates t-PA, which enhances thrombosis.

Endothelial dysfunction plays an important pathophysiologic role in coronary artery disease (CAD) and myocardial ischemia. CAD is more than a mechanical obstruction or stenosis of the vessels, since the physiological functions of the arteries are also considerably altered. In both stable and unstable coronary syndromes, lesion severity does not correlate with the degree of symptoms, suggesting an underlying functional abnormality of the artery (20,21), which may be partially responsible for clinical manifestations of the disease. The artery may be unable to dilate, resulting in an exacerbation of ischemia from a fixed stenosis, or an atheromatous plaque may become active and susceptible to rupture. In addition, increased platelet aggregation and decreased fibrinolysis may promote thrombus formation. Thus, the supply of blood through an already narrowed coronary artery is further compromised by the dysfunctional status of the endothelium, leading to myocardial ischemia or infarction.

Endothelial function in the coronary arteries has been studied using acetyl-choline, a muscarinic agonist, which normally causes endothelium-dependent vasodilation. However, in patients with atherosclerotic risk factors but angio-graphically normal coronary arteries, acetylcholine results in paradoxical vasoconstriction of the coronary vessels. Furthermore, the more risk factors present, the more likely the artery is to constrict (22), suggesting that endothelial dysfunction occurs in patients with CAD risk factors in the absence of overt atherosclerosis. When acetylcholine is infused into coronary arteries with ob-structive and nonobstructive atherosclerotic stenoses, paradoxical vasoconstric-tion occurs at the same doses that cause vasodilation in normal coronary arteries. However, vasodilation with nitroglycerin is preserved, indicating an endothe-lium-dependent abnormality rather than a generalized impairment of smooth muscle relaxation (23,24). Endothelium-dependent dilation in response to other stimuli, such as increased flow, is also impaired in patients with CAD. Cox and colleagues (25) found that distal infusion of intracoronary adenosine results in increased flow and proximal vasodilation in normal coronary arteries. However, when it is infused distal to a stenosis, the proximal segment of the atherosclerotic artery fails to dilate.

Ischemia—Clinical Manifestations

The clinical manifestations of ischemia are quite variable. Ischemia may produce symptoms of typical angina or appear in a more vague presentation as dyspnea or fatigue. It is now widely accepted that the occurrence of angina is late in the sequence of observed pathophysiological consequences of ischemia. Inadequate perfusion of the myocardium due to alterations in either supply and/or demand will lead to diminished regional contractility, followed by electrocardiographic changes, and finally the occurrence of angina (26). Ischemia can manifest as ST-segment changes during exercise testing without accompanying angina. Data from the Framingham Heart Study demonstrates that greater than 25% of the myocardial infarctions occurring over a 30-year period were initially discovered by the presence of new diagnostic electrocardiographic changes on routine fol-low-up examination. Of these, more than half were completely silent, whereas the remainder were symptomatically atypical (27). Large trials evaluating exer-cise testing among patients with angiographically documented coronary artery disease have yielded remarkable findings. Weiner et al. (28) report that among 2982 patients in the Coronary Artery Surgery Study (CASS) registry, 424 demon-strated ischemic ST-segment depression during exercise testing without angina. Mark et al. (29) found that among 1698 consecutive symptomatic patients who underwent testing at Duke University Medical Center, 242 had painless exercise-induced ST deviation. These data confirm that ischemia without angina is not uncommon.

An important question remains: Why is ischemia sometimes silent and sometimes painful? Cabin and Roberts (30) have demonstrated no difference in the extent or severity of CAD between patients with and without angina prior to sudden death. Moreover, radionuclide studies confirm that major perfusion or wall-motion abnormalities can occur during ischemia without associated pain (31,32). There may be differences in pain thresholds or pain perception among individuals with CAD (33).

Angina is grouped into functional classes primarily based on the individual's ability to perform a given level of activity without the occurrence of angina. The most commonly used classification scheme is outlined in Table 1, with class I representing the least symptomatic patients and class IV representing the most limited group (34).

Exercise Testing for the Detection of Ischemia

Many diagnostic methods have been employed to detect myocardial ischemia. Foremost among these is the exercise test, which yields valuable information in the management of persons with either proven or suspected CAD. The exercise test plays a key role in exercise therapy and exercise prescription. Although various exercise test protocols are available, all share the common goal of creating a gradual increase in muscular activity, which will, in turn, increase myocardial oxygen demand. This increase in demand may provoke a supply/demand imbalance for oxygenated blood to the myocardium and thus precipitate ischemia. The treadmill and bicycle are the most commonly used exercise modalities. The pres-

TABLE I   New York Heart Association Classification

Class I	Patients with cardiac disease but without resulting limitation of physical activity. Ordinary physical activity does not cause undue fatigue, palpitations, dyspnea, or anginal pain.
Class II	Patients with cardiac disease resulting in slight limitation of physical activity. They are comfortable at rest. Ordinary physical activity results in fatigue, palpitations, dyspnea, or anginal pain.
Class III	Patients with cardiac disease resulting in marked limitation of physical activity. They are comfortable at rest. Less than ordinary physical activity causes fatigue, palpitations, dyspnea, or anginal pain.
Class IV	Patients with cardiac disease resulting inability to carry on any physical activity without discomfort. Symptoms of cardiac insufficiency or of the anginal syndrome may be present even at rest. If any physical activity is undertaken, discomfort is increased.

Source: From Ref. 34.

ence or absence of symptoms is noted, as well as the heart rate and blood pressure response to each given level of exercise. The electrocardiographic analysis of the ST-segment response to exercise remains the most widely accepted and employed marker of exercise-induced ischemia. Interpretation of the ST-segment shift during exercise testing involves a familiarity with sensitivity, specificity, and predictive value of this test in detecting CAD.

Bayesian analysis of test interpretation emphasizes the importance of the prevalence of disease in the population being tested. Consideration of the patient's age, sex, symptoms, and coronary risk factors will influence the pretest risk and thus affect how a "positive" or "negative" outcome is viewed. Thus, the likelihood that CAD is either present or absent will depend both on the outcome of the test and the pretest likelihood of coronary disease for the individual being tested. A positive test among subjects with a high pretest likelihood of disease (e.g., older men with definite angina) is highly predictive of coronary disease, whereas a negative test in this group is more likely to be a false negative. Alternately, a negative test among subjects with a low pretest likelihood of coronary disease (e.g., women with atypical chest pain) is highly predictive of the absence of coronary disease, whereas a positive test in this group usually represents a false-positive response (35). However, a test should not be considered negative unless the patient reaches an adequate level of exercise—usually considered to be at 85% of maximum predicted heart rate for age. Moreover, underlying resting electrocardiographic (ECG) abnormalities due to digitalis, hyperventilation, hypokalemia, left ventricular hypertrophy, or intraventricular conduction defects decrease the specificity of the ST-segment response to exercise. This increases the false-positive rate and weakens the validity of the test results. In such cases or when the ST-segment response is equivocal, exercise radionuclide or echocardiographic testing will provide additional sensitivity and specificity for diagnostic interpretation (36).

Exercise Testing with Imaging

Echocardiography can be combined with exercise ECG in an attempt to increase the sensitivity and specificity of stress testing as well as to determine the extent of myocardium at risk for ischemia. Echocardiographic images at rest are compared with those obtained while the patient pedals a cycle or immediately after treadmill exercise. Images must be obtained within 1–2 min after exercise, since abnormal wall motion begins to normalize after this point. Rest and stress images are then compared side by side in a cine loop display that is gated during systole from the QRS complex (37). Myocardial contractility normally increases with exercise, whereas ischemia causes hypokinesis, akinesis, or dyskinesis of the affected segments. Therefore, a test is considered positive if wall-motion abnormalities develop in previously normal territories with exercise or worsen in an already abnormal segment (38). The overall sensitivity and specificity of exercise echo-cardiography range from 74–97% and 64–88%, respectively, with higher sensitivities in patients with multivessel disease. Its advantages over nuclear imaging include the absence of exposure to ionizing radiation and the shorter amount of time required for testing. Limitations include dependence on the operator for obtaining adequate, timely images. In addition, approximately 5% of patients have inadequate echocardiographic windows secondary to body habitus or lung interference. Nevertheless, stress echocardiography provides an accurate assessment of CAD and yields important diagnostic and prognostic information in the majority of patients (38).

Imaging of myocardial perfusion can also be accomplished with nuclear agents in conjunction with exercise or with a pharmacological agent such as di-pyridamole. Technetium-99m sestamibi offers several advantages over thallium, which was previously the most commonly used tracer. Sestamibi has a half-life of 6 h, compared with 73 h for thallium, and it also has a higher photon energy. This permits higher dosing with less radiation exposure than thallium, resulting in improved images that are sharper and have less artifact and attenuation. An-other unique property of sestamibi is its relative lack of redistribution. Mitochon-drial membranes bind the tracer in proportion to blood flow, and minimal additional tracer is taken into the cells after ischemia has been alleviated. Therefore, two separate injections more than 3–4 h apart are required to obtain rest and stress images, which can be done on the same day or separate days. Sestamibi is the preferred agent for performing single-photon emission computed tomography (SPECT) imaging (39). Perfusion defects that are present during exercise but are not seen at rest suggest ischemia. Perfusion defects that are present during exercise and persist at rest suggest previous myocardial infarction. Exercise with ses-tamibi imaging has shown accuracy similar to exercise with thallium imaging in the detection of myocardial ischemia. For planar imaging, the sensitivity and specificity of sestamibi are 84 and 83%, compared with 90 and 67% for thallium; for SPECT imaging, they are 90 and 93%, compared with 83 and 80% for thallium (40). The limitations of sestamibi SPECT imaging include the exposure to ionizing radiation, the need for additional equipment and personnel for image acquisition, and the time requirement for obtaining rest and stress images.

Exercise Testing and Prognosis

Using a variety of ECG, hemodynamic, and symptomatic parameters, the exercise test can be used to guide further therapy or diagnostic testing. Important prognostic information can be gained in patients with known CAD or symptoms suggestive of ischemia. Probably the most important variable is exercise capacity, which is dependent on left ventricular systolic function, age, physical condition, and other comorbid illnesses. Exercise-induced ischemia also provides crucial prognostic information and manifests as ST-segment depression, ST-segment elevation, and angina. Less important variables include the number of leads with ST-segment depression, downsloping versus upsloping or horizontal ST-segment depression, and total duration of ST-segment depression. This has been confirmed in several important studies of exercise testing. Using the Duke Cardiovascular Disease Databank, McNeer and colleagues found that ST-segment depression during the first two stages of the Bruce protocol predicted a group of patients at high risk for future coronary events. Patients able to exercise into stage four were found to be at low risk, even if ST-segment depression was present (41). Weiner and colleagues came to similar conclusions after studying medically treated patients with CAD. Patients who could exercise only to stage I of the Bruce protocol and had ST-segment depression had an annual mortality rate of 5%. In contrast, patients who exercised to stage IV with no ST-segment depression had an annual mortality rate of less than 1% (42).

Several studies have addressed the issue of exercise-induced silent ischemia with regard to prognosis. Callaham et al. (43) evaluated 1747 patients referred for exercise testing at a Veterans Administration Hospital. Some 60% of individuals with abnormal exercise-induced ST-segment depression has no accompanying pain. Ischemic ST-segment depression conferred an adverse 2-year prognosis among those with or without exercise-induced angina. The prevalence of exercise-induced silent ischemia was found to increase with age. Bonow et al. (44) and Weiner et al. (28) have also reported that patients with exercise-induced ischemia share the same adverse prognosis whether or not angina was present. Mark et al. (29) also found that exercise-induced silent ischemia conferred a worse prognosis, although the survival rates among these patients were better than those with exercise-induced angina. In addition, exercise-induced silent ischemia in the Coronary Artery Surgery Study demonstrates that patients with either silent or symptomatic ischemia during exercise testing among medically treated patients with documented CAD have a similar 7-year risk of developing acute myocardial infarction or experiencing sudden death (45). Moreover, among patients with exercised-induced silent ischemia and three-vessel disease and left ventricular dysfunction, survival was enhanced by coronary artery bypass surgery. This survival benefit is similar to that observed among patients in similar groups who have symptomatic exercise-induced ischemia. Therefore, it is the presence or absence of ischemia during exercise testing which influences prognosis, whether ischemia is silent or not.

Ischemic Threshold

The reproducibility of the exercise ischemic threshold is of particular interest, especially when exercise tests are used to formulate an exercise prescription for exercise training. Several studies have addressed this issue, and most agree that the heart rate–blood pressure product at onset ischemic ST-segment depression is fairly constant when serial testing using the same protocol is performed (46). Importantly, when differing protocols are used, the exercise-induced ischemic threshold may vary. Differences in exercising limbs (47), exercise position (48), and whether or not a warm-up precedes the exercise (49) all appear to influence the heart rate–blood pressure product at onset ischemia.

EFFECTS OF EXERCISE ON MYOCARDIAL OXYGEN SUPPLY/DEMAND RELATIONSHIPS

The physiological responses to exercise are detailed in a separate chapter in this text; however, the specific effects of acute and chronic exercise on myocardial oxygen supply and demand relationships are addressed here.

Acute Effects of Exercise

During acute endurance exercise, the cardiac output rises in response to the metabolic needs of the exercising muscles. Factors that influence this rise in cardiac output include an increase in sympathetic tone, which increases the heart rate and left ventricular contractility—both indices of myocardial oxygen consumption. Stroke volume rises because of increases in venous return of blood from exercising muscles. During exercise, blood flow is redistributed from the renal, splanchnic, and cutaneous circulation to the exercising muscles. The accumulation of metabolites in the actively contracting muscles causes a vasodilation in muscle arterioles. This increases skeletal muscle blood flow up to four times that of the resting level while reducing the overall aortic outflow impedance. This reduction in impedance allows for a more complete systolic ejection, thereby further increasing stroke volume. Systolic blood pressure increases primarily because of the augmentation of the cardiac output, whereas diastolic blood pressure either remains constant or falls (50). The size and location of the exercising muscle group may affect hemodynamic responses to exercise. Dynamic arm exercise elicits greater responses in heart rate and systolic and diastolic blood pressure during any given workload than does leg exercise. Differences in sympathetic output, peripheral vasodilation, venous return, and metabolic requirements of the exercising muscle mass may account for the greater heart rate–blood pressure product during arm work as compared with leg work (50).

Isometric work (heavy resistance, low repetition) generates an increased sympathetic response with a resulting increase in the heart rate. Venous return, especially during straining, may decrease. Therefore, the rise in the cardiac output (relatively small compared with that in dynamic exercise) is primarily due to increases in the heart rate. External compressive forces on muscle capillaries during isometric exercise lead to an elevated peripheral resistance. This rise in resistance and cardiac output yields an increase in both the systolic and diastolic pressures. Elevations in the systolic blood pressure from rest to exercise are proportionally greater than those in heart rate (51). Therefore, during both dynamic and isometric exercise, myocardial oxygen demand increases owing to rises in the heart rate, blood pressure, contractility, and left ventricular wall stress.

Coronary blood flow increases during exercise in response to neurohumoral stimulation (primarily sympathetic β-receptor) and endothelial substances that are released (e.g., EDRF). Thus, during acute exercise, coronary blood flow is augmented in response to the increases in myocardial oxygen demand. Among patients with atherosclerotic coronary artery disease, the demand may exceed the supply, and thus ischemia ensues. The flow reduction from a fixed stenosis is exacerbated by endothelial dysfunction. Gage and coworkers (52) found that in patients with stable angina, stenotic arteries constrict with exercise, whereas angiographically normal arteries dilate. The failure of atherosclerotic arteries to dilate with appropriate stimuli, such as increased flow during exercise, has the potential to decrease further the supply of blood in the setting of increased demand. In addition, stimulation of the sympathetic nervous system, along with the accumulation of metabolic by-products that normally accompany exercise, results in increased coronary blood flow. However, patients with atherosclerosis appear to be more sensitive to the vasoconstrictor effects of catecholamines (53).

Chronic Effects of Exercise

A regular program of exercise training yields a number of physiological adaptations that affect the oxygen supply/demand relationship. Consistent observations among individuals with and without coronary artery disease include changes in autonomic tone at rest and during exercise; central cardiac adaptations; and peripheral changes in muscle capillary density, myocyte mitochondrial number, and enzymes involved with the metabolism of glycogen and fat. A complex interrelationship among these factors leads to:

Resting bradycardia.
Decreased heart rate and systolic blood pressure response at any submaximal workload.
Increases in exercise capacity (maximal oxygen consumption).
Increase in maximal cardiac output—mostly observed in normal, healthy persons.
More rapid return to recovery hemodynamics after exercise.
Decrease in lactic acid concentration during submaximal exercise.
Increase in blood flow in exercising skeletal muscles.

Increased arteriovenous oxygen differences due to greater extraction of oxygen by the exercising muscles. This makes possible an increased oxidative metabolism of muscle fuels and the generation of more high-energy phosphates for muscle contraction (54).

The major product of these adaptations is increased functional capacity, which can be employed in numerous domestic, occupational, and leisure/recreational athletic activities. However, intuitive analysis would also argue that reduction in the heart rate–blood pressure product (an index of myocardial oxygen demand) at submaximal exercise levels translates to an improvement in the myocardial oxygen/supply demand relationship at that workload. Indeed, this appears to be the case, as many investigators have demonstrated a diminution of the ischemic response at a given submaximal workload in cardiac patients after training (55–61). However, several provocative studies have reported a decrease in the ischemic response—angina (56), ST-segment depression, (55,57) nuclear and positron emission tomography (PET) scanning perfusion defects (58–61)—at a given heart rate–blood pressure product after training as compared with the pretrained state. These findings suggest that there is an improvement in myocardial oxygen supply (i.e., coronary blood flow) at a given level of myocardial oxygen demand.

There are many mechanisms or combinations thereof that may explain these findings. Pathological studies in animals reveal that endurance training causes an increase in the size of the superficial coronary arteries and increased myocardial capillary density. However, angiographic studies to date have not confirmed this finding in humans (62). Importantly, three studies to date have demonstrated angiographic evidence of regression of atherosclerosis as well as reduction in the progression of atherosclerosis among patients who are actively involved in a multifactorial risk-reduction program that which includes exercise training, (63–65). However, the observed absolute measures of atherosclerotic change are small. Improved myocardial perfusion may be due to changes in coronary vasomotor reactivity. Animal studies suggest that one important consequence of chronic exercise is an improvement in vasomotor function. This is manifest by increased endothelium-dependent vasodilation in response to increased blood flow and EDRF agonists (66,67). High-resolution brachial artery ultrasound has been used to assess flow-mediated dilation of peripheral arteries and is a means for the evaluation of endothelial function (68,69). Using this method, Clarkson et al. (70) showed that exercise training improved endothelium-dependent flow-mediated dilation in healthy men. This effect was present in patients with and without CAD risk factors and was not related to lipid levels.

There is mounting evidence that hemostatic parameters are important cardiovascular risk factors, and emerging evidence suggests that exercise training favorably affects the fibrinolytic system. This may, in turn, help to explain the reduction in cardiac events observed in those who are more physically active. Strenuous endurance exercise for 6 months in healthy older patients resulted in a significant improvement in hemostatic parameters with a reduction in plasma fibrinogen levels, an increase in mean tissue plasminogen activator (t-PA), an increase in active t-PA, and a reduction of plasminogen activator inhibitor (PAI-1) (71). In contrast, younger patients, whose baseline fibrinolytic variables were lower than those of the older group, had no significant change in fibrinogen, t-PA, or PAI-1 activity. However, other studies have shown favorable effects of fibrinolytic enzymes after exercise training in younger subjects (73) and in patients after myocardial infarction (73).

There is also evidence that acute and chronic exercise affects platelet activation, which plays an important role in the pathophysiological mechanisms of unstable coronary syndromes and acute myocardial infarction. Kestin et al. (74) studied the effects of treadmill exercise on platelet activation in sedentary and physically fit individuals. After acute strenuous exercise of similar duration and intensity, platelet activation and hyperreactivity were increased in sedentary subjects but unchanged in physically fit subjects. Rauramaa et al. (75) demonstrated that 12 weeks of regular, moderate-intensity physical activity in middle-aged, overweight, mildly hypertensive men results in decreased platelet aggregation. Thus, it appears that although acute exercise can lead to increased platelet activity, especially in sedentary individuals, regular exercise may abolish or improve this response. Thus exercise training affects several of the factors that influence coronary blood flow.

Effects of Cardiac Medications on Training

Many patients with documented ischemic CAD take medications that influence autonomic tone, vascular smooth muscle tone, myocardial contractility, and many other parameters involved with physiological response to acute exercise. It is clearly the purpose of these medications to reduce or eliminate the occurrence of myocardial ischemia. However, do these medications affect the beneficial responses to long-term exercise training by interfering with mechanisms involved with the attainment of a training effect? This topic is addressed in detail in a separate chapter of this text; however, a few points here need to be made. β-Adrenergic blockers have been the most widely evaluated in this regard. It appears that these agents, in reducing exercise-induced ischemia, allow the patient to work at higher levels than would have been achieved without medications. Moreover, exercise capacity has been shown to increase in individuals who have completed an exercise training program and are taking β-blocking agents. However, this improvement appears to be relatively attenuated as compared with that in those individuals taking placebo (76–78). The influence of calcium-channel blocking agents on training has been less well evaluated, although studies to date have demonstrated no negative effects on the training response as compared with placebo (79,80).

RECOMMENDATIONS FOR EXERCISE TRAINING OF PATIENTS WITH ISCHEMIC HEART DISEASE

Exercise therapy among patients with ischemic heart disease should be prescribed as any form of treatment would be, such that the effectiveness of therapy is optimized and the risks are minimized. The goals of exercise therapy, when used as such, should be individualized to meet the patient's needs in domestic, occupational, and leisure-time activity. One must also take into account the limitations that may have ensued from a patient's cardiac condition and preexisting disease.

Medical Screening

Any patient with ischemic heart disease who is considering or being considered for an exercise program should undergo medical evaluation by a qualified physician. The medical history, with particular reference to cardiovascular status, is essential. Symptoms of angina, dyspnea, palpitations, and syncope should be sought. The patient should be questioned regarding the previous occurrence of myocardial infarction, coronary angioplasty, or bypass surgery. A complete list of medications and dosing intervals must be reviewed, as these may affect the responses to exercise. Patients taking insulin or oral hypoglycemics will require particular attention and monitoring for signs and symptoms of hypo-or hyperglycemia. Associated illnesses—including pulmonary, neurological, and musculoskeletal conditions—must also be considered in the evaluation. A social and detailed occupational history will yield valuable information, such that program training and goals are tailored to meet individual needs. Physical examination should focus at least on the heart rate, blood pressure, and pulmonary, cardiac, vascular, and musculoskeletal area. Signs of congestive heart failure and valvular disease should be evaluated with further workup if deemed appropriate.

Prior to beginning each exercise session, the patient should be questioned regarding new or worsening symptoms suggesting cardiovascular instability. Patients should also be instructed to be aware of these issues and to address them to the appropriate medical personnel. Any changes in medications should be reported, as these may affect the exercise prescription. A resting ECG and physician-supervised exercise test are integral to the medical evaluation and the exercise prescription itself. Exercise testing can be used to detect ischemia—whether symptomatic or silent—with particular reference to the workload and heart rate–

blood pressure product at which ischemia begins. Risk stratification using these parameters will greatly assist in determining the adequacy of current therapy as well as the level of supervision and monitoring necessary in a given patient. Serial exercise testing can be useful to monitor functional capacity, evaluate the training effect, and assess changes in the ischemic threshold. Should medication changes occur that might affect training parameters, it is prudent to repeat the exercise test so that the exercise prescription can be adjusted accordingly. Exercise testing is also useful in the evaluation of new or changing symptoms of chest pain or dyspnea, particularly when the etiology is not clear.

The Training Program

The exercise prescription is formulated based on the evaluation as detailed above. Important components should include the type of exercise; limbs being used; and intensity, duration, and frequency of exercise sessions. Optimal training effects will occur when exercise is performed three to five times per week for 30–40 min at a specified heart rate. The training heart rate should be determined from the results of the exercise test. Using the peak heart rate achieved on the exercise test, at least two methods of target-range formulation can be used (81):

1. From 60–90% of maximum heart rate achieved
2. From [(peak heart rate − resting heart rate) × 45%] + resting heart rate to [(peak heart rate − resting heart rate) × 85%] + resting heart rate (Karvonen method)

If angina or ischemic ST-segment depression occurs during testing, then the peak heart rate should be at least 10 beats below the heart rate at which ischemia begins (ischemic threshold). It is important to note that the use of the Karvonen method generates the target heart range, which is usually not far from the peak heart rate. This occurs particularly among patients taking medications that blunt the peak heart-rate response. If the heart rate at ischemia is employed as the peak heart rate in this situation, patients may be exercising at a range near the ischemic threshold. Careful monitoring and caution should be used here, particularly among patients who demonstrate ischemia at a low heart rate and low workload. Serious consideration for optimization of medical therapy and/or revascularization should be entertained in this latter groups of high-risk patients prior to exercise therapy. Exercise training at lower intensity is appropriate in this group.

As the physiological and ischemic responses to different types of exercise vary according to limbs used, body position, and relative amounts of dynamic and isometric work (47,48,51), one must consider that the ischemic threshold and functional capacity measured during one type of exercise testing may not translate to another type of exercise. Exercise prescription should be formulated using a testing protocol that reflects the major type of exercise modality to be used during exercise therapy sessions. It appears that during arm ergometry (47) and isometric exercise (51), the ischemic threshold is higher than it is during treadmill testing. Therefore it is unlikely that an individual will exceed his or her ischemic threshold when performing either arm ergometry or weight training within a given target heart rate range as determined from treadmill testing.

Alternate methods of training should be incorporated into exercise therapy. Specifically, arm ergometry (82) and circuit weight training (83–85) have been shown to yield benefits of both strength and endurance in patients with cardiac disease while being relatively safe modalities of training. Patients with ischemic heart disease whose occupations or activities involve upper extremity and/or isometric (lifting) work would particularly benefit from such a program. Stretching exercises and low-resistance warm-up and cool-down should be employed in each exercise session.

Safety of Exercise Therapy in Patients with Ischemic Heart Disease

There is evidence that heavy exertion may trigger acute myocardial infarction. Two studies (86,87) have found that the relative risk of myocardial infarction within 1 h after strenuous physical exertion was increased two to six times over that of patients who were sedentary or less active during that hour. However, the risk was inversely related to the amount of leisure-time physical activity performed by the subjects. Thus, the more active the individual, the lower the risk for development of acute myocardial infarction during strenuous exertion.

Exercise training among patients with cardiac disease has been found to be relatively safe. VanCamp and Peterson (88) have accumulated important data from 167 outpatient cardiac rehabilitation programs involving a total of 51,000 patients. In this survey the incidence of cardiac arrest was 1 per 112,000 person-hours (86% of patients being successfully resuscitated); the incidence of myocardial infarction was 1 per 294,000 person-hours (all myocardial infarctions were nonfatal); and the incidence of death was 1 per 784,000 person-hours. No difference in event rate was found between programs that employed continuous ECG (telemetry) monitoring versus those who used intermittent monitoring.

Monitoring by continuous telemetry would be most appropriate among individuals designated as being at high risk based on their exercise test results, low ejection fraction, symptom class, history of syncope, or malignant arrhythmias or history of cardiac arrest. Telemetry monitoring would also be useful among patients who are unable to monitor their own pulse. However, application of the Borg scale of perceived exertion (89) should be emphasized to maintain exercise training intensity—as well as outside, unmonitored activities—below the exercise-induced threshold.

CONCLUSIONS

Recent years have witnessed an impressive growth in the understanding of ischemic heart disease and exercise therapy. These knowledge bases intersect on many levels, including pathophysiology, clinical testing, and therapeutic application. Exercise therapy among individuals with ischemia should be prescribed with a full understanding of the methodologies available to maximize outcome and minimize risk. Realizing that significant ischemia can occur without presenting symptoms, medical personnel responsible for prescribing and administering exercise therapy must be astute in their management of patients with CAD. Familiarity with the methods of detecting ischemia and appraising risk in these patients provides essential information necessary to guide treatment.

REFERENCES

1. American Heart Association, *Heart and Stroke Statistics.* American Heart Association, Dallas, Texas (1996).
2. Balady, G.J., Fletcher, B.J., Froelicher, E.S., Hartley, L.H., Krauss, R.M., Oberman, A., Pollock, M.L., and Taylor, C.B., *Circulation,* 90: 1602–1610 (1994).
3. Ganz P., Braunwald, E., in *Heart* Disease: *A Textbook of Cardiovascular Medicine* (E. Braunwald, ed.). Saunders, Philadelphia, pp. 1161–1183 (1997).
4. Kitamura, K., Jorgensen, C.R., Gobel, F.L., Taylor, H.L., and Wang, Y., *J. Appl. Physiol.,* 23: 516–522 (1972).
5. Brown, B.G., and Smith, B.H., in *Silent Myocardial Ischemia and Angina* (B.H. Singh, ed.). Pergamon Press, New York, pp. 16–27 (1998).
6. Nademanee, K., in *Silent Myocardial Ischemia* and *Angina* (B.H. Singh, ed.). Pergamon Press, New York, pp. 223–233 (1988).
7. Herzel, H.O., Leutwyler, R. and Krayenbuehl, H.P., *J. Am. Coll. Cardiol.,* 6: 275–284 (1985).
8. Rubanyi, G.M., *J. Cardiovasc. Pharmacol.,* 22: S1–S14 (1993).
9. Furchgott, R.F., and Zawadzki, J.V., *Nature,* 288: 373–376 (1980).
10. Ignarro, L.J., Buga, G.M., Wood, K.S., Byrns, R.E., and Chaudhuri, G., *Proc. Natl. Acad. Sci. U.S.A.,* 84: 9265–9269 (1987).
11. Palmer, R.M., Ferrige, A.G., and Moncada, S., *Nature* 327: 524–526 (1987).
12. Palmer, R.M., and Ashton, D.S., Moncada, S., *Nature,* 333: 664–666 (1988).
13. Ignarro, L.J., *F.A.S.E.B.J.,* 3: 31–36 (1989)
14. Bredt, D.S., and Snyder, S.H., *Proc. Natl. Acad. Sci. U.S.A.,* 87: 682–685 (1990).
15. Furchgott, R., *Circ. Res.,* 35: 557–573 (1983).
16. Rubanyi, G.M., Romero, J.C., and Vanhoutte, P.M., *Am. J. Physiol.,* 250: H1145–H1149 (1986).
17. Moncada, S., and Vane, J.R., *Pharmacol. Rev.,* 30: 293–331 (1979).
18. Levin, E.R., N. Engl. J. Med., 333: 356–363 (1995).
19. Feletou, M., and Vanhoutte, P.M., *Br. J. Pharmacol.,* 93: 515–524 (1988).

20. Ambrose, J.A., Tannenbaum, M.A., Alexopoulos, D., et al., *J. Am. Coll. Cardiol.,* 12: 56–62 (1988).
21. Folland, E.D., Vogel, R.A., Hartigan, P., et al., *Circulation,* 89: 2005–2014 (1994).
22. Vita, J.A., Treasure, C.B., Nabel, N.G., et al., *Circulation,* 81: 491–497 (1990).
23. Ludmer, P.L., Selwyn, A.P., Shook, T.L., et al., N. Engl. J. Med., 315: 1046–1051 (1986).
24. Gordon, J.B., Ganz, P., Nabel, E.G., et al., *J. Clin. Invest.,* 83: 1946–1952 (1989).
25. Cox, D.A., Vita, J.A., Treasure, C.B., et al., *Circulation,* 80: 458–465 (1989).
26. Rozanski, A., Berman, D.S., *Am. Heart. J.,* 114: 615–626 (1987).
27. Kannel, W.B., *Adv. Cardiol.,* 37: 202–214 (1990).
28. Weiner, D.A., Ryan, T.J., McCabe, C.H., Luk, S., Chaitman, B.R., Sheffield, L.T., Tristani, F., and Fisher, L.D., *Am. J. Cardiol.,* 59: 725–729 (1987).
29. Mark, D.B., Hlahtky, M.A., Califf, R.M., Morris, J.J., Sisson, S.D., McCants, C.B., Lee, K.L., Harrel, F.E., and Pryor, D.B., *J. Am. Coll. Cardiol.,* 14: 885–892 (1989).
30. Cabin, H., and Roberts, W., *Am. J. Cardiol.* 46: 754–763 (1980).
31. Deanfield, J.E., Shea, M., Ribiero, P., DeLAndsheer, C.M., Wilson, R.A., Horlock, P., and Selwyn, A.P., *Am. J. Cardiol.* 54: 1195–1200 (1984).
32. Cohn, P.F., Brown, E.J., Wynn, J., Holomon, B.L., and Adkins, H.L., *J. Am. Coll. Cardiol.* 1: 931–933 (1983).
33. Glazier, J.J., Chierchia, S., Brown, M.J., and Maseri, A. *Am. J. Cardiol.,* 58: 667–672 (1986).
34. Goldman, L., Hashimoto, B., Cook, E.F., and Loscalzo, A., *Circulation,* 64: 1227–1234 (1981).
35. Weiner, D.A., Ryan, T.J., McCabe, C.H., Kennedy, J.W., Schloss, M., Tristani, F., Chaitman, B.R., and Fisher, L.D., *N. Engl. J. Med.,* 302: 230–235 (1979).
36. Gibbons, R.A., Balady, G.J., Beasely, J.W., Bricker, J.T., Duvernoy, W.F.C., Froelicher, V., Mark, D.B., Marwick, T., McCallister, B.D., Thompson, P.D., Winters, W.L., and Yanowitz, F.G., *J. Am. Coll. Cardiol.,* 30: 260–315 (1997).
37. Zoghbi, W., in *Myocardial Perfusion Imaging* (A.S. Iskandrian, ed.). Am J Cardiol Continuing Education Series Cahners Publishing, New York, pp. 17N23 (1993).
38. Armstrong, W., and Marcovitz, P.A., *Stress Echocardiography: Heart Disease Updates* (E. Braunwald, ed.). Saunders, Philadelphia, pp. 1–10 (1993).
39. Garcia, E.V., in (*Cardiac Imaging: A Companion to Braunwald's Heart Disease* M.L. Marcus, H.R. Schelbert, D.J. Skorton, et al. eds.). Saunders, Philadelphia pp. 977–1005 (1991).
40. Berman, D.S., Kiat, H., and Leppo, J., et al., in *Cardiac Imaging: A Companion to Braunwald's Heart Disease* (Marcus, M.L., Schelbert, H.R., Skorton, D.J., et al. eds.) Saunders, Philadelphia, pp. 1097–1109 (1991).
41. McNeer, J.F., Margolis, J.R., Lee, K.L., Kisslo, J.A., Peter, R.H., Kong, Y., Behar, V.S., Wallace, A.G., McCants, C.B., and Rosati, R.A., *Circulation,* 57: 64–70 (1978).
42. Weiner, D.A., Ryan, T.J., McCabe, C.H., Chaitman, B.R., Sheffield, L.T., Fergusen, J.C., Fisher, L.D., and Tristani, F., *J. Am. Coll. Cardiol.,* 3: 772–779 (1984).
43. Callaham, P.R., Froelicher, V.F., Klein, J., Risch, M., Dubach, P., and Friis, R., *J. Am. Coll. Cardiol.,* 14: 1175–1180 (1989).

44. Bonow, R.O., Bacharach, S.L., Green, M.V., LaFreniere, R.L., and Epstein, S.E., *Am. J. Cardiol.,* 60: 778–783 (1987).

45. Weiner, D.A., Ryan, TJ, McCabe, C.H., Chaitman, B.R., Sheffield, L.T., Ng, G., Fisher, L.D., and Tristani, F.E., *J. Am. Coll. Cardiol.,* 62: 1155–1158 (1988).

46. Waters, D., McCans, J.L., and Crean, P.A., *J. Am. Coll. Cardiol.,* 6: 1011–1015 (1985).

47. Balady, G.J., Weiner, D.A., McCabe, C.H., and Ryan, T.J., *Am. J. Cardiol.,* 55: 37–39 (1985).

48. Whetherbe, J.N., Banrah, V.S., Ptacin, N.J., and Kalbfleish, J.H., *J. Am. Coll. Cardiol.,* 11: 330–337 (1988).

49. Pupita, G., Kaski, J.C., Galassi, A.R., Vejar, M., Crea, F., and Maseri, A., *Am. Heart. J.,* 118: 539–544 (1989).

50. Clausen, J.P., *Prog. Cardiovasc. Dis.,* 18: 459–495 (1976).

51. Wilke, N.A., Sheldahl, L.M., Tristani, F.E., Hughes, C.V., and Kalbfleish, J.H., *Am. Heart J.* 110: 542–545 (1985).

52. Gage, J.E., Hess, O.M., and Murakami, T., et al., *Circulation,* 73: 865–876 (1986).

53. Vita, J.A., Treasure, C.B., and Yeung, A.C., et al., *Circulation,* 85: 1390–1397 (1992).

54. Smith, M.L., and Mitchell, J.H., in *American College of Sports Medicine Resource Manual for Exercise Testing and Prescription.* Lea & Febiger, Philadelphia, pp. 75–81 (1993).

55. Ehsani, A., Heath, G.W., Hagberg, J.M., Sobel, B.E., and Holloszy, J.O., *Circulation,* 64: 1116–1124 (1981).

56. Ben-Ari, E., Kellermann, J.J., Rothbaum, D.A., Fisman, E., and Pines A., *Am. J. Cardiol.,* 59: 231–234 (1987).

57. Rogers, M.A., Yamamoto, C., Hagberg, J.M., Holloszy, J.O., and Ehsani, A.A., *J. Am. Coll. Cardiol.,* 10: 321–332 (1987).

58. Todd, I.C., Bradnam, M.S., Cooke, MBD, and Ballantyne, D., *Am. J. Cardiol.,* 68: 1593–1599 (1991).

59. Froelicher, V., Jensen, D., Genter, F., Sullivan, M., McKirnan, M.D., Witzum, K., Scharf, J., Strong, M.L., and Ashburn, W., *J.A.M.A.,* 252: 1291–1297 (1984).

60. Gould, K.L., Ornish, D., Scherwitz, L., Brown, S., Edens, P., Hess, M.J., Mullani, N., Bolomey, L., Dobbs, F., Armstrong, W., Merritt, T., Ports, T., Sparler, S., and Billings, J., *J.A.M.A.,* 274: 894–901 (1995).

61. Schuler, G., Schierf, G., Wirth, A., Mautner, H.P., Scheurlen, H., Thomm, M., Roth, H., Schwartz, F., Johlemeier, M., Mehmel, H.C., and Kubler, W., *Circulation,* 77: 172–181 (1988).

62. Scheuer, J., *Circulation,* 66: 491–495 (1982).

63. Hambrecht, R., Niebauer, J., Marburger Grunze, M., Kalberer, B., Hauer, K., Schlierf, G., Kubler, W., and Schuler, G., *J. Am. Coll. Cardiol.,* 22: 468–477 (1993).

64. Haskell, W.L., Alderman, E.L., Fair, J.M., Maron, D.J., Mackey, S.F., Superko, R., Williams, P.T., Johnstone, I.M., Champagne, M., Krauss, R.M., and Farquhar, J.W., *Circulation,* 89: 975–990 (1994).

65. Ornish, D., Scherwita, L.W., Doody, R.S., Kesten, D., McLanahan, S.M., Brown, S.E., Depuey, E.G., Sonnemaker, R., Haynes, C., Lester, J., McAllister, G.K., Hall, R.J., Burdine, J.A., and Gotto, A.M., *J.A.M.A.,* 249: 54–59 (1983).

66. Sessa, W.C., Pitchard, K., Seyedi, N., Wang, J., and Hintze, T.H., *Circ. Res.,* 74: 349–353 (1994).

67. Muller, J.M., Meyers, P.R., and Laughlin, H., *Circulation,* 89: 2308–2314 (1994).

68. Uehata, A., Lieberman, E.H., Meredith, I., Anderson, T., Polak, J., Creager, M., and Yeung, A. Noninvasive assessment of flow-mediated dilation in brachial arteries. Circulation 1992; 86: I–620.

69. Celermajer, D.S., Sorensen, K.E., Gooch, V.M., and Deanfield, J.E., *Lancet,* 340: 1111–1115 (1992).

70. Clarkson, P., Montgomery, H., Donald, A., Powe, A., Bull, T., and Dollery, C., *J. Am. Coll. Cardiol.,* 27(Suppl. A): 288A (1996).

71. Stratton, J.R., Chandler, W.I., Schwartz, R.S., Cequeira, M.D., Levy, W.C., Kahn, S.E., Larson, V.G., Cain, K.C., Beard, J.C., and Abrass, I.B., *Circulation,* 83: 1692–1697 (1991).

72. de-Geus, E.J., Kluft, C., de-Bart, A.C., and van-Doornen, L.J., *Med. Sci. Sports Exerc.,* 24: 1210–1219 (1992).

73. Suzuki, T., Yamauchi, K., Yamada, Y., Furumichi, T., Furui, H., and Tsuzuki, J., *Clin Cardiolo.,* 15: 358–364 (1992).

74. Kestin, A.S., Ellis, P.A., Barnard, M.R., Errichetti, A., Rosner, B.A., Michelson, A.D., *Circulation,* 88: 1502–1511 (1993).

75. Rauramaa, R., Salonen, J.T., Seppanen, K., Salonen, R., Venalainen, J.M., Ihanainen, M., *Circulation,* 74: 939–944 (1986).

76. Ewy, G.A., Wilmore, J.H., Morton, A.R., Stanforth, P.R., Constable, S.H., Buono, M.J., Conrad, K.A., Miller, H., Gatewood, C.F., *J. Cardiac Rehabil.,* 3: 25–29 (1983).

77. Sable, D.L., Brammell, H.L., Sheehan, M.W., Nies, A.S., Gerber, J., and Horwitz, L.D. *Circulation,* 65: 679–684 (1982).

78. Pratt, C.M., Welton, D.E., Squires, W.G., Kirby, D.E., Hartung, G.H., and Miller, R.R., *Circulation,* 64: 1125–1129 (1981).

79. Duffey, D.J., Horwitz, L.D., and Brammell, H.L., *Am. J. Cardiol.,* 53: 908–911 (1984).

80. Stewart, K., Effron, M.B., Valenti, S.A., and Keleman, M.H., *Med. Sci. Sports Exerc.,* 22: 192–198 (1989).

81. U.S. Department of Health and Human Services: U.S. Department of Health and Human Services, Centers for Disease Control and Prevention, National Center for Chronic Disease Prevention and Health Promotion, Atlanta (1996).

82. Franklin, B.A., Hellerstein, H.K., Gordon, S., Timmis, G.C., in *Exercise in Modern Medicine* (B.A. Franklin, S. Gordon, and Timmis G.C., eds.). Williams & Wilkins, Baltimore, p. 44–80 (1989).

83. Kelemen, M.H., Stewart, K.G., Gillilan, R.E., Ewart, C.K., Valenti, S.A., Manley, J.D., and Keleman, M.D., *J. Am. Coll. Cardiol.,* 7: 38–42 (1986).

84. McCartney, N., McKelvie, R.S., Haslam, D.R.S., and Jones, N.L., *Am. J. Cardiol.,* 67: 939–945 (1991).

85. Ghilarducci, L.D.C., Holly, R.G., and Amsterdam, E.A., *Am. J. Cardiol.* 64: 866–870 (1989).

86. Siscovick, D.S., Weiss, N.S., Fletcher, R.N., et al., *N. Engl. J. Med.,* 311: 874–877 (1984).

87. Mittleman, M.A., Maclure, M., Tofler, G.H., Sherwood, J.B., Goldberg, R.J., and Muller, J.E., *N. Engl. J. Med.,* 329: 1677–1683 (1993).

88. VanCamp, S.P., and Peterson, RA., *J.A.M.A.,* 256: 1160–1163 (1986).

89. Borg, G., *Med. Sci. Sports Exerc.,* 14: 377 (1982).

13

Exercise Prescription in the Rehabilitation of Patients Following Coronary Artery Bypass Graft Surgery and Percutaneous Transluminal Coronary Angioplasty

CARL FOSTER
Milwaukee Heart Institute
Milwaukee, Wisconsin

KATHARINA MEYER
Herz-Zentrum
Bad Krozingen, Germany

LISA L. HECTOR
Memorial Hospital at Oconomowoc
Oconomowoc, Wisconsin

INTRODUCTION

Exercise and risk-factor education programs for patients following myocardial infarction have a generation-long history. Their beneficial effect on the clinical outcome of these patients, including hard clinical outcomes such as morbidity and mortality, is well accepted (1,2). Beginning about 25 years ago, significant numbers of patients began to be referred to rehabilitation programs following coronary artery bypass graft surgery (CABGS). As reviewed by Foster, the general clinical experience in this population has been favorable (3). Over the last 10–15 years, significant numbers of patients began to be referred following per-

cutaneous transluminal coronary angioplasty (PTCA). The overall clinical experience with this population has also been favorable.

The purpose of this chapter is to (a) review the overall clinical expectations
following CABGS and PTCA and how they might be influenced by participation
in risk factor and exercise based rehabilitation programs, (b) review the physiological sequelae of successful CABGS and PTCA and how they may be used to
evaluate the success of these procedures, and (c) discuss unique approaches to
exercise prescription and monitoring that we have developed which may be useful
in the CABGS/PTCA population.

CLINICAL EXPECTATIONS FOLLOWING CABGS AND PTCA

Symptomatic relief from exertional angina pectoris is usually a reliable measure
of outcome following CABGS and PTCA. CABGS extends survival in patients
with three-vessel or left main coronary artery disease (4) and in those with exercise-induced left ventricular dysfunction while they are receiving medical therapy
(5). There are surprisingly unfavorable statistics on the likelihood of returning
to work following either CABGS or PTCA (6,7); previous work status and the
nature of the occupation seem to have a significant impact on this. Additionally,
job classification, concurrent myocardial infarction, and self-efficacy all influence
the likelihood of returning to work following CABGS or PTCA.

Solymoss (8) demonstrated that 15–25% of saphenous vein grafts close
during the first postoperative year. This is generally attributed to thrombosis secondary to endothelial damage at the time of surgery (9). After the first year,
bypass grafts close at the rate of 0.5–3.0% of grafts per year through year 7.
After year 7, the rate of closure increases to 1.5–9.0% per year. Internal mammary
artery grafts have a greater rate of sustained patency than saphenous vein grafts.
The risk of closure of grafts is related to a number of variables, including mechanical problems with the graft and conventional risk factors for atherosclerosis.
Both postoperative dyslipidemia and smoking (9) increase the risk of graft closure. There are no randomized clinical trials documenting the effect of participation in rehabilitation programs on the fate of bypass grafts or on hard clinical
endpoints following CABGS or PTCA. Common sense argues for favorable effects of exercise and risk-factor reduction in this patient population, similar to
that seen in post-MI patients.

The 1-year risk of restenosis following PTCA varies between 15 and 50%
(10); the rate is somewhat more favorable in the presence of stenting. The risk
is increased in patients with narrow coronary vessels, in the presence of total
occlusion prior to PTCA, or in the presence of dissection associated with balloon

inflation. There are no appropriately controlled data regarding the influence of participation in rehabilitation programs on the long-term fate of dilated vessels. Smoking increases the risk of restenosis from approximately 38% in nonsmokers to 55% in continuing smokers (11). Other data suggest that the restenosis rate is increased in patients with hypercholesterolemia.

In patients with coronary artery disease (CAD), a multifactoral intervention trial including exercise training and a low-fat diet resulted in significant improvement in lipoprotein levels and physical work capacity at 6-year follow-up. In the control group, these variables remained essentially unchanged. In the intervention group, coronary stenoses progressed at a significantly slower rate than in controls. As only physical activity correlated independently with the angiographic findings, the beneficial effects appear to be due largely to chronic physical exercise (12).

CONSEQUENCES OF MYOCARDIAL REVASCULARIZATION

Responses during exercise testing before and after CABGS and PTCA have been reviewed by Dubach et al. (13). They observed that although CABGS patients had a much greater incidence of multivessel disease than PTCA patients, the relief of anginal symptoms was similiar, and the reversal of exercise-induced ST-segment depression was also similar. The investigators pointed out that direct comparison of the interventions is complicated by the usual time course of exercise testing following the procedures. Although patients can safely perform symptom-limited exercise testing by the time of hospital discharge following CABGS (14), they most often are not tested until 2–3 months after surgery, when grafts that are destined to close early have already closed. Alternatively, PTCA patients are more commonly tested within days of the procedure.

Exercise capacity usually improves following both CABGS and PTCA, although the time course following surgery is often delayed secondary to recovery from the surgical procedure. In Fig. 1 we present schematic recovery curves for several variables of clinical interest during participation in a rehabilitation program for post-CABGS patients (15). No comparable data for PTCA patients are available, although it is reasonable to expect a grossly accelerated time course of recovery. Studies in our laboratory have demonstrated that even patients who are not assigned to exercise therapy demonstrate considerable improvement in exercise capacity, although the time course and magnitude of recovery are slowed (16). At the present time, there are no data on the time course of recovery following the new minimally invasive CABGS procedure. Common sense suggests that eliminating the trauma associated with the sternotomy should greatly accelerate the time course of recovery. As is evident from Fig. 1, some of the subjective

Time Course of Rehabilitation

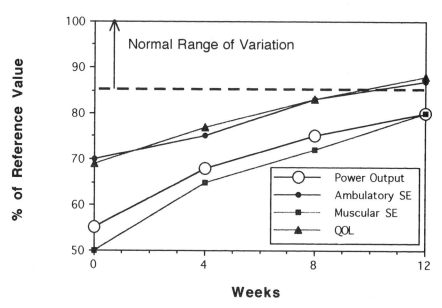

FIGURE I   Schematic time course of recovery of objective and subjective indices of exertional tolerance in patients following CABGS. Although self-efficacy and quality of life measures are not ordinarily scaled as a percent of predicted, results have been normalized to the percentage of possible points on the scales available in order to provide a conceptually simple way of understanding the relative time course of recovery of the various markers of exertional tolerance. (Adapted from data in Ref. 15.)

markers of exercise capacity recover more rapidly than the objectively measured exercise capacity. Since it is known that a patient's lifestyle is as dependent on perceived exercise capacity as on what he or she is objectively capable of doing, these data suggest that the greatest need for structured rehabilitation is in the very early weeks after surgery. In this regard, we have, for the past 20 years, had patients return to the rehabilitation center as soon as possible, certainly within the first week after discharge. We have felt and continue to feel that this practice encourages earlier resumption of activities of daily living (ADLs), allows the patient early access to staff to discuss questions or concerns, and provides optimal patient surveillance. It also has the value of keeping the patient from "crying wolf" to the doctor several times during the early weeks after discharge for bothersome but ordinary complaints. These complaints can, instead, be addressed by the rehabilitation staff. Even without exercise testing prior to program entry, the availability of electrocardiographic (ECG) monitoring allows sufficient surveillance, so that we have had virtually no complications attributable to early program entry.

Although exercise capacity improves significantly following PTCA, we have seen comparatively small changes when exercise testing is conducted relatively soon following PTCA; moreover, we have noted similar improvement in functional capacity in patients with unsuccessful PTCA (not requiring emergency surgery) versus those with angiographically successful procedures (17). In view of the presumed importance of coronary blood flow as a factor limiting exercise cardiac output, the failure to note bigger differences between successful and unsuccessful PTCA was surprising and perhaps hints at the poorly recognized importance of skeletal muscle factors in this population.

Following CABGS exercise testing without a preoperative control study is generally disappointing; there are a substantial number of normal tests despite the continued presence of anatomically significant disease (18). Observation of abnormal ventricular function during exercise testing using either radionuclide (16) or echocardiographic (19) methods following surgery is better correlated with angiographic evidence of incomplete revascularization. We feel that normal exercise test results, particularly normal exercise LV function, suggest that revascularization is effectively complete, even in the presence of anatomically apparent residual disease.

Peak-exercise left ventricular (LV) ejection fraction usually improves significantly following successful CABGS (16). If exercise studies are conducted at the time of hospital discharge, the magnitude of improvement in ejection fraction may be overestimated (16). Exercise LV function is improved following successful PTCA, based on the results of both radionuclide (20) and echocardiographic (21) studies. Although there appears to be a tendency for participants in rehabilitation programs following PTCA to have higher values for resting ejection fraction as compared with usual-care patients, there are no appropriately controlled data to address this issue.

As demonstrated in the Coronary Artery Bypass Surgery Study, CABGS improves survival only in patients with three-vessel disease, exertional ischemia, and limited exercise capacity (5). Other studies have demonstrated that survival in medically treated patients is good as long as exercise LV function remains normal (6). In patients who become symptomatic after CABGS, the prognostic information available from exercise testing is low, although, like nonsurgical patients, patients with a good exercise capacity in relation to the magnitude of ischemia have a better prognosis (22,23). To the degree that exercise capacity and heart rate reserve measure the same thing as exercise LV ejection fraction, the overall message is that "good pump performance makes for a good prognosis."

EXPERIENCE WITH POSTSURGICAL/
ANGLOPLASTY PATIENTS

In general, post-CABGS patients may be treated more aggressively than post-myocardial infarction patients, and post-PTCA patients may be treated more aggressively than post-CABGS patients. As long as there is appropriate monitoring for early restenosis, the presence of exercise-induced catastrophic events is related mostly to the presence of myocardial ischemia during exercise training (24). In the revascularized patient, this risk factor is largely absent. Beyond this, we have recently demonstrated that even mild ischemia may be relatively well tolerated, at least in terms of LV function (25). Thus, the primary limitation of the postoperative patient is related to sequelae of the sternotomy, which may limit upper extremity exercise for some weeks and may hamper ventilatory efforts up to 6 months postoperatively (26). At the present time there are no systematically collected data regarding how much more aggressively one can treat CABGS patients if the chest incision is made via a minimally invasive intercostal approach rather than by the sternal approach. One would presume that the reduced trauma would allow more aggressive therapy. However, despite the possibilities of being more ''aggressive'' with revascularized patients, we have felt that accelerating the entry into the program rather than necessarily increasing the intensity or duration of the exercise program is the critical issue.

There are generally fewer medical problems during rehabilitation of postsurgical patients as compared with patients after myocardial infarction (MI), despite the more aggressive approach usually taken with the postsurgical population (27). Several studies have demonstrated a high frequency of dysrhythmias following surgery (28–30), although these dysrhythmias are often not severe and may not require intervention. Despite the lack of serious medical problems, rehabilitation programs have an important and continuing role in providing for physician surveillance and identifying early postoperative problems before they evolve into situations that require urgent intervention. Given the high rate of restenosis following PTCA, it makes sense that similar surveillance would be appropriate following PTCA.

EXERCISE PRESCRIPTION

The basic concept of exercise prescription for post-CABGS and post-PTCA patients is the same as for any other individual. In general, exercise effects and side effects follow a dose-response curve, as do pharmacological agents. The prescriptive markers for exercise can be remembered by the acronym FIT, meaning frequency, intensity, and time. The combination of frequency, intensity, and time necessary to provoke physiological adaptations in healthy individuals is well documented (31). As a general rule, more debilitated patients cannot tolerate either the intensity or time of exercise that healthy individuals can, but they may tolerate very frequent small exercise bouts (three to four times daily). As the patient recovers, the exercise prescription is modified, first by increasing the time of exercise bouts and later by increasing the intensity of effort, eventually evolving to maintenance guidelines. For the post-PTCA patient, an exercise prescription not unlike that for healthy, sedentary controls may be appropriate, with the understanding that surveillance for ischemia secondary to early restenosis is crucial. Given our emphasis on the critical importance of early program entry after hospital-discharge, the initial exercise sessions are often comparatively mild—little more than extensions of the inpatient program. However, we feel that early program entry is so important to a well-organized convalescence that it supersedes any special details of exercise prescription.

In our inpatient program, we employ a modification of the step approach of Wenger (31). During the last decade, with the progressive reduction in the duration of hospitalization, we have given our inpatient staff great latitude in adjusting the step schedule and responding to the patient's present clinical condition and needs. This has included the administration of a routine lifting task for all suitable patients in order to familiarize them with the practical implications of the 10–16 lb. lifting limitation that we recommend at the time of hospital discharge (32). In our experience, patients seem surprised at how light 10 1b feels; i.e., they have a low self-efficacy for lifting at the time of hospital discharge. Thus, in addition to providing clinical guidelines, lifting completed during the inpatient phase may help to improve self-efficacy and remove one of the primary impediments to return to work in post-CABGS and post-PTCA patients (7,8).

FUNCTIONAL TRANSLATION OF EXERCISE TEST RESULTS

We have long felt that many patients were fairly unskilful at taking exercise pulse rates, despite extensive instruction and practice. Frequently, they have asked specific questions about exercise, such as how fast to walk, how hard to ride the ergometer, or whether they could participate in recreational activities such as tennis or skiing. For patients in our outpatient program, it is relatively easy to titrate appropriate exercise loads. However, for patients who are seen only at the time of hospital discharge or in single-visit consultations, the process is more difficult. Accordingly, we have developed a method for "translating" exercise test information into specific exercise guidelines. We have the patient perform a standard exercise protocol on either the treadmill or the cycle ergometer. The heart-rate (HR) responses during the test are then plotted (Fig. 2). From the experimentally observed relationship between the time HR relationship during exercise testing and the ambulatory velocity-HR relationship during exercise training (which is built into the structure of the nomogram), we can predict an appropriate pace for level-ground ambulation during exercise training (33). This approach also works well for cycle ergometry. Originally we anticipated that we might be able to cross-translate this approach to common recreational activities based on their published aerobic requirements. However, subsequent studies (34) demonstrated that many patients could participate successfully in recreational activities even when the functional translation algorithm predicted that the activity would be too strenuous for them. This is probably because the aerobic requirements of recreational activities were established on young and comparatively athletic physical education students who, additionally, were performing the recreational activity in a manner organized to allow steady-state measurements of respiratory metabolism. Ordinary breaks in activity were eliminated, leading to a spurious elevation of the "real world" aerobic requirements of these activities. With older

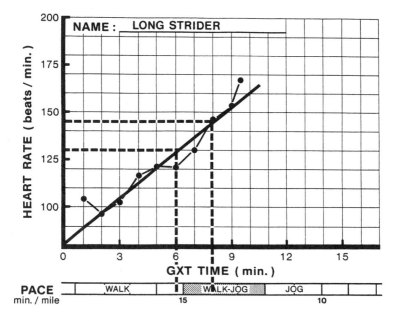

FIGURE 2   Functional translation algorithm demonstrating the relationship between the heart-rate response during a standard graded exercise test (Bruce treadmill protocol) and the speed of level walking necessary to produce a desired target heart rate during exercise training. (Adapted from data in Ref. 33.)

or less fit participants who are willing to ''let the ball do the running,'' it appears possible to modulate the aerobic requirements of even strenuous recreational activities. Thus, as long as there is no evidence of exertional ischemia, which might predispose the participants to complications (24), we do not discourage participation in reputedly strenuous recreational sports activities. At the same time we counsel patients to undertake appropriate conditioning to support the physical requirements of their chosen recreational activities.

A particular advantage of the functional translation approach is that patients can have their health status and exercise capacity determined in a single session. Then, after a brief rest, they can perform submaximal exercise at the intensity recommended by the functional translation algorithm. Once the patients' HR is in the target zone we can ask patients to note how the exercise feels. Thus, we can teach then perceptual cues to an appropriate exercise intensity, reducing the need to measure HR during exercise.

INTERVAL TRAINING

Some years ago, we became concerned that part of the exercise limitation in post-CABGS patients was as dependent on muscular weakness as on limitations of oxygen transport. We demonstrated that the use of interval training, a technique commonly applied with athletes, allowed a more rapid increase in exercise capacity than conventional steady-state aerobic training in post-CABGS patients (35). We noted that as long as the duration of the high-intensity phase was kept comparatively brief (≤ 30 s), even patients with severe congestive heart failure could tolerate bursts of fairly high-intensity activity with little metabolic disturbance (36). Given the frequent observation of skeletal muscle abnormalities in patients with heart failure and the low probability of significant central gas exchange improvements with training in this population, we have extended the concept of higher-intensity-interval training to patients with chronic heart failure (37, 38). Our results have been excellent and as beneficial as interval training in post-CABGS patients. We interpret these data as indicating that skeletal muscle weakness is a generally underrecognized component of exercise intolerance. Interval training, which allows high skeletal muscle loading while minimizing metabolic disturbance, may be an important future tool in the conditioning of post-CABGS and post-PTCA patients. We have developed a very brief cycle-ergometer exercise test (3 min of unloaded pedaling followed by increases of 25 W/10 s to muscular failure), which allows us to set useful interval training work rates. Power outputs 50% of the maximum observed during this test are very well tolerated when alternated (30 s:60 s) with recovery work rates of 10 W. If the resulting work rate is perceived as too strenuous, it can easily be modified by changing the time sequence to 25 s:65 s or 20 s:70 s. The shorter the "hard" segment the less the overall metabolic demand of the interval session.

MONITORING EXERCISE TRAINING

The exercise prescription is usually defined in terms of the frequency, intensity, and duration of training. The integrated product of frequency, intensity, and duration effectively represents the "input" to the system causing the physiological responses to training that effectively represent the "output" of the system. However, if exercise is to be compared to pharmacological therapy, there must be a single number that represents the overall "dose" of exercise, just as the patient who is on "Atenolol 50 mg bid" is on the same "dose" as a patient who is taking "Atenolol 25 mg quid." Although some authors (31) have recommended using total kilojoules of exercise as a single number, the essential equality of total energy expenditure at high and low exercise intensities means that it does not well represent the impact of exercise intensity on the exercise prescription.

Early studies by Bannister et al. (39, 40), using % HR reserve with a multiplier for exercise intensity and exercise duration, demonstrated an excellent ability to account for fitness changes associated with the total training impulse (TRIMPS). Preliminary studies by the same group have demonstrated that changes in blood pressure and serum cholesterol can be related to the TRIMPS. We have used a conceptually similar system based on multiplying the rating of perceived exertion for an entire exercise session by its duration (41). This system has demonstrated an excellent ability to account for the performance of athletes (42) and the likelihood of developing overtraining (43). Preliminary studies in patients show that this system is a useful method of partitioning exercise between home and the rehabilitation center (Fig. 3). It remains to be seen whether this simplification of the TRIMPS, which no longer requires measurement of HR during every exercise session, will be useful in monitoring long-term behavioral and risk-factor changes in patient populations. In any case, the active monitoring of behavior is an underutilized method in most cardiac rehabilitation programs.

CONCLUSIONS

Post-CABGS and post-PTCA patients may respond favorably to participation in a rehabilitation program based on exercise and risk-factor reduction. Although there are no hard data regarding the effect on subsequent morbidity/mortality, there is enough supporting evidence to hypothesize an effect as great as that documented in post-MI patients. The basic principles of exercise prescription are similar to those accepted following MI. Generally, post-CABGS and post-PTCA

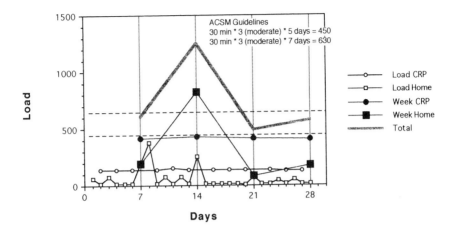

FIGURE 3   Schematic data for a representative patient during 4 weeks of exercise training, demonstrating the amount of exercise accomplished in both the cardiac rehabilitation program (CRP) and at home. Daily totals are presented along with summated weekly values. The patients' total exercise training load easily satisfies current American College of Sports Medicine recommendations.

patients may be progressed more aggressively than post-MI patients. Some care is required to adjust upper-extremity exercise in post-CABGS patients until the sternotomy has healed. Surveillance for the reemergence of ischemia secondary to graft closure and, particularly, restenosis of dilated arteries remain important features of the rehabilitation program in this population. Given the negative impact on compliance from patients thinking that they are ''cured,'' aggressive use of compliance-enhancing strategies such as self-monitoring is particularly important following CABGS and PTCA.

REFERENCES

1. Oldridge, N.B., Guyatt, G.H., Fischer, M.E., and Rimm, A.A., *J.A.M.A.,* 260: 945–950 (1988).
2. O'Connor, G.T., Buring, J.E., Yusuf, S., Goldhaber, S.Z., Olmstead, E.M., Paffenbarger. R.S., and Hennekens; C.H., *Circulation,* 80: 234–244 (1989).
3. Foster, C., in *Exercise and Sport Sciences Reviews,* Vol. 14 (K. Pandolf, ed.). Macmillan, New York, pp. 303–323 (1986).
4. Weiner, D.A., Ryan, T.J., McCabe, C.H., Chaitmen, B.R., Sheffield, L.T., Fisher, L.D., and Tristani, F., *J. Am. Coll. Cardiol.,* 8: 741–748 (1986).

5. Jones, R.H., Floyd, R.D., Austin, E.H., and Sabiston, D.C., *Ann. Surg.,* 197: 743–754 (1983).
6. Gutmann, M.C., Knapp, D.N., Pollock, M.L., Schmidt, D.H., Simon, K., and Walcott, G., *Circulation,* 66 (Suppl. III): 33–42 (1982).
7. Fitzgerald, S.T., Becker, D.M., Celentano, D.D., Swank, R., and Brinker, J., *Am. J. Cardiol.,* 64: 1108–1112 (1989).
8. Solymoss, B.C., Nedeau P., Millette, D., and Campeau, L., *Circulation,* 78: 140–143 (1988).
9. Angelini, G.D., and Newby, A.C., *Eur. Heart J.* 10: 273–280 (1989).
10. McBride, W., Lange, R.A., and Hillis, L.D., *N. Engl. J. Med.,* 318: 1734–1737 (1988).
11. Galan, K.M., Deligonnul, V., Kern, M.J., Chaitman, B.R., and Vandromeal, M.B., *Am. J. Cardiol.,* 61: 260–263 (1988).
12. Niebauer J., Hambrecht, R., Velich, T., Hauer, K., Marburger C., Kalberer B., Weiss, C., von Hodenberg, E., Schlieft, G., Schuler, G., Zimmermann, R. and Kubler, W., *Circulation.* In press.
13. Dubach, P., Lehmann, K.G., and Froelicher, V.F. *Am. J. Cardiol.,* 64: 1039–1040 (1989).
14. Rod, J.L., Squires, R.W., Pollock, M.L., Foster, C., and Schmidt, D.H., *J. Cardiopulm. Rehabil.,* 2: 199–205 (1982).
15. Foster, C., Oldridge, N.B., Dion, W., Forsyth, G., Grevenow, P., Hansen, M.A., Laughlin, J., Plichta, C., Rabas, S., Sharkey R.E., and Schmidt, D.H., *J. Cardiopulm. Rehabil.,* 15: 209–215 (1995).
16. Foster, C., Pollock, M.L., Anholm, J.D., Squires, R.W., Ward, A., Dymond, D.S., Rod, J.L., Saichek, R., and Schmidt, D.H., *Circulation.* 69: 748–755 (1984).
17. Rod, J.L., Foster, C., and Schmidt, D.H., *J. Cardiopulm. Rehabil.* 4: 70–73 (1984).
18. Pollock, M.L., Foster, C., Anholm, J., Rod, J.L., Wolf, F., Akhtar, M., Al-Nouri, M., and Schmidt, D.H., *Cardiology,* 69: 358–365 (1982).
19. Sawada, S.G., Judson, W.E., Ryan, T., Armstrong, W.F., and Feigenbaum, H., *Am. J. Cardiol.,* 64: 1123–1129 (1989).
20. O'Keefe, J.G., Layre, A.C., Holmes, D.R., Gibbons, R.J., *Am. J. Cardiol.,* 61: 51–59 (1988).
21. Labovitz, A.J., Lewen, M., Kern, M.J., Vandormeal, M., Mroesk, D.G., Beyers, S.L., Pearson, A.C., and Chaitman, B.R., *Am. Heart. J.,* 117: 1003–1008 (1989).
22. Dubach, P., Froelicher, V.F., Klein, J., and Detrano, R., *Am. J. Cardiol.,* 63: 530–533 (1989).
23. Mark, D.B., Shaw, L., Harrell, F.E., Hlatky, M.A., Lee, K.L., Bengtson, J.R., McCants, C.B., Califf, R.M., and Pryor, D.B., N. Engl. J. Med., 325: 849–853 (1991).
24. Hossack, K.F., and Hartwig, R., *J. Cardiopulm. Rehabil.,* 2: 402–408 (1982).
25. Foster, C., Gall, R.A., Murphy, P., Port, S.C., and Schmidt, D.H., *Med. Sci. Sports. Exerc.,* 29: 297–305 (1997).
26. Foster, C., Pollock, M.L., Anholm, J.D., Squires, R.W., Ward, A., Rod, J.L., Lemberger, K., Rasansky, M., Oldridge N.B., and Schmidt, D.H., *Circulation,* 72: III-268(1070) (1985).
27. Sennett S.M., Pollock, M.L., Pels, A.E., Foster C., Dolatowski, R., and Patel, S., *J. Cardiopulm. Rehabil.* 7: 458–465 (1987).

28. Dion, W.F., Grevenow, P., Pollock, M.L., Squires, R.W., Foster, C., Johnson, W.D., and Schmidt, D.H., *Heart Lung,* 11: 248–255 (1982).

29. Silvidi, G.E., Squires, R.W., Pollock, M.L., and Foster, C., *J. Cardiopulm. Rehabil.,* 2: 355–362 (1982).

30. Dolatowski, R.P., Squires, R.W., Pollock, M.L., Foster, C., and Schmidt, D.H., *Med. Sci. Sports Exerc.,* 15: 281–286 (1983).

31. Pollock, M.L., Pels, A.E., Foster, C., and Ward, A., in *Heart Disease and Rehabilitation,* 2nd ed. (M.L. Pollock and D.H. Schmidt, eds.). Wiley, New York, pp. 477–515 (1985).

32. Grevenow, P., Foster, C., Dion, W., Adashek, M., and Schmidt, D.H., *J. Cardiopulm. Rehabil.,* 9: 409(Abstr.) (1989).

33. Foster, C., Lemberger, K., Thompson, N.N., Sennett, S.M., Hare, J., Pollock, M.L., Pels, A.E., and Schmidt, D.H., *Am. Heart. J.,* 112: 1309–1316 (1986).

34. Foster, C., and Thompson N.N., *J. Cardiopulm. Rehabil.,* 11: 373–377 (1991).

35. Meyer, K., Lehmann, M., Sunder, G., Keul, J., and Weidemann, H., *Clin. Cardiol.,* 13: 851–861 (1990).

36. Meyer, K., Samek, L., Schwaibold, M., Westbrook, S., Hajric, R., Lehmann, M., Ebfeldt, D., and Roskamm, H., *Eur. Heart. J.,* 17: 1040–1047 (1996).

37. Meyer, K., Schwaibold, M., Westbrook, S., Beneke, R., Hajric, R., Gornandt, L., Lehmann, M., and Roskamm., H., *Am. J. Cardiol.,* 78: 1017–1022 (1996).

38. Volterani, M., *Eur. Heart J.* 15: 801–809 (1994).

39. Morton R.H., Fitz-Clarke, J.R., and Banister, E.W., *J. Appl. Physiol.* 69: 1171–1177 (1990).

40. Fitz-Clarke, J.R., Morton, R.H., and Banister, E.W., *J. Appl. Physiol.,* 71: 1151–1158 (1991).

41. Foster, C., Hector, L.L., Welsh, R., Schrager, M., Green, M.A., and Snyder, A.C., *Eur. J. Appl. Physiol.,* 70: 367–372 (1995).

42. Foster, C., Daines, E., Hector, L., Snyder, A.C., and Welsh, R., *Wisc. Med. J.,* 95: 370–374 (1996).

43. Foster, C., *Med. Sci. Sports Exerc.* in press.

14

Exercise in the Prevention and Management of Diabetes Mellitus and Blood Lipid Disorders

ARTHUR S. LEON
University of Minnesota
Minneapolis, Minnesota

INTRODUCTION

Diabetes mellitus (DM) is the most common endocrine disorder in the United States. It is a serious systemic disease, which affects over 5% of the general population (or currently about 16 million Americans), about half of whom are unaware that they have this condition (1). The prevalence rate is much higher in African-American, Hispanic, and certain Native American groups as compared with non-Hispanic Caucasians. The incidence of the disease also progressively increases with aging at a rate of 0.5 to 1.0% per year after age 65, as compared to 0.2% per year at ages 24–44. DM is an important contributor to morbidity and premature mortality, directly causing about 10 deaths per 100,000 population or about 55,000 deaths per year, making it the seventh leading cause of mortality in the United States. However, this represents only the tip of the iceberg, since most deaths in the diabetic population are attributed to secondary complications, particularly cardiovascular disease (CVD). About 200,000 to 300,000 deaths per year directly or indirectly due to DM is a more realistic figure. DM also is the principal cause of nontraumatic lower limb amputations, which result from peripheral vascular disease, a not uncommon CVD complication. Further, it is a major contributor to visual impairment and new blindness, renal failure requiring chronic renal dialysis and kidney transplants, and many different forms of central and peripheral neuropathies. The disease accounts for at least 10% of all acute hospital days. The gross overall economic impact of DM in this country is estimated to be currently over $100 billion per year, a substantial part of the total health care expenditures in the United States.

Exercise has both potential benefits and some risks for prediabetic and diabetic individuals as well as for nondiabetic people with blood lipid disturbances (dyslipidemias). This chapter is designed to provide physicians and other health care practitioners with guidelines to help integrate exercise into the overall management of patients with these conditions while minimizing associated risks. This requires an understanding of the pathophysiology of DM and other modes of management of DM and blood lipid disorders, reviewed here.

The chapter begins with a discussion of the etiology and pathophysiology of the two major forms of diabetes and their associated microvascular and macrovascular (or atherosclerotic) complications. The contribution of dyslipidemias to atherosclerosis and coronary heart disease (CHD), the most common cardiovascular complication of both diabetes and dyslipidemias, is discussed in detail, along with dietary and pharmacological treatment of lipid disorders in addition to the contributions of exercise. Guidelines for the diagnosis of diabetes and its management by dietary modifications and glycemic control with insulin and oral hypoglycemic drugs are provided in addition to the role of exercise. The section on exercise therapy includes a discussion of the role of metabolic and endocrine adaptations during acute aerobic exercise in glycemic control of diabetic individuals and the additional physiological and psychological benefits of exercise training. Guidelines also are provided on how to make recreational exercise or competitive sports safer for the individual with DM. These include measures to help avoid possible adverse effects of exercise, particularly aggravation of hyperglycemia, episodes of hypoglycemia in those receiving insulin therapy, triggering of myocardial ischemia, aggravation of proliferative retinopathy, and complications from lower extremity injuries (particularly a problem among those with peripheral neuropathy and peripheral vascular disease, two common complications of DM).

Pathophysiology and Classification

Diabetes mellitus is not a single disease entity; rather, it is a metabolic syndrome of heterogeneous origin with hyperglycemia the principal hallmark. Hyperglycemia and the associated metabolic derangements stem *primarily* from either an absolute deficiency of circulating insulin or a relative insufficiency of insulin in terms of its ability to normalize blood glucose levels (1). Insulin is a small protein consisting of two amino acid chains attached via sulfydryl groups and by a short connecting peptide, C-peptide. It is synthesized and released by the beta cells of the pancreas along with C-peptide, which can serve as a marker for insulin secretion. Circulating insulin binds to specialized-cell plasma membrane receptors to stimulate uptake and oxidation of glucose as a fuel substrate by the liver, muscle, adipose tissue, and other tissues. In addition, insulin affects specific rate-limiting cell enzymes, such as tyrosine kinase, promoting multiple anabolic biosynthesis processes while inhibiting catabolic ones. These include storage of glucose as glycogen in muscle and the liver, cell amino acid uptake and protein synthesis, and fatty acid synthesis and triglyceride store in adipocytes, as well as inhibition in the liver of glycogen breakdown and release of its glucose building blocks into the circulation. Furthermore, insulin inhibits triglyceride lipolysis in adipocytes, thereby reducing the release of free fatty acids (FFA) from adipocytes into the blood stream.

Thus, an absolute deficiency of insulin or cell insulin resistance (a relative insufficiency) results in hyperglycemia because of both failure of tissues to clear glucose from the blood and excess glucose release from the liver. In addition, insulin deficiency or resistance initiates a series of other catabolic processes. These include accelerated lipolysis of triglycerides in adipocytes with an increased FFA release into the circulation and their accelerated utilization by tissues for fuel. Formation of ketone bodies and subsequent ketoacidosis result from an inability by the liver to utilize all the excess acetyl coenzyme A generated from metabolism of the excess FFA. Insulin insufficiency also results in a reduced cell uptake of amino acids, increased cell proteolysis, and increased conversion of circulating amino acids to glucose by the liver (gluconeogenesis). Dehydration and electrolyte disturbances may result from an excess loss of fluid and electrolytes in the urine owing to the diuresis accompanying hyperglycemia, glycosuria, and ketoacidosis. DM also is accompanied by an excess secretion of hormones that antagonize the action of insulin, i.e., the so-called counterregulatory hormones, which contributes significantly to the metabolic derangements. These hormones include cortisol, epinephrine, growth hormone, and particularly glucagon, from the alpha islet cells of the pancreas.

DM is a heterogeneous condition commonly classified into at least four clinically and pathologically distinct clinical types (1,2): (a) idiopathic insulin-dependent or type I diabetes (IDDM), formerly referred to as juvenile-onset DM; (b) non-insulin-dependent or type II diabetes (NIDDM), formerly referred to as adult- or maturity-onset DM; (c) malnutrition-related DM; and (d) secondary forms of DM. The secondary forms result from specific conditions and syndromes that reduce the availability of insulin, such as destructive diseases of the pancreas or syndromes resulting from excess secretion of hormones antagonistic to insulin (e.g., Cushing's disease or acromegaly). In addition, gestational diabetes is a form of DM initially recognized during pregnancy, which, if it persists after pregnancy, is subsequently reclassified into type 1 or 2 DM. Further, impaired glucose tolerance (IGT) describes the condition in which there is a moderate elevation in plasma glucose in the postprandial state or following an oral or intravenous glucose challenge in the presence of a normal or slightly elevated fasting plasma glucose level. However, IGT is not a benign condition, since it is associated with an increased future risk of NIDDM as well as of future cardiovascular complications.

Insulin-Dependent (Type 1) Diabetes Mellitus

The underlying pathophysiology of the two major types of diabetes, IDDM and NIDDM, are quite different (1–4). IDDM accounts for about 10% of all cases of DM in the United States. This form of DM is believed usually to result from a physical destruction of pancreatic beta cells by an autoimmune process in which antibodies to islet cells cause or contribute to their destruction. It is hypothesized that an "environmental trigger," which damages beta cells (e.g., an enterovirus or toxic chemicals), causes antigen release that initiates the progressive autoimmune destructive process in genetically susceptible people (1,5,6). Supporting evidence for this hypothesis is the demonstration of antibodies to beta islet cells in the blood of prediabetic individuals and newly diagnosed patients with IDDM; this hypothesis is further supported by the facts that IDDM is much more likely to occur in people with certain inherited major classes of human histocompatibility leukocyte antigen (HLA) complexes (i.e., HLA types DR3 and DR4), and the reported effectiveness of experimental immunosuppression with cyclosporine in enhancing and preserving beta cells function in newly diagnosed patients with IDDM (1). The effect of prophylactic insulin therapy on prevention of IDDM in susceptible individuals with high titers of islet cell antibodies also is currently under investigation. Although hyperglycemia in IDDM is primarily due to insulin deficiency, it also is commonly contributed to by a defect in insulin-stimulated glucose uptake—i.e., cell resistance to insulin effects—which may be caused by hyperglycemia.

Commonly, IDDM first becomes clinically evident with an abrupt onset of classical symptoms and signs before age 30 and particularly during childhood or adolescence (1,3); however, it may occur at any age. The incidence of IDDM is about 15 per 100,000 in those under 20 years old with no gender predominance. Victims are usually of normal weight or underweight and often have a family history of type 1 DM, suggesting a genetic predisposition. The risk of IDDM is about 1 in 20 to 50 in the offspring of someone with this condition as compared to 1 in 400 in the general population (1).

Non-Insulin-Dependent (Type 2) Diabetes Mellitus

NIDDM accounts for about 90% of all cases of diabetes in the United States (1,4). It generally presents insidiously after age 40 with less severe symptoms than type 1 diabetes and a higher incidence in women than men. It also often is discovered in asymptomatic individuals by the finding of an elevated blood glucose level or glycosuria. It is usually associated with obesity and physical inactivity as well as with a strong family history of type 2 DM, suggesting at least in some cases an autosomal dominant trait. In contrast to IDDM, antibodies to islet cells are not present in the plasma of patients with NIDDM, and there is no association with any particular HLA type. Thus, hyperglycemia with NIDDM is not secondary to autoimmune destruction of insulin-secretor cells, and there is no absolute insulin deficiency, at least early in the course of their disease. However, reduced beta cell mass and function appear to be contributing factors, and beta cell failure may develop later, particularly in obese individuals (1). Not only is circulating insulin always detectable at least initially in patients with type 2 DM, but plasma insulin levels often are higher than in nondiabetic individuals, i.e., hyperinsulinemia may be present at least in the early stages of the disease. The implication of these findings is that the primary defect exists in the ability of insulin to maintain glucose hemostasis—i.e., the liver and peripheral tissues are insensitive or resistant to insulin. Although a great deal of experimental evidence supports this conclusion, the cellular mechanisms responsible for the insulin resistance are as yet unclear. It appears that defects may exist in both cell insulin receptor binding and in postreceptor effector activity in liver, muscle, and other insulin-sensitive tissues (1,4,7). These defects may include a deficiency or reduced functional activity of cell glucose transporter proteins. In addition, a defect in insulin-mediated glycogen synthesis by skeletal muscle may contribute to the pathophysiology of NIDDM. Furthermore, a delayed or relatively insufficient responsiveness of beta cells to an increase in blood glucose generally coexists with peripheral insulin resistance, particularly in older patients with NIDDM (1). Although insulin administration may be required to control severe hyperglycemia and associated symptoms, it is extremely unusual for patients with this form of DM to develop ketoacidosis in the absence of medication. However, insulin is often required for glycemic control, particularly under special stressful circumstances, such as acute injuries, infections, surgery, pregnancy, or when there is an allergic response to oral hypoglycemic agents (4).

Although a genetic predisposition appears to play a more important role in the etiology of NIDDM than in IDDM, there is strong evidence that lifestyles also are very important in the etiology of this condition. This is a hopeful finding in terms of the potential for primary prevention. Both epidemiological and experimental data indicate that obesity commonly plays a critical role in the pathogenesis of type II DM (1,4). About 80% of individuals with NIDDM are obese, with a body mass index (BMI) exceeding 27 kg/m^2, and the incidence of this disease is extremely low in lean populations. Recent research has shifted attention from obesity per se to the differential distribution of body fat. A central or abdominal-type of fat storage predominance is indicated by a waist-to-hip ratio of >1.0 in men or >0.8 in women and is often accompanied by excess intra-abdominal visceral fat. This central obesity pattern is commonly associated with an increased incidence of a metabolic syndrome consisting of hyperinsulinemia, disorders of glucose metabolism, disorders of lipid metabolism, and increased risk of hypertension, cardiovascular complications, and premature death (8,9). This syndrome is less common in obese individuals with a peripheral predominance of fat storage (i.e., the gluteofemoral phenotype). Experimentally, overeating and weight gain in both animals and humans have been demonstrated to cause insulin resistance, associated with a loss of insulin receptor activity in distended adipocytes (7,10). The resulting insulin resistance with obesity is not as severe as with NIDDM and it can be reversed by weight loss; however, in the presence of a genetic predisposition for type 2 DM, central obesity probably strongly contributes to the development of NIDDM and may serve a risk marker for its future development, particularly if associated with hypertriglyceridemia (11).

A sedentary lifestyle also appears to be an important risk factor for NIDDM in both men and women, independent of its relationship to weight gain and obesity (12–18). In fact, the syndrome of peripheral insulin resistance, hyperinsulinemia, and glucose intolerance can be induced experimentally in healthy volunteers by just a few days of bed rest (19,20).

In our society, the incidence of NIDDM is much greater in women than men; the risk increases with parity and aging (1,4,8), with the majority of victims being women over 40 years of age. The usual decline in physical activity and the associated weight gain that occurs after attainment of physical maturity, particularly in women, undoubtedly contribute to risk of this disease. A decline in lean body mass during aging may be another contributing factor that could be attenuated by regular exercise. Thus, a strong, consistent body of evidence suggests that weight maintenance or management and regular physical activity are the keys to delay the onset, help prevent, or reduce the severity of NIDDM. Such preventive measures are particularly important for overweight middle-aged women with a family history of type 2 diabetes and a tendency for central accumulation of fat, which generally follows the menopause because of estrogen deficiency.

CLINICAL COURSE AND LONG-TERM COMPLICATIONS

The natural clinical course of both types of DM is extremely variable. Many individuals (probably about 20–30%) with even severe IDDM remain free of major complications; however, as a rule, complications are common in people who have had diabetes for many decades (1). There usually is a lag period of several years before chronic complications occur, and the risk of complications increases with duration and severity of the disease. The late complications, elaborated on below, are the principal contributors to morbidity and premature mortality in the diabetic population. These are commonly classified as either microvascular complications, which affect the small vessels of the eyes, kidneys, peripheral and cranial nerves and the autonomic nervous system, or macrovascular/atherosclerotic cardiovascular complications, which affect the major arteries of the heart, brain and lower extremities. There is good evidence that "tight" glycemic control by multiple daily insulin injections or an insulin pump can reduce the incidence and severity of at least the microvascular complications. The landmark multicenter Diabetes Control and Complications Trial demonstrated a 7-year reduction in risk and severity of diabetic microvascular complications (i.e., retinopathy, nephropathy, and neuropathy) in the intensive treatment group (1,21). A brief review of major late complications of DM follows.

Ocular Complications

DM is the leading cause of significant visual impairment in the United States. Visual loss may result from diabetic retinopathy, premature cataracts, glaucoma, or optic neuropathy (1). Of these ocular conditions, retinopathy is the major contributor to blindness. Despite major recent advances in the management of diabetic retinopathy, it currently remains responsible for over 12,000 new cases of blindness annually in the United States. Diabetic retinopathy is a microvascular disorder specific for DM, which involves the capillaries and veins of the retina. The associated lesions include microaneurysms, small hemorrhages, intraretinal lipid infiltrates, and a proliferation of newly formed exudates. Accelerated retinopathy, consisting of a proliferation of microvascular abnormalities arising from the retinal veins, develops in about 5% of all diabetic individuals (1). Vitreous hemorrhages from the fragile new vessels result in scarring and retinal detachment, which can lead to blindness. It should be noted that proliferative retinopathy is generally considered an absolute contraindication for strenuous endurance or resistance exercise because of the fear that a marked increase in blood pressure can cause bleeding from friable vessels, leading to retinal separation (22). Treatment of proliferative retinopathy consists of photocoagulation of the new vessels by a xenon or argon laser light beam photocoagulator and vitrectomy to remove vitreous hemorrhages (1). Although some degree of visual impairment is common with long-term DM, less than 2% diabetic individuals become completely blind. The presence of ocular complications in patients with diabetes is associated with a reduced long-term survival rate.

Renal Complications

Renal failure is a significant cause of both morbidity and mortality among diabetic patients. About 30–40% of people with IDDM and 10% of those with NIDDM develop renal failure within 25 years after the onset of DM (1). Further, about 20–30% of all newly diagnosed cases of end-stage renal disease (ESRD) in the United States, requiring chronic hemodialysis and/or kidney transplant, is related to DM. The underlying cause of renal failure is usually diabetic nephropathy, often accompanied or preceded by diabetic retinopathy. The risk of diabetic ESRD appears to be much higher among blacks as compared with white diabetic individuals, particularly among those with NIDDM. The annual death rate from renal disease in the diabetic population is 18 times greater than that in the nondiabetic population. At the onset of hyperglycemia, even before any pathological lesions are evident, there often is an increase in the glomerular filtration rate, which may be accompanied by *microalbuminuria* and is detectable only by radioimmunoassay. The earliest morphological renal lesions visible under the microscope are microvascular changes involving both the afferent and efferent arterioles of the glomeruli (1,3,4). This is followed by diffuse intracapillary glomerulosclerosis, leading to glomerular obliteration and secondary interstitial fibrosis and tubular atrophy. As with retinopathy, these renal microvascular changes are believed to be related to vessel damage by hyperglycemia and associated metabolic disturbance, which accompany poor diabetic control, particularly the glycosylation of tissue proteins. The initial evidence of clinically significant renal lesions is progressive gross albuminuria detectable by ''dipstick'' methods. If renal insufficiency develops, this is followed by increased blood levels of creatinine and urea nitrogen. Urinary tract infections and pyelonephritis may contribute to the progressive development of renal insufficiency. Hypertension, a concomitant finding in most diabetic patients with renal insufficiency, accelerates the progression of the nephropathy.

At present, there is no known treatment to prevent the progression of proteinuria and renal failure; however, the investigational use of angiotensin-converting enzyme (ACE) inhibitor drugs appears promising as a preventive measure (1), and ACE inhibitors are the drugs of choice for management of concomitant hypertension. Vigorous endurance and resistive exercise should be avoided in people with progressive renal problems (22).

Neurological Changes

Diabetic neuropathy is another condition related to chronic hyperglycemia and its associated intracellular biochemical abnormalities. Multiple metabolic abnormalities similar to those contributing to the development of diabetic retinopathy, cataracts, and nephropathy are believed to promote nerve dysfunctions (1,3,4). Diabetic neuropathy usually occurs in patients with more than a 15-year history of DM and may affect the peripheral sensory and motor nerves, cranial nerves, and/or the autonomic nervous system. Although mononeuropathy may occur, symmetrical polyneuropathy is more common. The initial symptoms and signs of peripheral neuropathy, the most common neurological complication of DM, typically involve the lower legs and feet. These include a gradual loss of deep tendon reflexes and proprioception, and especially the development of disturbances in sensory functions. Accompanying sensory symptoms may include paresthesia, numbness, and burning or lancinating pain, particularly severe at night. Some patients also develop symmetrical muscular atrophy and weakness. Complications may include painless arthropathy with joint destruction (Charcot's joints) and plantar foot ulcerations, prone to secondary infections. Cranial neuropathies with motor deficits of nerves III, IV, and VI are less common than peripheral neuropathies. Older individuals with mild DM also may develop a progressive atrophy and weakness (amyotrophy) involving the muscles of the pelvic girdle and proximal thighs; however, this neuromuscular complication is uncommon.

Autonomic neuropathy usually occurs only in association with significant peripheral polyneuropathy and other major complications in patients with long-standing diabetes. Diabetic autonomic neuropathy can present with a wide variety of clinical manifestations. Symptoms may include postural hypotension and hypotension after vigorous exercise, gastrointestinal dysfunctions (especially of the stomach, esophagus, and small intestine) that cause a variety of gastrointestinal symptoms, a neurotropic or atonic urinary bladder, and impotence. Autonomic neuropathy is associated with a high morbidity rate and a poor prognosis. Complications resulting from the neuropathic bladder dysfunction include urinary tract infections, ureteral reflux, hydronephrosis, and pyelonephritis, all of which can contribute to loss of renal function. Abnormal sweating patterns, ranging from anhidrosis (absence of sweating) to hydrohidrosis (excess sweating), are other possible manifestations of autonomic dysfunction. Autonomic dysfunction may also reduce warning symptoms or awareness of hypoglycemia in patients on insulin therapy as well as symptomatic awareness of myocardial ischemia (1). The latter is one of multiple reasons to carefully evaluate a diabetic patient with neuropathy prior to prescribing an exercise regimen because of the risk of silent myocardial infarction and sudden death (22). Elevated resting heart rate and chronotropic insufficiency with a reduced maximal heart rate may be observed during exercise testing in those with autonomic neuropathy (22).

The Diabetic Foot

The foot is another common site of diabetic complications (1). Generally, serious foot complications are due to a combination of diabetic neuropathy, vascular impairment, and infection. Neuropathy makes the feet more vulnerable to damage and ulceration in response to injury or even normal pressure during walking. Absence of sweating and loss of sensation may be contributing factors. Atherosclerotic peripheral vascular disease and probably hyperglycemia itself make the injured foot more susceptible to infection. Because of the reduced or absent pain sensation, an infection may remain untreated and spread throughout the foot and up the leg. The associated increase in metabolic demands and blood flow requirements of the involved tissues may not be met because of associated vascular insufficiency, and the end result may be gangrene of the foot requiring amputation. Some 50–70% of all nontraumatic limb amputations in this country are attributed to DM (23). It is estimated that about 80 per 10,000 diabetic individuals per year require amputations, with the rate increasing to over 1000 per 10,000 in those over age 65 years. The potential for prevention of serious foot problems in diabetic individuals is illustrated by a preventive program reported by a large diabetic clinic (23). The amputation rate was halved simply by having all diabetic patients remove their shoes for foot inspection at each clinic visit and referring those with early evidence of potential foot problems or education and advice about proper foot care and shoe fitting.

Cardiovascular Complications

The advent of insulin replacement therapy more than 75 years ago was followed by a shift in the pattern of mortality accompanying type 1 DM. A marked decline in deaths from diabetic coma shortly after the onset of the disease, unfortunately, has been accompanied by a progressive rise in the proportion of deaths in diabetic people later in life from CVD. In part, this reflects the improved survival rate related to insulin therapy. However, a more important contributing factor to the high incidence of deaths from CVD in diabetic people is the increased prevalence of maturity-onset NIDDM with the aging of the population. About 75–80% of patients with NIDDM die of CVD. There also is a high rate of cardiac mortality with juvenile-onset IDDM with the risk increasing with the duration of the disease (1).

Observational epidemiological and necropsy studies have demonstrated that coronary atherosclerosis and clinical manifestations of CHD are more frequent, more severe, occur at an earlier age, and CHD is the principal contributor to CVD mortality in people with either major type of DM, as compared to matched nondiabetic individuals, and the disease affects men and women similarly (1,24, 25). In addition, diabetic individuals over age 35 are also more likely than matched nondiabetic individuals to have silent myocardial ischemia detected during an exercise tolerance test as well as silent myocardial infarctions. As mentioned above, it is suspected that silent ischemia is related to the absence or attenuation of myocardial ischemic pain owing to damage of cardiac nerves resulting from autonomic neuropathy. Further, diabetic individuals who sustain a myocardial infarction have a poorer prognosis and survival rate than matched nondiabetic individuals as a result of a higher incidence of congestive heart failure, cardiogenic shock, serious arrhythmias, and myocardial rupture and a higher recurrence of heart attacks as compared with nondiabetic patients.

Even in the absence of significant coronary artery atherosclerosis, individuals with DM are at increased risk for the development of cardiac problems. This is because they are susceptible to a specific type of cardiomyopathy presenting with enlargement of the heart, impaired left ventricular function, and congestive heart failure (26). This condition is apparently due to myocardial microangiopathy involving small coronary vessels, analogous to that found in the retinas and kidneys. Coexisting hypertension may be a contributing factor.

Occlusive atherosclerotic peripheral artery disease (PVD) is another important CVD complication with a markedly increased incidence in people with DM, which results in morbidity due to lower extremity intermittent claudication, gangrene, and amputation (1). About 8% of diabetic adults have evidence of PVD at the time of initial diagnosis of DM, and the prevalence increases with disease duration, peaking at about 45% after 20 years, generally in the sixth and seventh decades of life (27).

Mechanisms of Accelerated Atherosclerosis (Macrovascular Disease)

Multiple mechanisms appear to contribute to accelerated atherosclerosis and an increased incidence of acute myocardial infarctions and other CHD clinical events, as well as PVD and stroke, in diabetic individuals (28). These may be classified as (a) factors increasing injury and dysfunction of endothelium cells lining arteries, (b) blood lipid-lipoprotein disturbances, and (c) hemostatic disturbances. Injury or dysfunction of the vessel wall endothelium in diabetic individuals may be related to premature endothelial cell aging, increased permeability to plasma proteins, and osmotic damage due to the accumulation of abdominal metabolites (as with microvascular disease). In addition, endothelial damage is accelerated by elevated blood pressure levels commonly associated with diabetes. Diabetic individuals not only have a higher prevalence of hypertension but also, as a group, generally have higher blood pressure levels than matched nondiabetic individuals. Coexisting diabetic renal and renovascular disease can further contribute to the blood pressure elevations. In addition, obesity and hyperinsulinemia, both commonly associated with NIDDM, also contribute to blood pressure elevation (probably by increasing sodium reabsorption by the kidney tubules). Cigarette smoking is another important cause of endothelial damage which accelerates atherosclerosis, markedly increasing risk of CHD, PVD, and stroke. An abnormal blood lipid profile contributes to endothelial damage, which, in turn, increases lipid infiltration into the subendocardial space initiating the atherosclerotic process (Table 1).

Blood Lipid Abnormalities and Atherosclerosis

Abnormal blood lipid and lipoprotein concentrations as well as alterations of the structure of certain lipoproteins and altered metabolism of apolipoproteins appear to play important roles in accelerated atherosclerosis associated with DM (1,3,4). However, lipid and lipoprotein abnormalities are not inevitable consequences of

TABLE I   Possible Contributing Factors to Accelerated Atherosclerosis and Coronary Artery Occlusions in Diabetic Individuals

Injury and dysfunction of artery endothelial linings
    Premature endothelial cell aging
    Increased permeability to plasma proteins
    Osmotic damage and glycation
    Accumulation of abnormal metabolites
    Elevated blood pressure
    Excess smooth muscle proliferation at injury sites
    Elevated LDL cholesterol
Blood lipid-lipoprotein disturbances
    IDDM (type 1 diabetes mellitus)
        Hypertriglyceridema
        Elevated VLDL and IDL triglyceride and cholesterol levels
            (less common—increased total and LDL cholesterol levels)
        Reduced lipoprotein lipase activity
        Impaired removal of chylomicrons
        Reduced HDL-cholesterol (esp. HDL_2) levels
        Increased small, dense LDL particles
        Glycation of LDL (increases oxidation)
        Blood lipid abnormalities potentiated by nephropathy
        Possible normalization of blood lipid-lipoprotein profile with glycemic control
    NIDDM (type 2 diabetes mellitus)
        Variable abnormalities
          possible hypertriglyceridemia
          possible elevated VLDL cholesterol and triglyceride levels
          possible reduced HDL cholesterol levels
          possible elevated total cholesterol and LDL levels
        Blood lipid-lipoprotein abnormalities more likely in the presence of obesity, high waist-to-hip ratio, a high saturated fat diet, and physical inactivity
        Abnormal blood lipid-lipoprotein profile improved by glycemic control
Hemostatic abnormalities
    Increased platelet adhesiveness and aggregation in response to injury or physiological stimuli
    Increased ratio of thromboxane (TXA_2), to prostacyclin (PGI_2), promotes thrombosis and coronary spasm
    Increased plasma protein coagulation factors (factors VI and VIII, von Willebrand factor, and fibrinogen)
    Deficiency of certain coagulation inhibitors
    Diminished levels of tissue plasminogen activators and increased levels of platelet plasminogen activator inhibitor (PAI-1) reduce fibrinolytic activity

LDL = low-density cholesterol; HDL = high-density cholesterol; VLDL = very low density cholesterol; IDDM = insulin-dependent diabetes mellitus; NIDDM = non-insulin-dependent diabetes mellitus.

this disease. Variability in blood lipid and lipoprotein levels is understandable considering the heterogeneity of DM and the large number of biological and host factors that affect lipid metabolism. These factors include the type of DM, gender, body fatness and fat distribution, dietary habits, physical activity, alcohol consumption, cigarette smoking, the concomitant use of various types of medication, hormone replacement therapy, and extent of diabetic control. The prevalence and pattern of blood lipid and lipoprotein disturbances differ between IDDM and NIDDM (29–31). Patients with untreated insulin deficiency, particularly if it is associated with ketoacidosis, commonly present with moderate to severe hypertriglyceridemia. This is primarily due to extreme elevation of very low density lipoprotein (VLDL) levels. Increased intermediate-density lipoprotein (IDL) particles also may be a contributing factor. An elevation in chylomicron levels also sometimes is present in the fasting state and gives the plasma a lactescent or creamy appearance. An elevation in triglyceride-rich VLDL levels is generally due to overproduction of triglycerides by the liver. This results from the excess release of FFA by adipocytes and their uptake by the liver, associated with a deficiency in insulin and an excess of counterregulatory hormones. In addition, there often is an accompanying impairment in removal of VLDL (as well as of chylomicron) from the blood due to deficient activity of lipoprotein lipase (LPL) in tissue capillaries, another manifestation of insulin deficiency. Severe hypertriglyceridemia (>800 mg/dl) can initiate acute pancreatitis; therefore its management by diet plus antilipemic drugs is urgently required. Elevated VLDL levels also may cause a small increase in level of total cholesterol.

The excess production of VLDL and deficient activity of LPL are believed to contribute to a reciprocal reduction in levels of high density lipoprotein (HDL), especially the cholesterol-rich HDL_2 fraction. HDL is believed to be a lipid scavenger (particularly its HDL_2 fraction) that helps prevent or reverse atherosclerosis by transporting cholesterol away from peripheral tissues (including artery walls) to the liver for excretion into the gut directly or as bile salts. Numerous epidemiological studies have confirmed the inverse relationship between plasma HDL cholesterol levels and the risk of CHD—i.e., a low HDL cholesterol is associated with increased risk while a high concentration appears cardioprotective (32,33).

The scientific evidence is overwhelming that low-density lipoprotein (LDL), which delivers cholesterol to tissue cells, is at "center stage" in atherogenesis (33–35). High levels of LDL are strongly related to the severity of atherosclerosis and the risk of CHD, while reduction in levels by diet and/or medications can stop the progression and partially reverse the severity of atherosclerosis, stabilize the plaques, improve endothelial cell function, and reduce risk of initial or recurrent CHD events. Although elevated levels of total and LDL cholesterol are inconsistently found in people with poorly controlled IDDM, it is not uncommon for such individuals to have elevated levels of the more atherogenic, small, dense apolipoprotein B–rich LDL particles (33). This fraction is often associated with elevated levels of triglycerides and VLDL cholesterol. Further, it has been postulated that elevated levels of plasma VLDL and chylomicrons promote atherosclerosis by formation of cholesterol-rich remnants after lipolysis; these become incorporated into the artery wall, stimulating atherosclerotic lesion formation in a manner similar to LDL.

Another factor that may contribute to accelerated atherogenesis is impaired removal of LDL from the plasma in the presence of poor glycemic control of DM (30). The major pathway for LDL removal from the plasma is by binding to specific LDL receptors present on cell membranes of the liver and various other tissues initiating cellular uptake. The LDL receptor recognizes apoprotein B-100, present on the LDL surface. After receptor binding, LDL is taken up by the tissues for degradation by an endocytotic process to free its cholesterol, which is subsequently stored as cholesterol ester (33). A deficiency of LDL receptors or chemical alterations of apoprotein B-100 or of other LDL particle components results in a decreased rate of LDL clearance and catabolism. Elevated levels of blood sugar cause glycosylation or glycation of LDL by the binding of glucose to amino acids on apoprotein B-100 molecules. This reduces "recognition" of LDL by cell receptors and decreases cellular uptake and degradation. Glycation of LDL–apoprotein B also is believed to promote LDL oxidation and subsequent uptake by arterial wall macrophages to form foam cells involved in initiating atherogenic lesions (30).

Diabetic nephropathy may further contribute to disturbances in lipid-lipoprotein metabolism with elevated plasma levels of triglycerides; total, LDL, and VLDL cholesterol; and reduced levels of HDL cholesterol, thus increasing severity of atherosclerosis (30). Dietary and insulin therapy may help normalize these blood lipid abnormalities through maintenance of good or at least moderate glycemic control (30).

Although patients with NIDDM are more likely than those with IDDM to have lipid and lipoprotein disturbances, blood concentrations in these patients are highly variable for similar reasons as outlined for type 1 diabetic individuals. The most common lipoprotein abnormalities with type 2 DM is elevation of fasting levels of plasma VLDL cholesterol and associated triglyceride level, resulting primarily in hypertriglyceridemia (22,30,31). This may be a consequence of excess levels of circulating endogenous insulin due to peripheral insulin resistance and may precede the appearance of type 2 DM. The levels of HDL cholesterol in NIDDM generally vary inversely with those of VLDL cholesterol and triglycerides and the presence of hypertriglyceridemia and low HDL cholesterol levels are "classical findings" with this disease (31). Slightly to moderately increased levels of plasma total and LDL cholesterol also may be present in patients with NIDDM. However, in some studies the prevalence of hypercholesterolemia in type 2 diabetic patients was similar to that in matched nondiabetic controls.

Improved diabetic control by loss of excess weight, a reduced dietary lipid intake, exercise, insulin, or oral antidiabetic drugs all may favorably affect the blood lipid-lipoprotein profile in diabetic patients (30,31). For many patients however, antilipidemic drug therapy will be required.

Table 2 lists lipid-lowering pharmacological agents currently available in the United States and their expected actions on blood lipid and lipoprotein levels. These may be used as single agents or in combination along with diet, exercise, and improved glucose control by medication for management of dyslipidemic patients. It is beyond the scope of this chapter to discuss in detail the indications, details for administration, safety precautions, and adverse reactions associated with the use of these lipid-lowering agents. The reader is referred elsewhere for this information (31,36,37). In brief, the fibric acid drug gemfibozil or short- or long-acting nicotinic acid preparations are the initial agents of choice for management of severe hypertriglyceridemia or combined lipid disorders. Of these, nicotinic acid, which is the lowest priced of the antilipid drugs and is available without a prescription, requires the most clinical skill in its progressive administration to minimize multiple possible adverse effects, including flushing, hyperuricemia,

TABLE 2 Drugs Currently Available in the United States for Lipid Management

Drug	Usual therapeutic dose	Indications
Nicotinic acid (niacin)	3 to 6 g/day in divided doses	Elevated TG or LDL-C. Also markedly increases HDL-C (25–50%)
Fibric acid derivatives		Elevated TG (also reduces LDL-C
Gemfibrozil	600 mg bid	10% and increases HDL-C 10%)
Clofibrate	1000 mg bid	
Bile acid sequestrants		Elevated LDL-C [also slightly raises
Cholestyramine	16 g bid	HDL-C, but *increases* TG (10–
Colestipol	10 g bid	20%)]
HGM-COA reductase inhibitors ("statin" drugs)		Elevated LDL-C (also raises HDL-C and lowers TG)
Lovastatin	10–80 mg/day	
Pravastatin	10–40 mg/day	
Fluvastatin	10–80 mg/day	
Simvastatin	10–80 mg/day	
Atorvastatin[2]	10–80 mg/day	
Cerivastin	0.2–0.3 mg/day	

[a]The most potent "statin drug" (can lower LDL-C 60% as compared to 30–40% by the others; also it is the only statin drug approved by the FDA for management of elevated TG). LDL-C = plasma low density lipoprotein cholesterol; HDL-C = plasma high density lipoprotein cholesterol; TG = plasma triglycerides.

and aggravation of glycemic control in diabetic patients. For management of elevated LDL cholesterol levels, the "statin" drugs currently are the agents of choice. They are easy to administer (usually once daily at bedtime) and rarely have adverse effects. They can also be used in combination with a fibric acid drug or niacin in individuals with combined hypertriglyceridemia and hypercholesterolemia. The bile sequestrant drugs, which may also be used to lower blood cholesterol, are contraindicated in the presence of hypertriglyceridemia because they may aggravate the condition.

It also is recommended that vitamin E (400 IU of alpha tocopherol) be administered daily to patients with lipid disorders to help prevent LDL oxidation and reduce risk of CHD events (38). Consideration also should be given to the use of estrogen replacement therapy in postmenopausal women to help normalize blood lipids and reduce risk of CHD (31,37). Estrogen raises plasma HDL cholesterol and may reduce LDL cholesterol levels; however, it can aggravate hypertriglyceridemia and should be used in minimal dose with careful follow-up evaluation in patients with elevated triglycerides. Because of estrogen-induced increased risk of endometrial cancer, a progestational agent should be included in hormonal replacement therapy for women with an intact uterus.

The optimal goals for lipid management of the diabetic patient with dyslipidemia through intervention with diet, exercise, and drugs are to maintain level of plasma total cholesterol below 200 mg/dl, LDL cholesterol below 100 mg/dl, HDL cholesterol above 45 mg/dl for men and above 55 mg/dl for women, and triglycerides below 250 mg/dl (35,36). It is hoped that the careful management of these lipid disorders will reduce the risk of CVD in patients with DM, as it has in nondiabetic individuals. Although this remains to be confirmed by definitive, randomized controlled clinical trials, strong suggestive evidence of reduction of major coronary events in NIDDM individuals with LDL cholesterol reduction comes from subgroup analysis of major drug primary and secondary CHD trials, particularly the Scandinavian Simvastatin Survival Study (4S trial) (30,37,38).

Hemostatic Abnormalities.   A "hypercoagulable state" appears to contribute to the high incidence of occlusive arterial disease accompanying DM (39,40). An array of hemostatic abnormalities appear to be involved, an understanding of which requires a general review of hemostatic mechanisms (41).

The initial coagulation response to injury is rapid adhesion of platelets to areas of endothelial damage. A platelet-fibrin plug occurs at the injury site as a result of a sequence of complex physiochemical changes in which platelets, endothelial cells, clotting factors, and inhibitors all make important contributions. Normal hemostasis depends upon the proper interaction of these systems, and an alteration in any one of them can increase the tendency for either vascular thrombosis or hemorrhage. In addition, there appears to be a relationship between both altered platelet activity at an injury site and platelet adherence to areas of denuded endothelium to development of atherosclerosis (37,42). Injured or dysfunctional endothelial cells release chemicals that promote macrophage adhesion and uptake into the endothelium. The injured cells also have a reduced synthesis of nitric oxide (NO) and prostacyclin (PGI_2), which are potent vasodilators, and an increased secretion of potent vasoconstrictors, endothelin, angiotensin II, and, under certain conditions, thromboxane A_2(TXA_2) (43). This results in increased platelet aggregation and reduced blood flow, which promote thrombus formation. Furthermore platelets at the injury site release chemicals which further promote vasoconstriction and their own aggregation (43). The most potent of these substances is TXA_2. Other substances released by platelets stimulate smooth muscle cell migration from the media to the subendothelial area. Both smooth muscle cells and macrophages have a great avidity for the uptake of modified LDL and in the presence of elevated plasma LDL they are converted to foam cells, the focal elements in atheromata formation. The smooth muscle cells are also the source of connective tissue deposits, thereby contributing to the ''sclerosis'' component of atherosclerotic lesions.

In vitro studies have found increased platelet adhesiveness and aggregability in response to usual chemical agonists, such as catecholamines, in some but not all diabetic individuals as well as in experimental animal models of DM. Diabetic individuals including children often have elevated plasma levels of β-thromboglobulin (BTG), a specific protein released from platelets during aggregation, believed to be a marker for increased in vivo platelet activation. Particularly high levels of BTG are found in diabetic patients with either atherosclerosis or microangiopathy. Furthermore, glycemic control in newly diagnosed diabetic patients reduces blood levels of this platelet protein.

Prostaglandin synthesis by platelets and endothelial cells also plays a role in hemostasis. As mentioned, platelet and dysfunctional endothelial cells synthesize and secrete TXA_2, which is a prostanoid derivative of the polyunsaturated fatty acid arachidonic acid. TXA_2 is an extremely potent but short-lived promoter of platelet aggregation as well as of vasoconstriction. Its generation is believed to be one of the principal mechanisms for the platelet aggregation response to endothelial injury. The activity of TXA_2 is counteracted by another prostanoid metabolite of arachidonic acid, PGI_2, which is generated by endothelial cells. PGI_2, as mentioned, is a potent naturally occurring inhibitor of platelet adhesion and aggregation, as well as a potent vasodilator, as is NO. In patients with both type 1 and 2 DM, there is evidence of the increased production of TXA_2 by platelets and reduced synthesis of PGI_2 and probably of NO by endothelial cells (40–42). However, controversy exists as to whether the excess production of TXA_2 in patients with DM is the result rather than the cause of vascular complications.

In addition to platelet abnormalities, a number of other coagulation factor dysfunctions can contribute to the hypercoagulable state in DM (40,43,44). These include increased blood viscosity due to hypertriglyceridemia; increased plasma concentrations of coagulation factors VII, VIII, fibrinogen, and of the von Willebrand factor, necessary for binding of platelets to subendothelium in the process of platelet adhesion; a deficiency of antithrombin II and of other physiological inhibitors of coagulation; diminished levels of plasminogen activators in blood vessels, required to activate plasmin in order to initiate fibrinolytic activity; and an increased concentration in platelets of patients with type 2 diabetes of plasminogen activator inhibitor 1 (PAI-1), the main inhibitor of the fibrinolytic system of the blood.

Much additional work is required to better understand the relationship of disturbances of blood platelet and endothelial cell function, coagulation factors, and fibrinolytic activity to vascular complications of DM. Such studies should include assessment of the effects of improved metabolic control of DM by diet, exercise, and drugs on platelet reactivity and the TXA_2 to PGI_2 balance, endothelial NO activity, bleeding time, fibrinolysis, and subsequent rate of diabetic complications. As mentioned, there also is growing evidence that a myocardial infarction is usually triggered by an obstructive thrombus forming in a coronary artery at a site of rupture of a vulnerable, lipid-laden atherosclerotic plaque with associated mural hemorrhage and vasospasm (34,35,42). Thus, reducing the risk of thrombosis also may reduce the risk of a myocardial infarction in a diabetic individual with coronary atherosclerosis. Intensive management of glycemia and other risk factors and the use of aspirin as an antiplatelet agent are being promoted for these purposes (40).

MANAGEMENT OF DIABETES MELLITUS

Initial Evaluation

General steps involved in the management of DM are summarized in Table 3. Traditionally, the initial diagnosis of DM has been made in a nonpregnant adult by the presence of classic symptoms and unequivocally persistent elevated plasma glucose levels of >140 mg/dl or a 2-h postprandial plasma glucose level of 200 mg/dl (1–4). If the fasting glucose concentration is increased but less than diagnostic (i.e., a fasting plasma glucose level between 115 and 140 mg/dl), an oral glucose tolerance test (OGTT) may confirm the diagnosis. The finding of two elevated plasma glucose levels (i.e., ≥200 mg/dl) during the glucose tolerance test, including the 2-h specimen, also has been considered diagnostic of DM. It should be noted that recently the International Expert Committee has recommended lowering the fasting blood glucose cut point for the diagnosis of DM to repeated fasting plasma glucose levels of *126 mg/dl* or a random or 2-h

TABLE 3   Steps in Management of Diabetes Mellitus

Initial evaluation
  Rule out secondary causes and contributing factors
  Classification
  Evaluate for diabetic complications
  Screen for additional atherogenic risk factors, including blood lipids and
    lipoproteins
Glycemic control/normalization of metabolic state by nonpharmacological and
    pharmacological intervention
Nonpharmacological and pharmacological intervention on other risk factors
Prevention and management of microvascular and macrovascular complications

plasma glucose reading of 200 mg/dl after an oral glucose challenge in order to detect DM at an earlier stage to help prevent or delay the onset of complications (45). Further, impaired glucose now is considered to be fasting plasma glucose level between 110 and 125 mg/dl, and impaired glucose tolerance an abnormal but less than diagnostic OGTT.

The determination of glycosylated hemoglobin, particularly the Hgb A_{1c} fraction at baseline, is useful for monitoring metabolic control (1,3,4). This test is based on the glycosylation reaction between the terminal amino acid of red blood cell hemoglobin and the number 2 carbon of glucose. This reaction increases with the blood glucose concentration. Since the reaction is irreversible and persists for the life of the red blood cell (about 120 days), the glycosylated hemoglobin concentration reflects the average blood glucose control for the previous 120 days, and serial changes have been shown to be useful for monitoring the adequacy of long-term glycemic control during subsequent treatment to improve metabolic control (46). Normal glycosylated hemoglobin values range from 3.5–8.5% (1,3,4). Poor control is generally associated with values greater than 12%.

Radioimmunoassay for levels of plasma insulin and determination of serum or urinary C-peptide levels at the time of diagnosis of DM may help distinguish an absolute deficiency of pancreatic insulin secretory activity (type I DM) from a relative insulin deficiency state (type II DM) (1). In addition, pancreatic islet cell antibodies generally are present in the blood of a majority of patients with IDDM at the time of initial diagnosis, although this may only be a transitory phenomenon.

Medical evaluation of the diabetic patient should include ruling out secondary causes or contributing factors for the metabolic abnormalities. These may include obesity (particularly the central or abdominal phenotype), other endocrine disturbances, pancreatic disease, and diabetogenic drugs such as glucocorticoids or thiazide diuretics. Evaluation should also include screening for evidence of diabetic complications, accelerated atherosclerosis, and other risk factors for CHD. As a minimum, in addition to a general physical examination, the evaluations should include ophthalmological and neurological examinations; careful inspection of the feet and skin; assessment of peripheral pulses; auscultation for carotid, abdominal, and femoral bruits; complete urinalysis; blood for determination of urea nitrogen, creatinine, total cholesterol, triglycerides, and HDL cholesterol; a resting electrocardiogram (ECG); and a chest x-ray. Relative weight for height and desirable weight should be determined as well as the waist-to-hip circumference ratio. Patients should also be questioned about smoking habits, alcohol consumption, and dietary and physical activity habits. Current American College of Sports Medicine guidelines advise a progressive exercise stress test to screen for myocardial ischemia in patients with type 1 diabetes over age 30 or type 2 diabetes over age 35 as well as younger patients with a history of DM for 15 years or longer, particularly if they have one or more risk factors for CHD, known or suspected CHD, or microvascular complications (47). The exercise test also provides information on functional capacity and exercise tolerance useful in order to give appropriate exercise advice. This testing is particularly important for those who are physically active on the job or during leisure time or who plan to initiate a strenuous exercise program.

Glycemic Control and Prevention of Complications

The two major therapeutic goals in the management of DM are the following: (a) to achieve glycemic and metabolic control of the disease and (b) to prevent, slow the progression, or attenuate microvascular and atherosclerotic complications. Three major treatment approaches act in concert toward accomplishment of these two goals. These are dietary modification (including a weight-management program for overweight individuals with type II diabetes), increased physical activity, and pharmacological intervention with insulin or an oral hypoglycemic agent. As previously indicated, it is hoped that good metabolic control by these approaches will reduce the rate of diabetic complications, as is supported by the results of the Diabetes Control and Complications Trial (21).

Multiple risk factor intervention in conjunction with metabolic control of DM also is crucial to reduce the risk of atherosclerotic CVD complications. This includes smoking cessation, loss of excess weight, reduced dietary lipid intake, and control of hypertension and blood lipid disorder. In addition, regular exercise may not only improve glycemic control but also reduce blood pressure levels and improve the blood lipid profile, as discussed further on in more detail. Finally, the addition of drug therapy is indicated if these nonpharmacological measures fail to achieve glycemic control, sufficiently reduce blood pressure levels, and/or correct blood lipid abnormalities. An intensive patient education program is the cornerstone for successfully carrying out these lifelong diabetic management requirements.

The Diabetic Diet

General nutritional objectives for management of DM are listed in Table 4 and discussed below. With the exception of the symptomatic patient with IDDM and ketosis requiring immediate insulin therapy, nutritional management is usually the initial treatment and cornerstone for management of hyperglycemia as well as for the associated blood lipid disorders (1,3,4). Generally, dietary therapy is attempted for at least a month alone or in combination with exercise for glycemic control prior to the initiation of insulin or an oral hypoglycemic agent in patients with type 2 DM. It is estimated that nutritional therapy alone will control hyperglycemia in about one-third of ketoacidosis-resistant diabetic patients (1). In ketosis-prone type 1 patients for whom insulin is required, a diabetic diet generally is begun simultaneously with insulin therapy, and insulin dosage is adjusted to balance the glycemic effects of meals (1,3). Timing of the IDDM patient's meals and snacks is influenced by the type(s) and dosage of insulin prescribed.

Food Exchange System

The basic meal structure, usually required for the IDDM patient after attaining glycemic control with insulin is three main meals a day plus snacks at midmorning, midafternoon, and bedtime. A food-exchange system is an excellent educational tool commonly employed for making dietary recommendations (1,3,4,48). This system involves selection of food choices for daily menus from lists of six different food types: (a) milk, (b) vegetables, (c) fruit, (d) bread, (e) meat, and (f) fat. In addition, lists are provided of specific food items that should generally

TABLE 4   General Objectives of Nutritional Care of the Diabetic Patient

Provide an adequate intake of essential nutrients throughout the life cycle.
Adjust energy intake (and physical activity) to achieve or maintain proper body weight.
Restore blood glucose, blood lipids, and blood pressure levels to normal.
Maintain a consistent timing of meals and snacks (and physical activity) in patients receiving insulin therapy to prevent large fluctuations in blood glucose levels.
Individualize the patient's eating (and physical activity) plan to fit his or her lifestyle.

be avoided and of items permitted in unlimited quantities. Selection of a properly prescribed number of food items from each of the food-exchange lists will provide a proper blend of essential vitamins, minerals, and protein to meet recommended dietary allowances as well as to meet the average, moderately active person's daily energy requirements.

Desirable Body Weight and Energy Requirements

Two other basic considerations necessary for designing a nutritional program are to determine the individual's "desirable" body weight and daily energy requirements for achieving or maintaining desirable weight. A number of standards for desirable weight for height have been proposed. The National Institute of Health's Consensus Conference on obesity and health (49) recommended the 1959 Metropolitan Life Insurance Tables (50), based on the mortality survival rate in an insured population. A commonly used rule of thumb for estimating desirable body weight, which approximates values from the Metropolitan Life tables, is to allow for adult men 106 lb for the first 60 in. of height and 6 lb for each additional inch. For women, 100 lb is allowed for the first 60 in. and 5 lb for each additional inch. Adjustments can be made for body frame size by subtracting or adding 10% to the above estimated weight for those with small and large frames.

Energy needs are affected by body weight and height, age, gender, and most importantly, physical activity habits. Approximate energy expenditure values for adults are based on estimates of the resting metabolic rate for age and usual physical activity status for average-sized men and women. Roughly sedentary people require 25 kcal/kg per day and moderately active people 35 kcal/kg per day (4). Another rule of thumb that can be used to estimate daily energy requirements for adults is as follows: resting energy requirement (kcal/day) = desirable body weight (DBW) in pounds $\times$ 10 (51). Then add the following in kilocalories for the estimated usual physical activity status as follows:

Sedentary	DBW $\times$ 3
Moderately active	DBW $\times$ 5
Very active	DBW $\times$ 10

For example, the estimated daily energy requirement for a moderately active 150-lb DBW man would be $150 \times 10 = 1500$ kcal + 750 kcal for a total of 2250 kcal/day. For women over age 50 years, subtract 200 kcal from the total and for men under age 50 years add 200 kcal per day. For patients who are underweight, an additional intake of 500 kcal per day will provide for a weight gain of 16 lb per week or a similar addition will meet the requirement for pregnancy or lactation. On the other hand, if the patient is overweight, a 500-kcal deficit per day should provide for approximately a pound a week weight loss.

An alternative system for estimating adult energy needs, which takes DBW and physical activity status into consideration is as follows (51):

Estimated Daily Energy Needs by Physical Activity Classification in Kilocalories per Kilogram of Actual Body Weight

Weight Status	Sedentary	Moderate	Very Active
Above DBW	20–25	26–30	31–35
At DBW	25–30	31–35	36–40
Below DBW	30–35	36–40	41–45

Table 5 lists the usual range of energy requirements for age and gender for adolescents and adults based on the National Research Council recommendations (50). For children, energy recommendations can be estimated as follows:

Age 4–6 years   90 kcal/kg
Age 7–10 years   80 kcal/kg

The following is a brief review of current recommendations for macronutrient intake by diabetic individuals.

Protein Requirements

The ADA (52) recommends that the diabetic person's eating plan contain a daily protein intake for adults of 0.8 g/kg of body weight, the same as recommended for nondiabetic individuals. For most diabetic adults, this allowance means that protein will contribute about 10–20% of the total daily energy requirements. In

TABLE 5   Usual Range of Daily Energy Requirements by Gender and Age

Gender and age group	Kilocalories per day
Males	
Adolescents	2000–3000
19–50 years	2500–3300
51–75 years	2000–2800
Females	
Adolescents	1500–3000
19–50 years	1700–2500
51–75 years	1400–2200

patients with diabetic nephropathy, the protein intake should be kept at about 10% in an attempt to slow the progression of the disease. In general, protein sources should be provided by foods that are relatively low in total fat, saturated fat, and cholesterol. This is because of the well-documented relationship of these dietary lipids to levels of plasma total and LDL cholesterol, severity of atherosclerosis, and risk of CVD (37,53). Thus, animal sources of protein should be limited to 6 oz or less daily and should consist of leaner types of red meat, fish, and poultry (without skin). Complementary plant sources of protein also should be used as often as possible in place of animal sources—e.g. a combination of beans and a grain or corn.

Carbohydrate Intake

The place of carbohydrates in the diet of diabetic individuals has long been a subject of controversy. Substantial data support previous recommendations by the ADA for a diet high in complex carbohydrates (i.e., 55–70% of calories) and in dietary fiber (about 20 to 35 g/day). Fiber should be obtained by an increased consumption of whole-grain cereals and bread, starchy roots, legumes and other vegetables, and fruits. The basis of these recommendations are research findings from both epidemiological and short-term metabolic experiments. These studies have shown the *adverse effects* on glucose tolerance (as well as on blood lipid levels) of a diet low in complex carbohydrates and dietary fiber and high in fat (54). Conversely, glucose tolerance and insulin sensitivity are generally improved and blood cholesterol levels are significantly reduced with no long-term adverse effects on plasma triglyceride levels by a diet high in complex carbohydrate and fiber and low in fat; however, because of the possibility that a high carbohydrate intake will aggravate hypertriglyceridemia, current ADA recommendations are to individualize the intake of complex carbohydrates (52). Although most of the reduction in total and LDL blood cholesterol levels with such an eating plan is due to the reduced saturated fat intake, soluble components of dietary fiber can also make a modest independent contribution (31,53).

Further support for such a dietary plan comes from population studies, which show that diabetic individuals who habitually consume low-fat diets with carbohydrates contributing up to 70% of calories, such as those in Japan, have an extremely low incidence rate of CHD even in the presence of DM (54–56). However, when Asian adults adopt a western-style diet (e.g., Japanese diabetic men living in Hawaii) their CHD rates increase markedly. Furthermore, there is evidence in nondiabetic patients with CHD who have had coronary artery bypass surgery that a diet high in complex carbohydrates and low in saturated fats can reduce the progression or cause partial regression of atherosclerotic lesions on serial coronary arteriogram (37). Additional studies are required to determine if similar beneficial dietary effects on atherogenesis occur in diabetic individuals.

Another recommendation by ADA is to *liberalize* the consumption of sucrose and fruit-containing simple carbohydrates by diabetic individuals. The basis for this is that the postprandial glycemic effects of sucrose and certain types of starch—for example, from potatoes—are similar when these are consumed as part of a meal by individuals with type 1 or 2 diabetes. However, a high intake of sucrose (17–35% of total calories) may have at least short-term adverse metabolic effects in some diabetic and nondiabetic individuals. These include the possibility of at least transient impaired insulin receptor binding and sensitivity and increases in the plasma levels of fasting triglycerides and VLDL cholesterol, as well as a significant reduction in the levels of HDL cholesterol. Thus, the current consensuses that sucrose and other glucose-containing disaccharides should not account for more than 10% of the total dietary energy. Since the average American usually obtains 16% of his or her calories from sucrose, the recommendation will require a reduction in sucrose intake for most diabetic individuals.

Fat Intake

The ADA also currently recommends that the saturated fat content of the diabetic diet should provide less than 10% of the daily energy intake, since this is the principal dietary contributor to plasma LDL cholesterol levels. The ADA further recommends that the quantity of polyunsaturated and monounsaturated fats be individualized depending on baseline plasma lipid levels and that dietary cholesterol consumption be limited to less than 300 mg/day.

For NIDDM patients with hypertriglyceridemia, total dietary fats should be restricted to 20% of total energy intake and of dietary cholesterol to 100–150 mg/day. This level of reduction in dietary fats and cholesterol intake requires a restriction in sources and quantities of animal flesh products, limiting egg yolk consumption to only a few per week, using only low-fat dairy products, and avoiding commercially prepared baked goods and other products containing animal fat, hydrogenated oils, or tropical oils (palm and coconut), all rich in saturated fatty acids. Good sources of omega-6 polyunsaturated oils, which lower blood cholesterol levels, are safflower, sunflower, corn, and soybeans. In addition, olive and canola oils are good sources of monounsaturated fatty acids, which have a neutral effect on blood cholesterol levels, while being low in saturated fatty acids (37,53). Soft margarines containing these oils as their principal ingredients are excellent substitutes for butter and hard (hydrogenated) margarines. Hydrogenated margarines are high in *trans*-fatty acids, which raise total and LDL cholesterol levels, but not as much as saturated fatty acids.

In individuals who do not tolerate a high carbohydrate intake or in whom it results in at least a temporary worsening of hypertriglyceridemia, it is possible to substitute more monounsaturated fat. An intake of monounsaturated fatty acids (such as oleic acid) up to 18% of total calories does not adversely affect the cholesterol-lowering power of the AHA Step 1 Diet (37). In addition, the consumption of a monounsaturated fat-enriched diet may prevent the decrease in plasma concentration of HDL cholesterol, which frequently occurs with a marked reduction in total or saturated fat intake (37).

Another dietary issue related to lipid ingestion for the diabetic patient pertains to the appropriate dietary content of the essential omega-3 polyunsaturated fatty acids (n-3 PUFA) and their possible role in the prevention of diabetic complications. Fish oils are a rich source of two of these highly unsaturated fatty acids; i.e., eicosapentaenoic acid (EPA, C22:5) and docosachexenoic acid (DHA, C22:6). In addition, another n-3 PUFA, alpha-linolenic acid (C16:3), present in certain vegetable oils, particularly canola and soybean oils, can be converted in the body to EPA and DHA.

Epidemiological studies have reported that a high intake of seafood rich in n-3 PUFA is associated with a reduced risk of CVD (37,57). Most of the earlier studies performed in the 1970s involved Greenland Eskimos, who consumed a diet composed predominately of seafood. However more recently, in a retrospective study from the Netherlands (The Zutphen Study), Kromhout et al. (57) reported that middle-aged men who consumed on the average 30 g of fish per day also had a reduced death rate from CHD as compared to non-fish eaters. To put this quantity of fish in perspective, the mean daily per capita consumption of fish in the United States is about half that amount. These and a number of other such epidemiological observations in the United States and Europe in nondiabetic individuals have stimulated animal and human feeding trials using either fatty fish, fish oils, or purified n-3 PUFA to examine the metabolic and biochemical effects related to the development of atherosclerotic CVD. A number of these findings, discussed below, may have relevance to the diabetic patient, although the amounts of n-3 PUFA required for these beneficial effects would require the administration of fish oil or n-3 PUFA supplements, since the quantity of fatty fish that would have to be consumed regularly to achieve these desirable physiological effects is not commonly practiced in western societies.

There is consistent evidence that 5–10 g/day supplement of n-3 PUFA (EPA + DHA) can reduce elevated plasma triglycerides and VLDL cholesterol levels with no change or at least a transient increase in HDL cholesterol levels (36,37,58). Some of these studies included preliminary observations in patients with NIDDM. However, the above changes may be associated in hyperlipidemic patients with an undesirable actual *increase* in the levels of plasma LDL cholesterol and LDL-apoprotein B. The possibility also exists that n-3 PUFA may have adverse effects on glycemic control in some NIDDM patients (37,59).

In addition to their effects on blood lipid levels, n-3 PUFA have a profound influence on platelet aggregation and blood coagulability (58). Decreased platelet aggregation in response to usual stimuli has been demonstrated in both animal and human feeding studies with n-3 PUFA, apparently due to their ability to reduce platelet TXA_2 formation. This results in prolongation of bleeding time. Such blood platelet changes theoretically should help counteract increased platelet aggregability and increased TXA_2 release often found in patients with DM, thereby reducing risk of thrombosis in narrowed atherosclerotic arteries; however, these possibilities remain to be proven.

A large dietary supplementation trial also has demonstrated the effectiveness of 6 g/day of EPA and DHA in reducing elevated blood pressure levels in nondiabetic hypertensive individuals (60). Furthermore, a fish oil supplement (cod liver oil) has been shown in IDDM patients to reduce the rate of renal transcapillary escape rate of albumin, independent of its effect on blood pressure (61). These intriguing observations of the potential beneficial effects of n-3 PUFA in reducing diabetic renal complications require confirmation. In the meantime, the routine use of n-3 PUFA supplements for diabetic patients is not currently being recommended beyond encouraging fish consumption several times a week.

A modest restriction of sodium intake to less than 3 g/day also is generally recommended for diabetic patients to reduce the propensity for high blood pressure and perhaps of diabetic nephropathy (1). Sodium intake can be minimized by the avoidance of table salt and grossly salty foods and by reducing the intake of processed foods.

Although alcohol raises plasma HDL cholesterol levels and reduces risk of CHD, it has potential adverse effects in some diabetic individuals. Alcohol should be avoided by individuals whose blood glucose is out of control and by those who have hypertriglyceridemia or hypertension. In other diabetic individuals, it can be used prudently, i.e., up to two alcoholic beverages per day with proper adjustments for the additional energy intake (52). However, because of the possibility of alcohol-induced hypoglycemia in diabetic individuals receiving insulin or an hypoglycemic drug, it should be consumed only at meals along with food.

In summary, nutritional management is a major pillar in the control of DM and in the prevention and management of associated blood lipid disorders and elevated blood pressure levels. Its potential role in the prevention of atherosclerosis and thrombotic complications appears promising but remains to be confirmed by clinical trials. In patients receiving insulin therapy, the timing and distribution of meals and snacks is crucial for the prevention of hypoglycemia, particularly in physically active individuals, as is discussed in greater detail further on in this chapter.

Insulin Therapy

Candidates

About one-third of all diabetic individuals in the United States require insulin for treatment (1). Patients with IDDM, characterized by a near absolute deficiency in endogenous insulin, require daily insulin replacement to treat or avoid keto-acidosis. Insulin therapy is also useful in both type 1 and 2 diabetic patients to control symptoms accompanying marked hyperglycemia (i.e., fasting plasma glucose levels of >250 to 300 mg/dl) in the absence of ketoacidosis and for glycemic control even in asymptomatic type 1 or 2 diabetic patients. Further, insulin also is being more widely used routinely in an attempt to reduce risk of future chronic complications in type 1 diabetic patients and for initial pharmacological intervention in type 2 diabetic patients as an alternate to oral hyoglycemic agents if diet and exercise fail to normalize blood glucose levels. It also may be prescribed if oral hypoglycemic agents are ineffective or contraindicated because of allergic problems or in the presence of significant renal or hepatic disease. In addition, it can serve as a short-term measure to control the exacerbation of diabetic metabolic dearrangements accompanying the stress of trauma, surgery, infections, pregnancy, or myocardial infarction. It should be noted that large doses of insulin (i.e., >100 U/day) are likely to be required for glycemic control in obesity-related type 2 diabetic patients due to their usual marked peripheral insulin resistance (1–4).

Goals

The immediate goals of insulin therapy are to alleviate diabetic symptoms and correct metabolic disorders while returning blood glucose and glycosylated hemoglobin levels to as normal levels as possible and avoiding hypoglycemia due to overdosage. As mentioned, improved metabolic control in type 1 diabetic individuals with insulin therapy generally is accompanied by a reduction of associated blood lipid abnormalities, including an increase in plasma HDL levels (30, 31).

Details on Insulin Administration

Insulin therapy is usually initiated in a hospital setting with insulin doses related to body weight and physical activity status and correlated with the patient's blood glucose response. The usual starting dose for a normal-weight sedentary adults 0.5 U/kg of body weight of a form of insulin with an intermediate duration of action (e.g., NPH insulin) administered subcutaneously usually in an arm (1). Adolescents usually require a larger initial dose. In the present of ketoacidosis, the initial dose may be as high as 2–4 U/kg. Following hospital discharge, subsequent management of insulin dosage is based on self-monitoring at home of capillary blood glucose levels in drops of blood obtained by a fingerstick using an automated lance. Details for self-monitoring of DM control have been extensively reported elsewhere (1,3,48). As previously mentioned, periodic glycosylated hemoglobin determinations are useful in gauging the adequacy of long-term glycemic control during therapy. Suggested algorithms for insulin dosage adjustments based on blood glucose levels are available (1,3).

Most commercial insulin preparations consist of a mixture of beef and pork insulins obtained by pancreatic extraction; however, pure pork insulin, which is usually less antigenic than beef insulin because of an amino acid sequence closer to that of human insulin, is also available. In addition, human insulin is now manufactured by recombinant deoxyribonucleic acid (DNA) techniques or by chemical modification of the pork insulin molecule. Although this product is less antigenic than pure pork insulin, the subcutaneous administration of human insulin preparations may still elicit some antibody response. The purified pork and human preparations are much more costly than the mixture of beef and pork insulin and are generally prescribed only to patients who develop significant immunological or local skin complications (1).

A complete list of insulins currently available in the United States has been published (1,3). In general, insulins may be classified by their duration of action as short-, intermediate-, and long-acting. The longer-acting preparations have had certain materials added in order to prolong their pharmacological activity in order to reduce the required number of daily injections for glycemic control.

Table 6 lists the expected duration of action of representative animal insulins from each duration class; however, since the actual rates of absorption may vary up to 25% from day to day, owing to variations in local subcutaneous tissue conditions and other factors influencing insulin pharmacokinetics, the clinician should not rely too heavily on textbook descriptions of insulin activity. Adjustments of insulin dosage should be based on actual blood glucose values obtained by self-monitoring by the patient of blood glucose levels before and after meals and exercise and during the night. Frequent self-monitoring of glucose levels is particularly important when initiating or intensifying insulin therapy or adjusting dosage because of the possibility of hypoglycemic reactions. A variety

TABLE 6   A Comparison of Time Course of Action of Different Classes of Insulins of Animal Origin After Subcutaneous Administration

Insulin type	Preparation	Onset, hours	Peak, hours	Duration, hours
Short-acting (rapid onset)	Iletin II Regular	0.5–1	2–4	6–8
Intermediate	NPH[a]	1–4	6–8	10–16
	Lente			
	Globin			
Long-acting	Ultralente	4–6	14–16	24–36

[a]NPH = Neutral Protamine Hagedorn.

of products are available for self-monitoring of blood glucose (1,48). As mentioned, insulin therapy is usually initiated in a nonemergency situation with a dose of an intermediate-acting insulin well below the amount likely to be required for glycemic control. The dose then is increased gradually in order to minimize the risk of hypoglycemia. For example, a usual safe starting dose of insulin is 15–20 U of NPH or lente (U–100 containing 100 U/ml) given subcutaneously 30 min before breakfast. The maximal blood glucose–lowering effect with intermediate-acting insulins is about 8 h after administration, with its ability to lower blood glucose concentration waning overnight and reaching a nadir in the early morning hours. A 2- to 5-day observation period is recommended prior to adjustments in the dose of intermediate-acting insulin because of the variability in the rate of insulin absorption and the day-to-day variation in food intake and physical activity. Optimal glycemic control is unlikely with a single daily insulin dose. Generally two or more doses of intermediate-acting insulin or of a combination of regular insulin with the intermediate-acting insulin are required. An advantage of using regular insulin in combination with an intermediate-acting insulin is that the peak effect of regular insulin (2–4 h after administration) may abort midmorning hyperglycemia, which is common when an intermediate-acting insulin is used alone. However, regular insulin should be added only after the appropriate dose of intermediate-acting insulin has been established. Usually 5–10 U of regular insulin is then administered in the same syringe with the intermediate-acting insulin. If postprandial hyperglycemia persists, additional doses of regular insulin alone may be administered 30 min before meals. In general, 1 U of regular insulin will lower the blood glucose level 40–50 mg/dl when the blood glucose concentration is in the range of 150–200 mg/dl. For example, 2 U of regular insulin would be expected to reduce a plasma glucose level of 200 mg/dl to 100–120 mg/dl.

A typical multidose regimen might consist of an injection of a mixture of NPH or lente insulin and regular insulin in the morning, a half hour prior to breakfast, and a second injection of the same mixture in the evening, a half hour before the evening meal. The recommended ratio of intermediate-acting to regular insulin in the morning is 2:1 and in the evening 1:1. Adjustments of the dosage and amounts of each type of insulin can be made to further reduce blood glucose levels at appropriate times of the day; however, the clinician should be aware that mixing different types of insulin may alter the time of the peak effect and duration of action of insulin, especially when regular insulin is mixed with lente insulin (1,3).

Goals for plasma or capillary glucose concentrations considered to reflect excellent or "tight" glycemic control are 70–120 mg/dl in the fasting state or before meals and 100–140 mg/dl 1 h after meals. Control is considered poor if the fasting and preprandial glucose levels are >150 mg/dl or if the postprandial level is greater than 200 mg/dl (1,3).

Usual sites for the subcutaneous administration of insulin include over either the quadriceps muscle, the deltoids, the abdominal muscle, or the gluteal regions. Injection of insulin into a region of the body (upper or lower extremities) soon to be involved in physical activity should be avoided because of the resulting accelerated absorption of insulin during muscular activity (22). This can cause a rapid onset of insulin action, resulting in a greater reduction than expected of blood glucose levels during exercise, increasing the risk of hypoglycemia as well as reducing the duration of insulin activity. Avoiding exercise for an hour immediately after insulin injection or using the abdominal region for insulin administration usually alleviates these problems. Using a single anatomical site for all insulin injections rather than rotation of anatomical sites was recently reported to reduce the variability in blood glucose levels in type 1 diabetic individuals (62).

Side Effects

Side effects of insulin therapy include a loss of subcutaneous fat at injection sites, local skin reactions, systemic allergic reactions, insulin resistance (with >100 U of insulin required daily), and hypoglycemia (insulin reaction) (1,48). In actuality, hypoglycemia (blood glucose level <60 mg/dl) is actually considered an exaggerated therapeutic response and occasional mild episodes are unavoidable during intense insulin therapy, especially in someone who exercises regularly. The symptoms and signs of hypoglycemia include one or all of the following: anxiety, tremulousness, tachycardia, sweating, tingling of the digits, dizziness, headache, and hunger (1,48). Sympathoadrenal system stimulation is primarily responsible for these initial warning symptoms, and the suppression of these symptoms by the concomitant use of β-adrenergic blocking drugs for the management of hypertension or CHD may mask the onset of hypoglycemia. Hypoglycemic symptoms also may occur in some diabetic individuals with normal or even elevated glucose levels as a result of a rapid insulin-induced reduction of hyperglycemia. The presence of true hypoglycemia constitutes a medical emergency, since cerebral dysfunction may result if it is not corrected by prompt glucose administration. Symptoms at the stage of advanced hypoglycemia may include faintness, visual disturbances, mental disturbances, slurred speech, coordination problems, personality changes or bizarre behavior, drowsiness, and unconsciousness or coma (1,48). Because of the resemblance of these cerebral symptoms to alcohol or drug intoxication, it is imperative for a diabetic individual receiving insulin to wear a medical alert identification. Delayed or skipped meals or an unexpected increase in physical activity uncompensated for by extra food intake or reduced insulin dosage can contribute to the development of hypoglycemia.

Every diabetic individual receiving insulin therapy should be cognizant of their individualized early warning symptoms of hypoglycemia and respond to them by promptly checking their capillary blood glucose level, and have an existing plan for combating low blood glucose levels. Food containing 10–15 g of simple carbohydrates, such as 1 cup (8 oz) of orange juice, or 7 to 8 hard candies (such as hard candies) may be sufficient to abort a mild insulin reaction. This should be repeated within 20 min if symptoms persist. Since avoiding hypoglycemia is a major concern of the diabetic individuals participating in sports or on an exercise program, additional discussion of this topic is included in the section of this chapter on exercise for the diabetic individual.

External or implantable battery-powered insulin infusion devices are recent developments that can significantly improve the metabolic control for the diabetic individual receiving insulin and make life easier and nearer normal (1,3). Insulin pumps are refillable reservoirs that deliver short-acting regular insulin subcutaneously, usually into the abdominal wall, by means of a small needle-like catheter or a flexible plastic catheter (inserted with a needle). The external pumps are worn on a belt and require refilling and a catheter change every 2 days. These pumps offer the opportunity for tight diabetic control and great flexibility of lifestyle for well motivated patients. Potential serious risks with either type of infusion device can result from pump damage or malfunction. In addition, there is the possibility of catheter-related problems, infections, and severe hypoglycemia.

Another important development that holds great promise for the future control of IDDM is the progressive improvement in the success of transplanting in diabetic individuals of a whole or partial pancreas or islet beta cells.

Oral Hypoglycemic Drug Therapy

Types of Agents

Oral hypoglycemic agents (OHAs) are commonly prescribed for NIDDM, with about 40% of diabetic patients in the United States receiving one of these drugs. Table 7 lists those currently in use in the United States with their usual dose range, frequency of administration, and usual duration of action (1,48). It will be noted that all but three of these drugs are sulfonylurea derivatives, three of which—chlorpropamide, glyburide, and glypizide—account for the majority of OHAs prescribed. In recent years metformin, a biguanide, was approved for marketing by the FDA (63,64). Another recently marked nonsulfonylurea OHA is troglitazone. The last drug listed, acrobose, is an alpha-glucosidase inhibitor that has been in clinical use for several years in Europe. Its effectiveness and safety have been confirmed in clinical trials in the United States and Canada, and it is expected to be approved for marketing by the FDA in the near future (63). As is true with the different insulin preparations, the duration of action of these drugs varies from short (e.g., 6 to 10 h for tolbutamide) to long-acting (e.g., 27 to 72 h for chlorpropamide).

TABLE 7   Currently Available Oral Hypoglycemic Agents by Usual Dosages Duration of Action

Drug	Daily dose range, milligrams	No. of doses per Day	Duration of action, hours
Sulfonureas			
Tolbutamide (Orinase)	500–3000	2–3	6–10
Acetohexamide			
(Dymelor)	250–1500	2	12–18
Tolazamide (Tolinase)	100–1000	1–2	16–24
Glipizide (Glucotrol)	2.5–40	1–2	16–24
Glipizide long-acting			
(Glutorol XL)	5–20	1	24–48
Glyburide (Micronase,			
DiaBeta)	1.25–20	1–2	18–24
Glyburide micronized			
(Glynase pres tab)	1.5–12	1	18–24
Chlorpropamide			
(Diabinese)	100–500	1–2	17–72
Others			
Metformin (Glucophage)	1000–2550	2–3	18–24
Troglitazone (Rezulin)	200–600	1	16–34
Acarbose (Precose)	75–300	3	6–10

Pharmacological Actions

The principal pharmacological action of the sulfonylurea drugs is stimulation of pancreatic beta islet cells to release more insulin, apparently by increasing their sensitivity to glucose (1,63,64). High-affinity sulfonylurea receptors have been demonstrated on pancreatic beta cells. The order of potency of binding of these drugs to beta cells approximates their potency in stimulating the release of insulin. Sulfonylurea drugs may also inhibit the secretion of the counterregulatory hormone glucagon from the pancreatic alpha islet cells. Possible extrapancreatic effects of these drugs include improved peripheral tissue sensitivity to insulin and reduced clearance of insulin from the blood by the liver. The net result of these actions is increased effectiveness of available endogenous insulin.

The newly approved biguanide, metformin, can be used alone or in combination therapy with a sulfonylyrea or alpha-glucosidase inhibitor drug in patients with NIDDM (63). It improves cell insulin sensitivity and oral glucose tolerance primarily by decreasing hepatic glucose output and enhancing peripheral glucose uptake and oxidation by muscle and adipose tissue. It also appears to promote muscle glycogen formation and adipose tissue lipogenesis. In addition, it may increase intestinal utilization of glucose as a fuel and delay glucose absorption. A moderate decrease in plasma triglycerides, a small decrease in plasma total and LDL cholesterol, and a small increase in HDL cholesterol also have been noted in some studies evaluating long-term therapy with metformin. Troglitazone acts primarily by improving muscle and adipose tissue sensitivity to insulin, but it also reduces gluconeogenesis and hepatic glucose output. In clinical trials it is reported to increase both LDL and HDL cholesterol levels and to reduce fasting triglyceride levels (-13–26%). The proposed mechanism of action of alpha-glucosidase inhibitors, such as acarbose, reduce postprandial glucose levels and resulting glycemia by delaying the breakdown and absorption of carbohydrates in the gut (63).

Candidates

OHDs are primarily used to treat patients with type 2 DM who fail to adhere to or respond to nonpharmacological measures, including diet, weight reduction, and exercise therapy. These drugs generally are contraindicated as sole therapy in most patients with type 1 DM, especially those prone to ketoacidosis. However, some patients with mild type 1 DM, capable of some endogenous insulin production, may also be suitable candidates for sulfonurea therapy alone or in combination with small doses of insulin (1,3). The rationale for this combination is that the sulfonylurea drugs may improve insulin sensitivity, which may potentiate the effectiveness of concomitant insulin administration. Factors involved in the selection of specific OHAs have been described elsewhere (3,48) and are beyond the scope of this chapter.

OHA therapy should begin with the lowest dose possible with increases as necessary at weekly intervals until satisfactory glycemic control is attained or the highest recommended dose is reached. Patients who respond satisfactorily to OHA therapy should undergo periodic reassessments to determine whether the drug dose can be reduced. A "bonus" associated with long-term improved glycemic control with sulfonylurea drugs, metformin, and troglitazome, is an improvement in the blood lipid profile. This generally includes a decrease in plasma levels of total and LDL cholesterol, triglycerides, VLDL triglycerides and cholesterol, and either no change or a small to moderate increase in HDL cholesterol levels (63).

Side Effects

Sulfonylurea drugs are generally well tolerated, with only about 2% of patients having to discontinue therapy because of adverse effects (1). The most common serious side effect of sulfonylurea therapy is an insulin-like hypoglycemic reaction. Its frequency seems to be related to the potency and duration of drug action. The highest incidence has been reported with glyburide and chloropropamide and the lowest with tolbutamide. The hypoglycemia produced may be prolonged and require intravenous glucose infusions for several days to correct it. Severe sulfonylurea-induced hypoglycemia is associated with about a 1% mortality rate. Other less common side effects, occurring with a similar frequency with all of the available agents, include gastrointestinal disturbances, skin rashes, bone marrow suppression, hyponatremia, mild intolerance to alcohol (a disulfram-like reaction), and interactions with other drugs including their potentiation of the action of sulfonylurea drugs (1,4). Weight gain is common in patients who improve glycemic control, but this also occurs with insulin therapy and is presumably the result of reduced energy loss with clearing of glycosuria. However, the weight gain, in turn, may cause secondary therapeutic failure in patients with initial good glycemic control with sulfonylurea drugs. Weight gain appears less likely with metformin than with the sulfonylurea drugs (63). Sulfonylurea drugs also cross the placental barrier in pregnant women and can cause severe hypoglycemia in the fetus or newborn. Lactic acidosis is a rare but potentially serious adverse effect in metformin-treated patients, with an incidence of only about 0.03 cases per 1000 patient years but a reported mortality rate of 50%. The risk of death from lactic acidosis in metformin-treated patients in actuality is similar to that due to severe hypoglycemia in sulfonylurea-treated patients (64). The risk of lactic acidosis was 10–20 times higher with another biguanide, phenformin, than with metformin, leading to its withdrawal from use in this country in the 1970s. Rare cases of hepatocellular injury have been reported with troglitazone.

Exercise Therapy

Introduction

A consensus now exists—including the recent Surgeon General's Report on Physical Activity and Health (15), and a report from the recent NIH consensus conference on Physical Activity and Cardiovascular Health (18)—that regular moderate-intensity aerobic or endurance exercise plays a key role in both the prevention and management of type 2 diabetes and in the improvement of cardio-respiratory fitness and psychological well-being of people with both types of diabetes. Strong evidence also exists that regular exercise can improve an abnormal blood lipid profile and provide other favorable physiological and metabolic adaptations, contributing to reduced risk of CHD in physically active people (15,65–67).

Metabolic Effects of Acute Aerobic Exercise

Exercise conditioning has been promoted since ancient times as a treatment for DM. Evidence of the role of exercise in the management of this disease has previously been reviewed (1,18,22,68–71). A review of the metabolic effects of acute aerobic exercise on substrate utilization is helpful to better understand its potential usefulness for glycemic control as well as for the understanding of the potential hazard of hypoglycemia during exercise for patients with DM receiving insulin therapy.

Most of the metabolic benefits of regular exercise, which contribute to improved glycemic control, appear to be due more to the overlapping effects of acute bouts of aerobic exercise than to chronic adaptations to exercise training. During physical exertion, the energy demands of muscular work necessitate an accelerated delivery of fuels and oxygen to the contracting skeletal muscles. These demands are met by major metabolic, hormonal, and cardiovascular adjustments. The principal fuels or substrates utilized by the contracting muscles are carbohydrates (i.e., muscle glycogen and blood-borne glucose) and circulating FFA, derived primarily from the lipolysis of triglycerides in adipose tissue (22,71,72). The relative contribution of carbohydrates and FFA to energy production depends both on the intensity and duration of muscular exertion. The more strenuous the exercise—i.e., the greater the percentage of one's maximal oxygen uptake achieved per minute—the greater the dependence of the participating muscles on carbohydrates for fuel. Strenuous high-intensity exercise also results in a transient increase in the blood glucose level, since glucose production and release by the liver initially exceeds peripheral utilization. Light- to moderate-intensity dynamic endurance exercise that can be sustained for long intervals of time—such as walking, running, cycling, and swimming—results in an orderly sequence of fuel utilization. During the first few minutes of exercise, muscle glycogen provides the chief source of energy for muscle contraction. After about 5–10 min, blood glucose and FFA become increasing more important as substrates. Glucose utilization during exercise may increase 20-fold over the basal rate and contribute 25–40% of the total oxidative fuel requirements in both diabetic and nondiabetic people. An acute increase in blood flow to the exercising muscle contributes to this increased glucose uptake; however, skeletal muscle contraction itself also has a proinsulin effect on facilitating glucose uptake by muscle, even in the absence of circulating insulin, which continues for several hours postexercise (22,71). An acute exercise-induced increase in activity of glucose transporters, especially the GLU 4 isomer in the muscle sarcolemma, appears to be involved with this increased glucose uptake by exercised muscle. An increase in insulin receptor number after acute exercise also has been reported in both diabetic and nondiabetic people (71).

Diabetic individuals are more effective than nondiabetic people in maintaining glucose homeostasis by hepatic gluconeogenesis and subsequent glucose release into the circulation. Substrates for gluconeogenesis include blood-borne lactate, pyruvate, glycerol, ketone bodies, and alanine and other amino acids. Eventually after several hours of endurance activity, this process begins to fail and blood glucose levels fall. However, this decline in blood glucose is accompanied by a progressive compensatory shift from dependence on carbohydrates to FFA for oxidative metabolism. Diabetic individuals show a superior efficiency for utilization of FFA as fuels as compared with nondiabetic individuals. Exercise conditioning further improves the ability to use FFA as a fuel, thereby sparing muscle glycogen. Despite this shift during prolonged exercise to the increased use of FFA for fuel, the continued utilization of muscle glycogen for fuel remains essential to maintain muscle contractions. Preexercise stores of muscle glycogen are thereby an important limiting factor for performing prolonged dynamic exercise. This can prove to be a problem for diabetic individuals, who generally have reduced muscle glycogen synthesis and stores. A further reduction of muscle and liver glycogen during exercise stimulates activity of glycogen synthetase, an enzyme essential for glycogen synthesis. Increased activity of this enzyme appears to be related, along with increased cell insulin receptor number, to the accelerated, non-insulin-dependent uptake of glucose by muscle and liver, which can persist at least 24 h following prolonged exercise, while glycogen stores are being replenished (22). These metabolic adaptations result in a temporary postexercise improvement in glucose tolerance and insulin sensitivity in both diabetic and nondiabetic individuals, as well as reduced exogenous insulin replacement requirements in those with IDDM. As mentioned, authorities now generally believe that improved glycemic control of DM in people who regularly exercise is primarily due to an overlapping of metabolic changes resulting from acute exercise sessions. However, exercise conditioning also improves the ability of muscle to store glycogen and to take up and oxidize glucose, as will be discussed further on.

A number of hormones contribute to the regulation of fuel availability, the rate of its utilization, and maintenance of glucose hemostasis during exercise. Of these, insulin plays the critical role in promoting glucose uptake and its metabolic utilization by muscle. However, an important adaptation to prolonged exercise (90 min or more) in both nondiabetic and type 2 diabetic individuals is a decline in circulating endogenous insulin levels. Increases in activity of insulin cell receptors and cell membrane glucose transport proteins (particularly of GLU 4) and in the blood flow to exercising muscle appear to contribute to increased uptake of glucose despite the reduction in plasma insulin concentration. As previously indicated, this improved insulin sensitivity and increased muscle glucose uptake may persist for 24 h or more following a single acute, prolonged exercise session.

A consequence of reduced levels of circulating endogenous insulin during prolonged exercise is stimulation of hepatic glycogenolysis and gluconeogenesis with an increase in glucose release by the liver. However, diabetic individuals receiving insulin replacement therapy do not experience this physiological decline in blood insulin levels during prolonged exercise. Persistence of exogenous insulin plasma concentration during and following prolonged exercise thus limits the liver's ability to release glucose in response to the decline in blood glucose levels which increases the risk of hypoglycemia. This translates into the necessity of having diabetic individuals receiving insulin therapy either to reduce their usual dosage of insulin prior to exercise or to increase their intake of carbohydrates before, during, and after prolonged physical exertion in order to avoid hypoglycemia. This important topic of prevention of hypoglycemia during exercise for diabetic individuals receiving insulin therapy is discussed in more detail further on in this chapter.

The usual decline in circulating insulin levels during prolonged exercise in both the nondiabetic and type 2 diabetic individuals also promotes lipolysis of adipose tissue triglycerides with increased release of FFA. A concomitant increase in blood levels of epinephrine and glucagon and other counterregulatory hormones during exercise also profoundly affects carbohydrate and lipid availability. The contributions of these hormones to substrate availability for energy are the opposite of those associated with insulin—i.e., increased secretion of these hormones promotes the release of glucose by the liver and of FFA from adipose tissues, potentiating the metabolic effects of reduced circulating insulin levels.

The metabolic response to acute exercise is also profoundly influenced by the adequacy of preexercise diabetic control, particularly in those with type 1 DM. With poorly controlled DM (fasting plasma glucose levels >250 mg/dl with or without ketoacidosis), there is an excess secretion of these counterregulatory hormones at rest, which is potentiated during exercise. The end result may be a worsening of metabolic dysfunctions with aggravation of hyperglycemia and ketoacidosis. In contrast, if exercise is performed when blood glucose levels are relatively low or when exogenous insulin level or the activity of an OHA is at its peak, a hypoglycemic reaction may result either during or more commonly several hours following exercise.

In summary, acute aerobic exercise increases glucose uptake and oxidation by muscle in diabetic and nondiabetic people. Increased glucose uptake by muscle appears to be due to both increased cellular insulin sensitivity and a direct effect of muscle contraction. Transient increases in insulin receptor number and GLU 4 transporter protein activity appear to be primarily responsible. The resulting enhanced insulin sensitivity and glucose uptake generally persists for at least a day post-exercise. Diabetic individuals receiving insulin therapy are at risk of hypoglycemic episodes during prolonged exercise lasting several hours, as well as during the proceeding 24 h. This is because of the absence of the usual physiological drop in blood exogenous insulin levels during exercise with the resulting elevated insulin levels suppressing glucose release from the liver. This increases the possibility of hypoglycemia during exercise and the recovery period in the absence of adequate carbohydrate replacement.

TABLE 8   Possible Beneficial Effects of Dynamic Exercise
Training in Patients with Diabetes Mellitus

Primary prevention of NIDDM in susceptible people
Improved glucose-insulin dynamics and glycemic control
Prevention or reduction of obesity
Improved physical fitness
Improved blood lipid profile
Reduced blood pressure and risk of coronary heart disease
Psychosocial benefits

Regular Physical Activity and Exercise Training in Diabetic Management

The basis of the common recommendation of regular physical activity and aerobic exercise for the prevention of NIDDM and adjunctive therapy for patients with DM is summarized in Table 8. Supporting data for each of these proposed benefits are discussed below.

Primary Prevention of NIDDM

Biological factors, particularly a strong genetic predisposition and advanced age, clearly are strongly implicated in the etiology of NIDDM. However, as indicated in the recent Surgeon General's Report on Physical Activity and Health (15), there is now a consensus supporting the relationship of physical inactivity to increased risk of NIDDM. This is based on a considerable body of epidemiological evidence recently extensively reviewed (15,16) and the demonstration of plausible biological mechanisms from experimental studies discussed below.

Initial suggestions of a relationship between inactivity and NIDDM emerged from observations that societies that had discontinued their traditional physically active lifestyles, such as the Pima Indians in Arizona, experienced major increases in the prevalence of NIDDM, which is generally preceded by development of obesity. Many but not all cross-sectional epidemiological studies also found physical inactivity to be significantly associated with NIDDM or glucose intolerance. Further, during the present decade there have been three landmark large-scale prospective cohort studies in the United States, involving female registered nurses (12), male college alumni (13), and male physicians (14) and two additional large cohort studies involving middle-aged European men (73,74), all strongly supporting the postulated protective effects of physical activity against NIDDM. For example, in the College Alumni Study (13), men at high risk for developing NIDDM (as indicated by either a parental history of NIDDM, increased BMI, and/or high blood pressure) had a reduced risk of NIDDM if they were physically active. Each increment of 500 kcal per week in leisure-time physical activity (between 500 and 3500 kcal per week) consisting of walking, stair climbing, and/or sports was associated with a 6% reduction in risk of developing NIDDM (after adjustments for age, BMI, history of hypertension, and parental history of diabetes). Further, the incidence of diabetes was 24% lower in the most-active as compared with the lowest-active subgroup. In addition, there appeared in this study to be a more pronounced reduction of risk of DM associated with vigorous sports than for the less intensive activities surveyed. Further support of the exercise-NIDDM prevention hypothesis is provided by two intervention studies during this decade in different areas of the world; these demonstrated that physical activity along with dietary intervention cut in half the 5- to 6-year rates of developing DM in adults with impaired glucose tolerance (75,76).

Improved Glucose-Insulin Dynamics

Historically, the demonstration that exercise can improve glycemic control of DM actually preceded the discovery of insulin. As mentioned, acute exercise potentiates the effect of insulin on glycemic control in IDDM as a result of enhanced glucose uptake and utilization by working skeletal muscle both during exercise and for a prolonged period of exercise recovery. In addition, an exercise-induced increased rate of absorption of an insulin dose recently injected into an exercising limb can contribute to blood glucose reduction (71,72).

Further, it is well documented experimentally, including studies in our laboratory (77), that exercise conditioning can improve insulin sensitivity and reduce hyperinsulinemia and/or glucose intolerance in nondiabetic individuals. Mechanisms involved include, in addition to a loss of adipose tissue, increases in skeletal muscle mass, capillary density and blood flow, and its mitochondrial oxidative capacity and its ability to synthesize glycogen (22,71). However, there is a paucity of controlled clinical studies to determine whether exercise conditioning has any long-term beneficial effects on glucose-insulin dynamics and glycemic control in either type 1 or type 2 diabetes beyond those resulting from repeated bouts of acute exercise or an accompanying weight loss.

Most of the limited number of studies involving children and adolescents with type 1 DM have demonstrated substantially improved glycemic control with regular, vigorous dynamic exercise (22,71). In these successful studies, exercise was performed at least 30 min at a time, three times a week for up to 12 weeks and was associated with a significant improvement in $\dot{V}_{O_2max}$ ($>15\%$). Exercise conditioning in these studies was shown to either substantially reduce the youngsters' daily insulin requirements and lower fasting blood glucose and glycosylated hemoglobin concentrations or improve insulin sensitivity as measured by the euglycemic clamp technique. Variability in metabolic responses in these exercise training studies appears related to the extent of control of DM prior to the exercise program, changes in energy intake to compensate for the exercise program, extent of improvement in $\dot{V}_{O_2max}$, and whether there was an accompanying increase in lean body mass.

On the other hand, at least eight reported controlled exercise studies involving adults with type 1 DM, reviewed in detail by Champaign (71) and Schneider and Morgado (78), yielded mixed results. In these studies, training generally consisted of moderate-intensity exercise sessions performed three to four times a week on a cycle ergometer for 12 weeks to 6 months. None of these eight studies were able to demonstrate improved long-term glycemic control by reduced glycosylated levels. Increased energy intake, primarily as carbohydrates, on exercise days is postulated to have contributed to the failure to improve glycemic control with exercise training in these studies, despite the acute glucose-lowering effect with each exercise session. Other factors mentioned above, which contributed to the variable response in the juvenile diabetic exercise studies, may also have contributed to the lack of response in adults with type 1 diabetes.

Thus, it is concluded that exercise training programs have not been demonstrated to independently improve *long-term* glycemic control in adults with IDDM. The apparent discrepancy between the better glycemic responsiveness to exercise training in children with IDDM as compared with adults has been attributed to differences between adults and children in duration of DM and the greater potential for residual beta-cell insulin production among the younger diabetic individuals and in those with recent onset of IDDM (22). Despite the absence of ability to demonstrate improved long-range glycemic control in adults, the ADA continues to advocate exercise programs for individuals of all ages with IDDM because of the associated benefits of improved cardiorespiratory fitness and psychological well-being and the opportunity provided for social interaction and recreation (52).

There have been only about a dozen generally small-scale studies evaluating the effects of exercise training on metabolic control in young and middle-aged men and women patients with NIDDM or impaired glucose tolerance (22, 69–71,78–81). In these studies, exercise was performed generally for 6 to 24 weeks at a moderate to high intensity 3 to 7 days per week for 20 to 60 min per session. These studies, like those involving adults with IDDM, also yielded contradictory results. Less than half of the studies reported reductions in glycosylated hemoglobin levels while even fewer documented improved peripheral insulin sensitivity, and oral glucose tolerance tests (OGTT) generally showed no improvement. For the most part, younger NIDDM people (both obese and lean) appeared more likely in these studies than older patients to obtain improved metabolic control in response to regular exercise regardless of whether body weight was reduced with training. However, in participants showing improvement in glycemic control and/or glucose-insulin dynamics, these changes rapidly regressed to pretraining levels within several days after exercise was discontinued.

In the largest controlled exercise training study involving adults with DM, which was performed in our laboratory (79), 48 mildly overweight, sedentary, middle-aged men with mild or moderately severe NIDDM or glucose intolerance who were not receiving glucose-lowering medications, participated in a supervised exercise program for 12 weeks. Exercise consisted of moderate-intensity treadmill walking for 30 to 60 min per sessions two or four times a week. Body weight was purposely kept constant in order to differentiate the effects of exercise from those of weight reduction; however, a significant reduction in skinfold thickness did occur with training, while $\dot{V}_{O_2max}$ showed a mean increase of 5.5%. This training program failed to significantly improve levels of either fasting glucose, glycosylated hemoglobin, glucose tolerance after an oral challenge, fasting insulin, or the insulin response to oral glucose, all measured 48 h after the last exercise session.

Inconsistency in changes in glucose-insulin dynamics with endurance exercise conditioning in people with type 2 DM may be related to a number of factors. These include (a) the heterogeneity of study populations; (b) baseline differences in disease severity and degrees of insulin resistance; (c) differences in relative weight, body fatness, fat distribution, and initial physical fitness of study participants; (d) the variability in control of energy intake and diet composition; (e) the presence or absence of weight and body composition changes; (f) the type, intensity, frequency, and duration of exercise sessions and duration of the training; (g) the magnitude of the resulting improvement in $\dot{V}_{O_2max}$; and (h) how long after the last exercise session the metabolic measurements were made. None of the few studies reporting metabolic benefits with exercise could exclude the possibility that the observed changes may have at least partially been due to the last bout of exercise, since most measurements were made 36–48 h after the last exercise session. Additional research is needed to clarify these discrepancies among exercise studies involving type 2 diabetic individuals, taking the above variables into consideration. However, a combined intensive 26-day residential program that included a 5-day-a-week 40- to 50-min sessions of walking or stationary cycling and a diet high in complex carbohydrates and low in fats was associated with a 4.3-kg loss of body weight. This program resulted in a marked improvement in glycemic control (as well as improvement in blood lipids) in 652 people with NIDDM attending the Pritikin Longevity Center (82).

It is concluded that moderate to vigorous endurance exercise is a little more likely to improve insulin resistance and blood glucose control in adults with type 2 DM than in those with type 1, with or without associated weight loss. However, these changes are rapidly reversible if exercise training is discontinued. There is also some suggestive evidence that regular aerobic exercise may help to prevent the progression of glucose intolerance to NIDDM. More research is clearly needed in these areas. Nevertheless, a combined program of exercise, diet, and loss of excess weight clearly can improve the control of type II diabetes substantially.

Prevention or Reduction of Obesity

The contributions of obesity, particularly central obesity, to insulin resistance and to the etiology of type 2 DM as well as to increased blood lipids and blood pressure levels and risk of CHD were referred to earlier in this chapter. Physical inactivity is clearly a major contributor to prevalence of both childhood and adult obesity in modern societies. Increased physical activity, particularly regular aerobic exercise, theoretically should reduce the susceptibility to DM by weight maintenance, in addition to its independent contribution to improved glucose-insulin dynamics. Regular walking is the most popular form of physical activity for people of all ages in the United States. The value of exercise for helping to normalize body weight and reduce adiposity and in helping maintain the loss in obese women and men has been demonstrated alone or combined with reduced energy intake (67,83–87). The loss of lean body mass commonly associated with dieting does not occur or is minimized during weight reduction by exercise alone or exercise combined with mild to moderate caloric restriction in obese individuals (67,85–88). In addition, with exercise, body fat may be lost more rapidly from the abdominal region and around the viscera of the body than elsewhere (88). It will be recalled that fat distribution in these regions is associated with an excess risk of DM, hyperlipidemia, hypertension, CVD, and premature mortality. Exercise training also may attenuate the reduction in resting metabolic rate associated with weight reduction (85–87). However, despite these potential contributions of an exercise program to weight reduction and maintenance, there are no prospective studies demonstrating the long-term effectiveness of exercise alone in managing obesity in people with or without NIDDM. A more feasible weight-reduction plan for most obese type 2 diabetic patients is a combination or a moderate increase (30–60 mm/day) in daily moderate-intensity physical activity at least 5 days per week, a reduction in energy and fat intake, and lifelong behavioral changes.

Improved Physical Fitness

Physical fitness has been defined as the ability to carry out daily tasks with vigor and alertness without fatigue and with ample reserve energy to enjoy leisure-time pursuits and to meet unforeseen emergencies as well as to respond to physical and emotional stress without an excessive increase in heart rate and blood pressure (89). The measurable components of physical fitness may be derived into two major groups; one related to *health* and the other related to *skills* primarily pertaining to athletic performance.

Cardiorespiratory endurance or aerobic power, the most important health-related component of physical fitness, is defined as the maximal ability of the circulatory and respiratory systems to supply oxygen and fuels to the skeletal muscles and other organs and to eliminate metabolic waste products. It is determined by measuring or estimating $\dot{V}_{O_2max}$ during all-out exercise on the treadmill or cycle ergometer. An increase in $\dot{V}_{O_2max}$ not only enhances the maximal capacity for endurance types of physical exertion but also reduces fatigue and the level of perceived exertion during performance of sustained moderate-intensity activities. This can greatly enhance the quality of life, particularly in people with a chronic disease such as DM. As discussed in Chapter 2 of this book, in order to increase $\dot{V}_{O_2max}$, it is necessary to perform regular dynamic endurance-type physical activities that increase the heart and respiratory rates, such as walking, running, cycling, or swimming. It has been repeatedly demonstrated that to obtain a significant improvement in $\dot{V}_{O_2max}$ (typically 5–30%), 20–60 min of such training activities are required at least three times a week at an intensity of 50–85% of a person's baseline $\dot{V}_{O_2max}$ as recommended by the ACSM for diabetic exercisers (47). This intensity level corresponds to about 60–90% of maximal heart rate. A similar intensity and volume of dynamic exercise appear to be required to improve carbohydrate and lipid metabolism in both diabetic and nondiabetic people. An inverse relationship also exists between the intensity and duration of exercise necessary to improve $\dot{V}_{O_2max}$. In other words, to obtain improved $\dot{V}_{O_2max}$ with moderate-intensity exercise at 60% $\dot{V}_{O_2max}$ requires a longer duration and frequency of exercise sessions than is required with higher-intensity exercise. A trade-off is that moderate exercise is less likely to result in musculoskeletal injury or a serious CHD event as compared with high-intensity exercise, and long-term adherence is generally better with regular lower-intensity exercise. Attention should also be directed to the fact that the relative improvement in aerobic power after a training program is inversely related to levels of baseline $\dot{V}_{O_2max}$. Hemodynamically, improvement in $\dot{V}_{O_2max}$ with exercise training results from increases in either the maximal arteriovenous oxygen exchange, the maximal stroke volume of the heart, or both. To maintain one's existing or attained level of $\dot{V}_{O_2max}$, only twice-a-week endurance exercise is generally required; however, this may not be of sufficient frequency to maintain the other physiological and metabolic benefits of exercise described below.

Improved Blood Lipid Profile

The effects of acute exercise and exercise training on plasma lipoprotein levels have been extensively reviewed (66,90–92); only the highlights are summarized here, along with data from some of the few training studies involving diabetic individuals (22,78,79,91,92). Cross-sectional observational studies report a dose-response association between habitual physical activity and plasma HDL cholesterol levels, ranging from extreme inactivity associated with quadriplegia to the high volume of training required for marathon running (93). The increase in HDL cholesterol levels with activity status parallels the usual mean levels of $\dot{V}_{O_2max}$ expected for the various activity groups. For example, men and women athletes trained for endurance exercise, such as long-distance runners and Nordic skiers, generally have plasma HDL cholesterol levels 20–35% higher than the values for matched, healthy, sedentary individuals (94). Higher levels of HDL_2 cholesterol subfraction generally account for most of the differences in HDL cholesterol levels between endurance athletes and sedentary people, although in some studies higher levels of both HDL_2 and HDL_3 cholesterol were observed in the athletes. In contrast, strength-trained athletes, such as weight lifters, as a group have been reported to have HDL cholesterol levels similar to those of nonathletes (94). Further, American men and women selected from the general population for the Lipid Research Clinic Prevalence Study who reported regular vigorous occupational or recreational physical activity were found to have about 5 mg/dl higher HDL cholesterol levels than those who reported no such heavy activities (95).

In respect to other blood lipid components, cross-sectional comparison studies show that plasma triglyceride and VLDL cholesterol levels are generally significantly lower in more active people, especially endurance athletes, as compared with matched, inactive individuals. Typically, endurance athletes in these studies had triglyceride levels below 100 mg/dl but had either similar or only slightly lower LDL cholesterol levels as compared with sedentary subjects. In general, a major problem in interpreting cross-sectional comparisons of athletes versus nonathletes is the failure of most of these studies to adjust for potential confounding variables, which can contribute to differences in blood lipid levels between athletes and nonathletes (i.e., differences in body weight and composition, dietary habits, cigarette usage, alcohol consumption, and the use of oral contraceptives and other drugs as well as other variables).

Experimentally, *acute* prolonged endurance exercise generally results in significant changes in blood lipid levels, probably related to increased energy needs by working muscles (65). These changes include reductions from baseline levels in plasma triglycerides and VLDL and LDL cholesterol and a substantial (10–17.5%) increase in HDL cholesterol levels. These changes generally persist for several days following prolonged exercise. Thus, at least some of the reported effects on blood lipid levels of chronic exercise training may actually reflect acute changes remaining from the last exercise session, reminiscent of the postexercise effects on glucose metabolism.

Experimental studies to determine the effects of endurance exercise conditioning on blood lipid levels have yielded mixed results in both nondiabetic and diabetic groups. Differences in responses probably reflect differences in confounding variables affecting blood lipids, including differences in the exercise program, baseline fitness and fatness levels, life habits (particularly diet, cigarette smoking, and other physical activity), drug use, accuracy of the laboratory measurements, seasonal fluctuations in blood lipid levels, the phase of the menstrual cycle in eumenorrheic women, how long after the last exercise session blood was drawn for lipid assays, and the extent of control of diabetes.

In nondiabetic individuals, there is relatively consistent evidence that endurance exercise conditioning can significantly reduce *elevated* levels of fasting and postprandial plasma triglycerides, on the average of about 18%, but generally exercise training does not affect triglyceride levels in the normal range (66,67, 91–93). Reductions in fasting and postprandial triglyceride levels reflect the increase during exercise in lipoprotein lipase (LPL) activity in skeletal muscle and adipose tissue capillary linings, with a resulting increase in the rate of catabolism of triglyceride-rich lipoproteins both in the fasting and postprandial state. The relevance of these changes to the risk of CHD is the possible atherogenicity of catabolic products of remnants of these triglyceride-rich lipoproteins.

Only about half of all published endurance exercise training studies involving nondiabetic men have demonstrated a significant exercise-induced increase in plasma HDL cholesterol concentration. In most of the positive studies, the increase in HDL cholesterol levels generally ranged from 3–8 mg/dl or 5–16%. Theoretically, based on epidemiological data, an increase in plasma HDL cholesterol levels of this magnitude should reduce the risk of CHD by 15–40%. One of the largest reported studies was a 1-year randomized trial involving 48 previously sedentary middle-aged men. In this study, Wood et al. (96) observed a significant increase in plasma HDL and HDL_2 cholesterol levels in only 25 (52%) of the participants. These responders performed at least 4.8 km (8 m) per week of running for at least 9 months. Their reported average increase in HDL cholesterol levels was 4.4 mg/dl, or about 9%. Statistically significant correlations were also observed between weekly self-selected running mileage and both the increase in plasma HDL cholesterol levels and an associated reduction in body fatness. However, surprisingly, the men who self-selected the higher volumes of running generally had higher pretraining baseline levels of plasma HDL cholesterol as well as significantly lower baseline levels of triglycerides as compared with the less active runners. This raises the intriguing possibility that unmeasured factors, such as higher tissue LPL activity (generally associated with elevated HDL cholesterol levels), improve the ease of participation in endurance activities, perhaps by reducing perceived exertion levels, which thereby enhances compliance (97). Based primarily on data from this 1-year exercise study, it has been postulated that the lowest threshold of energy expenditure to produce an increase in HDL cholesterol values for healthy but previously sedentary men over a 9- to 12-month period is 1000 kcal/week of exercise (66).

In our laboratory, we have consistently demonstrated increases in plasma HDL cholesterol concentrations of 15% or more in previously sedentary and overweight nondiabetic men within 12–16 weeks of high-volume, brisk treadmill walking with or without accompanying weight loss. In these studies, exercise was distributed over 4–5 days per week and the weekly energy expenditure was 2000–5000 kcal. In the best-controlled of these studies (98), diet composition was kept constant, with all meals and exercise provided in the laboratory. One group of men walked 5 days a week on a treadmill (about 14 km/week) at an approximate energy cost of 3500 kcal/week, with body weight kept constant by increasing food energy intake. This group experienced a 12% mean increase in HDL cholesterol concentration over a 15-week training period. A similar increase in mean HDL cholesterol level was achieved by a physically inactive second group, which lost 6.1 kg of body weight over a 12-week period by dietary restrictions followed by 3 weeks of weight stabilization by increasing food intake. A third group performed a similar amount of exercise per week as group 1 but were not provided additional food and lost a similar amount of weight as the group that lost weight by dieting. This third group, which lost weight by exercising, experienced a more rapid rate of increase in HDL cholesterol levels than the other two groups; the total increase in plasma HDL cholesterol levels was 22% above baseline levels, almost twice the increase found in the other two treatment groups. These findings suggest an additive effect of exercise and weight reduction on HDL cholesterol levels. Schwartz (99), in an uncontrolled study, essentially confirmed our findings. Wood et al. (100) also compared weight loss through dieting and exercise in a less well controlled experiment than in our laboratory and found that a 7.8-kg weight loss by either dieting or exercise was accompanied by similar increases (11–12%) in the HDL cholesterol level. The reason for the discrepancies between studies is uncertain. The increase in the HDL cholesterol level with exercise training appears to regress to baseline levels within 4 weeks after cessation of training or with regaining of lost weight (98).

Endurance exercise training appears less likely to increase plasma HDL cholesterol levels in nondiabetic, normolipidemic women than men (66,92,101–104). In our laboratory, we were unsuccessful in increasing plasma HDL cholesterol levels in previously sedentary women age 20–40 years with four different modes of moderate-intensity endurance exercise training (i.e., treadmill walking or jogging, minitrampoline rebounding, and simulated cross-country skiing) for periods of 16–40 weeks. In one of these studies (103), women either walked or jogged on a treadmill 19.2 km/week divided into four weekly sessions for 20 weeks at exercise intensities of 52% or 70% $\dot{V}_{O_2max}$ and a weekly energy cost of about 1400 kcal. No mean changes in plasma lipid or lipoprotein levels were found with either mode of exercise as compared with the sedentary control group, despite marked improvements in $\dot{V}_{O_2max}$ levels with both walking and jogging. Body weight and composition also were unaltered during training in this study, which probably contributed to the stability of the blood lipid levels. A subsequent 40-week treadmill-walking program, using a similar population and exercise prescription as in the 20-week study, likewise failed to increase the mean HDL cholesterol concentration or significantly alter body weight or composition (101).

However, more recently we have observed a small (about 6%) but significant increase in HDL cholesterol levels (primarily in the HDL_2 fraction) in young and middle-aged previously sedentary women with 20 weeks of stationary cycling in the multicenter HERITAGE Family Study, similar to the increase in HDL cholesterol in male participants (unpublished data). The reasons for the gender difference in responsiveness of HDL cholesterol levels to exercise are uncertain but may reflect the following: (a) a lower volume of exercise achievable in training studies in sedentary women as compared to sedentary men, (b) the higher baseline concentrations of HDL cholesterol in sedentary women as compared to sedentary men, (c) greater body weight and composition changes during exercise training in women adipocytes compared to men, and (d) perhaps the gender differences in body-fat distribution and associated lipase activity.

A few but not all of the small number of studies involving resistive or strength exercise training have reported an increase in plasma HDL cholesterol levels as well as lower LDL cholesterol levels in nondiabetic men (66,91). These observations are contrary to what would be expected from lipid levels of weight lifters in cross-sectional observational studies (66,94).

It is concluded that acute and chronic endurance exercise generally has beneficial effects on the blood lipid profile in nondiabetic sedentary men, but these effects appear less likely to occur in nondiabetic women. Observed lipid changes with exercise include a marked improvement in both fasting and postprandial hypertriglyceridemia related to an increase in LPL activity and associated accelerated catabolism of VLDL and chylomicrons as well as an increase in levels of the antiatherogenic lipoprotein HDL, especially if training is accompanied by a significant weight loss. However, the volume of exercise needed for such improvements may prove excessive for many sedentary and usually overweight individuals. Nevertheless, based on the available data, the National Cholesterol Education Program guidelines (105) recommend exercise along with dietary changes, weight loss, and, if necessary, medications for the management of dyslipidemias.

In contrast to the relatively large number of exercise studies in nondiabetic populations, there is a paucity of well-controlled studies involving individuals with DM. The most consistent finding with endurance exercise training in the few reported studies is a reduction in elevated levels of plasma triglycerides of up to 25% in adolescents and adults with type 1 DM and in young and middle-aged adults with type 2 DM (22,79,80,91,92). A small reduction in total cholesterol levels (and presumably LDL cholesterol levels, which generally were not measured) was also commonly noted in these studies. In addition, small increases in HDL cholesterol levels were reported in over half of the studies involving type 2 diabetic individuals but in none of the studies to date involving type 1 diabetic people, even in the presence of a significant reduction in triglycerides. In the large study in our laboratory previously referred to involving normolipidemic middle-aged men with type 2 DM or glucose intolerance, exercise training for 12 weeks with body weight held stable also failed to significantly alter the group's mean plasma lipid profile. The reader is reminded that improved control of diabetes alone by diet, weight loss, OHAs, and/or insulin administration as well as smoking cessation should all contribute to raising HDL cholesterol levels and in normalizing of the blood lipid profile. A great deal of additional research is needed to better establish the contributions of exercise to the blood lipid profile of diabetic patients, including the dose-response relationship and differentiation between the acute and chronic effects of exercise.

Reduced Blood Pressure and Risk of CHD

There are other ways, briefly reviewed below, in which exercise can potentially reduce the severity of atherosclerosis and the risk of CHD in addition to its effects on body weight, adiposity, and blood lipids. These include a blood pressure–reducing effect, as demonstrated by both observational and interventional studies, in predominately nondiabetic populations (15,90,106,107). Some but not all epidemiological studies have documented an inverse association between physical activity or physical fitness and blood pressure levels. Acute endurance exercise 30 min or more duration has been shown to significantly decrease both systolic and diastolic blood pressures for 8–12 h during recovery. This appears to result primarily from vasodilatation, although reduced cardiac output may be a contributing factor in older individuals.

Hagberg (107) recently reviewed 47 endurance exercise studies published in English and found that about 70% of them reported reductions in mean systolic and diastolic blood pressure levels of about 10 mmHg each in hypertensive individuals. From the available data, it appears that 30 to 60 min of low- to moderate-intensity exercise training at 40–60% $\dot{V}_{O_2max}$ at least every other day for 10 or more weeks may be effective in reducing blood pressure levels in nondiabetic individuals. The resulting blood pressure reduction with exercise may occur in the absence of weight loss, but an associated weight loss should provide an additive blood pressure–reducing effect. Whether similar changes occur in diabetic people with hypertension remains to be proven.

At present the mechanisms by which exercise training reduces blood pressure in hypertensive individuals is unclear. The most plausible mechanism for this apparent antihypertensive effect, aside from a reduction in body fat, is attenuation of sympathetic nervous system activity (90,106). Reduced adrenergic activity would be expected, in turn, to reduce renin-angiotensin aldosterone system activity, to reset baroreceptor reflexes, and to result in arterial vasodilatation, thereby reducing elevated peripheral vascular resistance commonly associated with essential hypertension. Furthermore, in adolescents with early or reactive hypertension, exercise training may attenuate a hyperactive adrenergic system and reduce the associated elevation in heart rate and cardiac output contributing to blood pressure elevation. Improved insulin sensitivity and the associated reduction in circulating insulin levels with exercise training also conceivably may contribute to blood pressure reduction by reducing insulin-mediated sodium reabsorption by the renal tubules (87).

Exercise may also lower a diabetic individual's risk of coronary thrombosis. Endurance exercise conditioning attenuates increased coagulability of the blood associated with physical exertion by reducing platelet aggregation, apparently through an alternation in the prostaglandin balance between platelets and endothelial cells—i.e., by reducing platelet TXA_2 and increasing endothelial cell PGI_2 activity (108,109). In addition, fibrinolysis may be enhanced by exercise through a reduction in endothelial cell PAI-1 activity and an increase in tissue plasminogen activators (109). Physical activity also may reduce elevated fibrinogen levels, another risk factor for coronary occlusions in both healthy and diabetic people (109). However, these conclusions are preliminary and need to be confirmed in diabetic patients along with determination of dose-response relationships.

There are other proposed mechanisms by which exercise may protect against major CHD events in both diabetic and nondiabetic individuals (110–112). These include an increase in myocardial vascularity and improved cardiovascular efficiency through a reduction in the heart rate and systolic blood pressure levels during submaximal exertion, thereby decreasing myocardial oxygen demands and vulnerability to ventricular fibrillation and sudden death. A reduction in catecholamine secretions or an increased rate of their clearance may contribute to the reduced vulnerability to ventricular fibrillation with exercise training.

Documentation of the apparent independent protective effects of regular physical activity and improved physical fitness against CHD has mainly come from large cohort studies generally involving nondiabetic individuals (15,110–113). Over two-thirds of published observational studies show an inverse association between physical activity and CHD. In the "better" studies reviewed in metaanalyses by Powell et al. (114) and by Berlin and Colditz (115), the relative risk of CHD for physically inactive people was almost twice that of active people. In the Multiple Risk Factor Intervention Trial (MRFIT), involving over 12,000 middle-aged men at high risk of CHD because of elevated blood cholesterol and blood pressure levels and cigarette smoking (and thereby with undoubtedly advanced coronary atherosclerosis), it was observed that 30 min or more daily of predominately moderate-intensity leisure-time physical activity was associated with one-third fewer CHD deaths as compared to less than 15 min per day of activity (116). Statistical adjustments for other risk factors only slightly weakened the inverse association between physical activity and CHD in this and most other cohort studies, suggesting an independent protective effect of physical activity against CHD. Thus, the MRFIT study provides supporting evidence that exercise can reduce death from CHD probably even in the presence of suspected advanced coronary atherosclerosis. This possibility is further substantiated by a metaanalysis of pooled data on over 4000 patients who participated in controlled cardiac rehabilitation studies, which included an exercise component (117). Analysis of these pooled data revealed that active intervention participants had about 25% fewer *fatal* recurrent coronary events as compared with control subjects, consistent with the findings from the MRFIT. In addition, it has been demonstrated that an exercise training as part of a comprehensive lifestyle modification program can reduce the progression or even slightly reduce the severity of angiographically documented coronary artery disease after only 1 year intervention (118,119). Whether exercise conditioning can offer similar protection against CHD in diabetic individuals remains to be proven.

Psychosocial Benefits

It is widely believed among health professionals that regular exercise provides psychosocial benefits that improve the quality of life; however, this is difficult to substantiate by controlled studies (120). Improved feelings of well-being, health consciousness, self-confidence, self-control, and self-esteem provided by an exercise program are especially important for patents with a chronic disease such as DM and is one of the principal reasons given by the ADA for encouraging exercise as part of a health care plan. Exercise may also prove helpful in relieving muscular tension and mental depression, and in promoting sound sleep (121). In order to achieve such benefits, physical activities should be selected that are fun and enjoyable and can easily be incorporated into one's lifestyle.

Exercise Hazards and Precautions

There are special problems and hazards associated with exercise for diabetic individuals, particularly for those requiring insulin for metabolic control (1,22,47,48, 52,71,77,81). These are summarized in Table 9 and discussed below. Even de-

TABLE 9   Potential Adverse Effects of Exercise in Diabetes Mellitus

Worsening of the metabolic state
Hypoglycemia in patients receiving insulin or hypoglycemic
  drug therapy
Complications from proliferative retinopathy
Musculoskeletal or soft tissue injuries
Complications from superficial foot injuries
Myocardial infarction or sudden death

tractors who feel that exercise is merely a "perturbation that makes treatment of diabetes difficult," agree that the "present knowledge and technology allow the well-informed and cooperative patients with IDDM to exercise and even to reach the elite level."

Worsening of the Metabolic State

As previously mentioned, individuals with DM should not perform vigorous or prolonged exercise if their fasting blood glucose level exceeds 250 mg/dl, particularly if ketoacidosis is present, since exercise may result in a worsening of their metabolic state. Consequently, an exercise program should not be recommended until at least moderate metabolic control is obtained by diet, and, if necessary, by insulin or an OHA.

Hypoglycemia. For the diabetic individual receiving insulin therapy, an insulin reaction or hypoglycemia is a common problem associated with prolonged exercise and is the major exercise risk in people with IDDM. For example, one study reported hypoglycemic episodes related to exercise in 16% of 300 young people with IDDM over a 2-year period of observation (122). This problem also is of concern in patients on OHAs, but is much less common. The risk of hypoglycemia is most marked in exercisers receiving intensive, multidose insulin therapy or continuous insulin infusion delivery by pump. Even if hypoglycemia does not occur during the exercise itself, the possibility remains for a delayed episode of hypoglycemia for many hours after prolonged exercise owing to the common decline in blood glucose levels as depleted glucogen stores in muscle and liver are replenished. In the study referred to above involving 300 young people with IDDM, episodes of hypoglycemia were most commonly reported 6 to 15 h after exercise and occurred up to 31 h postexercise (122). Therefore, a diabetic individual receiving insulin should avoid sports that place him or her or the public in jeopardy if hypoglycemia occurs—e.g., scuba diving, parachute jumping, hang gliding, or automobile racing. Certain guidelines and precautions are required to avoid or minimize hypoglycemia during other forms of prolonged exercise. These have been reviewed in detail elsewhere (1,48,52,123); they are summarized in Table 10 and briefly reviewed below.

First, it is important for all diabetic individuals receiving insulin or oral hypoglycemic agents to try to maintain as much consistency in their life habits as possible. This is particularly important for those who are participating in organized sports. For example, diabetic exercisers should keep as constant as possible the time of day for getting up and going to bed, for meals and snacks and their energy content, for the administration of insulin or an OHA, the dose(s) and form(s) of the medication, the time of day for exercise, and the volume and

TABLE 10   General Precautions to Reduce Risk of Exercise-Induced Hypoglycemia in Diabetic Individuals on Insulin Therapy

Maintain consistency in life habits.

Careful self-monitoring of blood glucose levels.

Avoid using extremities involved in exercise as injection sites for insulin within an hour of exercising.

Avoid exercising during time of peak insulin or oral hypoglycemic agent activity.

Best time to exercise is following a light meal or after a carbohydrate snack.

Take carbohydrate snacks during and following prolonged exercise.

Inform others about diabetic condition and risk of hypoglycemic and usual associated symptoms, and the proper response to hypoglycemic episodes.

Be alert for symptoms of hypoglycemia both during and several hours after exercise.

Promptly cease exercise upon experiencing symptoms of hypoglycemia and take a carbohydrate snack.

Take sufficient fluid intake before, during, and after exercise to prevent dehydration.

intensity of the exercise performed. Such consistency simplifies the process of regulating blood glucose levels. It also helps with the decision making for adjusting food intake and insulin or oral hypoglycemic medication dosage in response to changes in physical activity levels as the need arises. These adjustments have to be accomplished on an individualized basis because of the marked variability in responsiveness of each diabetic individual to exercise. Quantifiable or easily reproducible forms of recreational exercise—such as walking, jogging, bicycling, and lap swimming—simplify adjustments in food intake and/or medication dosage to properly regulate blood glucose and avoid hypoglycemia on an exercise program.

A major breakthrough for both improving metabolic control of DM and helping to avoid hypoglycemia related to exercise is the availability of simple self-monitoring techniques, such as finger-stick methods of determining blood glucose levels by visual or glucose meter readings of color changes of chemically treated tape strips. These techniques permit blood glucose levels to be checked by the patient receiving insulin several times during the day—for example, upon arising, before meals, 90 min following meals, at bedtime, and perhaps at 3 A.M. for those on intensive therapy as well as before, during, and following prolonged exercise. For those diabetic athletes participating in team sports, these techniques also make it possible to measure capillary blood glucose levels between periods of sporting events or whenever hypoglycemia is suspected.

When a diabetic individual receiving insulin first initiates an exercise program or sports participation, it is advisable, at least initially, to reduce the basal insulin requirements 10–40% to avoid hypoglycemia until a new balance between food intake, physical activity, and insulin levels is established. A conservative approach is to first decrease the dose of the form of insulin with peak activity during the period of the day that the exercise is performed (123). For example, let us consider the hypothetical case of a man with type 1 DM planning strenuous prolonged exercise in midmorning. He is on a combination of regular and NPH insulin with divided doses administered before breakfast and before the evening meal for a total daily insulin requirement of 40 U/day. His usual morning breakfast dose of insulin consists of 8 U of regular insulin plus his usual 12 U of NPH. The dose of his regular morning insulin should be reduced by at least 10% of his *total daily insulin dose requirement,* or in this case 4 U. Since he is planning midmorning exercise, at which time the pharmacological activity of regular insulin is at its peak, his adjusted morning insulin combination would then consist of 4 U instead of 8 U of regular insulin plus his usual 12 U of NPH. On the other hand, if the strenuous activity were planned for the afternoon, the 10% reduction in the 40 U daily insulin dosage would be applied to the morning dose of NPH insulin. The morning insulin combination would then still consist of 8 U of regular insulin, but the NPH dose would be reduced from 12 to 8 U, since the peak action of the NPH insulin is in the afternoon. If strenuous prolonged activities were planned for the entire day, such as backpacking or skiing, the morning dose of *both* types of insulin should be decreased by 10% or 4 U. The morning insulin combination would then be 4 U of regular insulin and 8 U of NPH. In such a situation, it would also be particularly important for the individual to monitor blood glucose levels closely throughout the day, including during and following exercise. It may be necessary, based on blood glucose determination, for the individual also to decrease the evening dosage of his insulin combination as well as to eat extra food. Additional adjustments of insulin dosages or extra food intake should be based on records of self-monitored glucose levels.

An alternative approach to reducing insulin dosage when initiating an exercise program, if the DM is under good control, is to consume extra food prior to, during, and following prolonged exercise. Requirements for extra food energy intake are based on the intensity and duration of the intended physical activity and the patient's preexercise blood glucose level (123). Table 11 provides guidelines for increasing food intake based on these variables.

Another approach to determining the amount of extra food in the form of carbohydrate to consume to compensate for anticipated prolonged physical activity is to base the estimated needs for extra carbohydrates on the approximate energy cost of the anticipated activity. The energy cost can be estimated by the type of physical activity, its intensity and duration, and the body weight of the individual (123). For activities considered light to moderate (an intensity of 5 kcal/min or 300 kcal/h or less for a 70-kg person), no additional food is required prior to exercise unless the activity is to exceed 30 min. A snack containing 5 g of simple carbohydrates is recommended for every additional 30 min of moderate exercise. For higher-intensity prolonged, strenuous activities, one-half of the esti-

TABLE 11   General Guidelines for Increasing Food Intake Prior to and During Exercise

Intensity (type of exercise)	Blood glucose (mg/100 dl)	Quantity of extra carbohydrates
Low to moderate (e.g., walking)	<100	None before exercise (if <30 min duration and/or leisurely cycling) 10–15 g/h during more prolonged exercise
	>100	None
Moderate (e.g., tennis, swimming, jogging)	<100	20–50 g before exercise and 10–15 g/h during exercise
	100–180	None before exercise but 10–15 g/h during exercise
	180–250	None
	<250	No exercise until blood glucose is under better control
Strenuous (e.g., contact team sports, basketball, competitive running, cycling, swimming, or heavy physical labor)	<100	50 g before exercise and subsequent amounts based on monitoring of blood glucose
	100–180	25–50 g before exercise and 10–15 g/h during exercise
	180–250	None before exercise and 10–15 g/h during exercise
	>250	No exercise until blood glucose is under better control

mated caloric expenditure should be taken as a snack in advance of the exercise and followed with 10 to 15 g/h of simple carbohydrates during exercise, examples of which are shown in Table 12. It is important to reiterate at this point the need for the diabetic individual to monitor his or her blood glucose level at 1- to 2-h intervals *following* heavy exercise and to make appropriate adjustments in insulin and food intake based on actual blood glucose levels. Furthermore, at least a small carbohydrate-rich snack should be consumed immediately following prolonged strenuous exercise to prevent hypoglycemia because of the accelerated glucose uptake by recovering muscle during this period.

It is commonly believed that insulin should not be administered subcutaneously in extremities directly participating in the activity within an hour prior to exercise, making the abdominal wall the preferred site of administration for the exerciser immediately prior to exercise. This is because of the accelerated rate of insulin absorption from the active limbs. A reason in favor of the habitual use of the abdominal wall for insulin administration is the recent demonstration by Bantle et al. (62) that limiting insulin injections to this region of the body rather

Table 12   Commonly Available Sources of Simple
Carbohydrates for Management of Insulin or Oral
Hypoglycemic Drug-Induced Hypoglycemia

Source	Serving size to provide 10–15 g of carbohydrate
Fruit	
Apple (size: 3 per pound)	3/4
Orange	1
Peach	2
Pear	1/2
Raisins	2 tsp
Dried fruit roll-up	1/4 cup[a]
	1
Beverages	
Fruit juices	
Apple	1/4 cup
Cranberry	1/4 cup
Grape	1/2 cup
Lemonade	1/2 cup
Orange	1/2 cup
Milk	1 cup
Soft drinks	
Cola type	1/2 cup
Ginger ale	3/4 cup
Candy/sugar	
Chocolate	1 oz
Corn syrup	2 tsp
Glucose tablets	2–3
Honey	2 tsp
Lifesavers	7–8
Sugar cubes	2 large or 5 small
Table sugar	5 tsp

[a] 1 cup = 8 fl oz.

than rotating anatomical regions, as is a common clinical practice, markedly reduces day-to-day fluctuations in blood glucose levels due to variations in the rate at which insulin is absorbed from different subcutaneous sites. Such fluctuations in blood glucose levels expose patients to increased risks of both hypoglycemia and hyperglycemia.

The time of day selected for exercise also is an important consideration. If possible, heavy physical exertion should be avoided during the time of peak action of the form of insulin used; e.g., the peak action for NPH insulin is approximately 6–16 h after injection and it is 2–4 h after administration of regular insulin. A particularly good time to exercise in terms of glycemic control is about 1–2 h after meal, since postprandial blood glucose levels are generally at a peak at this time. This is particularly true after breakfast, when the blood glucose level tends to be at its peak for the day. This, of course, is not always practical. If exercise is performed in the afternoon, during the period of peak activity of intermediate-acting insulins, a blood glucose test should be performed prior to exercise and the guidelines previously discussed followed in terms of decision making on the need for extra food and/or subsequent adjustments in the morning dose of intermediate-acting insulin.

Type 1 diabetic individuals on divided doses of insulin who exercise in the evening should take their usual predinner insulin injection, eat dinner, and then exercise an hour or so after eating. The blood glucose should then be tested following exercise and before their usual evening snack. If necessary, extra food should be added to the snack. It also is extremely important for diabetic individuals on insulin who exercise in the afternoon or evening to have a bedtime snack to compensate for the delayed fall in blood glucose level hours after prolonged or strenuous exercise.

Diabetic individuals on insulin or OHAs who exercise regularly or are athletes should wear adequate medical identification, be aware of their usual prodromal symptoms accompanying an insulin reaction, have available a source of easily ingested simple carbohydrates, and have a plan in place for aborting or treating a hypoglycemic reaction. While exercising, the following guidelines should be included in their plan of action (123):

1. Exercise should be promptly discontinued at the first suspicion of an insulin reaction.
2. Blood glucose should be immediately measured (if feasible).
3. A snack providing 10–15 g of simple carbohydrates should be consumed (see Table 11 for examples).
4. The athlete should rest long enough to allow glucose absorption.
5. Blood glucose levels should be reassessed, and exercise should only be resumed when the blood glucose level is above 100 mg/dl.

Furthermore, an athlete participating in team sports should make certain that his or her teammates, coaches, and athletic trainer are aware of their diabetic state, of their usual symptoms and signs of hypoglycemia, of the remedy provided for its management, and of the location of the athlete's reserve carbohydrate supply for responding to hypoglycemic episodes.

Guidelines are also available for avoiding hypoglycemia during exercise for individuals with IDDM who use a portable continuous subcutaneous insulin injection system (124,125). It appears possible to regulate the rate of insulin administration using such a pump to provide excellent glycemic control during exercise. Nevertheless, prior to prolonged exercise, it is prudent to reduce both the basal insulin infusion rate as well as the usual premeal bolus of insulin. Another potential problem is that the catheter infusion sites may be susceptible to disruption during exercise. Implantable pumps, as they become more widely available, should help eliminate this problem. An alternative approach is for the athlete to remove the portable pump prior to exercise and substitute a small dose of regular insulin for glycemic control. This approach is not feasible with the "closed loop" pumps, which have intravenous lines. This latter type of pump is also too large and cumbersome for use during vigorous exercise.

The concomitant use of β-adrenergic blocking drugs is generally contraindicated in diabetic athletes receiving insulin. These drugs may mask the symptoms of hypoglycemia, which are primarily related to the increased activity of the sympathetic adrenalmedullary system. In addition, β-blocking agents interfere with the cardiovascular response to exercise by markedly reducing the heart rate, cardiac output, and thereby functional capacity.

Complications from Proliferative Retinopathy

Simple or background retinopathy with microaneurysms of the small arteries of the retina and associated small retinal exudates or hemorrhages is not generally considered a contraindication to exercise; however, contact sports with acceleration-deceleration trauma to the head and perhaps resistive or static exercise should be avoided. In a minority of diabetic individuals, this condition progresses to proliferative retinopathy with formation of new retinal vessels. These new vessels are friable and can easily rupture, causing large retinal and vitreous hemorrhages, retinal detachment, and sometimes blindness (1). Since blood flow and blood pressure acutely increase during exercise, there is concern that vigorous endurance or resistive exercise may promote retinal hemorrhage, causing retinal separation in such individuals. Therefore, in addition to the precautions with simple retinopathy, people with active proliferative retinopathy should avoid strenuous exercise, resistive exercise, the use of standard weight-lifting machines, and other exercises that require Valsalva-like maneuvers. Recent vitreous or major retinal hemorrhages and recent photocoagulation and eye surgery are absolute contraindications to all types of exercise (1).

Musculoskeletal or Soft Tissue Injuries

The potential for musculoskeletal injuries is always present while exercising. There is no evidence that diabetic individuals are more prone to injuries of muscle and joints and their attaching structures; however, to reduce the possibility of such injuries, similar precautions are advised as for nondiabetic individuals. These include warm-up and cool-down periods incorporating flexibility exercises and initiating a physical conditioning program at a relatively low intensity, duration, and frequency of exercise and progressing gradually (22).

Contact sports were formerly prohibited for all diabetic individuals because of the fear that soft tissue injuries would not heal well. This is generally not true in diabetic persons whose diabetes is under reasonably good control, and such sports are now permitted for young diabetic individuals in the absence of significant retinopathy.

Complications from Superficial Foot Injuries

Proper foot care is extremely important for all diabetic individuals, especially for those who are athletes, since infections and ulcerations of the feet are a major cause of morbidity. Gangrene, amputation, and death may ultimately result from such foot problems. This is of particular concern to those over age 40 years, who are more likely to have coexisting circulatory problems. In general, serious foot problems in diabetic individuals who are exercising regularly are related to three factors: (a) neuropathy, which decreases the ability to perceive pressure and pain, making the diabetic individual unaware of repeated trauma; (b) impaired circulation in the feet due to peripheral vascular disease, which delays healing; and (c) poorly controlled DM, which increases susceptibility to infections (1).

It is especially important that the feet of diabetic individuals over the age of 40 years and those who have had DM for 20 years or more be examined regularly by a physician or podiatrist. Those with peripheral vascular insufficiency or insensitive feet should avoid high-impact activities, such as running or high-impact aerobics; for such individuals, walking, cycling, or swimming would be more suitable forms of recreational exercises. Calluses and corns are other important signs of potentially serious problems, since most foot ulcers start under these pressure areas. Such lesions should be pared off routinely by a podiatrist or physician. The source of the pressure causing their formation (e.g., ill-fitting shoes, foot deformities, or flat feet) should also be identified and corrective measures taken. Preventive measures may include softer or better-fitting shoes, prosthetic inserts for dress and sport shoes, and prophylactic surgery to correct foot defects.

Other important foot hygiene measures include careful trimming of the toenails; proper care of the skin, including the use of talcum power to remove excess moisture; special medicated powders to treat fungal infections between the toes (athlete's foot); and lanolin or other lubrication agents to lubricate dry skin.

Myocardial Infarction or Sudden Death

As previously indicated, CHD is the most common cause of death in diabetic adults. Even asymptomatic diabetic individuals over the age of 30 are likely to have significant underlying coronary atherosclerosis (including possible left main coronary artery disease), particularly if they have an abnormal blood lipid profile, elevated blood pressure, and/or smoke cigarettes (1). Therefore, medical evaluation is imperative before a diabetic individual over age 30 or even younger, if other risk factors are present, starts a vigorous exercise program. Selected clinical assessment studies in such persons may help rule out silent myocardial ischemia. This evaluation should include a standard multistage exercise ECGs, echocardiography, or thallium scintigraphy test using a treadmill or cycle ergometer protocol. In a study in our laboratory asymptomatic men aged 33–69 years with type 2 diabetes or glucose intolerance, 11 out of 48 (23%) had ischemic ECG changes during a symptom-limited treadmill exercise test (79). Exercise test results, in addition to unmasking silent or latent ischemia, also provide objective information for prescription of exercise intensity and training heart rate levels. If silent ischemia is uncovered on an exercise test, the training heart rate should be kept to at least 15–20 beats per minute below the level causing ischemic changes during the exercise test. All of the diabetic men in our study, referred to above, who had ischemic exercise ECG changes were able to complete a 12-week supervised treadmill walking program safely by taking such precautions.

SUMMARY AND CONCLUSIONS REGARDING THE ROLE OF EXERCISE IN THE MANAGEMENT OF DIABETES AND BLOOD LIPID DISTURBANCES

There is growing evidence that regular, moderate-intensity endurance exercise can reduce the risk of NIDDM, even in genetically susceptible individuals. It also can play a role in the management of types 1 and 2 diabetes and perhaps reduce the risk of atherosclerotic complications, including CHD. Both excess body weight and low levels of physical activity independently contribute to cellular insulin resistance and are important risk factors for NIDDM, the most prevalent form of DM in the United States. Exercise has been proposed as therapy for DM since ancient times. Currently, it is widely used as an adjunct to dietary therapy and glucose-lowering drugs in diabetic management. Acute prolonged, rhythmic exercise involving large muscle groups lowers blood glucose levels and improves insulin sensitivity for at least 24 h postexercise in both diabetics and nondiabetic individuals. Regular endurance exercise, if not compensated by excess energy intake, may further contribute to improvements in glycemic control, glucose tolerance, and insulin sensitivity in patients whose diabetes is at least under fair control by diet and/or medications. A minimum of 30–60 min of dynamic exercise at an intensity of 50–85% $\dot{V}_{O_2max}$ or peak heart rate at least 3 or 4 times a week is required to improve fitness. Strength training may also help to improve glucose-insulin dynamics as well as the blood lipid profile. Mechanisms for improved glycemic control with aerobic exercise training include the overlapping effects of the last exercise session, apparently related to the prolonged proinsulin effect of muscular contractions, improved insulin sensitivity, replenishment and augmentation of muscle glycogen stores, and improvements in skeletal muscle mass, blood supply, metabolic capacity, and cellular glucose transporter activity. However, these adaptive changes contributing to improving glycemic control apparently persist for less than 1 week after cessation of exercise.

Other potential beneficial effects of an exercise conditioning program to the diabetic individual are the following: (a) loss of excess fat, particularly visceral abdominal fat, which can further improve insulin sensitivity and glucose tolerance in individuals with NIDDM; (b) the reduced risk of atherosclerotic complications; and (c) improved quality of life.

A number of possible mechanisms exist by which exercise conditioning may reduce the severity of atherosclerosis and the risk of common cardiovascular complications often contributing to premature mortality in patients with long-term diabetes. These include a favorable effect of aerobic exercise on the blood lipid profile, particularly decreases in elevated levels of triglycerides and their principal lipoprotein carriers (VLDL and chylomicrons), and a possible increase in HDL cholesterol, particularly in younger diabetic individuals. An additional improvement in the blood lipid profile results from improving glycemic control by diabetic diet and drugs, by the loss of excess weight, smoking cessation, and by the use of antilipidemic drugs. Exercise training also may help correct elevated blood pressure levels and hypercoagulability of the blood, both often associated with diabetes. Modification of such risk factors as cigarette smoking should further reduce the severity of coronary atherosclerosis and help prevent thrombosis in narrowed coronary arteries. In addition, endurance exercise conditioning can reduce adrenergic system activity, which, in turn, decreases myocardial oxygen requirements by lowering the heart rate and systolic blood pressure levels during physical exertion, making it less likely for an individual to reach their ischemic threshold. Animal research also strongly suggests that vigorous aerobic exercise training may increase the myocardial blood supply. These favorable effects of exercise conditioning on myocardial oxygen balance, along with decreased adrenergic activity, should substantially reduce vulnerability to ventricular fibrillation and sudden death in the presence of significant coronary atherosclerosis. The quality of life also can be significantly enhanced by an exercise program through improved physical fitness and psychosocial benefits.

There are, however, potential risks accompanying strenuous exercise in diabetic individuals, which should be taken into consideration in planning an exercise program. These include aggravation of metabolic dysfunctions, if strenuous exercise is performed in the presence of markedly uncontrolled diabetes. On the other hand, in patients whose diabetes is well controlled by insulin or an oral hypoglycemic agent, hypoglycemia is a common problem during and following prolonged exercise. Frequent self-monitoring of blood glucose levels is crucial for the diabetic athlete and the recreational exerciser in order to properly adjust insulin or OHG dosage and food intake. This is required to compensate for the increase in energy expenditure and glucose utilization for fuel to help avoid hypoglycemic episodes. Consistency in eating, and exercise as well as in the administration of diabetic medications and other habits also is important. A diabetic individual on insulin, when initiating a vigorous exercise program, must either reduce his or her insulin dose, increase food intake, or both. Insulin should also not be administered in an active extremity for at least an hour prior to exercise because of the associated increased rate of insulin absorption from the site. An alternative is to routinely use the abdominal wall as a site for insulin administration. Prolonged exercise should be preceded by a light meal or carbohydrate snack. Based on self-monitored blood glucose levels, supplementary carbohydrates then should be administered regularly during and following prolonged exercise to prevent hypoglycemia.

Vigorous exercise, resistive exercise, and contact sports should be avoided in the presence of uncontrolled proliferative retinopathy or recent eye surgery because of the danger of retinal hemorrhage and retinal separation. Well-fitting footwear and careful foot care and hygiene are crucial to the diabetic exerciser in order to avoid complications, which can lead to gangrene and limb amputation, particularly in those with peripheral neuropathy and peripheral vascular disease.

In addition, careful cardiovascular screening, including exercise testing, is required in all diabetic individuals over age 35 years of age or younger individuals with over a 10-year history of diabetes or with other risk factors for CHD or with microvascular complications who wish to perform vigorous exercise in order to rule out latent manifestations of myocardial ischemia and to establish a baseline fitness level for exercise prescriptive purposes. A prescribed exercise program should be commensurate with the severity of diabetes, fitness status, and recreational interests of the individual in order to minimize the risk of musculoskeletal and cardiovascular problems and promote compliance and psychosocial benefits. Exercise should be initiated at low-intensity and short-duration levels and progressed gradually to prescriptive levels. Warm-up and cool-down periods are of importance to minimize the risk of musculoskeletal injuries.

ACKNOWLEDGMENT

The author thanks Ms. Marilyn Borkon for her invaluable assistance in preparation of this manuscript.

Dr. Leon is supported in part by the Henry L. Taylor Professorship in Exercise Science and Health Enhancement and a grant from the NHLBI, 2RO1-HL47323-06A1.

REFERENCES

1. Haire-Joshv, D. *Management of Diabetes Mellitus: Perspectives of Care Across the Life Span.* Mosby, St. Louis, pp. 1–894 (1996).
2. World Health Organization Study Group. *Diabetes Mellitus, Report of WHO Study Group.* Technical Report Series 727. WHO, Geneva, pp. 1–13 (1995).
3. American Diabetes Association. *Physician's Guide to Insulin-Dependent (Type I) Diabetes: Diagnosis and Treatment,* 2nd ed. American Diabetes Association, Alexandria, Virginia, pp. 1–150 (1988).
4. American Diabetes Association. *Physician's Guide to Non-Insulin-Dependent (Type II) Diabetes: Diagnosis and Treatment,* 2nd ed. American Diabetes Association, Alexandria, Virginia, pp. 1–93 (1988).
5. Nerup, J., Mandrup-Poulsen, J., Movig, S., et al. *Diabetes Care,* 11 (Suppl 1): 16–23 (1988).
6. Hyot, H., Hiltumen, M., Knip, M., et al. *Diabetes,* 44: 652–653 (1995).
7. Garvey, W.T. *Pathogenesis of Non-Insulin-Dependent Diabetes Mellitus* (V. Grill and S. Eflendic, eds.). Raven Press, New York, pp. 171–199 (1988).
8. Kaye, S.A., Folsom, A.R., Sprafka, J.M., et al. *J. Clin. Epidemiol.,* 44: 329–334 (1991).
9. Pouliot, M.-C., Despres, J.-P., Nadeau, A., et al. *Diabetes,* 41: 826–834 (1992).
10. Truglia, J.A., Livingston, J.N., and Lockwood, D.H. *Am. J. Med.,* 79 (Suppl): 13–22 (1985).
11. Sane, T., and Taskinen, M.-R. *Diabetes Care,* 16: 1494–1501 (1993).
12. Manson, J.E., Rimm, E.B., Stampfer, M.J., et al. *Lancet,* 338: 774–778 (1991).
13. Helmrich, S.P., Ragland, D.R., Leung, R.W., and Paffenbarger, R.S. Jr. *N. Engl. J. Med.* 325: 147–152 (1991).
14. Manson, J.E., Nathan, D.M., Krolewski, A.S., et al. *J.A.M.A.,* 268: 63–67 (1992).
15. *Physical Activity and Health: A Report of the Surgeon General.* Superintendent of Documents, Pittsburgh, pp. 85–172 (1996).
16. Kriska, A.M., Blair, S.N., and Pereira, M.A. *Exerc. Sports Sci. Rev.,* 22: 121–143 (1994).
17. Helrich, S.P., Ragland, D.R., and Paffenbarger, R.S. Jr. *Med. Sci. Sports Exerc.,* 26: 824–830 (1994).
18. Schwartz, R.S. In: *Physical Activity and Cardiovascular Health: A National Consensus* (A.S. Leon, ed.). Human Kinetics, Champaign, Illinois, pp. 105–111 (1997).
19. Lipman, R.L., Schnure, J.J., Bradley, E.M., and LeCocq, F.R. *J. Lab. Clin. Med.,* 76: 221–230 (1970).
20. Lipman, R.L., Raskin, P., Love, T., et al. *Diabetes,* 21: 101–107 (1972).
21. American Diabetes Association. *Diabetes Care* 16: 1517–1520 (1993).
22. Campaigne, B.N., and Lampman, R.M. *Exercise in the Clinical Management of Diabetes.* Human Kinetics, Champaign, Illinois, pp. 1–211 (1994).
23. Brand, P.W., and Coleman, W.C. In: *Diabetes Mellitus: Theory and Practice.* 4th ed. H. Rifkin and D. Ponte Jr., eds. Elsevier, New York, pp. 792–811 (1990).
24. Kannel, W.B., and McGee, D.L. *J.A.M.A.* 241: 2035–2038 (1979).
25. Davidson, M.B. *J. Chronic Dis.* 34: 5–10 (1981).
26. Borow, K.M., and Jaspan, J.B. *Primary Cardiol.,* 17(6): 38–48 (1991).

27. Kilo, C., and Dudley, J.D. *Geriatr. Med. Today,* 7(1): 63–79 (1988).

28. Jacoby, R.M., and Nesto, R.W. *J. Am. Acad. Cardiol.,* 20: 736–744 (1992).

29. Lithel, H.O.L. In: *Biochemistry of Exercise* (B. Saltin, ed.). Champaign, Illinois, Human Kinetics, pp. 280–309 (1986).

30. Nikkila, E.O. In: Metabolic Aspects of Cardiovascular Disease: Diabetes and Heart Disease (R.J. Jarrett, ed.). Elsevier, New York, pp. 133–167 (1988).

31. Gylling, H., and Miettinen, T.A. *Curr. Opin. Lipidol.,* 8: 342–347 (1997).

32. Gordon, J.G., and Rifkind, B.M. *N. Engl. J. Med.,* 1311–1316 (1989).

33. Dominiczak, M.H., In: *Handbook of Lipoprotein Testing* (N. Rifai, G.R. Warnick, and M.H. Dominizak, eds.). AACC Press, Washington, D.C., pp. 1–24 (1997).

34. Leon, A.S. In: *Heart Disease and Rehabilitation,* 3rd ed. (M.L. Pollock and D.H. Schmidt, eds.). Human Kinetics, Champaign, Illinois, 1996, pp. 116–147.

35. Grundy, S.M. *Arch. Intern. Med.,* 157: 1177–1184 (1997).

36. Stone, N.J., Blum, C.B., and Winslov, E. *Management of Lipids in Clinical Practice.* Professional Communications, Cado, Oklahoma, pp. 1–286 (1997).

37. Fishman, W.H. *Medical Management of Lipid Disorders: Focus on Prevention of Coronary Heart Disease.* Futura, Mount Kisco, New York, pp. 3–328 (1992).

38. Pyorala, K., Pedersen, T.R., Kjekshus, J., et al. *Diabetic Care,* 20: 614–620 (1997).

39. Greaves, M., and Preston, F.E. In: *Diabetes and Heart Disease* (K.J. Jarrett, ed.). Elsevier, New York, pp. 47–80 (1984).

40. Colwell, J.A., Cisinger, C., and Klein, R. In: *Hyperglycemia, Diabetes, and Vascular Disease* (N. Ruderman, J. Williamson, and M. Brownlee, eds.). Oxford University Press, New York, pp. 30–47 (1992).

41. Ogston, D. *The Physiology of Hemostasis.* Harvard University Press, Cambridge, Massachusetts, pp. 1–378 (1983).

42. Charo, S., Gokce, B., and Vita, J.A. *J. Cardiopulm. Rehabil.,* 18: 60–67 (1998).

43. Alessandrini, P., McRae, J., Feman, S., and Fitzgerald, G.A. *N. Engl. J. Med.,* 319: 208–212 (1988).

44. Davi, G., Catalano, I., Averna, M., et al. *N. Engl. J. Med.,* 322: 1769–1774 (1990).

45. The Expert Committee on the Diagnosis and Classification of Diabetes Mellitus. *Diabetes Care,* 20: 1183–1197 (1997).

46. Larsen, M.L., Horder, M., and Mogensen, E.F. *N. Engl. J. Med.,* 323: 1021–1025 (1990).

47. Albright, A.L. In: *ACSM's Exercise Management for Persons with Chronic Diseases and Disabilities.* Human Kinetics, Champaign, Illinois, pp. 94–105 (1997).

48. Franz, M.J., Etzwiler, D.E., Joynes, J.O., and Hollander, P.M. *Learning to Live Well with Diabetes.* DCI, Minneapolis, Minnesota, pp. 1–511 (1991).

49. National Institute of Health Consensus Development Conference Statement. *Ann. Intern. Med.,* 106 (6, suppl, part 2): 1073–1077 (1985).

50. *Build and Blood Pressure Study,* vol. I. Society of Actuaries, Chicago, pp. 1–530 (1959).

51. Zeman, F.J., and Ney, D.M. *Application of Clinical Nutrition.* Prentice-Hall, Englewood Cliffs, New Jersey, pp. 222–256 (1988).

52. American Diabetes Association. *Diabetes Care,* 18 (suppl 1): 1–96 (1995).

53. Leon, A.S., and Hartman, T. In: *Coronary Heart Disease Prevention* (F.G. Yanowitz, ed.). Marcel Dekker, New York, pp. 149–187 (1992).

54. Bieman, E.L. In: *Nutrition and the Killer Diseases* (M. Winick, ed.). Wiley, New York, pp. 153–164 (1981).
55. Keys, A., Menotti, A., Karvonen, M.J. et al., *Am. J. Epidemiol.,* 124: 903–915 (1986).
56. Stamler, J. In: *Nutrition, Lipids, and Coronary Heart Disease* (R. Levy, B.M. Rifkind, B.H. Dennis, and M.D. Ernst, eds.). A Global View. Raven, New York, pp. 25–88 (1979).
57. Kromhout, D., Bosschieter, E.B., and Coulander, C.D.L. *N. Engl. J. Med.,* 312: 1205–1209 (1985).
58. Herold, P.M., and Kinsella, J.E. *Am. J. Clin. Nutr.,* 43: 566–598 (1986).
59. Hedra, T.J., Britton, M.E., and Roper, D.R. *Diabetes Care,* 13: 821–829 (1990).
60. Bonaa, K.H., Bjerve, K.S., Straume, B., et al. *N. Engl. J. Med.,* 322: 795–801 (1990).
61. Jensen, T., Stender, S., Goldstein, K., et al. *N. Engl. J. Med.,* 321: 1522–1527 (1989).
62. Bantle, J.P., Weber, M.S., Rao, S., et al. *J.A.M.A.,* 263: 1802–1806 (1990).
63. Hollander, P.A. *Postgrad. Med.,* 98: 110–125 (1994).
64. Bailey, C.J., and Turner, R.C. *N. Engl. J. Med.,* 334: 574–579 (1996).
65. Stefanick, M.L., and Wood, P.D. In: *Physical Activity, Fitness and Health: International Proceedings and Consensus Statement* (C. Bouchard, R.J. Shephard, and T. Stephens, eds.). Human Kinetics, Champaign, Illinois, pp. 417–431 (1994).
66. Durstine, J.L., and Haskell, W.L. *Exerc. Sports. Sci. Rev.,* 22: 477–521 (1994).
67. Leon, A.S. In: *Physical Activity and Cardiovascular Health: A National Consensus* (A.S. Leon, ed.). Human Kinetics, Champaign, Illinois, pp. 57–66 (1997).
68. Jensen, M.D., and Miles, J.M. *Mayo Clin. Proc.,* 61: 813–819 (1986).
69. Giacca, A., Shi, Z.Q., Marliss, E.B., et al. In: *Physical Activity, Fitness, and Health. International Proceedings and Consensus Statement* (C. Bouchard, R.J. Shephard, and T. Stephens, eds.). Human Kinetics, Champaign, Illinois, pp. 656–668 (1994).
70. Gudat, U., Berger, M., and Lefebvre, P.J. In: *Physical Activity, Fitness, and Health. International Proceedings and Consensus Statement* (C. Bouchard, R.J. Shephard, and T. Stephens, eds.). Human Kinetics, Champaign Illinois, pp. 669–683 (1994).
71. Champaign, B.M. In: *Exercise for Prevention and Treatment of Illness* (L. Goldberg and D.L. Elliot, eds.). FA Davis, Philadelphia, pp. 173–188 (1994).
72. Zinman, B. In: *Biochemistry of Exercise VI* (B. Saltin, ed.). Human Kinetics, Champaign, Illinois, pp. 241–253 (1996).
73. Perry, I.J., Wannamethee, A.G., Walker, M.K., et al. *Br. Med. J.* 310: 560–564 (1995).
74. Lynch, J., Helmrich, S.P., Lakka, T.A., et al. *Arch. Intern. Med.,* 156: 1307–1314 (1991).
75. Eriksson, K.-F., and Lindgarde, F. *Diabetologia,* 34: 891–898 (1991).
76. Pan, X., Li, G., and Hu, Y. *Clin. J. Intern. Med.,* 34: 108–112 (1995).
77. Leon, A.S., Conrad, J., Hunninghake, D.B., and Serfass, R. *Am. J. Clin. Nutr.,* 32: 1776–1787 (1979).
78. Schneider, S.H., and Morgado, A. *Diabetes Rev.,* 3: 378–407 (1995).
79. Leon, A.S., Conrad, J., Casal, D.E., et al. *J. Cardiac Rehabil.,* 4: 278–286 (1984).
80. Ruderman, M.B., and Schneider, S.H. In: *Biochemistry of Exercise VI* (B. Saltin, ed.). Human Kinetics, Champaign, Illinois, pp. 255–277 (1986).

81. Zierath, R.J., and Wallberg-Henriksson, H., *Sports Med.,* 14(3): 171–189 (1992).
82. Barnard, R.J., Jung, T., and Inkeles, S.B. *Diabetes Care,* 17: 1469–1472 (1994).
83. Gwinup, G. *Arch. Intern. Med.,* 135: 676–680 (1975).
84. Leon, A.S. In: *Sports Medicine,* 2nd ed. (J.A. Ryan and F.L. Allman Jr., eds.). Academic Press, San Diego, California, pp. 593–617 (1989).
85. Stefanick, M.L. *Exerc. Sports Sci. Rev.,* 21: 363–396 (1993).
86. DiPietro, L. *Sports Sci. Rev.,* 23: 275–302 (1995).
87. Wallace, J.P. In: *ACSM's Exercise Management for Persons with Chronic Diseases and Disabilities.* Human Kinetics, Champaign, Illinois, pp. 106–111 (1997).
88. Despres, J.-P. *Exerc. Sports Sci. Rev.,* 25: 271–298 (1997).
89. Caspersen, C.J., Powell, K.E., and Christenson, G.M. *Public Health Rep.,* 100: 126–131 (1985).
90. Leon, A.S. *J. Cardiopulm. Rehab.,* 11: 46–56 (1991).
91. Goldberg, L., and Elliot, D.L. In: *Exercise for Prevention and Treatment of Illness* (L. Goldberg and D.L. Elliott, eds.). F.A. Davis, Philadelphia, pp. 189–210 (1994).
92. Stefanik, M.L. In: *Physical Activity and Cardiovascular Health: A National Consensus* (A.S. Leon, ed.). Human Kinetics, Champaign, Illinois, pp. 98–104 (1997).
93. LaPorte, R., Brenes, G., and Dearwater, S., *Lancet,* 1: 1212–1213 (1993).
94. Ferrell, P.A., Maksud, M.G., Pollock, M.L., et al. *Eur. J. Appl. Physiol.,* 48: 77–82 (1982).
95. Haskell, W.L., Taylor, H.L., Wood, P.D., et al. *Circulation,* 62 (suppl 4): 51–59 (1980).
96. Wood, P.D., Haskell, W.L., Blair, S.N., et al. *Metabolism,* 32: 31–39 (1983).
97. Williams, P.T., Wood, P.D., Haskell, W.L., and Vranizan, K. *J.A.M.A.,* 247: 2674–2679 (1982).
98. Sopko, G., Leon A.S., Jacobs, D.R. Jr., et al. *Metabolism,* 39: 227–236 (1985).
99. Schwartz, S., *Metabolism,* 36: 15–171 (1987).
100. Wood, P.D., Stefanik, M.L., Dreone, D., et al. *N. Engl. J. Med.,* 319: 1173–1179 (1988).
101. Taylor, A., and Ward, A. *Arch. Intern. Med.,* 153: 1178–1184 (1993).
102. Pronk, N.P. *Sports Med.,* 16: 431–448 (1993).
103. Santiago, M.C., Alexander, J.F., Stull, G.A., et al. *Scand. J. Sports Sci.,* 9: 33–39 (1987).
104. Santiago, M.C., Leon, A.S., and Serfass, R.C. *Can. J. Physiol.,* 20: 417–428 (1995).
105. Expert Panel on Detection, Evaluation and Management of High Cholesterol in Adults. *Circulation,* 89: 1329–1445 (1994).
106. Faagard, R.H., and Tipton, C.M. In: *Physical Activity, Fitness, and Health: International Proceedings and Consensus Statement* (C. Bouchard, R.J. Shephard, and T. Stephens, eds.). Human Kinetics, Champaign, Illinois, pp. 633–653 (1994).
107. Hagberg, J.M. In: *Physical Activity and Cardiovascular Health: A National Consensus* (A.S. Leon, ed.). Human Kinetics, Champaign, Illinois, pp. 57–66 (1997).
108. Rauramaa, R., Salonen, J.T., Serpanen, K., et al. *Circulation,* 74: 939–944 (1986).
109. Eichner, E.R. In: *Physical Activity and Cardiovascular Health, A National Consensus* (A.S. Leon, ed.). Human Kinetics, Champaign, Illinois, pp. 120–126 (1997).
110. Blair, S.N., Kohl H.W. III, and Paffenbarger, R.S. Jr., et al. *J.A.M.A.,* 262: 2395–2401 (1989).

111. Leon, A.S., and Norstrom, J. *Quest,* 47: 311–319 (1995).
112. Leon, A.S. In: *Physical Activity and Cardiovascular Health: A National Consensus* (A.S. Leon, ed.). Human Kinetics, Champaign, Illinois, pp. 120–126 (1997).
113. Lee I.-M., and Paffenbarger, R.S. Jr. In: *Physical Activity and Cardiovascular Health: A National Consensus* (A.S. Leon, ed.). Human Kinetics, Champaign, Illinois, pp. 67–75 (1997).
114. Powell, K.E., Thompson, P.D., Caspersen, C.J., and Kendrick, J.S. *Annu. Rev. Public Health,* 8: 253–287 (1987).
115. Berlin, J.A., and Colditz, G.A. *Am. J. Epidemiol.,* 132: 612–628 (1990).
116. Leon, A.S., Connett, J., Jacobs, D.R. Jr., and Rauramaa, R. *J.A.M.A.* 258: 2388–2395 (1987).
117. O'Connor, G.T., Buring, J.E., Yusaf, S., et al. *Circulation,* 80: 234–244 (1987).
118. Ornish, D., Brown, S.E., Scherwitz, L.W., Billings, J.H., et al. *Lancet,* 336: 129–133 (1990).
119. Schuler, G., Hambrecht, R., Schlierf, G., et al. *Circulation,* 86: 1–11 (1992).
120. Hughes, J.R. *Prev. Med.,* 13: 66–78 (1984).
121. Biddle, I.S. *Res. Q. Exerc. Sports,* 66: 292–297 (1998).
122. MacDonald, M.J., *Diabetes Care,* 10: 584–588 (1987).
123. Franz, M.J., and Norstrom, J. *Diabetes: Actually Staying Healthy—Your Game Plan for Diabetes and Exercise.* DCI Publishing, Wayzata, Minnesota, pp. 1–170 (1990).
124. Trovati, M., Carta, Q., Cavalot, F., et al. *Diabetes Care,* 7: 327–330 (1984).
125. Riza, R.A. *Mayo Clin. Proc.,* 61: 796–805 (1986).

15

Exercise Training in Patients with Heart Failure

L. KENT SMITH
Arizona Heart Institute and Foundation
Phoenix, Arizona

INTRODUCTION

Based on figures from the American Heart Association, the last quarter century has seen a steady decline in mortality and event rates from coronary artery disease as well as reduction in events in patients with risk factors for cardiovascular conditions [such as elevated levels of low-density lipoprotein (LDL) cholesterol and hypertension] (1). Regrettably, the prevalence and the incidence of chronic heart failure are steadily increasing and have exceeded 450,000 new cases annually in the United States. Furthermore, as the U.S. population ages, the age-related development of heart failure in both men and women will almost certainly lead to a steady increase in cases of heart failure into the next century. While the improved recognition and management of hypertension has reduced this condition as an etiological factor in the development of heart failure, the increase in survival rate from the modern management of myocardial infarction has led to an increase in cases of chronic heart failure (2). The total number of patients with heart failure in the United States is approaching 5 million; worldwide, it is 15 million (3, 4).

According to the Federal Clinic Practice Guideline on heart failure, the annual health care dollars spent in the United States on care for patients with this condition is at least $10 billion, with $7.5 billion of that total coming from hospitalizations costs (5). The average cost per hospitalization is approximately $6500, and heart failure represents the single most common diagnosis for Medicare (Health Care Finance Administration) payments for hospitalization. Emerging strategies in the management of patients with heart failure, including exercise training (to be discussed later in this chapter), hold promise for reducing health care costs related to heart failure management.

MEDICAL THERAPY

In the last decade, major advances in the medical management of patients with heart failure (specifically left ventricular systolic dysfunction) have occurred. Several well-designed and well-executed clinical trials have documented reduction in morbidity and mortality in patients with heart failure. Historically, the first study to document survival advantage was the first Veterans Administration Cooperative Study, which demonstrated reduction in mortality compared to placebo patients from 47–36% at 3 years (6). Even more impressive results in morbidity and mortality reduction resulted from a series of trials involving the angiotensin-converting enzyme (ACE) inhibitor class of drugs, including a 40% relative reduction in mortality in functional class IV heart failure patients with the ACE inhibitor enalapril (7). ACE inhibitor trials of more relevance to patients involved in cardiac rehabilitation included the SOLVD and SAVE trials (utilizing enalapril and captopril, respectively) in patients with New York Heart Association (NYHA) functional class II and III heart failure. These large clinical trials documented substantial reductions in cardiovascular event rates (both morbidity and mortality) and very impressive reductions in hospitalization rates and the subsequent potential for substantial cost savings (8, 9). In contrast, trials using calcium-channel blockers in patients with heart failure secondary to coronary artery disease documented either no benefit or a worsening of clinical outcomes. The more recent clinical trials evaluating the nonselective β-receptor antagonist carvedilol (which also blocks the α_1-receptor and has antioxidant effects), has demonstrated clinical outcome benefit in patients with mild, moderate, and severe heart failure (10, 11). These beneficial effects included a relative reduction of 48% in heart failure progression in patients with mild impairment. Furthermore, reduction in morbidity and mortality was documented, as well as a favorable impact on rates of cardiovascular hospitalization. These improvements were accompanied by increase in measurements of left ventricular ejection fraction but no improvement in exercise performance. The preponderance of the clinical trial data establishing the favorable role of ACE inhibitor prescription in patients with heart failure has led to the conclusion, in the Federal Clinical Practice Guideline, that ''patients with heart failure due to left ventricular systolic dysfunction should be given a trial ACE inhibitors unless specific contraindications exists'' (5). The guideline also states that digoxin should routinely be used in patients with more severe degrees of heart failure.

EXERCISE TESTING AND PHYSIOLOGICAL EFFECTS OF EXERCISE TRAINING

The role of exercise testing has been established to provide clinical and prognostic information above and beyond the additional assessment techniques of directly measuring systolic and diastolic ventricular function and, when appropriate, the presence and extent of coronary artery narrowing. Cardiopulmonary exercisetesting with direct measure of key metabolic parameters (oxygen consumption, production of carbon dioxide, minute ventilation, and onset of production of lactic acid) has provided important information to direct optimum management and also provides meaningful prognostic information. Specifically, peak exercise $\dot{V}_{O_2}$ values less than 14 ml/kg/min^{-1} are related to worsened prognosis in patients with heart failure, including those awaiting heart transplantation (12). In this subset of patients with severe heart failure, an ambulatory program including exercise training has been demonstrated to improve prognosis and allow approximately one-third of transplant candidates to be removed from the transplantation list (13). This raises the compelling question as to whether exercise training in patient with impaired left ventricular systolic function may result in an improved clinical outcome, including mortality reduction. Additionally, in patients with either ischemic or dilated cardiomyopathy (approximately 50% with each etiology) and principally NYHA functional class II and III heart failure participating in the Veterans Administration Heart Failure trial, baseline peak $\dot{V}_{O_2}$ measurement was a strong independent predictor of 1 year survival (14). Specifically, patients with $\dot{V}_{O_2max}$ less than 14.5 ml/kg/min^1 had a 59% survival at 1 year, compared with 94% in the patients with peak $\dot{V}_{O_2}$ greater than 14.5 ml/kg/min^{-1}.

Exercise training has been demonstrated to be associated with several beneficial physiological changes in patients with left ventricular systolic dysfunction. Measures of submaximal and maximal exercise performance, including 6-min walk tests, show improvement. Physiological measures following exercise training in patients with heart failure demonstrate improvement in peak oxygen consumption accompanying the increase in the duration of treadmill or bicycle exercise time. Furthermore, at submaximal workload, heart rates were reduced (15, 16). Beneficial changes are seen when using a low-intensity exercise training regimen in patients with heart failure (forty percent of peak $\dot{V}_{O_2}$), resulting in a 22% improvement in peak $\dot{V}_{O_2}$ levels following the training regimen (17). Furthermore, this beneficial effect of exercise training in improving peak oxygen consumption is still achieved in patients managed with β-blocker medication for heart failure (carvedilol or propranolol) (18).

EXERCISE TRAINING: PHYSIOLOGICAL BASIS AND SAFETY ISSUES

Patients with heart failure are at reasonably high risk for morbidity and mortality. Even in the active-treatment arms of the successful clinical trials utilizing ACE inhibitors or, more recently, β-blockers, the annual rate of mortality still remains greater than 10% in patients with NYHA functional class II and III heart failure. In the treatment arm of the CONSENSUS study in patients with functional class IV heart failure, the 1-year mortality rate was 36%. Furthermore, approximately 15% of patients with functional class II and III heart failure on active drug therapy required hospitalization for cardiovascular reasons on an annual basis. These rates of morbidity and mortality are considerably higher than those of the "usual" patient participating in outpatient cardiac rehabilitation programs. With this background of high-risk in heart failure patients, the important question regarding effects of exercise training on morbidity and mortality needs to be clearly addressed. Except for one study (see Ref. 30), there are no data regarding mortality in patients with diminished left ventricular function randomly assigned to exercise training compared with nontraining controls. Nevertheless, there is no evidence of increased mortality and several studies have evaluated the safety of exercise training appropriately applied to patients with stable heart failure and carefully conducted in the supervised setting of cardiac rehabilitation. Although an early nonrandomized trial of exercise training in patients with diminished left ventricular systolic function following myocardial infarction documented unfavorable outcomes regarding left ventricular remodeling (19), two larger, randomized, long-term studies of exercise training have documented no deterioration in measures of ventricular geometry or ventricular performance (20, 21). An additional study in postinfarction patients with mean ejection fraction of $32 \pm 6\%$ using relatively high peak exercise intensity during four weekly monitored stationary cycling sessions (in addition to 2 h of daily walking) over 2 months revealed no adverse outcomes in ventricular geometry or performance as measured by magnetic resonance imaging (22).

The specific adverse cardiovascular events that are reported in patients undergoing randomized controlled trials of exercise training are presented below. Specific information is documented in the outcomes column in Table 1. To summarize, patients with heart failure are at greater risk of adverse outcomes over time (compared with patients with coronary artery disease with preservation of ventricular function); however, this does not appear to occur more often in patients randomly assigned to exercise training versus control subjects.

EXERCISE TRAINING

In the final decade of this century, several well-designed and well-conducted clinical trials have addressed the issue of exercise training in patients with ventricular dysfunction. No fewer than 12 reports have appeared since 1991 describing randomized controlled trials, providing the scientific basis for establishing the beneficial outcomes of exercise training in patients with heart failure (23–34). Based upon these trials, a broad array of beneficial outcomes following exercise training in patients with left ventricular systolic dysfunction has been established. Although these patients experience cardiovascular adverse events more often than patients without heart failure, there was no greater likelihood of morbidity or mortality in comparing exercise training groups with randomized controls. The Specchia study provides evidence of a potential survival advantage for patients with left ventricular systolic dysfunction who participate in cardiac rehabilitation exercise training following an uncomplicated first myocardial infarction.

Two additional nonrandomized controlled trials have recently been published and have added to the data base documenting the safety and benefits of exercise training in heart failure patients (35, 36). These two nonrandomized controlled studies provide additional important information regarding the role of exercise training in patients with chronic heart failure. One study involving 27 patients documented beneficial training effects resulting from an 8-week regimen of cardiac rehabilitation exercise training utilizing low-intensity aerobic activity (40% of peak oxygen uptake) (35). The second nonrandomized controlled trial reports beneficial outcomes from 12 weeks of aerobic exercise training in heart failure patients who are treated with concurrent carvedilol or propranolol (in addition to ACE inhibitors, digoxin, and diuretics) for concomitant management of heart failure.

COST BENEFIT AND REIMBURSEMENT ISSUES

There have been no exercise training or cardiac rehabilitation studies that have directly addressed the issue of cost-effectiveness or cost-benefit. There are data from the large placebo-controlled clinical trials of ACE inhibitor therapy that document reduction in hospitalization rates with concomitant reduction in health care expenditures. However, no such data have been presented regarding exercise

TABLE I   Randomized Controlled Trials of Exercise Training in Patients with Heart Failure

Reference and year of publication	Patient description	Intervention program and follow-up	Outcomes
Jette et al., 1991 (23)	Sample size: 39 Gender: 100% male Age: 51 ± 8 years Category: anterior MI less than 10 weeks prior to study entry. Radionuclide ejection < 50%. Training group; 18 points (7 w/EF < 30%). Control group 18 points (8 w/ EF < 30%). No baseline differences in hemodynamic variables, radionuclide measurements or medications.	Intervention: 4-week inhospital, supervised aerobic exercise training (jogging/bibycle ergometry) at 70–80% maximum baseline exercise stress test heart rate. Follow-up: 4 weeks.	Significant increase in maximum work (17% increase) and peak oxygen consumption (22% increase) in training group with baseline EF under 30%. No significant changes in hemodynamic measurements. 3 of 7 training points with baseline EF under 30% had cardiovascular complications and were removed from study.
Coats et al., 1992 (24)	Sample size: 19 Gender: 100% male Age: mean 61.8 ± 1.5% Category: Coronary artery disease. LVEF 19.6 ± 2.3%. NYHA class II–III.	Intervention: Randomized crossover comparison trial. 8 weeks of rest against 8 weeks exercise training. Home exercise training on bicycle ergometer 5 days/ week × 20 min at 60–80% baseline maximum heart rate. Follow-up: 8-week intervals × 2.	77% compliance with home-based training regimen. Significant increase in total exercise time (19% increase) and peak oxygen consumption 18% increase following 8 weeks exercise training only. Significant reduction in resting and submaximum heart rate following exercise training only. Significant increase in submaximum and peak cardiac output. Significant reduction in systemic vascular resistence. Significant decrease in norepinephrine levels. 2 patients dropped out (1 death for worsening heart failure, 1 undergoing heart transplantation) during rest phase (and prior to participation in exercise training phase).

Study	Sample	Intervention	Results
Koch et al., 1992 (25)	Sample size: 25 Gender: 19/25 male Age: 55 ± 10 years Category: EF 26 ± 11%. NYHA class II-III. Dilated or ischemic (proportion not specified). No significant difference in medication treatment.	Intervention: Exercise training group: utilizing specialized equipment for 40 sessions over 90 days without incidents. Follow-up: 3 months.	Significant improvement in bicycle ergometry exercise test duration (34% increase) in rehab group only. Significant improvement in total muscle strength (45% increase) in exercise training group only. No significant change in echocardiographic measures, including EF at rest, in either group. One control group patient required cardiac transplantation.
Kostis et al., 1994 (26)	Sample size: 20 Gender: 14 male; 6 female Age: 54–77 years Category: CHF. LVEF 30–37%. NYHA class II-III (only 1 patient class III). All receiving background ACE-inhibitor therapy.	Intervention: Control 6 patients, digoxin 7 patients, multidiscipline rehab 7 patients (sodium restriction, smoking avoidance, stress management, and exercise training). Exercise training 1-hr/session 3–5 times/week at intensity of 40–60% of functional capacity occurring in supervised outpatient rehab facility. Baseline variables not statistically significantly different. Follow-up: 12 weeks.	Significant increase in echocardiographic EF (4.4% increase) digoxin group only. Significant increase in treadmill exercise duration (37% increase) rehab group only Significant improvement in measures of depression and anxiety (reduced by 39–52%) rehab group only. No adverse clinical events in rehab group.

(Table Continues)

TABLE I Continued

Reference and year of publication	Patient description	Intervention program and follow-up	Outcomes
Hambrecht et al., 1995 (27)	Sample size: 22. Gender: 100% male. Age: 51 ± 10 years. Category: Dilated cardiomyopathy 19 patients, ischemic cardiomyopathy 3 patients. EF 26 ± 9. NYHA class II 12 patients, class III 10 patients. No significant difference in medications.	Intervention: Training group 12 patients, control group 10 patients. Initial 3 weeks of daily supervised bicycle ergometry $6\times$/day for 10 min at 70% symptom-limited baseline maximal effort. Continued home-based bicycle ergometry at 70% peak workload twice daily for 40 min plus two supervised group training sessions for 60 min/week.	Significant increase maximum oxygen consumption (31%) treatment versus controls. Significant increase in maximum exercise cardiac output (18% increase) treatment versus controls. Increase in peak-leg oxygen consumption (45%) treatment versus controls. One rehab patient experienced sudden death not related to exercise training. One control patient experienced decompensated heart failure requiring hospitalization.
Belardinelli et al., 1995 (28)	Sample size: 55. Gender: 47 male, 8 female. Age: 55 ± 7 years. Category: Ischemic cardiomyopathy 37 patients, dilated cardiomyopathy 18 patients. EF 27 ± 5%. NYHA class II 38 patients, class III 17 patients. No significant differences in medication treatment. Training group 36 patients, controls 19 patients.	Follow-up: 6 months. Intervention: Supervised exercise training at 60% of peak $\dot{V}_{O_2}$ $3\times$/week for 8 weeks 40 min/session on cycle ergometer. Follow-up: 2 months for physiological measurements. 12 $\pm$ 6 months for cardiac events (death, heart failure, angina).	Significant increase in $\dot{V}_{O_{2}max}$(15%) exercise training group versus controls. Significant increase in lactic acid threshold (12%) training group versus controls. No change in LVEF in either group. No significant cardiovascular events during training sessions. Cardiac event rates not significantly different training versus control groups.

| Keteyian et al., 1996 (29) | Sample size: 40
Gender: 100% male
Age: 56 ± 11 years
Category: Ischemic cardiomyopathy 16 patients, dilated cardiomyopathy 24 patients. EF 21 ± 7. No significant difference in medications. Exercise training group 15, control group 14 dropouts, 11). | Intervention: Supervised exercise training 3×/week × 33 min at 60–80% heart-rate reserve.
Follow-up: 24 weeks. | Significant increase in peak $\dot{V}_{O_2}$ (16.3%) treatment versus controls (significantly greater increase in patients with idiopathic versus ischemic cardiomyopathy). Significantly greater increase in exercise duration training versus control group. In training group, 1 patient developed atrial fibrillation. No other cardiovascular complications. In control group, 1 patient developed atrial fibrillation, 1 patient had nonfatal myocardial infarction, 1 patient experienced sudden death. |
| Specchia et al., 1996 (30) | Sample size: 256
Gender: 91% male
Age: 53 ± 7 years
Category: 100% following first uneventful MI (12 × 4 days prior to study entry). 37% received thrombolysis. EF 51 ± 13% (51 patients at baseline LV angio w/EF < 41%; 24 in training group, 27 controls). Training group 125, control group 131. No baseline differences regarding comorbidity, risk factors, location and extent of MI, thrombolytic therapy between groups. | Intervention: All patients underwent educational sessions regarding secondary prevention, dietary changes, and smoking cessation. Training group only had 4 weeks supervised exercise training 30 min by cycle ergometry 5×/week at 75% maximum work capacity. Continued unsupervised training 30 min every 2 days recommended thereafter.
Follow-up: mean 34.5 months. | Cardiac deaths; 5 in training group, 13 in control group. EF only multivariate independent predictor of death. Significant interaction between exercise training and survival based on EF. Namely, relative risk of death control versus training patients with EF < 41% of 8.6 ($p = 0.04$). |

(Table Continues)

TABLE 1 Continued

Reference and year of publication	Patient description	Intervention program and follow-up	Outcomes
Meyer et al., 1997 (31)	Sample size: 18 Gender: 100% male Age: 52 ± 2 years Category: Ischemic cardiomyopathy 9 patients, dilated cardiomyopathy 9 patients. EF 21 ± 1% (half of patients listed for transplantation).	Intervention: Random-cross-over trial 3 weeks activity versus 3 weeks exercise training. Supervised cycle ergometry 5×/week × 15 min at 50% maximum workload plus 3×/week × 10 min treadmill walking plus 3 ×/week for 20 min flexibility, coordination, and strength exercise. Follow-up: before and after each 3-week session.	Significant increase in $\dot{V}_{O_2}$ at ventilatory threshold (23.7%) treatment versus controls. Significant increase in $\dot{V}_{O_2max}$ (19.7%) exercise training versus controls. No significant change in EF or cardiac index at rest. No significant cardiovascular adverse events occurred.
Giannuzzi et al., 1997 (32)	Sample size: 80 Gender: 76 male, 4 female Age: 53 ± 9 years Category: acute First MI (78% anterior wall). EF 34 ± 4%. NYHA class I and II. Training group 39 patients, control group 38 patients. No significant difference in presence in location or extent of MI, thrombolytic therapy (76 and 71%) interval since infarction (3.5 and 3.4 weeks) or medication usage.	Intervention; Supervised bicycle ergometry 3×/week × 30 min for 2 months at intensity of 80% peak maximum. Thereafter, home-based exercise training 30 min bicycle ergometry 3×/week for total exercise training of 6 months. Follow-up: 6 months.	Significant improvement in work capacity (28% increase) training versus control. Significant increase by echo of LV end-diastolic and end-systolic volume in control group; no significant change in training group. Significant increase in echocardiographic EF (4% increase) in training group versus control group. Significant increase in measures of anxiety and general well-being training versus control group. No cardiovascular adverse outcomes reported.

Dubach et al., 1997 (34)	Sample size: 25 Gender; 100% male Age: 56 ± 6 years Category: MI (and post-CABG in 20 patients). EF 32 ± 6%. NYHA class II and III. Exercise training group 12 patients, controls 13 patients. No significant differences regarding presence and extent of CAD, risk factors, CABG or medication therapy.	Intervention: Residential-based exercise training plus education and dietary management. Twice daily walking 1 hr/session plus monitored stationary ergometry training 4×/week × 45 min/session at 70–80% heart rate reserve for 2 months. Follow-up: 2 months.	At the lactate threshold, significant increases in oxygen uptake, minute ventilation, exercise time, and workload in watts for exercise group versus controls. Significant increase in maximum $\dot{V}_{O_2}$ baseline versus 2-month follow-up exercise training group only; but not statistically different from control group ($p = 0.13$). Significant increase in exercise time (29% increase) exercise versus control groups. No significant differences between groups in LV mass and end-systolic or end-diastolic volume or EF as measured by magnetic resonance imaging in either the infarct or noninfarct areas of the myocardium. No events during exercise testing or training.
Dubach et al., 1997 (35)	Sample size: 25 Gender: 100% male Age: 56 ± 6 years Category: MI and post-CABG in 20 patients). EF 32 ± 6%. NYHA class II and III. Exercise training group 12 patients, controls 13 patients. No significant differences regarding presence and extent of CAD, risk factors, CABG or medication therapy.	Intervention; Residential-based exercise training plus education and dietary management. Twice daily walking 1 hr/session plus monitored stationary ergometry training 4 ×/week × 45 min/session at 70–80% heart rate reserve for 2 months. Follow-up: 2 months.	At the lactate threshold, significant increases in oxygen uptake, minute ventilation, exercise time, and workload in watts exercise group versus controls. Significant increase in maximum $\dot{V}_{O_2}$ baseline versus 2-month follow-up exercise training group only, but not statistically different from control group (p = 0.13). Significant increase in exercise time (29% increase) exercise versus control groups. No significant differences between groups in LV mass and end-systolic or end-diastolic volume or EF as measured by magnetic resonance imaging in either the infarct or noninfarct areas of the myocardium. No events during exercise testing or training.

training versus control studies in patients with heart failure. Extrapolation from the established cost-benefit of cardiac rehabilitation of patients without heart failure does not appeared justified.

There do exist four studies of specialized management systems or programs for delivery of care in the outpatient setting to patients with heart failure. Four recent studies have been reported offering encouraging information pertaining to the cost-benefit of improved systems for delivering services, including exercise training, in the outpatient setting for heart failure patients (37–40). These programs utilize a specialized team of health care providers focusing on a clinical nurse specialist as case manager for patients with heart failure. The first to report results (37) utilized a prospective, randomized study design in elderly patients hospitalized for decompensation of heart failure. The program started with in-hospital education and continued in the outpatient setting utilizing a nurse management strategy. This trial reported a very impressive absolute (not relative) reduction in 90-day readmission rates of 13% (with admission rates in the control patients of 42%, compared with 29% in the treatment group). The cost of providing specialized care for 90 days was $262. This was offset by less utilization of health care services, resulting in $1058 average reduction in expenditures per patient. The net savings per patient to the health care system was $796. Extrapolating this per patient health care saving to the large potential pool of patients with heart failure (4 million in the United States) would effect major health care expenditure benefit. A second group reports similar benefits using historical controls (39). This study was carried out in patients with moderately severe heart failure with a mean ejection fraction of 21% and involved 214 patients who were accepted as potential candidates for heart transplantation. This program was carried out by a specialized multidisciplinary team of health care professionals, with the clinical nurse specialist having a key role. The program included maximizing the medication regimen as well as providing educational guidelines regarding dietary management, alcohol abstinence, and smoking cessation. The comprehensive program included home-based exercise training of 30–45 min per session four times weekly. At 6 months follow-up, relative reduction in hospital readmissions was 85%, and the patients' functional status improved to a significant degree. The estimated cost savings from reduction in hospital readmission was a net of $9800 per patient. An additional study utilizing a team approach to optimize outpatient management of patients with heart failure presented data on 51 patients with ejection fraction of 40% or less (40). This program sought to optimize medication treatment and included initial and follow-up education and management of dietary measures. Counseling regarding daily physical activity, smoking cessation, and alcohol limitation was also included. Beneficial outcomes included significant improvement in functional status and exercise capacity. Based on historical controls (6 months prior to the program and 6 months after it) a 31% reduction in cardiology visits and a 67% decline in emergency room visits for heart failure reasons occurred. Hospitalization rates for heart failure declined by 87%. No financial analysis was reported.

THE SCIENTIFIC EVIDENCE FOR EXERCISE TRAINING

The references and essential components of the important randomized controlled trials are detailed in Table 1. As review of the data in this table indicates the benefits of exercise training in patients with heart failure are very well established and include a suggestion of mortality reduction and a reduction in morbidity with concomitant cost savings to the health care system. It can reasonably be concluded from this evidence that the role of exercise training/cardiac rehabilitation in patients with heart failure is based on solid scientific study and results in a wide range of clinical and economic benefits. It remains for the professional health care community to apply these proven approaches more broadly to managing patients with heart failure and to work toward establishing such programs nationwide.

It appears that programs designed to optimize well-established treatments for patients with heart failure result in a wide array of clinical and cost benefits. The majority of well-designed clinical trials establishing this accumulating body of evidence have been published in the last decade. Regrettably, recognition of these multiple benefits by the health care reimbursement community has not kept pace. To help bridge this gap, all health care professionals with concern for the well-being and care of patients with heart failure need to take appropriate action based upon sound scientific documentation so that appropriate support for a wide array of treatment programs, including exercise training, can reach more patients with heart failure.

References

1. American Heart Association. *Heart and Stroke Facts: 1997 Statistical Supplement.* AHA, Chicago.
2. Kostis, J.B., Davis, B.R., Cutler, J., Grimm R.H. Jr., Berge, K.G., Cohen, J.D., Lacy, C.R., Perry, H.M., Blaufox, M.D., Wasserheil-Smoller S., Black, H.R., Schom, E., Berkson, D.M., Curb, J.D., McFate Smith, W., McDonald, R., and Applegate, W.B. for the SHEP Cooperative Research Group. *J.A.M.A.,* 278: 212–216 (1997).
3. American College of Cardiology/American Heart Association Committee on Evaluation and Management of Heart Failure, *J. Am. Coll. Cardiol.,* 26: 1376–1398 (1995).
4. Eriksson, H., *J. Interm, Med.,* 237: 135–141 (1995)
5. Konstam, M.A., Dracup, K., Baker, D.W., Bottorff, M.B., Brooks, N.H., Dacey,

R.A., Dunbar, S.B., Jackson, A.B., Jessup, M., Johnson, J.C., Jones, R.H., Luchi, R.J., Massie, B.M., Pitt, B., Rose, E.A., Rubin, L.J., Wright, R.F., and Hadom, D.C., Rockville, M.D.: U.S. Department of Health and Human Services, Public Health Service, Agency for Health Care Policy and Research, AHCPR Publication No. 94-0612 (1994).

6. Cohn, J.N., Archibald, D.G., and Ziesche, S., *N. Engl. J. Med.,* 314: 1547–1552 (1986).

7. CONSESUS Trial Study Group, *N. Engl. J. Med.,* 316: 1429–1435 (1987).

8. SOLVD Investigators, *N. Engl. J. Med.,* 325: 293–302 (1991).

9. Pfeffer, M.A., Braunwald, E., and Moye, L.A., *N. Engl. J. Med.,* 327: 669–677 (1992).

10. Colucci, W.S., Packer, M., Bristow, M.R., Gilbert, E.M., Cohn, J.N., Fowler, M.B., Krueger, S.K., Hershbeger, R., Uretsky, B.F., Bowers, J.A., Sacjer-Bemstein, J.D., Young, S.T., Holcslaw, T.L., and Lukas, M.A., for the U.S. Carvedilol Heart Failure Study Group, *Circulation,* 94: 2800–2806 (1996).

11. Packer, M., Colucci, W.S., Sackner-Bernstein, J.D., Liang, C., Goldscher, D.A., Freeman, I., Kukin, M.L., Kinhal, V., Udelson, J.E., Klaophoz, M., Gottileb, S.S., Pearle, D., Cody, R.J., Gregory, J.J., Kantrowitz, N.E., LeJemtel, T.H., Young, S.T., Lukas, M.A., and Shusterman, N.H., for the PRECISE Study Group, *Circulation,* 94: 2793–2799 (1996).

12. Pina, I.L., *J. Am. Coll. Cardiol.,* 26: 436–437 (1995).

13. Stevenson, L.W., Steimle, A.E., and Fonarow, G., *J. Am. Coll. Cardiol.,* 25: 163–170 (1995).

14. Cohn, J.N., Johnson, G.R., and Shabetai, R., *Circulation,* 87 (suppl VI): VI-5–VI-6 (1993).

15. Sullivan, M.J., Higginbotham, M.B., and Cobb F.R., *Circulation,* 78: 506–515 (1988).

16. Sullivan, M.J., Higginbotham, M.B., and Cobb, F.R., *Circulation,* 79: 324–329 (1989).

17. Belardinelli, R., Georgiou, D., and Scocco, V., *J. Am. Coll. Cardiol.,* 26: 975–982 (1995).

18. Demopoulos, L., Yeh, M., Gentilucci, M., Testa, M., Bijou, R., Katz, S.D., Mancini, D., Jones, M., and LeJemtel, T.H., *Circulation,* 95: 1764–1767 (1997).

19. Jugdutt, B.I., Michorowski, B.L., and Kappagoda, C.T., *J. Am. Coll. Cardiol.,* 12: 362–372 (1988).

20. Giannuzzi, P., Tavazzi, L., and Temporelli, U.C., *J. Am. Coll. Cardiol.,* 22: 1821–1829 (1993).

21. Giannuzzi, P., Temporelli, P.L., Corra, U., Gattone, M., Giordano A., and Tavazzi, L., for the ELVD Study Group, *Circulation,* 96: 1790–1797 (1997).

22. Dubach, P., Myers, J., Dziekan, G., Goebbels, U., Reinhart, W., Vogt, P., Ratti, R., Muller, P., Miettunen, R., and Buser, P., *Circulation,* 95: 2060–2067 (1997).

23. Jette, M., Heller, R., Landry, F., and Blumchen, G., *Circulation,* 84: 1561–1567 (1991).

24. Coats, A.J.S., Adamopoulos, S., Radaelli, A., McCance, A., Meyer, T.E., Bernardi, L., Solda, P.L., Davey, P., Ormerod, O., Forfar, C., Conway, J., and Sleight, P., *Circulation,* 85: 2119–2131 (1992).

25. Koch, M., Douard, H., and Broustet, J.P., *Chest,* 101: 231S (1992).
26. Kostis, J.B., Rosen, R.C., Cosgrove, N.M., Shindler, D.M., and Wilson, A.C., *Chest,* 106: 996–1001 (1994).
27. Hambrecht, R., Niebauer, J., Fiehn, E., Kalberer, B., Offner, B., Hauer, K., Riede, U., Schlierf, G., Kubler, W., and Schuler, G., *J. Am. Coll. Cardiol.,* 25: 1239–1249 (1995).
28. Belardinelli, R., Georgiou, D., Cianci, G., Berman, N., Ginzton, L., and Purcaro, A., *Circulation,* 91: 2775–2784 (1995).
29. Keteyian, S.J., Levine, A.B., Brawner, C.A., Kataoka, T., Rogers, F.J., Schairer, J.R., Stein, P.D., Levine, T.B., and Goldstein, S., *Ann. Intern. Med.,* 124: 1051–1057 (1996).
30. Specchia, G., DeServi, S., Scire, A., Assandri, J., Berzuini, C., Angoli, L., LaRovere, M.T., and Cobelli, F., *Circulation,* 94: 978–982 (1996).
31. Meyer, K., Gomandt, L., Schwaibold, M., Westbrook, S., Hajric, R., Peters, K., Beneke, R., Schnellbacher, K., Roskamm, H, Am. J. Cardiol., 80: 56–60 (1997).
32. Giannuzzi, P., Temporelli, P.L., Corra, U., Gattone, M., Giordano, A., and Tavazzi, L., for the ELVD Study Group, *Circulation,* 96: 1790–1797 (1997).
33. Dubach, P., Myers, J., Dziekan, G., Goebbels, U., Reinhart, W., Muller, P., Buser, P., Stulz, P., Vogt, P., and Ratti, R., *J. Am. Coll. Cardiol.,* 29: 1591–1598 (1997).
34. Dubach, P., Myers, J., Dziekan, G., Goebbels, U., Reinhart, W., Vogt, P., Ratti, R., Muller, P., Miettunen, R., and Buser, P., *Circulation,* 95: 2060–2067 (1997).
35. Belardinelli, R., Georgiou, D., Scocco, V., Barstow, T.J., and Purcaro, A., *J. Am. Coll. Cardiol.,* 26: 975–982 (1995).
36. Demopoulos, L., Yeh, M., Gentilucci, M., Testa, M., Bijou, R., Katz, S.D., Mancini, D., Jones, M., and LeJemtel, T.H., *Circulation,* 95: 1764–1767 (1997).
37. Rich, M.W., Vinson, J.M. and Sperry, J.C., *J. Gen. Intern. Med.,* 8: 585–590 (1993).
38. Rich, M.W., Becham, V., Wittenberg, C., *N. Engl. J. Med.,* 333: 1190–1195 (1995).
39. Fonarow, G.C., Stevenson, L.W., Walden, J.A., Livingston, N.A., Steimle, A.E., Hamilton, M.A., Moriguchi, J., Tillisch, J.H., and Woo, M.A., *J. Am. Coll. Cardiol.,* 30: 725–732 (1997).
40. West, J.A., Miller, N.H., Parker, K.M., Senneca, D., Ghandour, G., Clark, M., Greenwald, G., Heller, R.S., Fowler, M.B., and DeBusk, R.F., *Am. J. Cardiol.,* 79: 58–63 (1997).

16

Exercise Therapy in Cardiac Transplant Patients

TERENCE KAVANAGH
University of Toronto
Toronto Rehabilitation Centre
Toronto, Ontario, Canada

INTRODUCTION

With 3-, 6-, and 12-year survival rates of approximately 70, 60, and 35% respectively, there is no longer any doubt that cardiac transplantation is the treatment of choice for selected patients in the terminal stage of congestive heart failure. This, together with the fact that the incidence and prevalence of chronic heart failure is on the rise as our population ages, has led to an overall increase in the number of surgical units offering heart transplantation from 21 in 1984 (1) to 297 in 1996 (2). Unfortunately, the availability of donor hearts has become a limiting factor, and currently heart transplantation procedures have plateaued. Nevertheless, given the high survival rates, there is an increasing pool of patients who are potential candidates for exercise rehabilitation.

The transplantation procedure improves both the length and the quality of life, at least when we compare the postsurgical condition with the immediate presurgical state of severe invalidism. On the other hand, it also commits the patient to a lifelong rigorous medical follow-up protocol—one that can seriously strain vocational, family, interpersonal, and social relationships. In addition, severe deconditioning frequently follows months of debilitating ill health. Thus, one can readily appreciate the need for formal postsurgical rehabilitation. This should include not only physical training but also guidance in smoking cessation, a prudent diet, weight control, advice on the effects and side effects of medication, and psychological and vocational counseling. This chapter deals with the exercise training component of rehabilitation as well as relevant aspects of the pathophysiology of the transplanted heart.

PHYSIOLOGY OF THE DENERVATED HEART

Rarely have clinicians and basic scientists been presented with such a fertile common ground as in the field of organ transplantation. In the case of the heart, cardiovascular surgeons have drawn heavily on the work of immunologists, pharmacologists, and applied physiologists.

Orthotopic heart transplantation involves removing the native heart at the level of the atrioventricular junction, leaving an atrial cuff, and transecting the aorta and pulmonary artery just above the semilunar valves. The native atria remain innervated but there is no conduction across the suture line and the donor heart is denervated.

Immediately after surgery, the function of the denervated heart is slightly impaired as a result of myocardial anoxia associated with graft transfer. Right- and left-sided chamber filling pressures are elevated. However, within weeks the myocardium recovers, pulmonary hypertension regresses and the intravascular pressures normalize. Thereafter any significant return to these abnormalities is seen only after the onset of an episode of transplant rejection. The following description therefore pertains to the status of the patient who has recovered from surgery and is free from manifestations of rejection.

In general, resting systolic performance is within normal limits as measured by left ventricular ejection fraction, myocardial contractility, and contractile reserve (3–5). On the other hand, some impairment of diastolic function may persist in the long-term cardiac transplant patient (6). In such cases, there is increased myocardial stiffness resulting in incoordinated contraction and relaxation, possibly the result of repeated episodes of mild rejection, prolonged graft ischaemic time, accelerated coronary atherosclerotic disease or the side effects of immunosuppressant drugs (7,8). This may contribute, at least in some part, to the limited exercise capacity so typical of the heart transplant patient.

The most prominent clinical finding following surgery is the rapid resting heart rate, usually 15–25 beats per minute above that of age- and sex-matched controls (9–13). This is due to the intrinsic rate of the transplanted heart's sinoatrial node, now free from customary vagal inhibition (14,15). The heart rate does not alter in response to the Valsalva manuever, carotid sinus massage, or a change in body position from lying to standing (13). Any minor fluctuations in rate that may occur over a 24-h period are the result of variations in the levels of circulating catecholamines (16,17). The resting tachycardia is associated with a reduced stroke volume to give a normal (18,19) or only mildly impaired (4) cardiac output at rest.

Interpretation of changes in blood pressure responses after transplantation is difficult because both cardiac and peripheral vascular components are involved, and one cannot easily differentiate between the various potential mechanisms. Resting hypertension is a common finding (18). It is characteristically associated with an elevated peripheral vascular resistance; this may be a persistent response to the preoperative state of congestive heart failure and its resultant chronic elevation of plasma norepinephrine (5) or an increased myocardial sensitivity to circulating catecholamines (20,21). However, most authorities now agree that the major cause of hypertension in transplant patients is cyclosporine therapy (22,23). High dosages may be a factor, and some have suggested that the hypertensive effect is increased by the concomitant use of steroids (24,25).

Acute Response to Exercise

While the transplanted heart may perform adequately at rest and during the normal activities of daily living, its limitations become more obvious during a bout of exercise, largely as a result of its denervated state (Fig. 1). Beating at the high

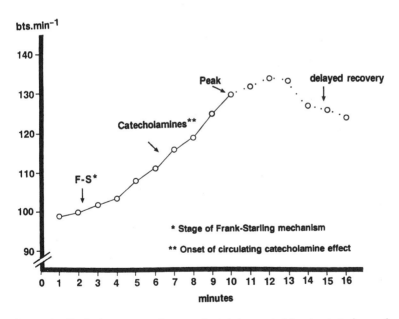

FIGURE 1   Typical response of a transplanted denervated heart rate to increasing effort. Note the high resting rate, the delayed rate of acceleration during effort, the tendency for the rate to continue to rise after the termination of effort (peak exercise), and the delayed deceleration during recovery.

intrinsic rate of the sinoatrial node and lacking any neural influence, it cannot respond to physical exertion by immediate acceleration, as is the case normally. Instead, in the beginning stages of exercise, it relies entirely on the Frank-Starling mechanism to augment cardiac output (11,12,19). Increased venous return results in an elevated left ventricular end-diastolic volume, which in turn results in an increase in stroke volume. With continuing effort, the heart rate, contractility, and ejection fraction increase in response to endogenously released catecholamines and their direct effect on the sinus node and myocardium (12,13,26). The tendency of the heart rate to continue to rise after the cessation of exercise and its tardy return to resting levels in the recovery period mirror the gradual fall in catecholamine concentrations (18,27). Thus, the heart transplant patient may be considered to be sequentially "preload-dependent" during the initial stages of effort and then "catecholamine-dependent" during prolonged exercise, unlike the normal response, in which both events occur simultaneously. The late phase of catecholamine dependency is clearly revealed by the use of β-blockers, which severely attenuate peak heart rate, systolic blood pressure, and exercise capacity (28).

Peak heart rate and peak systolic blood pressure are both reduced to approximately 80% of normal due to the loss of sympathetic stimulation of the sinus node and impairment of myocardial contractility (19,29,30). As a result, both peak rate pressure product and cardiac output are reduced, the latter by approximately 25%. The heart rate reserve ($HR_{max} - HR_{rest}$), normally 90–110 beats per minute, is reduced to 30–50 beats per minute (Table 1).

Peak work rate and oxygen intake are generally reported as being lower in heart transplant patients than in age-matched controls. This is probably due to a combination of central and peripheral limitations. The issue as to the degree to which central or peripheral factors limit exercise has been addressed by Kao and colleagues, who carried out upright exercise on the cycle ergometer on a group of cardiac transplant patients and age-matched controls at 3, 16, 24, and 72 months after surgery (4,6). The patients had a significantly reduced peak work rate, oxygen intake, and cardiac index. Pulmonary capillary wedge, right atrial, and mean pulmonary arterial pressures were elevated. The arteriovenous oxygen difference was 24% lower at peak effort in the transplant group. The authors attributed the limited exercise tolerance to a combination of chronotropic incompetence and diastolic dysfunction, which limited the appropriate compensatory use of the Starling mechanism. They also speculated that there is a peripheral abnormality in oxygen transport or utilization.

Abnormal pulmonary diffusion has been reported in some heart transplant patients (31); this may be due to cyclosporine therapy (32) or the residual effects of congestive heart failure. When present, it could account for at least some part of the reduction in peak oxygen intake (33).

If the reduction in exercise capacity were due to cardiac abnormalities, then

TABLE I   Initial Cardiorespiratory Response of Cardiac Transplant Patients ($N = 36$) and Age-Matched Normal Subjects ($N = 45$)

	Patients	Controls	Discrepancy from normal % of normal value	P value
Peak power output, W	101	219	-54	<0.001
Heart rate$_{rest}$, beats per minute	104	77	$+39$	<0.001
Heart rate$_{peak}$, beats per minute	136	176	-23	<0.001
Heart rate reserve, beats per minute	31	99	-69	<0.001
Systolic BP$_{rest}$, mmHg	138	129	$+7$	<0.001
Systolic BP$_{peak}$, mmHg	178	214	-17	<0.001
Diastolic BP$_{rest}$ mmHg	95	84	$+13$	<0001
Diastolic BP$_{peak}$, mmHg	100	96	$+4$	ns
Rate pressure product $_{peak}$, beats per minute/Hg^{-1}	18	19	-5	<0.001
$\dot{V}_{O_2max}$ml/kg/min^{-1}	22	34	-36	<0.001
Ventilatory threshold L/min	1.18	2.0	-41	<0.001
VE/$\dot{V}_{O_2}$	49.0	37.3	$+32$	<0.001
VE/$\dot{V}_{CO_2submax}$	43.8	33.5	$+36$	<0.001
Cardiac output$_{rest}$, L/min	5.4	5.1	$+6$	n.s.

the heart transplant recipient could be expected to regain full function shortly after surgery. In fact this is not the case, suggesting that the problem may reside in the periphery. As a result, increasing attention has been focused on the role of skeletal muscle. In our experience, the heart transplant patient has a 10–15% reduction in lean body mass, likely the result of a prolonged period of preoperative physical inactivity aggravated by the side effect of immunosuppressant steroid therapy (18). The ensuing weakness would discourage physical activity, leading to further muscle loss, greater weakness, and increasing disinclination to exercise. In fact, Braith and co-workers have demonstrated reduced leg strength in a group of heart transplant recipients and shown that this correlated highly ($R = 0.9$) with the reduction in peak oxygen intake (34).

The preexisting heart failure state is associated with abnormalities in skeletal muscle metabolism, and this may persist for some time after heart transplantation. Abnormalities include a reduced percentage of slow-twitch type I oxidative fibers and a higher percentage of type IIB fast-twitch fibers, a decreased oxidative enzyme activity, and an increased phosphocreatine depletion during exercise, indicating a greater reliance on anaerobic metabolism (35–38). Stratton and colleagues, using magnetic resonance spectroscopy, studied forearm exercise in groups of patients awaiting transplantation, and at approximately 4 and 15 months after surgery (39). Skeletal muscle abnormalities persisted up to 4 months post-transplantation. At 15 months, there was a significant improvement in phospho-creatine resynthesis rate and a trend to improvement in phosphocreatine concen-tration, but these did not reach normal levels. Bussières and coworkers took muscle biopsies from the vastus lateralis muscle in 12 patients at 3 and 12 months postsurgery and found that the ratio of type I to type II fibers did not change. However, cross-sectional area increased by 35% in all fiber types at 12 months, although dimensions still remained below normal. There was no change in the number of capillaries per fiber. Oxidative and glycolytic enzymes increased sig-nificantly at 12 months, as did peak oxygen intake, but the latter still remained less than normal (40).

There is clearly a similarity between the changes seen in skeletal muscle as a result of severe deconditioning and those associated with chronic heart failure (although they do differ in some aspects). This is not surprising, since the latter inevitably leads to a profound reduction in physical activity. Since these changes are only partially reversed by cardiac transplantation, there is a strong case for exercise training as soon as possible after surgery.

The early onset of anaerobiasis gives rise to higher-than-normal lactate levels during submaximal effort, with increased frequency of breathing. The ab-solute ventilatory threshold is lower than normal; but because of the reduced peak oxygen intake, the relative ventilatory threshold is similar to that of age-matched controls.

Evidence for Reinnervation

Early experiments established that, over time, reinnervation could occur in the denervated transplanted dog heart. Naturally, such an outcome in the human heart would be highly desirable, and a number of workers have addressed this issue over the years, only to arrive at the conclusion that the human transplanted heart remains denervated. Nevertheless, there is some evidence that autonomic rein-nervation may occur. Stark and colleagues were the first to report chest pain typical of angina in two cardiac transplantation patients who were subsequently discovered to have developed severe coronary atherosclerosis (41). Both were also found to have significant release of myocardial norepinephrine in response to a tyramine challenge, indicating some level of afferent sympathetic activity. As a result, various techniques have been employed to detect autonomic rein-nervation, including analysis of heart rate variability (42–44), positron emission tomography (45), measurement of myocardial norepinephrine release (46–48), and immunohistochemical examination of myocardial tissue for evidence of neu-ron growth (49). From these, one can conclude that, over a 2- to 8-year period following surgery, (a) there is evidence of limited sympathetic reinnervation in the transplanted heart but that it is inconsistent and (b) there is no evidence of vagal reinnervation. One study, however, suggests that when sympathetic reinnervation does take place, it may confer practical benefit in terms of improved exercise capacity. Lord et al., reported on eight orthotopic heart transplant patients in whom intracoronary injection of tyramine resulted in an increase in heart rate, an associated higher work rate and peak heart rate, and a more rapid recovery rate than in patients in whom response to tyramine was less marked. The authors concluded that sympathetic efferent sinus node reinnervation can occur and can result in an increased exercise time and total work rate, although not to normal levels (50).

Heterotopic Cardiac Transplantation

In heterotopic cardiac transplantation, the donor heart is implanted in the chest and parallel with the recipient heart. The arteries to both sinoatrial nodes are preserved as well as the nerves to the recipient heart but not those to the donor heart. Thus, the donor heart responds to acute exercise in the typically denervated manner but the recipient's heart still exhibits the effects of autonomic innervation. Occasionally there is persistence of anginal pain and/or dysrhythmias in the recipient's left ventricle. Apart from that, these patients share many of the features described for the orthotopic transplant recipient, including a loss of lean tissue, a low peak oxygen intake, and a low peak work output.

   Adoption of the heterotopic procedure has been very limited, with less than 1% of all cardiac transplants being heterotopic in type. Nevertheless, such cases are encountered from time to time, and reference is made below to their responses to an exercise rehabilitation program.

Heart-Lung Transplantation

Some 2000 combined heart-lung transplantation procedures have been carried out worldwide since 1982. The number peaked in 1990 and has declined since then, presumably because of increased use of single- and double-lung transplant procedures. Experience with heart-lung transplantation is less extensive than with cardiac transplantation: the 1-, 5-, and 10-year survival rates are approximately 60, 40, and 20%. Exercise capacity following surgery is restricted in a similar manner to that seen after a heart transplant, and therefore rehabilitation is indicated. In terms of responses to acute exercise, there are few differences from those of the orthotopic heart transplant recipient. Maximal work rate, peak heart rate, peak systolic blood pressure, and peak oxygen intake are all lower than normal, with reductions of the same order as for heart transplant patients. In response to submaximal effort, heart rate, systolic and diastolic blood pressures, and oxygen intake behave similarly in both types of patients. However, there is a tendency for respiratory minute ventilation and respiratory rate to be higher in the heart-lung group, possibly owing to a loss of negative feedback from the pulmonary afferent nerves (30). The slight difference in cardiopulmonary response to acute exercise does not appear to affect exercise training results.

THE EXERCISE PROGRAM

Inpatient

McGregor has recently described the early postoperative rehabilitation measures practiced at the Mayo Clinic (51). With minor variations, a similar regimen is followed in most units. After 24 to 48 h of intensive care monitoring, patients commence the customary breathing, postural, and mobilization exercises. These are carried out twice daily. Intensity of effort is monitored by heart rate (which should not exceed the resting rate by more than 30 beats per minute) and breathing frequency (which should not exceed 30 breaths per minute). Oxygen saturation should not fall below 90%. By the fifth day patients are walking in the ward, and they may then begin to use a cycle ergometer, pedaling at zero resistance for 3 to 5 min at a perceived exertion of 12–14 on the Borg scale (''fairly light'' to ''somewhat hard''). As performance improves, the duration of exercise and the power outputs on the ergometer are increased progressively. Corridor walking is also introduced, and by the time of discharge from hospital, usually about 3 weeks after surgery, a low-level incremental exercise test may be carried out on the cycle ergometer or the treadmill. This test allows for the prescription of a walking or stationary cycling program, which can be carried out during the early (4 to 8 weeks) outpatient phase.

Major concerns during the early postoperative weeks include problems of transplant rejection, infection, arrhythmias in the donor heart, neurological deficits, and renal dysfunction; in addition to intensive clinical monitoring for signs of cardiac rejection, there is also a need for frequent blood tests, serial electrocardiograms, echocardiographic and Doppler assessments of heart size and function, and repeat endomyocardial biopsies. All of these investigations must of necessity take precedence over an exercise rehabilitation program. Nevertheless, an enthusiastic therapist can do much in these weeks to attune the patient's mind to the restorative value of a long-term outpatient rehabilitation regimen.

Outpatient

An exercise training program for the heart transplant patient is no different from that prescribed for other cardiac patients in that the prescription comprises four components: the mode or type of exercise, the intensity, the duration, and the frequency of workouts. The most critical of these variables is exercise intensity, which is gauged from a preliminary exercise test. This can be carried out either on a treadmill or a cycle ergometer. The former test mode is almost standard in North America and the United Kingdom, but the latter remains the method of choice in Europe. Hospital cardiology departments also tend to favor the treadmill and respiratory laboratories the ergometer.

The advantages of the cycle ergometer are that the action is simple to perform and does not arouse anxiety, mechanical efficiency and work rate are largely independent of body mass, and the upper body remains stable, thus making it easier to obtain accurate metabolic and circulatory measurements. A possible disadvantage is early quadriceps fatigue, particularly in those unaccustomed to cycling. The treadmill employs a customary walking motion. However, in the absence of metabolic measurements, the use of the railings for support can reduce the energy cost of a given treadmill speed and slope, thus invalidating tables that relate exercise duration to oxygen intake. Alternatively, preventing the use of the railings for support introduces an element of fear for a severely deconditioned patient.

The protocol varies with the laboratory but in general calls for progressive increments in work rate of 1–2 metabolic equivalents or METs (3.5–7.0 mL/ kg/min^{-1}) until maximal effort is achieved, ideally within 10–14 min. A suitable treadmill protocol has been proposed by Savin; it uses 3-min stages, the first two at 3.2 km/h (2 mph) and then 4.8 km/h (3 mph) at 2.5% grade, with 2.5% increases in grade for each stage thereafter (52). Alternatively, modified Naughton or Bruce protocols can be used (53,54). A common incremental cycle ergometer protocol utilizes power outputs of 17 W (100 kpm/min) every minute or, in the case of the more severely deconditioned individual, 8.5 W (50 kpm/min) (18).

We have investigated the relative merits of progressive treadmill (1 MET increase per minute) and cycle (17 W increase per minute) testing in 12 chronic heart failure patients. Subjects performed two cycle ergometer tests and two treadmill tests at 4-day intervals according to a Latin square design. Neither peak oxygen intake nor ventilatory threshold measurements differed systematically between the two types of test. The patients preferred the cycle ergometer to the treadmill, and collection of expired gas was easier on seated patients (55).

At least during cycle ergometry, oxygen approaches a steady state more rapidly than does heart rate. If an attempt is made to predict maximal oxygen intake from a steady-state submaximal test following heart transplantation, then, because of the delayed exercise heart rate response, the prediction will overestimate $\dot{V}_{O_2max}$ by some 10%. Predictions based on a submaximal rapid progressive protocol give a gross overestimate of $\dot{V}_{O_2max}$. Therefore, direct measurement of oxygen intake at peak power output seems essential for accurate functional evaluation (56).

There has been some debate as to the relative merits of tests that employ rapid work-rate increments to reach peak effort and those using more prolonged stages. Gullestad and coworkers compared 1-min with 3-min stages on the cycle ergometer utilizing the same absolute work rates (57). Peak power output was higher during the 1-min versus the 3-min protocol, but peak heart rate and peak oxygen intake were the same. Olivari et al. compared a standard Naughton protocol with an individualized Naughton protocol, in which the slope of the treadmill at a given test stage was increased only after a steady state in heart rate and oxygen intake had been achieved and maintained for 30 s (58). At peak exercise, heart rate, oxygen intake, oxygen pulse, and minute ventilation were similar with the two protocols. However, at the ventilatory threshold, these measures were significantly higher when using the modified protocol. One can conclude that the more prolonged test gives higher cardiopulmonary values at submaximal levels of effort, whereas there is little difference in physiological response at peak effort.

Whatever the protocol, it is customary to monitor the exercise electrocardiogram continuously, and at every successive work stage the Borg (59) rating of perceived exertion (RPE) and the blood pressure. Expired air is collected and analyzed to measure ventilation, oxygen consumption, and carbon dioxide production. This permits a physiological determination of maximal effort as demonstrated by the achievement of an oxygen plateau—i.e., failure of oxygen intake to rise significantly despite an increase in work rate (60). It also allows measurement of the ventilatory threshold—the level of exertion at which there is a sharp rise in blood lactate—and exercise becomes increasingly anaerobic (61). The ventilatory threshold is usually attainable even by patients who are unable or unwilling to exert maximal effort (62). It is the preferred training intensity for cardiac patients and poorly conditioned subjects and occurs at an oxygen intake of between 50 and 65% of maximal oxygen intake. This relationship has been investigated by Brubaker and colleagues, who compared the invasive (blood lactates) and non-invasive (ventilatory) determination of anaerobic threshold in cardiac transplant patients and normal controls (63). There was no significant difference between the oxygen intake at which the ventilatory and lactate thresholds occurred in heart transplants. The same was true for normals, although the absolute values were higher than in the transplants. Neither was there any difference between the relative oxygen intake (percentage peak) at which lactate threshold and ventilatory threshold occurred in transplants and normals.

Determination of the ventilatory threshold has generally been defined in relation to a number of ventilatory variables. These include, in respect to a progressive increase in oxygen intake, a disproportionate increase in (a) the ventilatory equivalent for oxygen, (b) the minute ventilation, and (c) the carbon dioxide output; the data are expressed in terms of the oxygen intakes at which the upward "breakpoint" of each plot occurs (64–66) (Fig. 2).

In the event that respiratory gas analysis is not carried out, maximal effort

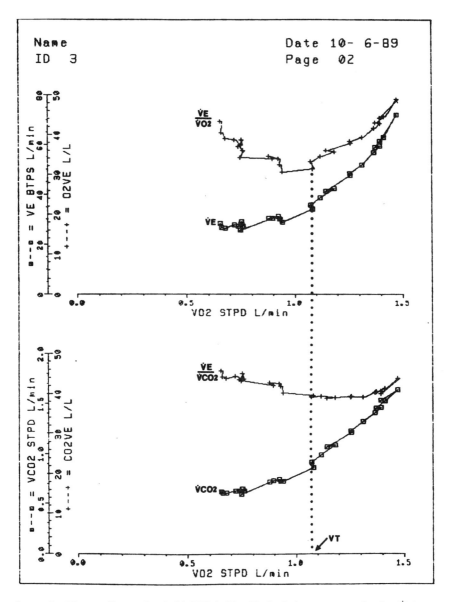

FIGURE 2 The ventilatory threshold (VT) is identified relative to oxygen intake ($\dot{V}_{O_2}$), at the upward inflection of the curves for the ventilatory equivalent for oxygen (VE/$\dot{V}_{O_2}$), the minute ventilation (VE), and the carbon dioxide output $\dot{V}_{CO_2}$). Note that the curve for the ventilatory equivalent for carbon dioxide (VE/$\dot{V}_{CO_2}$) is still flat at the VT.

can be assumed from a subjective rating of 18–20 on the Borg scale of perceived exertion and the ventilatory threshold from a Borg rating of 12–14.

An accelerated form of coronary atherosclerosis develops in a significant number of heart transplant patients (67). Unfortunately, one cannot rely on angina during the test as a symptom of myocardial ischemia. Furthermore, exercise in-duced ST-segment depression is frequently absent, despite angiographic evidence of severe coronary vasculopathy (68). Whether this is due to the typical lower heart rate attained by transplant patients on exercise testing or a difference in pathophysiology between transplant vasculopathy and native coronary athero-sclerosis remains unclear. Particular attention has to be paid, therefore, to the symptoms of dyspnoea, light-headedness, and faintness as well as to the develop-ment of ischemia-related arrhythmias. It is our practice in the Toronto laboratories to monitor the exercise electrocardiogram using three leads (aVF, V_1, and CM_5) (18). For heterotopic transplant recipients we use V_{6R}, V_5, V_1, and aVF; the QRS complex from the donor heart produces the dominant positive vector in V_{6R}, whereas that from the recipient heart produces a dominant positive vector in V_5 and aVF (69) (Fig. 3). As mentioned previously, the heterotopic patient may experience occasional persistence of anginal pain and/or dysrhythmias in the recipient's left ventricle.

Heart rate alone cannot be used to prescribe an intensity of exercise because of its atypical response to effort. The current recommendation is to identify the level of energy expenditure corresponding to the ventilatory threshold (measured directly or estimated from the RPE); this can be expressed, for example, in terms of walking pace, power output on the cycle ergometer, stair stepping cadence, etc.

Factors That May Modify Training

As pointed out previously, the development of hypertension is always a potential problem in the management of heart transplant patients. While there is good evidence that this is a side effect of immunosuppressant cyclosporine therapy, it may also be a persistent response to the preoperative state of congestive heart failure and its resultant chronic elevation of plasma norepinephrine. Braith, com-paring heart transplant patients with normal controls, found plasma norepineph-rine levels to be similar at rest and at an intensity of exercise below the anaerobic threshold (70). However, at intensities above the threshold, norepinephrine levels were significantly greater in the patients than in controls. If neuroendocrine hy-peractivity is a contributor to posttransplant hypertension, then exercise training should help, since it has been shown to reduce catecholamine levels (71) and to have an antihypertensive effect, particularly in hyperadrenergic individuals (72). In any event, a resting systolic blood pressure greater than 210 mmHg or a dia-

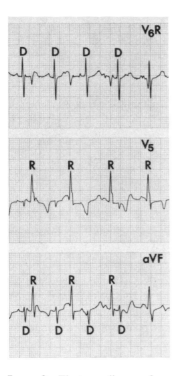

FIGURE 3   Electrocardiogram from a heterotopic cardiac transplantation patient showing separate identification of recipient (R) and donor (D) QRS complexes.

stolic pressure greater than 120 mmHg is a contraindication to exercise testing or training. Furthermore, an exaggerated inotropic exercise response in which the systolic pressure exceeds 260 mmHg or the diastolic pressure exceeds 115 mmHg (73) is enough to preclude entry into a training program, at least until the hypertension is controlled.

Rejection of the graft occurs most frequently in the first 6 months following surgery, affecting some 85% of all heart transplant recipients. Thereafter, the incidence drops. Nevertheless, acute episodes of graft rejection are an ever-present threat; they are detected most accurately by endomyocardial biopsy. Rejection may be accompanied by episodes of ventricular arrhythmias, particularly when there is concurrent coronary artery disease. Again, maintaining the training level at or below the ventilatory threshold should ensure that the arrhythmia threshold is not reached. Major rejection episodes are a contraindication to training. Intercurrent infections due to immunosuppression, particularly cytomegalovirus infection, are another hazard. Despite the formidable list of potential problems, total abstinence from physical activity is seldom required, and even then only for relatively brief interludes.

As mentioned previously, accelerated coronary atherosclerosis is a serious late complication after heart transplantation. By the fifth postoperative year, some 50% of patients show angiographic evidence of this condition. However, angiography may be less sensitive in detecting the form of atherosclerosis peculiar to the transplanted heart—i.e., a diffuse concentric intimal thickening rather than the classic asymmetrical and discrete atherosclerotic plaques (74,75). Anginal pain is absent in the orthotopic recipient with coronary artery disease, so one has to be particularly vigilant for such signs of ischemia as undue exertional breathlessness, light-headedness, and arrhythmias. The exact cause of the condition is unknown, although a likely theory is that it is a manifestation of cell-mediated or humoral immunological injury to the endothelium, with subsequent adhesion of platelets and monocytes, release of cytokines, and the chain of events that leads to occlusive disease (76,77). Some have suggested that it is due to prolonged use of cyclosporine and/or steroids (78), postoperative attacks of cytomegalovirus (79), or repeated bouts of rejection. The Harefield Transplantation Unit reports that the rate of coronary disease is lower in those patients who receive cyclosporine and azathioprine as opposed to those on prednisone and azathioprine (80). The Stanford group found a high association between elevated serum total and low-density-lipoprotein (LDL)-cholesterol levels and graft atherosclerosis, and they have advocated aggressive dietary, and if necessary, drug interventions (81). In support of that approach, a 1-year randomized trial of 97 heart transplant patients, 47 assigned to HMG-CoA reductase (pravastatin) and 50 controls, resulted in a significant reduction in the incidence of coronary disease in the treated group (82). The rehabilitation program will, therefore, pay close attention to serum lipid and glucose levels and will provide the necessary education to those who have problems in these areas.

From the viewpoint of exercise training, the transplant team's attitude toward the use of steroids as part of the postoperative immunosuppressant regimen is important. The long-term side effects of high-dosage oral steroids—which include osteoporosis, increased risk of infection, and adverse effects on glucose and lipid metabolism—can constitute problems during a prolonged training program. To date, the majority of transplant patients trained by the author's team have been receiving the customary Harefield immunosuppressant drug regimen, which utilizes cyclosporine in dosages sufficient to maintain a serum level of 100–200 nm/ml after the first month and azathioprine in the dosage of 2 mg/kg per day. Oral steroids are not used routinely, but they are used temporarily if the patient has recurrent or persistent rejection or develops post-operative renal dysfunction. Certainly this approach has certainly been associated with a successful use of a vigorous and effective training program. On the other hand, patients taking the more conventional dosage of prednisone have also benefited from training, although their progress has been slower.

Benefits of Exercise Training

Historically, cardiac exercise rehabilitation had its origins in the 1960s, with the care of the survivor of acute myocardial infarction. Since then, the spectrum of patients has broadened to include a variety of cardiac conditions. Heart transplant patients were not considered for such treatment until the early 1980s; consequently the number of reports dealing with the effects of exercise training in these individuals has been limited (Table 2). The earliest report was from Squires and coworkers, who demonstrated that the training regimen could be both effective and safe (83). Since that time there have been 12 reports (84–93). Of these, 10 have dealt with orthotopic transplant recipients, with only two devoted to patients who have undergone the far less common heterotopic procedure.

In the Toronto program, the initial exercise prescription calls for patients to cover a distance of 1.6 km five times weekly. The intensity or pace of the walk is based on 60% of peak oxygen intake, supported by the oxygen intake level at which the ventilatory threshold is determined, and a perceived exertion of 12–14 on the Borg scale. This usually results in an initial walking pace of between 11 and 14 min per kilometer. The distance is then increased by 1.6 km every 2 weeks, maintaining the same pace until, by 6 weeks, the patient is walking 4.8 km five times weekly. The pace is then quickened by 1 min/1.6 km until the 4.8 km is accomplished in 45 min (typically within 4 months of starting the program). Thereafter, 50-m bouts of slow jogging, paced at 7.5 min/km, are introduced at the start of every 800 m, then every 400 m, 200 m, 100 m, and so on, until ultimately the entire 4.8 km is completed in 36 min. Finally, the more highly motivated and compliant individuals are progressed to 6.4 km, or 32 km weekly, maintaining the same pace of 7.5 min/km. After the first 6 weeks, if the patient "sticks" at a given pace, then the exercise prescription is adjusted so as to obtain a training session which would last from 30 to 60 min.

Accurate pacing is emphasized, as well as thorough familiarity with the concept of perceived exertion, and correct interpretation of such symptoms of myocardial ischemia as excessive dyspnea, unusual fatigue, light-headedness, and extrasystoles. Rejection episodes or intercurrent infections may interrupt the training program from time to time, and patients should be advised of this possibility at the outset.

Initially, some patients may need regular supervision or even electrocardiographic monitoring during the exercise sessions, but these are a minority. Most will be able to train at home without risk, attending a supervised class only once a week or even once monthly. During the first 6–12 months there are frequent return visits to the transplant unit or the local hospital for routine follow-up test-

TABLE 2 Exercise Training After Cardiac Transplantation—Published Reports

Authors	No. of patients	Procedure	Exercise training protocol	Duration of training	Intensity of training	Benefits of training
Squires et al., 1983 (83)	2	Orthotopic	Treadmill walking and stationary cycling, 30 min., 2–3× weekly	8 weeks	12–14 RPE	Systolic BP↓, Borg RPE↓ at equivalent submax. work rates
Savin et al., 1983 (84)	5	Orthotopic	Cycling, 30 min, 5× weekly	16 weeks	≥75% peak heart rate	Peak: work rate↑, O_2 intake↑ Submax: HR↓
Sieurat et al., 1986 (85)	8	Heterotopic	Walking, calisthenics, stationary cycling	60 days	% (?) max heart rate	Peak work rate↑
Degré et al., 1986 (86)	3 2	Orthotopic controls	Cycle ergometer, 30 min, 3× weekly	5 months	60–80% exercise capacity	Peak: O_2 intake↑, work rate↑, respiratory equivalent for O_2↓ Submax: minute ventilation ↓, respiratory equivalent for oxygen↓
Niset et al., 1988 (87)	62	Orthotopic	Walking, cycling, calisthenics, 30 min, 5× weekly	12 months	30–50% of walking capacity	Peak: work rate↑, O_2 intake↑, HR↑, systolic BP↑, RER↓, respiratory equivalent for O_2↓ Submax: RER↓, respiratory equivalent for O_2↓, ventilation↓, breathing frequency↓
Kavanagh et al., 1988 (18)	36	Orthotopic	20 min stretching and warm up, 10 min cool-down, walk/jog, 5× weekly	24 months	Ventilatory threshold, 50–60% $\dot{V}_{O_2max}$ 12–14 RPE	Resting: lean body mass↑, HR↓, systolic BP↓, diastolic BP↓ Submax: HR↓,[a] diastolic BP↓, minute ventilation↓, RPE↓, VT (absolute)↑ Maximal: HR↑, work rate↑, O_2 intake↑, minute ventilation↑, systolic BP↑, diastolic BP↓

Study	n	Transplant	Protocol	Duration	Intensity	Results
Kavanagh et al., 1989 (69)	10	Heterotopic	20 min stretching and warm-up, 10 min cool-down; walk/jog, 5× weekly	18 months	Ventilatory threshold 50–60% $\dot{V}_{O_2,max}$, 12–14 RPE	Peak work rate↑, peak O_2 intake↑, absolute ventilatory threshold↑, training bradycardia achieved in native heart
Keteyian et al., 1990 (88)	19	Orthotopic	5 min warm-up, 32 min of aerobic circuit training (treadmill, stationary cycling, rowing machine, arm ergometer, stair-stepping, 3× weekly)	8 weeks	12–14 RPE	Peak work rate↑, peak HR↑, peak O_2 intake↑
Keteyian et al., 1991 (89)	12 patients (5 controls)	All orthotopic	As above, 3× weekly	10 weeks	12–14 RPE	Peak work rate↑, peak O_2 intake↑, peak HR↑
Ehrman et al., 1992 (90)	11	Orthotopic	As above, 3× weekly	10 weeks	12–14 RPE	Peak O_2 intake↑, peak HR↑, absolute ventilatory threshold↑
Daida et al., 1996 (91)	17 / 17	Orthotopic / Controls (CABG patients)	Phase II rehab (treadmill and stationary cycle, 40 min, 3× weekly); then home exercise (walk, cycle, swim, 30–45 minutes, ≥3× weekly)	6–8 weeks → 1 year	12–14 RPE / 12–14 RPE	At 3 and 12 months peak O_2 intake↑, peak HR↑, but to lesser extent than in CABG patients.
Geny et al., 1996 (92)	7	Orthotopic	Stationary cycle, 45 min, 3× weekly	6 weeks	50–90% of peak work rate	Peak work rate↑, peak O_2 intake↑, resting HR↓, max lactates↓, max norepinephrine↓[ns]
Lampert et al., 1996 (93)	8	Orthotopic	Stationary cycle, 45 min, 3× weekly	6 weeks	80–85% peak heart rate	Peak power output↑, peak O_2 intake↑, exercise blood lactates↓

Key: BP = blood pressure; RPE = rating of perceived exertion; HR = heart rate; RER = respiratory exchange ratio; CABG = coronary artery bypass graft.
[a]Highly compliant patients.

ing, and this gives ample opportunity for the appropriate rehabilitation team to carry out exercise testing and to assess the patient's progress and adherence to the training regimen.

Response to Exercise Training

There is general agreement that an aerobic type of training program can result in significant improvement in cardiopulmonary fitness. Heart transplant patients compete regularly in the World Transplant Games; some have taken part in long-distance runs, from 20-km (94) to the 42-km marathon (95). Peak oxygen intake is increased, and the onset of anaerobiasis is delayed; the latter is reflected in an increase in the absolute ventilatory threshold and a reduction in blood lactates at equivalent submaximal work rates. A decrease in resting and submaximal heart rates has also been reported, together with an increase in maximal rate-pressure product, the extent of these changes depending to some degree on the intensity and duration of the training program. The shorter programs have all resulted in appreciable gains in cardiorespiratory fitness, but the reduction in resting heart rate and an increase in lean body mass have been noted only after a longer training period, as was reported by the Toronto/Harefield program. There have been no reports of a training-induced change in cardiac dimensions or function. All programs used a training intensity corresponding to 12–14 on the Borg rating scale of perceived exertion the ventilatory threshold, and/or 50–70% of peak oxygen intake.

In the author's experience, much of the training effect is due to an increase in lean body mass or an improved skeletal muscle metabolism. Braith and colleagues have reported a correlation between leg strength and peak oxygen intake in heart transplant recipients (34) and have also demonstrated the beneficial effect of biweekly sessions of resistance training for 6 months on steroid-induced bone loss (96). Horber and coworkers have demonstrated that renal transplant patients responded well to a isokinetic training program regimen, with an improvement in strength and cardiorespiratory fitness (97). Thus, there is a strong argument for the use of a muscle strength training regimen, either in association with aerobic training or alone, following heart transplantation. To date, there have been no published reports of such an approach.

CONCLUSIONS

The routine use of a comprehensive exercise rehabilitation program following heart transplantation is a safe and effective way to maximize the benefits of surgery. Published studies have shown that an exercise rehabilitation program can induce a good training effect, although complete restoration of physiological function may not be possible. However, the prescription of exercise must take into account the denervated heart's peculiar response to effort and must rely on perceived exertion and metabolic measurements rather than on target heart rates for defining the intensity of training.

It is tempting to speculate as to whether a comprehensive rehabilitation program that includes not only exercise training (resistive as well as aerobic) but also dietary advice for lipid and weight control might favorably influence long-term prognosis.

REFERENCES

1. Kaye, M.P., *Heart Transplant.,* III: 278–279 (1984).
2. Hosenpud, J.D., Bennett, L.E., Berkeley, M.K., Fiol, B., Novick, R.J. *J. Heart Lung Transplant.,* 16: 691–712 (1997).
3. Tischler, M.D., Lee, R.T., Plappert, T., Mudge, G.H., St. John Sutton, M., and Parker, J.D., *J. Am. Coll. Cardiol.,* 19: 60–66 (1992).
4. Kao, A.C., Van Tright III, P., Shaeffer-McCall, G.S., Shaw, J.P., Kuzil, B.B., Page, R.D. and Higginbotham, M.B., *Circulation,* 89: 2605–2615 (1994).
5. Borow, K.M., Neumann, A., Arensman, F.W., and Yacoub, M.H., *Circulation,* 71: 866–872 (1985).
6. Kao, A.C., Van Tright III, P., Shaeffer-McCall, G.S., Shaw, J.P., Kuzil, B.B., Page, R.D., and Higginbotham, M.B., *J. Heart Lung Transplant.,* 14: 11–22 (1995).
7. Hausdorf, G., Banner, N.R., Mitchell, A., Khaghani, A., Martin, M., and Yacoub, M., *Br. Heart J.* 62: 123–132 (1989).
8. Paulus, W.J., Bronzwaer, J.G.F., Felice, H., Kishan, N., and Wellens, F., Deficient acceleration of left ventricular relaxation during exercise after heart transplantation. *Circulation,* 86: 1175–1185 (1992).
9. Beck, W., Barnard C.N., and Schrire, V., *Am. J. Physiol.,* 218: 475–484 (1969).
10. Carleton, R.A., Heller, S.J., Najaf, H., and Clark, J.G., *Circulation,* 40: 447–452 (1969).
11. Campeau, L., Pospisil, L., Grondin, P., Dydra, I., and LePage, G., *Am. J. Cardiol.,* 25: 523–528 (1970).
12. Pope, S.E., Stinson, E.B., Daughters, G.T., Schroeder, J.S., Ingels, N.B., and Alderman, E.L., *Am. J. Cardiol.,* 46: 213–218 (1978).
13. Yusuf, S.A., Mitchell, A., and Yacoub, M.H., *Br. Heart. J.,* 54: 173–178 (1985).
14. de Marneffe, M., Jacobs, P., Haaradt, R., and Englert, E., *Eur. Heart J.,* 7: 662–672 (1986).
15. Jose, A., and Collison, D., *Cardiovasc. Res.,* 4: 160–167 (1970).
16. Bernardi, L., Keller, R., Sanders, M., Reddy, P.S., Griffith, B., Meno, F., and Pinsky, M.R., *J. Appl. Physiol.,* 67: 1447–1455 (1989).
17. Alexopoulos, D., Yusuf, S., Johnston, J.A., Bostock, J., Sleight, P., and Yacoub, M.H., *Am. J. Cardiol.,* 61: 880–884 (1988).

18. Kavanagh, T., Yacoub, M., Mertens, D.J., Kennedy, J., Campbell, R.B., and Sawyer, P., *Circulation.*, 1: 162–171 (1988).

19. Pflugfelder, P.W., Purves, P.D., McKenzie, F.N., and Kostuk, W.J., *J. Am. Coll. Cardiol.*, 10: 336–341 (1987).

20. Dempsey, P.J., and Cooper, T., *Am. J. Physiol.* 215: 1245–1249 (1968).

21. Yusuf, S., Theodoropoulos, S., Mathias, C.J., Dhalla, N., Wittes, J., Amitchell, A., and Yacoub, M., *Circulation,* 75: 696–704 1987.

22. Bantle, J.P., Nath, K.A., Sutherland, D.E.R., Najaran, J.E.S., and Ferris, T.F., *Arch. Intern. Med.,* 145: 505–508 (1985).

23. Thompson, M.E., Shapiro, A.P., Johnsen, A.M., Reeves, R., Itzkoff, J., Ginchereau, E., Hardesty, R.L., Griffith, B.L., Bahnson, H.T., and McDonald, R. Jr., *Transplant. Proc.,* 15: 2573–2577 (1983).

24. Jarowenko, M.V., Flechner, S.M., Van Buren, C.T., Lorber, M.I., and Kahan, B.D., *Am. J. Kidney Dis.,* 10: 98–103 (1987).

25. Loughran, T.P. Jr., Deeg, H.J., Dahlberg, S., Kennedy, M.S., Storb, R., and Thomas, E.D., *Br. J. Hematol.,* 59: 547–553 (1985).

26. Perini, R., Orizio, C., Gamba, A., and Veicsteinas, A., Eur. J. Appl. Physiol., 66: 500–506 (1993).

27. Schuler, S., Thomas, D., Thebken, M., Frei, U., Wagner, T., Warnecke, H., and Hetzer, R., *Transplant. Proc.,* 19: 2506–2509 (1987).

28. Bexton, R.S., Milne, J.R., Cory-Pearce, R., English, T.A.H., and Camm, A.J., *Br. Heart J.,* 49: 584–588 (1983).

29. Banner, N.R., Lloyd, M.H., Hamilton, R.D., Innes, J.A., Guz, A., and Yacoub, M.H., *Br. Heart J.,* 61: 215–223 (1989).

30. Quigg, R.J., Rocco, M.B., Gauthier, D.F., Creager, M.A., Hartley, L.H., and Colucci, W.S., *J. Am. Coll. Cardiol.,* 14: 338–344 (1989).

31. Braith R.W., Limacher, M.C., Mills, R.M., Leggett, S.H., Pollock, M.L., and Staples, G.D., *J. Am. Coll. Cardiol.,* 22: 767–776 (1993).

32. Casan, P., Sanchis, J., Cladellas, M., Amengual, M.J., and Caralps, J.M., *Heart Transplant.,* 6: 54–56 (1987).

33. Kraemer, M.D., Kubo, S.H., Rector, T.S., Brunsvold, N., and Denk, A.J., *J. Am. Coll. Cardiol.,* 21: 641–648, (1993).

34. Braith, R.W., Limacher, M.C., Leggett, S.H., and Pollock, M.L., *J. Heart Lung. Transplant.,* 12: 1018–1023 (1993).

35. Mancini, D.M., Coyle, E., Coggan, A., Beltz, J., Ferraro, N., Montain, S., and Wilson, J.R., *Circulation* 80: 1338–1346 (1989).

36. Sullivan, M.J., Green, H.G., and Cobb, F.R., *Circulation,* 81: 518–527 (1990).

37. Drexler, H., Riede, U., Münzel, T., König, H., Funke, E., and Just, H., *Circulation,* 85: 1751–1759 (1992).

38. Sullivan, M.J., Green, H.G., and Cobb, F.R., *Circulation,* 84: 1597–1607 (1991).

39. Stratton, J.R., Graham, J.K., Daly, R.C., Yacoub, M., and Rajagopalan, B., *Circulation,* 89: 1624–1631 (1994).

40. Bussieres, L.M., Pflugfelder, P.W., Taylor, A.W., Noble, E.G., and Kostuk, W.J., *Am. J. Cardiol.,* 78: 630–634 (1997).

41. Stark, R.P., McGinn, A.L., and Wilson, R.F., *N. Engl. J. Med.,* 324: 1791–1794 (1991).

89. Keteyian, S., Shepard, R., Ehrman, J., Fedel, F., Glick, C., Rhoads, K., and Levine, T.B., *J. Appl. Physiol.,* 70: 2627–2631 (1991).
90. Ehrman, J., Keteyian, S., Fedel, F., Rhoads, K., Levine, B., and Shepard, R., *J. Cardiopulm. Rehab.,* 12: 126–130 (1992).
91. Daida, H., Squires, R.W., Allison, T.G., Johnson, B.D., and Gau, G.T., *Am. J. Cardiol.,* 77: 696–700 (1996).
92. Geny, B., Saini, J., Mettauer, B., Lampert, E., Piquard, F., Follenius, M., Epailly, E., Schnedecker, B., Eisenmann, B., Haberey, P., and Lonsdorfer, J., *Eur. J. Appl. Physiol.,* 73: 259–266 (1996).
93. Lampert, E., Oyono-Enguéllé, S., Mettauer, B., Freund, H., and Lonsdorfer, J., *Med. Sci. Sports Exerc.* 28: 801–807 (1996).
94. Niset, G., Poortmans, J.R., Leclerq, R., Brasseur, M., Desmet, J.M., Degré, S., and Primo, G., *Int. J. Sports Med.,* 6: 340–343 (1985).
95. Kavanagh, T., Yacoub, M., Campbell, R., and Mertens, D., *J. Cardiopulm. Rehab.,* 6: 16–20 (1986).
96. Braith, R.W., Mills, R.M., Welsch, M.A., Keller, J.W., and Pollock, M.L., *J. Am. Coll. Cardiol.,* 28: 1471–1477 (1996).
97. Horber, F.F., Scheidegger, J.R., Grunig, B.F., and Frey, F.J., *J. Clin. Endocrinol. Metab.,* 6: 83–88 (1985).

17
Exercise and Hypertension

Charles M. Tipton
University of Arizona
Tucson, Arizona

INTRODUCTION

When Stephen Hales recorded the height of a pulsating column of arterial blood in a conscious mare in 1733 (1), little did he realize that 265 years later, a ''high'' blood pressure value would be of major importance to the health of the people of the world and especially to the population in the United States. Despite the progress that has been made in recent decades in reducing the number of individuals who have elevated arterial blood pressure (2,3), approximately one in four individuals over the age of 18 years in the United States have pressures that equal or exceed 140 mmHg systolic and 90 mmHg diastolic (2,4). Translated into numbers, approximately 50 million Americans are hypertensive (2). Using the standards from the fifth report of the Joint National Committee on Detection, Evaluation, and Treatment of High Blood Pressure (JNCV) (5), these values would be classified as stage I, hypertensive (Table 1). Beside a concern for prevalence per se, hypertension is a major contributor to atherosclerotic cardiovascular disease because it enhances atherogenesis, which encompasses coronary heart disease. With cardiovascular diseases continuing to be the nation's number one cause of death (2) and the disease of hypertension being closely associated (clustered) with familial background; dyslipidemia; insulin resistance; glucose intolerance; obesity; ventricular hypertrophy; consumption of calories, electrolytes, and alcohol; plus physical inactivity (3,5,6) it is not surprising that a large percentage of funding for cardiovascular and metabolic diseases is related to hypertension research and for educational outcomes (3). Since 20% or less of the individuals classified as hypertensive will exhibit manifestations of elevated arterial blood pressure (2), it is understandable that hypertension has been categorized as a

Table I Classification of Resting Blood Pressure Values for Children and Adults
Mean Values and 95th Percentiles for Children and Adolescents

Age	Mean: Males	95th	Mean: Females	95th
6	96/57	116/74	96/57	115/73
9	101/61	119/77	100/61	119/77
12	107/64	126/81	107/65	126/82
15	114/65	133/83	111/68	130/86
18	121/70	140/88	113/66	132/85

Category, adults	Systolic in mmHg	Diastolic in mmHg
Normal	<130	<85
High normal	130–139	85–89
Hypertension		
Stage 1	140–159	90–99
Stage 2	150–179	100–109
Stage 3	180–209	110–119
Stage 4	≥210	≥120

Sources: The data on children and adolescents were modified from NIH sources and the results of a task force to study blood pressure in children as published by Daniels and Loggie (92), while the information on adults was published in The Fifth Report of the Joint National Commitee on Detection, Evaluation and Treatment of High Blood Pressure [(JNC-V)(5)].

cardiovascular-metabolic disease risk factor requiring multifaceted approaches to investigate responsible mechanisms or to initiate management procedures that attempt to "normalize" resting blood pressure (3). Unlike most diseases, hypertension is a "silent condition" that can best be detected by measurement, and, despite the dedicated efforts of health educators, approximately 31% of the hypertensivive population are unaware of their status (2). For unexplained reasons, hypertensive populations are predisposed to unrecognized myocardial infarction with a 45% incidence rate for women and a 35% value for men (2). Consequently, ignorance is not bliss for a hypertensive individual.

Consistent with previous reports, arterial blood pressure increases with age. For example, in the Framingham Study, average increases in systolic and diastolic blood pressures for individuals between the ages of 30 to 65 years were 20 and 10 mmHg, respectively (2). Moreover, for women, the values for systolic blood pressures continued to increase into their eighth decade, whereas for men, this trend persisted until they were in their 70s. However, this profile did not occur with diastolic pressure, presumably because of a loss in arterial vessel compliance, and resulted in many individuals being classified as having isolated systolic hypertension (2). Besides age, there are ethnic, gender, and behavioral considerations. Specifically, the incidence of hypertension is 32.4% for non-Hispanic blacks, 23.3% for non-Hispanic whites, and 22.6% for Mexican Americans (4).

Although the percent differences were not large, the prevalence of hypertension was consistently higher in men as when compared to women. When compared with the two other groups, markedly lower percentages of Mexican Americans were aware that they were hypertensive, were being treated for elevated blood pressure, or had achieved normalization of their resting pressures. If we consider the statistic that approximately half of the treated hypertensive population will achieve normalization and couple that fact with the high percentage (31%) of individuals who are unable or unwilling to be evaluated for the presence of hypertension, it becomes apparent that economic factors must also be included in any initiative designed to manage the disease.

Overview

As noted earlier, impressive changes have occurred in recent decades in the detection, treatment, management, and education of hypertension. As far as exercise is concerned, it was not until recent times that exercise has been included as an important component in the "hypertension story" (3). However, it is gratifying to exercise physiologist that this fact has been repeatedly emphasized in recent reports, proceedings, and meetings of national and international scientific groups and societies (7–10). The focus of this chapter is on experimental and clinical findings that best define the role of exercise in the diagnosis, management, and in the possible prevention of hypertension, and the reader is encouraged to consult relevant review manuscripts on the subject (9,10).

Definition

Although we previously defined exercise as the disruption of physiological homeostasis by physical movements (11), the definition was too esoteric for functional purposes. Experts at the NIH Consensus Conference defined exercise as "a type of physical activity" that is "a planned, structured, and repetitively bodily movement done to improve or maintain one or more components of physical fitness" (7). However, they failed to emphasize that there are two categories of exercise; namely, acute and chronic. The former relates the physiological responses that occur with a single bout of exercise whereas the latter describes the responses that occur during a single bout of exercise by a human or animal that has a history of repeated bouts, or physical training. To illustrate, heart rate will increase with acute exercise at a given power condition, but the increase will be less in an individual or animal with a history of chronic exercise (training). The types of muscle contractions necessary to execute movement also categorize exercise. If contraction occurs with little detectable shortening of muscles, it is labeled *isometric;* whereas if shortening (concentric) or lengthening (eccentric) occurs in muscles, there is tendency to assume the tension to be the same and the process is called *isotonic* (12). In the past, many authors have used the terms *static exercise* for isometric exercise and *dynamic exercise* for movements caused by isotonic contractions. These distinctions are relevant because isometric contractions elicit greater pressor responses than isotonic ones and because the exercise prescription for hypertensive populations will emphasize activities that require concentric and eccentric contractions and minimize those that are isometric in nature. Since there is a propensity of health and clinical educators to use terminology that is "user friendly," the energy expenditure associated with exercise has been metabolically categorized as being aerobic or anaerobic in nature, the inferences being that at times we will utilize oxygen and at other times we will not. Actually, both processes are occurring in the complex chemical reactions in cells; but, their relationships are such that aerobic reactions predominate at rest. However, with exercise that becomes more strenuous with time, their relationships change and more anaerobic reactions and their metabolic products occur, resulting in the descriptive terms of *aerobic* and *anaerobic* exercise. *Resistive exercise* is also used in texts and in lay publications to describe physical activities that are similar to weight lifting. Not only is the load "heavy," the execution of the movement requires a high percentage of isometric contractions along with concentric and eccentric contractions. In such situations, the pressor response can be quite high; hence, resistive exercises have not been recommended for the hypertensive or the hypertensive prone or individuals with high risk factors for cardiovascular disease (3). When targeted groups who prefer weight lifting to aerobic activities have ignored this advice, the results have not been as dire as predicted (12).

Components of the Exercise Prescription

The value of exercise for the hypertensive loses its effectiveness if the individual is not cognizant of or fails to follow the principles of the exercise prescription. As in the case of the familiar pharmaceutical prescription, the most important principle is the one of specificity (11); meaning that the exercise performed must be specific and effective in modifying the blood pressure response. Unless there are documented reports that the exercise being performed will be associated with either lower or higher pressures, the exercise being prescribed is nonspecific and changes in the prescription are needed. It is possible that the *intensity (dosage)* of exercise is insufficient to elicit physiological adaptations or that the weekly *frequency* of the exercise being performed is too irregular for meaningful changes to occur. Coupled with the prescription is the *duration* of the exercise being performed, and it is conceivable that negative results are reported because the time devoted for the disruption of the various physiological systems is too brief for any changes to be observed. When the term *mode* is used, it is employed to denote whether the recommended activity is swimming, running, cycling, walking, gardening, stair climbing, etc. But the key for success in the use of exercise in the management of hypertension, and for the application of the exercise prescription, is measurement, and any attempt to minimize or eliminate its importance is a lesson in futility. The three most important measurements are resting blood pressure, exercise blood pressure, and the maximal response to exercise. For the latter, the maximal consumption of oxygen ($\dot{V}_{O_2max}$test) during a progressive exercise test is strongly recommended, although maximal heart rates are a practical substitute (8). Maximal oxygen consumption can be elicited by treadmill or by leg and arm ergometer tests. Because of the muscle mass involved, the treadmill is the recommended procedure to follow. Moreover, arm movement tests are discouraged because they elicit a higher pressor response at given power condition than leg movements (12).

Although it may be unnecessary to stress the point, it is prudent to remind readers that hypertensive populations are diseased individuals; hence their exercise prescriptions and expectations should differ from those of normotensive subjects. In a recent review of the exercise performance of hypertensive patients, Lim and associates concluded their exercise capacity was reduced by as much as 30%. When compared to age-matched controls (13). Not unexpectedly, the reduction increased with age and end-organ damage. Interestingly, they concluded the impairment could be traced back to an adolescent origin.

Acute Exercise

Summarized in Fig. 1 are blood pressure profiles of normotensive and hypertensive individuals performing an exercise test. Although detailed explanations are available concerning relevant mechanisms, (3,14,15), the following descriptive relationships best describe the relevant functions of the cardiovascular system that are occurring (15,16).

1. Mean blood pressure ($\overline{X}BP$) = cardiac output ($\dot{Q}$) × total peripheral resistance (TPR)
2. TPR = $\overline{X}BP/\dot{Q}$
3. $\dot{Q}$ = heart rate (HR) × stroke volume (SV)
4. $\overline{X}BP$ = diastolic blood pressure (DBP) + [0.333 (systolic blood pressure − DBP)]
5. Flow (F) = (change in blood pressure) $\pi R4/ 8$ × length of vessel × viscosity of blood
6. Maximum oxygen consumption ($\dot{V}_{O_2max}$) = oxygen consumption/ arterial oxygen content − venous oxygen content × 100

Consequently, blood pressure will be elevated with exercise because cardiac output is increased while total peripheral resistance is decreased. Heart rate,

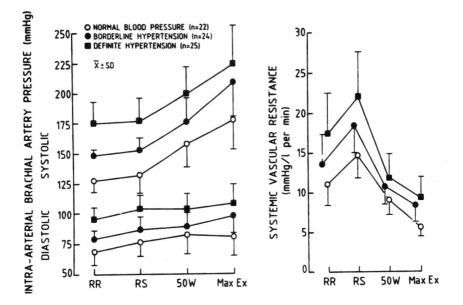

FIGURE I   Interarterial sytolic and diastolic pressures of normotensive, stage I hypertensive (borderline), and stage II hypertensive subjects during rest and during submaximal
and maximal exercise as performed on a cycle ergometer. Also shown are changes in
systemic vascular resistance RR = supine rest; RS = siting rest; W = 50-W exercise;
Max Ex = Maximal exercise. (From Ref. 14, with permission.)

oxygen consumption, and oxygen extraction will increase as the intensity of exercise (power) increases, while stroke volume will increase until approximately
50% of $\dot{V}_{O_2max}$ is reached, when it will begin to plateau (11,16). Systolic blood
pressure will increase with the intensity of exercise, while diastolic pressure will
exhibit modest changes. An example of interarterial changes in blood pressure
can be found in Fig. 1 (14).

Acute Exercise, Sudden Death, and the Detection of Hypertension

It is important to acknowledge that acute exercise will be associated with an
increased incidence of sudden death. Estimates of sudden cardiac death rates per
100,000 h of exercising range from 0 to 2.0 per 100,000 in the general population
and from 0.13 to 0.61 per 100,000 in cardiac rehabilitation programs (17). Moreover, it has been reported that for select individuals, an elevated pressor responses
during graded exercise will be identified with an elevated rate of cardiovascular
deaths (18). While a statistical reality and an argument advanced by skeptics of

exercise training programs for hypertensive populations (18), the probability is quite low and insufficient to support a position of non-exercise by individuals prone to hypertension or who are hypertensive.

The issue of whether exercise stress testing would be a useful diagnostic procedure to identify individuals with a propensity for hypertension is not new; in fact it was suggested almost 80 years ago (19). If the magnitude of the blood pressure response at a certain power condition or the slope of the pressure response during the test would reveal notable differences as compared with appropriate normotensive controls, this information would be extremely valuable to physicians performing the evaluation. Using this logic with children 8–10 years whose systolic blood pressures placed them higher than the 95th percentile, exercise testing did not reveal significant differences when comparisons were made with age-matched controls whose pressure values were lower than the 95th percentile (20). But when normotensive children have hypertensive parents, their systolic blood pressures with exercise were significantly exaggerated when the results were contrasted with age-matched normotensive children from normotensive parents (13). Lauer and coworkers reported in a 5-year follow up study in Muscatine, Iowa, that children who exhibited higher resting and exercise blood pressure responses would have a greater risk of becoming hypertensive than their normotensive controls (21). Although it has been hypothesized that children with a "hyperkinetic circulation" (higher cardiac index and heart rate with a normal stroke index and a normal TPR at rest in the supine position) would exhibit a propensity for hypertension that would be revealed during exercise testing, this hypothesis has not been confirmed (13). Fixler and coworkers conducted an interesting study in the Dallas, Texas, schools to determine whether the exercise testing of 16-year-old students with elevated resting pressures would be useful to predict the presence of hypertension 2 years later and whether the procedure [cycle ergometer and a hand-grip isometric contraction equal to 25% maximum (25% MVC)] would be useful in determining whether an individual should be allowed to participate in competitive athletics. From their results, they concluded the two exercise approaches were not helpful in identifying future hypertensives, but the testing was useful in determining whether a hypertensive high school student should participate in competitive athletics (22). In exercise testing investigations with young men or women (19 years of age) considered to be borderline hypertensives (Table 1), the results, when compared with those from normotensive controls, were not convincing enough to justify a view of exercise testing being superior to the use of resting values to identify a future hypertensive state (23). It was of interest that earlier they reached the same conclusion with men. Lim and associates reviewed several studies involving adults that used absolute systolic blood pressures of 200 mmHg or higher as "markers" for identifying future hypertensives from 1 to 14 years later; the procedure was able to identify from 11 to 40% of those who became classified as hypertensive (13). Benbassat and From evaluated 11 studies on the role of exercise testing as a predictor of hypertension. Even though the prevalence of hypertension among normotensive subjects who exhibited exaggerated pressor responses was 2.1 to 3.4 times higher than among individuals with normal responses, the variability of the responses and the wide percentage range (38–89%) of subjects with exaggerated values who did not exhibit evidence for hypertension from 0.5 to 15 years later forced the authors to conclude that exercise testing procedures for pressure responses had limited value as a predictor for hypertension (24).

Using subjects between the ages of 28 and 79 years and following their blood pressure changes during treadmill exercise and hand-grip dynamometer tests over a 14-year period, Chaney and Eyman reported that the best predictors of future hypertension were resting diastolic blood pressure, the hand-grip strength result, and the diastolic blood pressure values recorded during the treadmill test (25). Although Canadian fitness authorities believe that their bench-stepping testing procedures are effective predictors of future hypertension, they wait 30 s after the termination of the test before recording pressure changes which is a time interval when marked decreases in pressure are occurring (26). Tanji and associates used a stepping procedure to assess its merit for predicting hypertension in normotensive subjects over a 10-year period. At the onset, 43% of the 26 subjects had peak pressures that exceeded 200 mmHg and a decade later 10 were hypertensive, whereas only 1 of the controls ($N = 15$) could be classified as such (27). With untreated hypertensives, a systolic pressure higher than 200 mmHg with graded exercise testing is more the rule than the exception. Whether this response, considered to be "exaggerated," is correlated with end-organ damage is unclear as both positive and negative associations have been reported (13). If subjects are classified as having hypertensive heart disease (left ventricular hypertrophy, elevated myocardial fibrosis, accelerated atherosclerotic coronary artery disease), they have resting and exercise abnormalities of which an exaggerated systolic blood pressure response during exercise is a prominent feature. Since "white-coat hypertension" occurs in 7% of the population (elevated resting pressures in the presence of a physician), exercise testing has been advocated to improve the detection of an elevated blood pressure in this select group (13). However, the blood pressure responses are not sufficiently distinctive to suggest that this approach can eliminate the unknown factors responsible for this state. Since individuals with white-coat hypertension, when compared to normotensive controls, have elevated ventricular mass, larger atrial dimensions, poorer diastolic filling, lower high-density lipoprotein levels, and elevated plasma insulin, total cholesterol, and triglyceride concentrations, it is not, according to Lim et al. (13), "an innocuous condition." Fagard et al. reported on the prognostic value of invasive hemodynamic measurements of hypertensive men taken at rest and during exercise. Their data were collected from 143 hypertensive subjects and followed for 2186 patient years. The interesting finding was that exercise blood pressure did not significantly increase the prediction of cardiovascular morbidity or mortality events better than resting blood pressure, but the inclusion of systemic vascular resistance data with exercise blood pressure results significantly enhanced the prognostic value of their prediction equation (28).

In an attempt to gain additional insight on this topic, we used genetic hypertensive rats (SHR) and their controls (Wistar Kyoto rats, WKY) in a maximal treadmill test to determine the changes in the slope of the rise in systolic blood pressure during maximal exercise. Contrary to our hypothesis, the results did not exhibit a significant difference between the two groups (unpublished results).

Acute Exercise and Select Hemodynamic Changes with Hypertensive Subjects

In a study of untreated hypertensives men with limited target-organ damage (WHO Stages I and II) that were exercised to exhaustion, Farad et al. (29) concluded that maximum oxygen reduction in these subjects with high blood pressure was caused by a decrease in stroke volume. In addition, they felt that left ventrical function was impaired because of a possible reduction in compliance (29). Radionuclide angiography was used by Melin et al. (30) to study left ventricular function in normotensive and stage I hypertensives who had no evidence for coronary heart disease. They concluded that the reduction in ejection fraction was not due to an increased afterload but to an altered cardiac contractility caused by changes in intrinsic factors (30). Montain and cohorts (31) used a graded exercise test with older normotensive and hypertensive subjects and noted that during submaximal exercise, the hypertensives had lower cardiac outputs and reduced stroke volumes. As expected, at rest the older hypertensives had higher pressures and TPR values. Lund-Johansen (32) conducted a longitudinal study lasting 20 years involving 48 normotensive subjects and 93 hypertensive individuals (WHO stage I). His exercise test was one in which the subjects performed steady state exercise at 50-, 100-, and 150-W stages. When he compared the resting values of the two groups on a cross-sectional basis, the hypertensive subjects younger than 40 years of age had higher cardiac outputs and normal peripheral vascular resistance values, while those older than 40 years had higher cardiac output and resistance means. When the exercise results were evaluated, the younger hypertensives had lower cardiac outputs than their younger normotensive controls, which was attributed to a reduced stroke volume caused by a decrease in ventricular compliance. Ten years later, the resting and exercise blood pressures of the hypertensive group were slightly increased, but the exercise indices for stroke volume and cardiac output had diminished by 15% while their resistance value had decreased by 20%. After 20 years, most of the hypertensives were on medication, thus the investigator removed the drugs for 1 week before obtained resting and exercise data. He noted an immediate increase in peripheral resistance that was present at rest and during steady-state exercise. Resting and exercise heart rates, cardiac index, and the stroke index were markedly reduced with the cardiac and stroke values by as much as 20%. Lund-Johansen's results indicated that after two decades of hypertension, exercise would be associated with increases in systolic blood pressure and peripheral vascular resistance and a decrease in cardiac output (32).

When gender is considered, it is well recognized that men have higher absolute cardiac output and maximum oxygen consumption values than women. To study this matter in subjects with essential hypertension, Fagard et al. (33) matched 45 men and 45 women for age and blood pressure before having them perform submaximal (50-W) and maximal exercise. As expected, at maximal conditions, the men had significantly higher cardiac output and peak oxygen consumption values, but not heart rate, than the women. The submaximal results showed no significant gender differences in cardiac output or oxygen consumption values because the women had higher heart rates and a higher extraction of oxygen from arterial blood than the men (33).

Acute Exercise and Postexercise Hypotension

It is important for individuals concerned with the management of hypertension to be cognizant of the fact that immediately after the cessation of sustained exercise, the resting blood pressure will be lower than the preexercise value. This observation, noted almost a century ago by Hill (34) and McCurdy (35) in normotensive subjects after both aerobic and resistive exercise, also occurs in hypertensive individuals after aerobic exercise (3). The magnitude of the reduction and its duration is related to intensity of exercise as well as to its duration. From the published literature on the subject, it appears that an intensity level between 40–60% $\dot{V}_{O_2max}$ continued for 20 min or longer will be necessary to lower systolic and diastolic blood pressures by 10 and 5 mmHg respectively, although reduction of 25 mmHg have been reported (3). The effect can last from 1–4 h, depending upon the duration and intensity of exercise. When ambulatory data were measured for 12 h periods after 45 min of exercising at approximately 70% of the heart rate reserve ($\sim$60% $\dot{V}_{O_2max}$), no significant changes were noted when compared to the results obtained from a nonexercise day (14). Physiological and hemodynamic measurements obtained during the reduction in pressure have shown marked reductions in regional vascular resistance; decreases in cardiac output and stroke volume; reductions in epinephrine, dopamine, and cortical hormonal concentrations; inhibition of peripheral sympathetic nerve traffic and/or a reduction in α-adrenergic responses; a decline in plasma volume, or an increase in skin blood flow caused by thermoregulatory mechanisms (3,14). From their study, which demonstrated postexercise hypotension lasting for 2 h after aerobic exercise, Rueckert et al. (36) reported that a biphasic response pattern was occurring in which there was an initial decrease in peripheral resistance, with cardiac output remaining constant, that was followed by a decrease in cardiac output and an increase in peripheral resistance. In an interesting experiment, Boone and associates injected a bolus of naloxone into their subjects when they were experiencing postexercise hypotension and observed a rapid return of the blood pressure to preexercise values. They felt the result occurred because the drug had eliminated the effect of released opioids on the enkephin receptors which augment sympathetic responses (37).

Animal experiments with normotensive and hypertensive populations have also demonstrated the existence of postexercise hypotension after running exercise on activity wheels or treadmills. (10,38,39). Moreover, when anesthetized rats have had their sciatic nerves stimulated to simulate exercise, decreases in blood pressure were observed (40). Tipton and associates conducted numerous studies on this topic with normotensive and genetic hypertensive rats and found that the exercise intensity had to equal 50% $\dot{V}_{O_2max}$ for at least 20 min to have a postexercise hypotension that lasted 60 min or longer. When they used thermal dilution techniques to measure cardiac output before and after exercise, they found that reductions in both cardiac output and peripheral resistance were contributing to the postexercise hypotension (41) (unpublished data). The post-exercise hypotension review of Kenney and Seals (42) mentions a variety of experiments that used pharmacological agents having central and peripheral actions on opioid and serotonergic pathways. However, their results suggest an inhibition of the sympathetic nervous system. When Tipton and coworkers conducted their central and peripheral opioid experiments with SHR groups, they concluded that the action of the opiate was a peripheral rather than a central effect (10) (unpublished data). Opioid and serotonergic pathways are not the only possibilities to explain postexercise hypotension, as the release of peptides from the myocardium, endothelial factors, and the effects of calcium on the nucleus tractus solitarius (NTS) are other possible mechanisms (3).

Comments on Acute Exercise

To understand the role of exercise in the management of hypertension, it is essential that the patient, physician, and scientist understand the terminology of exercise as it relates to specificity, type, intensity, frequency, duration, and mode. Until this occurs, generalizations and misconceptions will prevail that will inhibit understanding and implementation. Intuitively, it would seem that the exercise profile of a hypertension prone individual to aerobic exercise would exhibit an exaggerated pressor response that could be useful for predictive purposes and as a diagnostic procedure. Surprisingly, the experimental evidence does not support such an impression, and the blood pressure results from such a test must be interpreted with caution. Moreover, the magnitude of the blood pressure response to exercise (e.g., > 200–250 mmHg) has not been as effective as a marker for the detection of hypertension prone individuals, causing investigators to consider hemodynamic changes related to cardiac output, stroke volume, and peripheral vascular resistance. However, their predictive value comes from longitudinal rather than cross-sectional approaches. Acute aerobic exercises performed at an intensity of 50% V_{O_2max} or greater for as little as 20 min will be associated with a postexercise hypotension that can persist for 60 min or longer. Reductions in cardiac output, peripheral vascular resistance, and stroke volume are consistent hemodynamic changes, although the specific sequence and time course of their alterations are unclear. Since acute exercise causes increases in pressure and cessation results in marked decreases, wide "swings" in pressure may cause anatomical and physiological changes that would influence baroreceptor functions in the regulation of blood pressure. While this statement will require more substantiation, it does indicate that the blood pressure response to acute exercise has many dimensions.

Epidemiological Investigations on Populations with Different Fitness and Energy Expenditure Levels

Epidemiological studies are useful in examining and defining relationships between various parameters, establishing research and clinical directions and for establishing the foundations for experimental studies designed to test various scientific hypotheses. Besides difficulty in controlling many of the confounding variables such as age, weight, and fat content, genetic and self-selection factors are design problems with planners of epidemiology experiments. When fitness levels of individuals between the ages of 7 and 17 ($N = 270$ boys and girls) were evaluated, children with higher fitness scores had lower systolic and diastolic pressures than those with lower scores (43). Panico et al. (44) used Harvard Step Test scores from 1341 (N of girls = 600) school children between 7 and 14 years of age and noted that systolic blood pressure was lower in the boys, who had higher fitness scores. This relationship was independent of age, height, and body mass but, was not present in girls or was related to the measurement of diastolic pressure. Interestingly, the pressure differential was 7 mmHg. Harvard Step Test scores were used with more than 2000 fourth graders in New York City. The authors reported that the students with the lowest values had the highest pressure (45). In addition, after a 1 year follow-up, those individuals who experienced a decrease in fitness scores had the highest increases in blood pressure. From a population of 289 tenth-graders, Fripp and coworkers (46) selected 37 for the Cooper run-walk fitness test to examine select relationships. They reported that the students with the lowest scores had the highest systolic and diastolic pressures. The differential between the low-fitness and the moderately fit group was approximately 9 mmHg. Harshfield et al. measured blood pressure and maximal oxygen consumption in a bi-racial population of 175 individuals ($N = 95$ girls) between the ages of 10 and 17 years (47). In addition they monitored blood pressure during the day and night. There were no relationships between the fitness scores and the pressures recorded for the Caucasian students regardless of the time of measurement. On the other hand, the "less fit" black male or female students had markedly higher systolic blood pressures than the "more fit" black student when awake or asleep. Since black populations have a higher prevalence of hypertension than non-Hispanic whites or Mexican Americans (4), these findings are of interest to health educators and professionals. Blair et al. used a treadmill and heart rate test to assign fitness scores to more than 6000 individuals ($N = 1219$ women) between the ages of 20 and 65 years. Later (median time $= 4$ years), 240 new cases of hypertension were identified. After statistical adjustments for age, gender, baseline values, and body mass, the subjects that had the lowest fitness ratings had a greater relative risk of becoming hypertensive than those individuals with higher ratings. Unfortunately, the racial and socioeconomic characteristics were not assessed (48).

Studies with athletic populations show similar trends. Lehman and Keul measured resting blood pressures from 810 athletes (14–69 years of age) who participated in a variety of aerobic and resistive events they reported that the incidence of individuals with "high normal" pressures (Table 1) was 11% while the percentage of athletes with hypertension was 5%. At that time, they expected incidence rates for both categories to be increased by twofold (48). Paffenbarger et al. followed blood pressure changes in approximately 15,000 men who were alumni of Harvard University (49). They were differentiated on the basis of participating in vigorous athletics when undergraduates. Despite the inability to control for lifestyles or their changes, the "nonathletes" had a 35% greater risk of becoming hypertensive than the "athletes." Darga and associates studied the exercise habits of 1269 members of the American Medical Joggers Association who averaged 10 mi/week and 683 members of the American Medical Association who were not joggers (jogging is generally assumed to require an energy expenditure between 25 and 50% $\dot{V}_{O_2max}$(50). According to the survey, 93% of the joggers and 81% of the nonjoggers had normal resting blood pressures. Of interest was the finding that five times as many nonjoggers than joggers had been or were taking antihypertensive medication. In 1933, Steinhaus concluded, after a thorough review of the national and international literature, that the majority of sportsmen would have lower resting blood pressures than their nonsportsmen controls (52). Consequently, it is time for investigators to accept this concept and to devote more energy to studies that explain why.

Epidemiological investigations of occupations that require different levels of energy expenditure have provided insights on the relationship between physical activity and resting blood pressure. Montoye et al. examined the relationships between physical activity and blood pressure in a Tecumseh, Michigan, community (population = ~10,000) and found the more active individuals had significantly lower systolic blood pressures (~2–3 mmHg) (53). It is of interest that when railroad workers were differentiated by the physical requirements of their duties, resting blood pressures were not significantly different (54). When Pappenbarger et al. compared cargo handlers and less active longshoremen, it was apparent that an elevated blood pressure was an important risk factor for coronary heart disease; however, it was not evident that the cargo handlers had lower resting pressures than their fellow workers (55). Buck and Donner examined the prevalence of hypertension in Canadian occupations that required repeated isometric exercise at the worksite. There were 4273 employees who were classified as having to perform low or high amounts of daily isometric exercise. After controlling for age, social class, alcohol consumption, and body mass index, they concluded that daily performance of isometric exercise prevented rather than induced the incidence of hypertension (56).

CHRONIC EXERCISE

Overview

There have been a plethora of longitudinal investigations pertaining to the effects of aerobic endurance training on the resting blood pressure of normotensive and hypertensive populations. Previous reviews by Tipton (3,19) and by Fagard and Tipton (10) have carefully evaluated the published data on the subject. In the 1994 presentation (10), they discussed the results from 48 separate groups in which control conditions were maintained. The collective evidence is sufficiently clear to indicate that aerobic training of an endurance nature will significantly reduce resting blood pressure. The critical issues are (a) the magnitude of the changes, (b) whether the changes noted have biological importance for hypertensive populations, (c) the exercise prescription that should be advocated for diseased population, (e) exercise contraindications, and (f) the relationships between the exercise and pharmacological prescription. Although several professional organizations (8, 57) have published official statements endorsing the concept that chronic exercise will lower resting blood pressure and should be incorporated within a management strategy for individuals with a hypertensive classification (Table 1), not all investigators familiar with the exercise literature believe the evidence is sufficiently supporting to warrant such a generalization (18). After a critical review of the literature in 1984 (19), I concluded that such a position was justified, and believe that the publications and data evaluations since that time are confirmatory.

The Meta-Analysis Approach

In recent years, biologists have used advanced statistical approaches to collectively evaluate trends in numerous studies with multiple results. Hagberg (9) used the meta-analysis statistical approach with 25 studies that examined the blood-pressure-lowering effect of endurance exercise training with subjects that had essential hypertension. Most of the subjects were men; they ranged in age from 15 to 70 years; the number of subjects/groups ranged from 4 to 66; training was from 4 to 52 weeks; and their adjusted initial systolic blood pressure was 150 mmHg. After training, the adjusted mean reduction was 10.8 mmHg for systolic blood pressure and 8.2 mmHg for diastolic blood pressure. Using the same approach with a smaller subset of training studies featuring women subjects, Hagberg (9) noted a greater reduction with training: namely, -19 and -14 mmHg for systolic and diastolic pressure respectively. Fagard and Tipton (10) reported on the results of 36 publications that contained 48 experimental trained groups. Most of the subjects were men, they ranged in age from 16 to 72 years, and the training programs lasted from 4–68 weeks with a median of 16 weeks. Using a WHO classification system to evaluate changes according to pretraining pressures, 27 groups were normotensive (140/90 mmHg), 7 were borderline or stage I (Table 1) hypertensives, and 7 were hypertensive, as they had pressures of 160/95 mmHg or better. After analysis and adjustment, the normotensive experienced a mean net reduction of $-3.2/-3.1$ mmHg; the stage I individuals had a decrease of $-6.2/-6.8$ mmHg, while the hypertensive subjects exhibited a decline of $-9.9/-7.6$ mmHg, respectively. When all the studies were combined to yield a single value for SBP and DBP, the net weighted means were $-5.3/-4.8$ mmHg. Kelley and McCellan published meta-analysis results from 9 exercise-trained and 8 control groups and indicated that the controls exhibited reductions of $-3/-3$, whereas the trained demonstrated declines of $-7/-6$ mmHg (58). Fagard and Amery (14) further analyzed the original data of Fagard and Tipton (10) from the 48 trained groups and indicated that a decrease of SBP by 7.2 mmHg and a decline of DBP by 6.2 mmHg would be statistically significant at the 5% level. Since a small reduction of blood pressure will have a significant effect on cardio-vascular mortality and morbidity (19), it is essential that health professionals include exercise training in the prevention and management strategy for the hypertensive or hypertension prone individual.

The effect of exercise training on resting blood pressure was extensively studied in normotensive and genetic hypertensive rats (SHR) by Tipton and colleagues (3,10,19). They measured caudal artery systolic blood pressure by a calibrated tail-cuff method as well as from the carotid artery by direct methods. Training was consistently associated with significantly lower resting arterial pressures and when they used a meta-analysis approach on 16 studies lasting 8 weeks or longer (10), the nontrained SHR groups had a mean blood pressure that was 10.5 mmHg higher than the trained hypertensive rats. Moreover, during the training period, the nontrained exhibited an increase of 74.6 mmHg while the trained demonstrated a rise of 63.6 mmHg. Tipton and associates also demonstrated that in older hypertensive rats that were kept inactive for 42 weeks before being exposed to a training program, training kept the pressures from rising, whereas their controls continued to show an increase with time (59). Last, when trained SHR groups were detrained, the effect of chronic activity on resting blood pressure was lost by the third week. The salient features from these animals' studies were a training effect of approximately 10 mmHg, training of older rats with established hypertension "prevented" the rise in pressure that occurs with time, and the effects of training will be lost after 3 weeks of inactivity (59). Since the trends and the magnitude of the pressure change follow the profile noted for humans, we believe the SHR is a useful model to gain insights on the effects of exercise with hypertensive humans.

Last, the fact that the results from various normotensive populations exhibit only slight changes in resting blood pressure with training is not an alarming statistic or one to cause health officials to be hesitant about implementing an exercise training program, because the critical issue is whether individuals who are at risk with elevated pressures will respond to a program of endurance training. They will.

Training and Ambulatory Blood Pressure

Fagard critically evaluated 10 frequently cited training studies that have used monitors to record day- and nighttime pressures (60). However, six of the investigations involved subjects whose initial pressures were less than 140 (systolic) / 90 (diastolic) mmHg. None of these selected investigations exhibited a reduction in systolic blood pressure during the day- or nighttime hours and one demonstrated a significant change in diastolic pressure during the day hours. On the other hand, the subjects with pressures higher than 140/90 mmHg in the four remaining studies showed significant reductions (-5 to -17 mmHg in systolic blood pressure, and in three studies, significant reductions in diastolic blood pressure (-5 to -8 mmHg) were noted during the daytime hours. Only one study showed significant changes during the nighttime hours and that change was a -5 mmHg reduction in diastolic pressure. The lack of a significant effect during the night is attributed to the fact that sympathetic tone is low or absent during those hours.

Resistive Training and Resting Blood Pressure

Included within this section is information pertaining to activities such as weight lifting or to those that require predominately isometric contractions. Until recently (3), health organizations and medical authorities strongly discouraged individuals with cardiovascular risk factors, and especially hypertensive populations, from performing such activities. Since maximum isometric contractions will elicit markedly elevated pressor and elevated peripheral resistance responses (61) and maximum weight lifting events can increase systolic blood pressure well in excess of 200 and occasionally to 300 mmHg (62), this recommendation was medically prudent and conservative. However, for a variety of reasons, many individuals who were at risk ignored this advice and performed resistive exercises with no or limited professional supervision and experienced no marked increase in mortality or morbidity events. In fact, several investigators have advocated resistive exercises alone or in combination with circuit training for normotensive and hypertensive populations (3,63). More than two decades ago, Kiveloff and Huber (64) prescribed isometric exercises for elderly patients and reported changes that ranged from -2 to -42 mmHg. Wiley and coworkers (65) demonstrated that isometric training (5 to 8 weeks) using handgrips prescribed at 30 and 50% of the subjects' maximum isometric contraction (MVC) resulted in decreases of -10 to 15 mmHg in measurements of systolic and diastolic blood pressure. When six adolescents performed weight-lifting activities for 20 weeks, reductions in systolic and diastolic blood pressure were 17 and 7 mmHg, respectively (66). Weight-training activities were practiced by normotensive subjects who had cardiac risk factors and their pressure reductions were similar to the values noted for the controls (67). Ten stage I hypertensive subjects (see Table 1) lifted weights in their circuit program for 9 weeks. At that time, they exhibited an increase of 1 mmHg in systolic blood pressure and a decrease of 5 mmHg in diastolic blood pressure (68). Their 16 controls had pressures similar to their initial values. Hypertensive subjects were assigned to a weight-training with flexibility exercise group (aerobic exercise and controls were the others) by Blumenthal et al. (69). At the end of the study, they reported that all groups exhibited similar reductions and concluded that neither aerobic or resistive exercise was able to significantly lower resting pressures. Running was incorporated within the circuit training program of 50 individuals with stage I hypertension and decreases of 14 mmHg systolic and 13 mmHg diastolic blood pressure were reported after 10 weeks. Unfortunately, this study had no control subjects, which limits the value of the investigation (63).

   Tipton and his assistants trained stroke prone genetic hypertensive rats to perform isometric hanging exercises for 16 weeks (70). Tests with subgroups indicated the exercise would elicit an increase in mean carotid artery blood pressure of ~60 mmHg. All the rats in the study had resting caudal artery systolic blood pressure in excess of 200 mmHg. Contrary to the expectations when comparisons were made with their trained controls, the trained rats did not exhibit significantly higher resting pressures, nor did they experience a higher incidence of strokes. Since a careful subsequent study demonstrated that endurance training between 50 and 70% $\dot{V}_{O_2max}$ would not increase the incidence of strokes in genetic hypertensive rats (SHR-SP) (71), we concluded that it was unlikely that moderate aerobic or isometric exercises would induce strokes in these animal models.

While the evidence is far from complete, the results to date suggest that the performance of moderate resistive exercises by "at risk" subjects will not be associated with elevated pressures or an increase in mortality or morbidity statistics. Although we believe aerobic activities should be prescribed for hypertensive subjects, an acceptable prescription would be to use a resistance that is between 40 and 50% of an individual's maximum capacity (3).

The Exercise Prescription

The overwhelming scientific evidence concerning the role of exercise in the management of elevated blood pressure endorses the concept of prescribing aerobic exercise. Thus it is not surprising that this theme is repeated in the statements of professional organizations (8, 57). Since a high percentage of the American population has a sedentary lifestyle or a poor compliance record in structured exercise programs, there has been an attempt by advocates of physical activity to make exercising more "user friendly" in order to increase continued participation. Hence, walking, hiking, stair climbing, jogging, bicycling, swimming, rowing, tennis, soccer, racquetball, basketball, or touch football have been recommended on a regular basis (7,8). While these activities have the aerobic specificity to be effective in the management of hypertension, it is difficult to achieve the necessary progression of frequency, duration, and intensity.

From the pioneering studies of Pollock and others, it is evident that the frequency of chronic exercise should be between three and five times per week (11,72). More is not necessarily better because of the problems associated with increases in muscle soreness, connective tissue tears, overuse injuries, and overtraining disorders. With regard to duration, an exercise period lasting between 30 and 60 min per session is strongly advocated (8). Inherent in this recommendation is the principle of progression, which is essential for individuals whose fitness levels are low because of an existing inactive lifestyle. The most important component of the exercise prescription is the intensity. Since descriptive terms such as *light, moderate, heavy,* or *severe* are relative and have different meanings for different individuals, it is essential that an objective assessment be obtained of one's exercise capacity before an exercise program is implemented. This is accomplished by scheduling a maximum oxygen consumption test at a reputable health, fitness, or medical center. Although not advocated by the author, many authorities will recommend a maximum performance test that uses heart-rate rather than oxygen-consumption data to assess maximum aerobic performance. With oxygen results, light exercise represents an aerobic requirement of 25%, moderate exercise denotes 50%, heavy exercise means a demand of 75%, and severe exercise reflects a performance level between 90 and 100% of $\dot{V}_{O_2max}$ (11).

After a critical evaluation of the factors within a training program that would influence changes in the resting blood pressure of hypertensive subjects, I concluded that exercise intensity was the most important factor. Although sedentary individuals with very low fitness levels will exhibit improvements in $\dot{V}_{O_2max}$ with walking programs that are classified as light exercise, a prescribed intensity level lower than 25% $\dot{V}_{O_2max}$ will produce minimal changes. On the other hand, exercise prescriptions that contain features followed by elite performers (sessions > 90% $\dot{V}_{O_2max}$) ignores the fact that hypertensive individuals have a disease and do not respond as do normal subjects (13). Consequently, we advocate using an exercise intensity level between 40 and 70% of $\dot{V}_{O_2max}$, a range that is in agreement with the recommendations of professional organizations (8, 57). While the availability of treadmills, cycle ergometers, and rowing machines facilitates the prescription of walking, running, cycling, and rowing programs, this is not the case for swim training, which also has been shown to be associated with lower resting pressures (73), because so few testing centers have swimming flumes. In such situations, extrapolations from the treadmill or cycle ergometer tests should be followed for prescription purposes (73). Inspection of the prescribed intensity levels that have been successful in lowering resting blood pressure of hypertensive subjects will indicate that the majority of aerobic training studies were within the recommended range. Although seldom cited in the American literature, it was the 1974 study of Shindo et al. that convincingly demonstrated that a training stimulus of approximately 50% of $\dot{V}_{O_2max}$ would be effective in lowering resting blood pressures (74). Although there is some dispute among investigators concerning the time course for a reduction in blood pressure to occur with a training program, the initial changes will generally appear after 3 and before 12 weeks have elapsed (3).

The issue of a training stimulus was carefully evaluated in genetic hypertensive rats (SHR) by Tipton and coworkers (59). When they prescribed a training program that required rats to run between 70 and 90% of $\dot{V}_{O_2max}$, the resting pressures increased more in the trained animals than in their sedentary controls, presumably because of an increase in resting sympathetic tone. However, when they changed the intensity level to 40–70% $\dot{V}_{O_2max}$, the rats that were being trained by this schedule exhibited significantly lower resting caudal artery pressures than their nontrained controls. As with most human studies, the reductions were noted after 4–6 weeks of training.

MECHANISMS FOR A TRAINING EFFECT BY HYPERTENSIVE SUBJECTS

With hypertension being a multifactorial disease and blood pressure being regulated by redundant systems, it is not surprising that a variety of mechanisms have been proposed to be responsible for lower resting values. Since the topic pertains to hypertensive subjects, mechanisms known to influence normotensive populations will not be discussed or used for extrapolation purposes. When hemodynamic data were evaluated, conflicting results have been reported concerning whether increases or decreases were noted with respect to cardiac output and to systemic vascular resistance (75–77). Since these investigators employed different methodologies, it is possible this explanation accounts for the uncertainty in the scientific community. On the other hand, trained hypertensive rats (SHR) had significantly lower resting cardiac output and carotid artery mean pressure with elevated resistance units than their nontrained controls (78). For more than 100 years, the sympathetic nervous system has been implicated in the etiology of hypertension (3). Since the activity of the sympathetic nervous system is decreased at night, this fact has been used to explain why trained subjects exhibit reductions during the day but not at night (14). However, not all the hypertensive trained groups showed significantly lower circulating levels of plasma catecholamines when comparisons were made with nontrained controls (10,14). Although microneurography studies have been conducted on normotensive subjects to denote the influence of training on sympathetic nerve traffic to the periphery (79), data have not been reported on the use of this technique with hypertensive subjects participating in a training study. When hypertensive rats (SHR) were chemically sympathectomized and trained, it was evident that ''elimination'' of the sympathetic nervous system would normalize resting blood pressure and that training could significantly lower resting pressures in sympathectomized animals (80).

It is well known that baroreceptors are ''reset'' with the disease of hypertension and the possibility that training could alter this process is an attractive but unproven possibility (3,81). While numerous investigators have studied baroreflex changes in normotensive human and animal subjects and noted attenuated blood pressure responses with the trained groups (3), these changes have interactions that involve fluid-balance and blood-volume regulatory mechanisms. Although we have postulated that the repeated hypotensive effect of acute exercise will reset baroreceptors, there is no experimental evidence from the exercising of hypertensive subjects to support this view point. The renin-angiotensin system also deserves consideration because of its importance to both fluid balance and blood pressure regulation. As noted by Fagard and Amery, endurance training by hypertensive subjects had no significant influence on the plasma concentrations of renin or on angiotensin II, even though positive results were reported for normotensive subjects (14).

It has been documented that an increase in body fat leads to obesity, elevations in plasma insulin concentrations, glucose intolerance, and insulin resistance; hence metabolic mechanisms deserve attention, because hypertension is included within Syndrone X (82,83). Creative investigations have demonstrated that insulin will increase the reabsorption of sodium by the kidney tubules (84) and enhance the activity of the sympathetic nervous system (85). It has been reported that endurance training by obese hypertensive subjects will decrease resting levels of plasma insulin and facilitate an increase in insulin sensitivity when blood pressures were being lowered (3,86). This metabolic explanation deserves consideration when blood pressure is normalized in stage I hypertensives by weight reduction (3). However, not all hypertensive subjects who lose weight become normotensive (87), indicating the complex nature of the disease.

For some time, the management of hypertension has included a reduction in the daily consumption of sodium (3,5). Although physical training has been included with salt reduction in several studies involving hypertensive subjects, the results have been incomplete or sufficiently confusing to conclude there is an interaction effect with the two interventions (14). The same conclusion is warranted for salt-sensitive hypertensive rats that have been exercised-trained (88). Although the supplementation of calcium to the diet of hypertensive subjects has been advocated by select investigators to facilitate a reduction in pressure, the epidemiological evidence does not support the practice (3,5,89). Moreover, its interaction with endurance training by humans is unknown.

EXERCISE TRAINING AND ANTIHYPERTENSIVE MEDICATION

As a result of the recommendations of the Fifth Report of the Joint National Committee on the Detection, Evaluation, and Treatment of High Blood Pressure (JNC-V), the terminology of the management of hypertension has been changed from non-pharmacological and pharmacological to lifestyle modifications and pharmacological treatment (5). As for the lifestyle modifications, they include weight reduction, moderation in alcohol consumption, reduction of sodium intake, smoking cessation, and participation in regular physical activity (3,5,6). However, if the lifestyle modifications are unsuccessful or the resting pressures remain elevated, pharmacological treatment is advocated (14,90). Initially, diuretics and β-blockers were recommended because their use significantly reduced the incidence of morbidity and mortality from hypertension (5). Usually, one drug is prescribed and evaluated before a second medication is used in combination. After suggesting the use of diuretics and beta-blockers, the JNC-V report (5) is very cautious concerning other drugs to prescribe because of an absence of supporting morbidity and mortality data with their use. The report does list ACE inhibitors, calcium channel inhibitors, α-receptor-blocking agents, and drugs that block both α and β receptors. However, their use is advocated only after careful evaluation of the subject's health and pressure status. Since the details are beyond the scope of this chapter, it is essential that the health professional prescribing the exercise, as well as the subject ''taking'' the medication, become familiar with the topic by reading the JNC-V report and related literature on the subject (5,14,90).

There are experimental results from exercising hypertensive subjects and animals which show that chronic exercise will reduce the amount of medication required during a training program (59,91). However, certain drugs will impair the exercise response and complicate the nature of the exercise prescription. Consequently, individuals who prescribe exercise should consult the material by Fagard and Amery (14) and by Swain and Kaplan (90) before combining training and medication interventions. For example, according to Swain and Kaplan (90), thiazide diuretics, β-blockers, α_2 agonists, short-acting calcium channel blockers, and direct vasodilators are not recommended for hypertensive patients who will be participating in an endurance-type training program.

SUMMARY

Hypertension is a complex and a multifactorial disease that continues to be a major health problem in the United States and elsewhere because of its impact on morbidity and mortality statistics. Despite the improvements in detection, evaluation, treatment, and management of the disease in recent decades, approximately 50 million Americans are currently afflicted with the disorder. At present, there is more progress being made in the management of the disease than in its prevention, although this relationship could be altered by more advances in genetic molecular biology. Health organizations concerned with the consequences of cardiovascular and metabolic risk factors recommend that the management of hypertension include numerous lifestyle modifications, of which exercise is one, and, if necessary, the use of appropriate drugs.

The exercise to be prescribed should be progressive and aerobic in nature, performed at an intensity level between 40 and 70% of a subject' $\dot{V}_{O_2max}$, should last between 30 and 60 min a day, and be repeated from three to five times per week. Because many individuals have poor compliance records in following their exercise prescriptions, certain groups encourage hypertensive subjects to participate in generic aerobic activities. This approach is not "championed" by the author because it fails to quantify or control the essential features of the exercise prescription. Consequently, we recommend an objective exercise evaluation session in a health, fitness, or medical center before undertaking a walking, running, cycling, or swimming program. While resistive exercise programs for the hypertensive will definitely increase muscular strength, the process has a minimal effect in lowering arterial pressures and, with a maximal effort, could elevate systolic pressures to levels considered "dangerous" because they can approach or exceed 300 mmHg.

Multiple mechanisms appear to be responsible for the changes in resting pressure; these include a reduction in cardiac output, decreases in the activity of the sympathetic nervous system, alterations in baroreceptor functioning, and an increase in insulin sensitivity coupled with a decrease in insulin resistance. Since lifestyle modification will be unable to normalize resting pressures in many hypertensives, these individuals will require one or more pharmacological agents. However, the hemodynamic response to exercise and the effects of drugs on select physiological systems by hypertensive subjects is not identical to the profile reported for normotensive individuals; hence, the exercise prescription for active patients must take these factors into consideration.

REFERENCES

1. Ruskin, A., *Classics in Arterial Hypertension*. Charles C Thomas, Springfield, Illinois, pp. 5–29 (1956).
2. Kannel, W.B., *J.A.M.A.,* 275: 1571–1576 (1996).
3. Tipton, C.M., in *Exercise and Sport Sciences Reviews* (J.O. Holloszy, ed.). Williams & Wilkins, Baltimore, pp. 447–505 (1991).
4. Burt, V.L., Whelton, P., Roccella, E.J., Brown, C., Cutler, J.A., Higgins, M., Horan, M.J., and Labarthe, D., *Hypertension,* 25: 305–313 (1995).
5. Joint National Committee on Detection, Evaluation, and Treatment of High Blood Pressure, *Arch Intern Med.,* 153: 154–183 (1993).
6. National High Blood Pressure Education Program Working Group, *Arch. Intern. Med.,* 153: 186–208 (1993).
7. NIH Consensus Conference, *J.A.M.A.,* 276: 241–246 (1996).
8. World Hypertension League, *J. Hypertens.,* 9: 283–287 (1991).
9. Hagberg, J.M., in *Exercise, Fitness, and Health: A Consensus of Current Knowledge* (C. Bouchard, R.J. Shephard, T. Stephens, J.R. Sutton and B.D. McPherson, eds.) Human Kinetics, Champaign, Illinois, pp. 455–466 (1990).
10. Fagard, R.F., and Tipton, C.M., *Physical Activity, Fitness, and Health: International Proceedings and Consensus Statement* (C. Bouchard, R.J. Shephard, and T. Stephens, eds.) Human Kinetics, Champaign, Illinois, pp. 633–655 (1994).
11. Scheuer, J., and Tipton, C.M., *Annu. Rev. Physiol.,* 39: 221–251 (1977).

12. Astrand, P.-O., Ekblom, B., Messin, R., Saltin, B., and Stenberg, J., *J. Appl. Physiol.,* 20: 253–256 (1965).

13. Lim, P.O., MacFadyen, R.J., Clarkson, P.B.M., and MacDonald, T.M., *Ann. Intern. Med.,* 124: 41–55 (1996).

14. Fagard, R., and Amery, A., in *Hypertension, Pathophysiology, Diagnosis, and Management,* 2d Ed. (J.H. Largah and B.M. Brenner, eds.). Raven Press, New York, pp. 2669–2681 (1995).

15. Rowell, L.B., *Human Cardiovascular Control.* Oxford University Press, New York, pp. 162–370 (1993).

16. McArdle, W.H., Katch, F.I., and Katch, V.L. *Exercise Physiology: Energy, Nutrition, and Human Performance,* 4th ed Human Kinetics, Baltimore, pp. 266–312 (1996).

17. Fletcher, G.F., Blair, S.N., Blumenthal, J., Casperson, C., Chaitman, B., Epstein, S., Falls, H., Froelicher, E.S.S., Froelicher, V.F., and Pina, I.L., *Circulation,* 86: 340–344 (1992).

18. Puddey, I.B., and Cox, K., *J. Hypertens.,* 13: 1229–1233 (1995).

19. Tipton, C.M., *Exerc. Sport. Sci. Revs.,* 12: 245–306 (1984).

20. Hansen, H.S., Hyldebrandt, N., Nielsen, J.R., and Froberg, K., *J. Hypertens.,* 7 (Suppl): S41–S42 (1989).

21. Lauer, R.M., Burns, T.L., Mahoney, L.T., and Tipton, C.M., in *Perspectives in Exercise Science and Sports Medicine,* vol. 2 (C.V. Gisolfi, and D.R. Lambs, eds.). Benchmark Press, Indianapolis, Indiana, pp. 431–463 (1989).

22. Fixler, D., Laird, W.P., and Diana, K., *Pediatrics,* 75: 1071–1075 (1985).

23. Drory, Y., Pines, A., Fisman, E.Z., and Kellermann, J.J., *Chest,* 97: 298–301 (1990).

24. Benassai, J., and Froom, P.F., *Arch. Int. Med.,* 146: 2053–2055 (1986).

25. Chaney, R.H., and Eyman, R.K., *Am. J. Cardiol.,* 62: 1058–1061 (1988).

26. Jette, M., Landry, F., Sidney, K., and Blumchen, G., *J. Cardiopulm. Rehab.,* 8: 171–177 (1988).

27. Tanji, J.L., Champlin, J.J., Yong, G.Y., Lew, E.Y., Brown, T.C., and Amsterdam, E.A., *Am. J. Hypertens.,* 2: 135–138 (1989).

28. Faggard, R.H., Pardens, K., Staessen, J.A., and Thijs, L., *Hypertension* 28: 31–36 (1996).

29. Fagard, R., Staessem, J., and Amery, A., *J. Hypertens.,* 6: 859–865 (1988).

30. Melin, J.A., Wijins, W., Pouleur, H., Robert, A., Nannan, M., De Coster, P.M., Bechers, C., and Detry, J.-M., *Int. J. Cardiol.,* 17: 37–49 (1987).

31. Montain, S.J., Jilka, S.M., Ehsani, A.A., and Hagberg, J.M., *Hypertension,* 12: 479–484 (1988).

32. Lund-Johansen, P., *J. Hypertens.,* 7(Suppl 6): S52–S55 (1989).

33. Fagard, R.H., Thijs, L.B., and Amery, A.K. *Med. Sci. Sports Exerc.,* 27: 29–34 (1995).

34. Hill, L., *J. Physiol.* (*London*), 22: xxvi–xxix (1898).

35. McCurdy, J.H., *Am. J. Physiol.,* 5: 95–103 (1901).

36. Rueckert, P.A., Slane, P.R., Lillis, D.L., and Hanson, P., *Med. Sci. Sports Exerc.,* 28: 24–32 (1996).

37. Boone, J.B., Levine, M., Flynn, M.G., Pizza, F.X., Kubitz, E.R., and Andres, F.F., *Med. Sci. Sports Exerc.,* 24: 1108–1113 (1992).

38. Overton, J.M., Joyner, M.J., and Tipton, C.M., *J. Appl. Physiol.,* 64: 748–752 (1988).

39. Shyu, B.C., and Thoren, P., *Acta Physiol. Scand.*, 128: 515–524 (1986).
40. Shyu, B.C., Andersson, S.A., and Thoren, P., *Acta Physiol. Scand.*, 121: 97–102 (1984).
41. Tipton, C.M., Hall, M.C., Monin, K.A., Sebastian, L.A., and Edwards, P.K., *Med. Sci. Sports Exerc.* 25 (Suppl): S63 (1992).
42. Kenney, M.J., and Seals, D.R. *Hypertension,* 22: 653–664 (1993).
43. Fraser, G.E., Phillips, R.L., and Harris, R., *Circulation,* 67: 405–412 (1983).
44. Panico, S., Celentano, E., Krogh, V., Jossa, F., Farinaro, E., Trevisan, M., and Mancini, M., *J. Chronic Dis.,* 40: 925–930 (1987).
45. Hoffman, A., Walter, H.A., Connelly, P.A., and Vaughan, R.D., *Hypertension,* 9: 188–191 (1987).
46. Fripp, R.R., Hodgson, J.L., Kwiterovich, P.O., Werner, M.C., Schuler, H.G., and Whitman, V., *Pediatrics,* 75: 813–818 (1985).
47. Harshfield, G.A., Dupaul, L.M., Alpert, B.S., Christman, J.B., Willey, E.S., Murphy, J.K., and Somes, G.W., *Hypertension,* 15: 810–814 (1990).
48. Blair, S.N., Goodyear, N.N., Gibbons, L.W., and Cooper, K.H., *J.A.M.A.,* 252: 487–490 (1984).
49. Lehmann, M., and Keul, J., *Zeits Chr. Kardiol.,* 73: 137–141 (1984).
50. Paffenbarger, R.S. Jr, Wing, A.L., Hyde, R.T., and Jung, D.L., *Am. J. Epidemiol.,* 117: 245–257 (1983).
51. Darga, L.L., Lucas, C.P., Spafford, T.R., Schork, M.A., Illis, W.R., and Holden, N., *Phys. Sportsmed.,* 17(7): 85–101 (1989).
52. Steinhaus, A.H., *Physiol. Rev.,* 13: 103–147 (1933).
53. Montoye, H.J., Metzner, H.L., Keller, J.B., Johnson, B.C., and Epstein, F.H., *Med. Sci. Sports,* 4: 175–181 (1972).
54. Taylor, H.L., Blackurn, H., Brozek, J., Parlin, R.W., and Puchne, T.P., *Acta Med. Scand.,* 460(Suppl): 55–115 (1966).
55. Paffenbarger Jr, R.S., Laughlin, M.E., Gima, A.S., Black, R.A., *N. Engl. J. Med.,* 282: 1109–1114 (1970).
56. Buck, C., Donner, A.P., *J. Occup. Med.,* 27: 370–372 (1985).
57. Hagberg, J., Blair, S., Ehsani, A., Gordon, N., Kapan, N., Tipton, C., and Zambraski, E., *Med. Sci. Sports Exerc.,* 25: i–x (1993).
58. Kelley, G.A., and McCellen, P., *Am. J. Hypertens.,* 7: 114–119 (1994).
59. Tipton, C.M., Matthes, R.D., Marcus, K.D., Rowlett, K.A., and Leininger, R.J., *J. Appl. Physiol.,* 55: 1305–1310 (1983).
60. Fagard. R.H., J., *Hypertens.,* 13: 1223–1227 (1995).
61. Asmussen, E., *Cir. Res.,* 48 (Part II): I3–I10 (1981).
62. MacDougall, J.D., Tuxen, D., Sale, D.G., Moroz, J.R., and Sutton, J.R., *J. Appl. Physiol.,* 56: 785–790 (1985).
63. Kelemen, M.H., *Med. Sci. Sports Exerc.* 21: 675–677 (1989).
64. Kivelof, B., Huber. O., *J. Am. Geriatr. Soc.* 19: 1006–1012 (1971).
65. Wiley, R.I., Dunn, C.L., Cox, R.H., Hueppchen, N.A., and Scott, M.S., *Med. Sci. Sports Exerc.* 24: 749–754 (1992).
66. Hagberg, J.M., Ehsani, A.A., Goldring, D., Hernandez, A., Sinacore, D.R., and Holloszy, J.H., *J. Pediatr.* 104: 147–151 (1984).
67. Hurley, B.F., Hagberg, J.M., Goldberg, A.P., Seals, D.R., Ehsani, A.A., Brennan, R.E., and Holloszy, J.O., *Med. Sci. Sports Exerc.,* 20: 150–154 (1988).

68. Harris, K.A., and Holly, R.G., *Med. Sci. Sports Exerc.,* 19: 246–252 (1987).
69. Blumenthal, J.A., Segal, W.C., and Appelbaum, M., *J.A.M.A.,* 266: 2098–2104 (1991).
70. Tipton, C.M., McMahon, S., Youmans, E.M., Overton, J.M., Edwards, J.G., Pepin, E.B., and Lauber, C., *Am. J. Physiol.,* 254: H592–H598 (1988).
71. Tipton, C.M., McMahon, S., Leininger, J.R., Pauli, E.L., and Lauber, C., *J. Appl. Physiol.,* 68: 1083–1085 (1990).
72. Pollock, M.L., Cureton, T.K., and Greninger, I., *Med. Sci. Sports,* 1: 70–75 (1969).
73. Tanaka, H., Bassett Jr., D.R., Howley, E.T. Thompson, D.L., Ashraf, M., and Rawson, F.L., *J. Hypertens.,* 15: 651–657 (1997).
74. Shinko, M., Tanaka, H., Ohara, S., and Tokuyama, I., *Rep. Res. Cen. Phys. Ed.,* 2: 139–152 (1974). (In Japanese, see Ref. 3.)
75. Seals, D.R., and Reiling, M.J., *Hypertension,* 18: 583–592 (1991).
76. Urata, H., Tanabe, Y., Kiyonaga, A., Ikeda, M., Tanaka, H., Shindo, M., and Arakawa, K., *Hypertension,* 9: 245–252 (1987).
77. Nelson, L., Jennings, G.L., Esler, M.D., and Korner, P.I., *Lancet,* 2: 473–476 (1986).
78. Tipton, C.M., Sebastian, L.A., Overton, J.M., Woodman, C.R., and Williams, S.B., *J. Appl. Physiol.,* 71: 2206–2210 (1991).
79. Grassi, G., Seravalle, G., Calhoun, D.A., and Mancia, G., *Hypertension,* 23: 294–301 (1994).
80. Tipton, C.M., Sturek, M.S., Oppliger, R.A., Matthes, R.D., Overton, J.M., and Edwards, J.G., *Am. J. Physiol.,* 247: H109–H118 (1984).
81. Krieger, E.M., *Clin. Exp. Pharmacol., Physiol.* 15(Suppl): 3–17 (1989).
82. Reaven, G.M., *Diabetes,* 37: 1594–1607 (1988).
83. Slater, E.E., *Hypertension,* 18(Suppl I): I-108–I-114 (1991).
84. DeFronzo, R.A., *Diabetologia,* 21: 165–171 (1987).
85. Anderson, E.A., Balon, T.B., Hoffman, R.P., Sinkey, C.A., and Mark, A.L. *Hypertension,* 19: 621–627 (1992).
86. Krotkiewski, M., Mandroukas, R., Sjostrom, L., Sullivan, L., Wetterqvist, H., and Bjorntorp, B., *Metabolism,* 28: 650–658, (1979).
87. Eliahu, H.E., Iaina, A., Gaon, T., Scochat, J., and Modon, M., *Int. J. Obesity,* 5(Suppl 1): 157–163 (1981).
88. Tipton, C.M., Overton, J.M., Pepin, R.B., Edwards, J.G., Wegner, J., and Youmans, E.M. *J. Appl. Physiol.,* 63: 342–346 (1987).
89. Cutler, J.A., and Brittain E., *Am. J. Hypertens.,* 3: 137S–146S (1990).
90. Swain, R., and Kaplan, B., *Phys. Sportsmed.,* 25(9): 47–50, 57–61 (1997).
91. Cade, R., Mars, R., Wagemaker, H., Zauner, C., Packer, D., Privette, M., Cade, M., Peterson, J., and Hood-Lewis, D., *Am. J. Med.,* 77: 785–790 (1984).
92. Daniels, S.R., and Loggie, J.M.H., *Phys Sportsmed.,* 20(3): 121–122, 125–128, 133–134 (1992).

18

The Role of Exercise in the Detection and Treatment of Peripheral Vascular Disease

R. James Barnard
University of California
Los Angeles, California

INTRODUCTION

Atherosclerotic peripheral vascular disease of the lower extremities (PVD) is a major clinical problem in most industrialized nations. The life expectancy of PVD patients is about 10 years less than that of the general population and PVD is commonly associated with coronary artery and cerebrovascular disease (1–3). In the large (18,388 subjects) Whitehall study, 17 years of follow-up showed that the death rates for coronary artery or cerebrovascular disease were approximately six times higher in PVD patients than in individuals with no signs of PVD (3). In a review of U.S. population-based studies, Vogt et al. (4) concluded that the prevalence of PVD rises sharply with age, from 3% in those under 60 years to over 20% in those over 75 years of age. These values may be an underestimation of the true incidence of PVD, as the diagnosis of PVD was based on the Rose questionnaire or the presence of rest pain and/or ulceration or gangrene.

Intermittent claudication is the only specific symptom of PVD. Like angina, claudicant pain is the result of inadequate delivery of oxygen to muscle cells. The term *claudication* comes from the Latin *claudicare,* which means to limp. This is a poor description of the symptoms of PVD, because limping is rarely observed. According to Friedman (5), claudication is variable. Some patients feel only a sense of aching or weakness in the legs with walking. In others, a tightening or pressing pain develops in the calves or buttocks, and yet others experience a sharp, cramping calf pain that may be excruciating. The interindividual variation in symptoms may make the diagnosis of PVD somewhat difficult, but thorough questioning by the physician can usually result in an accurate diagnosis. Diagnosis may become more difficult in older individuals, as some of the symptoms are the result of extreme deconditioning due to a lack of physical activity secondary to other medical problems.

Because PVD is a form of atherosclerosis, it is not surprising that risk factors for coronary or cerebrovascular disease such as hyperlipidemia, smoking, hypertension, and diabetes are also commonly associated with PVD (6–8). Diabetes mellitus seems to be the most prominent risk factor. PVD has been reported to be 4 to 11 times more common and gangrene 40 times more common in diabetic than in nondiabetic individuals (9–11).

A recent study by Mowat et al. (8) reported that PVD patients had high concentrations of triglycerides and very low density lipoprotein (VLDL) cholesterol and low concentrations of high-density lipoprotein (HDL) cholesterol, especially the HDL2b (large particles) commonly found in patients with insulin resistance and/or diabetes. Although mortality from cardiovascular disease has declined substantially in the United States since the 1950s due to a major decline in myocardial infarction and angina pectoris, the diagnosis of intermittent claudication has not declined in the Framingham cohort (7). In large population studies, questionnaires such as that of Rose have been used to diagnose PVD. In clinical practice, palpation of peripheral pulses has been a standard technique to detect PVD during routine screening. The posterior tibial pulse was found always to be present in normal individuals, but dorsalis pedis pulses were absent in up to 20% of normal individuals (11). Even in young individuals, the dorsalis pedis pulse may be absent in 5–12% of the population (5,11). Thus, the posterior tibial pulse is the one most commonly examined in clinical practice. However, this takes skill and practice. In 1961 Franklin et al. (12) described an ultrasonic flowmeter based on the Doppler effect, and in 1963 Watson and Rushmer (13) demonstrated that blood flow could be detected through human skin by pulsed ultrasound. Since then the transcutaneous Doppler flowmeter has proven far superior to simply palpating pulses (14), and it is now used extensively to evaluate patients with PVD. Taking measurements at various levels of the limb gives a better indication of the site of arterial obstruction. Colt (15) recommended measurements at the femoral popliteal, and both anterior and posterior tibial arteries in patients with PVD of the lower limb. According to Strandness (16), the transcutaneous Doppler flowmeter may be used in the clinical evaluation of patients with arterial disease at all levels of the upper and lower extremities.

The Doppler flowmeter provides an output that can be recorded as a flow-velocity waveform. The recorded velocity depends on many factors and thus is not a highly accurate measure of blood flow velocity. However, it is useful to record, because changes in waveform are obvious in patients with arterial obstruction (14). Analysis of the waveform has not provided precise information about the extent of vascular obstruction, only indicating whether or not obstruction is present. An attempt at evaluating the Doppler waveform by Laplace transformation also has been found to have major limitations (17).

The best use of the Doppler flowmeter in PVD patients is for the accurate measurement of blood pressure in the legs. According to Strandness, "the measurement of blood pressure at several levels of the limb is one of the simplest, most reliable and useful methods for the evaluation of arterial narrowing and occlusion." Standard clinical techniques for the diagnosis of PVD at rest, however, do not provide precise information as to the degree of hemodynamic impairment, and they underestimate the prevalence of PVD, since they provide information only in cases of severe blockage or complete occlusion (18,19).

EXERCISE TESTING IN PVD PATIENTS

In the 1960s it became apparent to Strandness (16) that better testing methods were needed for the detection and evaluation of PVD patients. Using the Doppler technique, he undertook a series of studies in normal individuals and in claudicant patients that led to the development of the Strandness Exercise Test. Subjects walked on a treadmill at 3.2 km/h, 12% grade until the development of claudication or for a maximum of 5 min. Immediately after the test, the subjects were asked to lie down and blood pressure was measured at the ankle. Pre- and postexercise measurements were compared. Strandness and his associates confirmed earlier observations by Leary and Allen in 1941 (20), Ejrup in 1948 (21), and Winsor in 1950 (22), who reported that following exercise in claudicant patients, pedal pulses either diminished or transiently disappeared. In normal individuals, ankle pressures increased at low work rates but fell at higher, more exhaustive work rates. Strandness and associates then used the test to evaluate the response of claudicant patients to exercise training and reconstructive surgery.

In 1950, Winsor (22) introduced the concept of the *blood pressure index,* the ratio of the ankle pressure to the arm (brachial) pressure (AAI or ABI). He found that in normal, healthy individuals, the ratio of systolic pressure in the lower extremity to systolic pressure in the upper extremity was always greater than 1.0. Blood pressure gradients less than 1.0 were found in 24% of patients with PVD in the lower limbs. In 1968, a more comprehensive study by Carter (23) found that the resting ankle systolic pressure was always ≥97% of the brachial systolic pressure in individuals without PVD. In claudicant patients with angiographically documented complete arterial occlusion, the ankle pressure was always less than 85% of the brachial pressure. In patients with mild to severe arterial stenosis, the ankle pressure ranged from 45–120% of the brachial pressure. Similar results were reported by Yao et al. (24) and by Carter (25), both in 1969. Thus, under resting conditions the ankle pressure may remain normal in patients with mild to severe atherosclerosis. Similar results have been obtained with blood flow measurements (16). May et al. (26) have suggested that in order to observe any consistent reduction in resting pressure or flow, a major artery must be stenosed by at least 80%. Thus, when PVD is detected by the resting Doppler, disease has already reached an advanced stage.

The value of exercise testing for the early detection of PVD was documented by Carter in 1972 (27). In 10 limbs with arterial stenoses $\geq 25\%$ of the lumen diameter, the resting pressure index was normal in six and abnormal in four instances. With exercise, abnormal indices were found in all 10 limbs. The exercise used by Carter consisted of up to 2.5 min of foot flexion and extension at a rate of one per second. Resistance was created during the first 30 s by the hand of the examiner. This test may be used for screening, but due to variations in the exact amount of work performed, it would not be appropriate for serial tests. We (28) reported similar results with a treadmill test in 25 cases with normal resting ankle pressures. In the San Luis Valley Diabetes Study (29), 113 PVD patients were identified by abnormal resting ankle pressures out of 950 individuals examined. Exercise testing identified an additional 14 cases. Although exercise testing can increase the detection rate of PVD, a recent International workshop (30) indicated that exercise testing is not recommended for use in the primary care setting.

For diagnosis and research purposes we (31) have used the approach outlined initially by Strandness, with some modification. Our patients are first given a symptom-limited progressive treadmill test, using a modified Bruce protocol that starts at 1.6 km/h, 0% grade. This test is given for two purposes. The first is to evaluate the cardiac status of the patient and to assign a maximum training heart rate. This is important, since many patients with PVD also have coronary disease. The second reason for the symptom-limited test is to determine the work rate to be used for the Doppler test. If the results of the symptom-limited test indicate that the patient can complete the Strandness test at 3.2 km/h, 12% grade, this test is used. If the patient cannot tolerate this work rate, we adopt a lower one that the patient can tolerate. Since it is sometimes difficult to pick a work rate for the Doppler test that the patient can maintain for 5 min and still develop claudication, we have developed a two-stage test, as outlined in Table 1. This two-stage test enables the technician to increase the work rate after 2.5 min if the patient has not started to develop signs of claudication. Using this approach, almost all patients can complete 5 min of exercise and most experience grade 2 claudicant pain in addition to a fall in ankle pressure. This approach also reduces the risk of electrocardiographic (ECG) or blood pressure abnormalities that might require termination of the test. Gardner et al. (32,33) have also utilized a progressive treadmill test, and they have emphasized the importance of not allowing the patients to use the hand rails for support.

Table I   Two-Stage Stress Test Protocol for Patients with
Peripheral Vascular Disease[a]

Max stress test MET level	Stage 1, 2.5 min		Stage 2, 2.5 min	
	km/h	% grade	km/h	% grade
≤3.5	1.6	0	2.4	2
3.6–5.5	2.4	2	3.2	6
5.6–7.5	2.4	4	3.2	8
7.6–9.5	2.4	6	3.2	12
<9.5	3.2	12	3.2	12

[a]After the first 2.5 min at stage 1, the workload is increased to stage 2 unless
the patient has developed grade 2 claudication pain, angina, or other contraindications.

Doppler testing should be done in a quiet room with the temperature at
approximately 23°C. On the day of testing, the patients are instructed not to
exercise for at least 6 h prior to test in order to preclude a warm-up effect (34)
and not to eat for at least 2 h prior to the test. On arrival at the testing room,
ECG electrodes are attached to monitor the resting and exercise ECG. During
5-min rest in the supine position, blood pressure cuffs are placed around the left
arm and both ankles. If the room temperature is cool, a blanket is placed over
the patient. At the end of the 5-min rest, branchial artery pressure is obtained by
standard auscultatory techniques. Ankle pressures are obtained by using a Parks,
Model 909, Ultrasonic Velocity Detector (Beverton, Oregon), or other Doppler
instrument in order to detect blood flow in the posterior tibial arteries.

Following resting measurements, the patient is instructed to inform the
technician about any symptoms that may develop during the Doppler exercise
test. Symptoms, both cardiac and leg, are graded on a scale of 1–4, 1 being the
onset of pain and 4 being the most severe. Patients are never taken beyond grade
2 anginal pain, but may be taken to grade 4 leg pain. The 5-min Doppler
exercise test is performed with continuous ECG monitoring. At the end of the
test, the patient is instructed to lie down quickly. Left brachial and right and left
posterior tibial artery pressures are taken immediately and are repeated each minute thereafter until ankle pressures return to resting levels. With practice, a skilled
technician can record all three pressures in less than 45 s. Two technicians are
preferable, one recording ankle pressures and the other brachial pressures. Using
this format, both ankle and brachial pressures may be recorded almost simultaneously.

Treadmill walking is the exercise of choice for Doppler testing of PVD patients for several reasons. First, it is an activity that most patients can undertake easily if the speed and grade are adjusted appropriately for the individual's work capacity. Second, walking uses primarily the calf muscles, so that there is a shunting of blood from the foot and other leg muscles to the gastrocnemius when ischemia produces vasodilation. This reduces the tibial artery pressure. Third, the work rate (speed and grade) can be controlled precisely and replicated for retest purposes following intervention.

Cycle ergometry is not recommended for claudicant patients because it uses primarily the thigh muscles. With ischemia, blood may be shunted from muscles in the upper leg, and the tibial pulse may not change appreciably. Alpert et al. (35) have also emphasized the importance of using upright exercise during testing. In one patient with claudicant symptoms and aortic occlusion, lower limb blood flow was normal during supine flexion-extension foot exercise but was clearly abnormal during walking.

Although treadmill walking is the preferable mode of exercise for testing PVD patients, lack of a treadmill should not discourage physicians from exercise testing patients with symptoms of PVD. Either foot flexion-extension as de-scribed by Carter (27) and earlier by Lassen et al. (36) or a simple exercise in which patients rise on their toes every few seconds can be used for screening. The main objective is to use the calf muscles.

EXERCISE TRAINING FOR PVD PATIENTS

Many modalities are available to treat PVD, ranging from lifestyle change (exer-cise and diet) through drug therapy to more aggressive procedures, including angioplasty and bypass surgery. In many cases, the medical approach to PVD treatment is short-lived or ineffective. In a recent analysis of the medical treat-ment of PVD in Maryland between 1979 and 1989, the rate of percutaneous transluminal angioplasty in the lower extremities rose from 1 to 24 per 100,000 population and that the use of bypass surgery rose from 32 to 65 per 100,000. Despite the dramatic increase in these invasive procedures, the rate of lower limb amputation remained stable at about 30 per 100,000 (37). These results may re-flect increased diagnosis of PVD or a lack of success from the invasive proce-dures. In another study, Veith et al. (38) reported a significant reduction in the number of amputations with increased angioplasty and bypass surgery. Based on a review of the literature, Coffman (39) discouraged the use of invasive treatment for PVD, stating "The treatment of patients with intermittent claudication alone should be conservative, because the prognosis for the limb is favorable, because surgical mortality from cardiovascular events is high among such patients, and because the use of interventions has not decreased the rate of amputation in many hospitals." The conservative treatments he suggested included exercise, smoking cessation, and controlling hyperlipidemia, hypertension, and diabetes mellitus.

Numerous studies have documented the value of exercise in the treatment of PVD. In 1994 this author (40) reviewed 41 human and 7 animal studies that showed an improvement in performance with regular exercise. In 1995 Regensteiner and Hiatt (41) reviewed nine randomized controlled studies, documenting the value of exercise rehabilitation in patients with PVD. In this same year, Gardner and Peohlman (42) reported a meta-analysis of 21 exercise rehabilitation programs. Although the general conclusion was the same (training increases performance), not everyone was able to achieve an increase. Some patients showed no change and the condition of a few worsened so that they had to undergo invasive procedures. In general there was an increase in exercise capacity before the onset of claudication as well as an increase in maximum performance capacity.

A wide variation in the amount of improvement is evident in the various studies. The meta-analysis by Gardner and Poehlman (42) indicated that both the amount of exercise and the intensity of exercise were important variables. Those studies with training sessions >30 min in duration achieved a much greater improvement than studies using ≤30 min. Frequency of training was also important, with studies using three or more sessions per week achieving greater improvement than those using fewer sessions. The intensity of training was also important. Those studies where patients were encouraged to exercise to near-maximal pain achieved far greater improvement than when patients exercised merely to the onset of pain.

The general conclusion seems that the more exercise the patient undertakes to near-maximal pain, the greater the increase in performance, but this response is not guaranteed. For example, Larsen and Lassen (43) studied seven PVD patients over a 6-month training program that consisted of 1 h of daily walking to the point of severe pain. At the end of 6 months, two patients showed no change in performance, and the remaining five showed improvements that ranged from 50–700%.

The long-term effects of regular exercise are not known. In a case report (44), we described a patient with severe claudication who undertook a walking program; after a few months, he advanced to a jogging program, and a year later he completed the Chicago Marathon. This patient continued regular training; when contacted several years later, he indicated that he was still running 5- and 10-km races but not marathons. Foley (45) reported that gangrenous feet healed faster when patients were placed on an exercise program. Twenty-two patients began a walking program in the hospital and were encouraged to walk on a daily basis following discharge. Follow-up ranged from 6 months to 6.5 years (mean ± SD 2.2 ± 1.7 years) and all but one patient, who stopped walking at discharge, reported healed feet. Many were able to return to work.

MODE OF EXERCISE TRAINING

Walking appears to be the exercise of choice. It is what patients naturally need to do, is inexpensive, and produces results. According to Gardner and Poehlman (42), supervised, intermittent walking to near-maximal pain results in improved performance that is only slightly better than a combination of home/supervised exercise.

Some patients with PVD may have to climb stairs at home or at work, so it is important to incorporate this type of activity into the training program. Jones et al. (46) compared training on a StairMaster versus treadmill for up to 12 weeks. Both groups showed significant improvements in performance, with some cross-over of gains when tested on the other apparatus than what had been used for training. However, peak performance was always less during crossover testing, indicating some specificity of training.

MECHANISMS OF ADAPTATION

Although there is no doubt that exercise training will increase performance in most cases, the precise mechanisms involved are not completely understood. Possibilities include increased blood flow, altered muscle metabolism, and increased mechanical efficiency, with a possible change in pain perception. Figure 1 shows changes in blood pressure at the ankle with only 3 weeks of intensive exercise and diet therapy. The improvement in the ankle/arm index clearly indicates physiological adaptation.

Increased Blood Flow

One human case report (44) and one animal study (47) have documented the development of collateral vessels following exercise training in subjects with arterial obstruction. If collateral vessels do develop as a result of exercise training, one would assume a resulting increase in blood flow and oxygen delivery to the ischemic limb. Nine studies in humans with PVD have reported an increase in maximum blood flow with training; however, eight studies found no change, and one study reported a decrease in maximum flow (40). In those studies where blood flow was increased, the percent increase was far less than the increase in performance. This might be due partly to difficulty in measuring limb blood flow in humans.

Another factor that might contribute to the increased performance and enhanced blood flow observed in some PVD patients with training is a decrease in blood viscosity. Ernst and Aartrai (48) reported that in a placebo-controlled, double-blind study, hemodilution over 3 weeks lowered hematocrit and blood viscos-

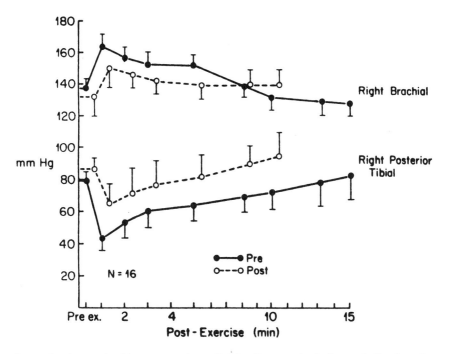

FIGURE 1   Arm and ankle pressures immediately after exercise before and after 3 weeks of daily exercise to the point of severe pain, combined with a very low fat diet. (From Ref. 31.)

ity but increased pain-free walking distance. They subsequently exercise-trained PVD patients for 2 months, finding a fall in both whole blood and plasma viscosity along with a significant increase in pain-free walking.

In animals where arterial insufficiency was created by ligation, training increased maximal blood flow in two studies but left flow unchanged in three other studies (40). One animal study reported an increase in capillarization of the ischemic limb with training; such a response could enhance oxygen delivery. Several observational studies in humans have reported an increase in the capillary-to-fiber ratio in the ischemic limb, but no training studies have yet been reported on human subjects (40).

Even if maximum blood flow does not increase, there is a possibility of a redistribution of flow to increase oxygen delivery to the ischemic area. Sorlie and Myhre (49) and Zetterquist (50) observed no change in maximal blood flow with training in PVD patients, but they did observe an increase in oxygen extraction, which suggests a redistribution of flow to the ischemic area of the limb.

Using an animal model, Yang et al. (51) documented a redistribution of flow from the proximal to the distal segments of the stenosed limb, as well as a greater oxygen extraction with training. Blood flow in control animals, as measured with radioactive microspheres, was almost equally distributed between the upper and lower limbs. With acute stenosis, flow to the distal bed was dramatically reduced. With chronic stenosis (approximately 6 weeks), flow to the distal limb had improved without any change in total blood flow; with exercise training, it was further improved but not normalized.

Mathien and Terjung (52) found a redistribution of flow within the distal limb muscle fiber types but no increase in maximal flow following training. Flow from the red portion of the gastrocnemius, mostly fast-twitch oxidative glycolytic fibers, was redistributed to the white portion, mostly fast-twitch glycolytic fibers. Although the oxidative capacity of the fast-twitch glycolytic fibers is low, increasing blood flow to these fibers in the face of severely depressed flow could enhance performance and reduce lactate formation at any given work rate. Thus, a redistribution of flow by mechanisms yet unknown could be, in part, responsible for the improvement in performance seen in patients with PVD.

Metabolic Adaptations

A reduction in lactate formation has been reported by Sorlie and Myhre (49) and by Ruell et al. (53), further supporting the view that blood flow and/or oxygen extraction are increased with training. In addition to this reduction in lactate, other metabolic adaptations have been reported. An increase in mitochondrial content and mitochondrial marker enzyme activity is commonly found in healthy individuals with intensive training (54). Several investigators have reported an increase in mitochondrial content or marker enzyme activity in PVD patients (40). However, others have reported a decrease in mitochondria with severe disease. With training, an increase in mitochondria has been reported in both PVD patients and animals with peripheral arterial insufficiency (40). Lundgren et al. (55) reported that the increase in cytochrome C oxidase after training was correlated much more closely with symptom-free walking distance than with maximum walking distance. They also found that cytochrome C oxidase decreased following bypass surgery but that this decrease could be prevented with regular training (56).

One might argue that because oxygen delivery is severely reduced by the disease, an increase in oxidative metabolic capacity should not be important. Yang et al. (51), however, have suggested two possible positive effects resulting from an increase in mitochondria in PVD patients. First, an increase in mitochondrial density could reduce the average path length for oxygen diffusion within the muscle. In addition, more mitochondria could reduce the cytosolic adenosine diphospate (ADP) concentration, which would reduce the rate of glycolysis and lactate production.

Abnormalities in lipid metabolism have been suggested in PVD patients. Hiatt et al. (58) found an increase in plasma acylcarnitines at rest and after only 10 min of exercise, whereas healthy subjects showed no accumulation after 18 min of exercise. However, at much higher work rates, acylcarnitines also increased in healthy subjects. Thus, the observed accumulation of acylcarnitines at lower work rates in PVD patients may be a response to hypoxia rather than an abnormality in lipid metabolism. Based on respiratory quotient measurements, Lundgren et al. (55) concluded that at the point of claudicant pain, the patients were oxidizing mainly fat in spite of a rising lactate output. Lundgren et al. also reported that training resulted in an increase in the activity of hydroxyacyl-CoA dehydrogenase, an enzyme involved in fat metabolism. Hiatt et al. (59,60) found a decrease in resting plasma acylcarnitines after exercise training. Unfortunately, no measurements were reported immediately after exercise in the trained patients. Thus, it remains to be determined whether or not there is any abnormality in lipid metabolism in PVD patients.

Walking Efficiency and Pain Perception

Another possible mechanism that could account for the reduced pain and increased performance with training in PVD patients is an improved mechanical efficiency. Hiatt et al. (60,61) reported a reduction in whole-body oxygen consumption at a given work rate with training. This type of adaptation is not generally seen in older people without PVD (62).

A change in the pain threshold for any level of ischemia has also been suggested, but it is something that is very difficult to quantitate in PVD (unlike coronary artery disease, where angina generally correlates well with changes in the electrocardiogram). Rosfors et al. (63), however, have recently reported that cognitive factors are important for improving performance with training in PVD patients.

COMPARISON OF TRAINING WITH INVASIVE PROCEDURES

Although there has been a tremendous increase in the use of surgical procedures to treat PVD, there has been little documentation of the benefits of surgery as assessed by increases in work capacity. In 1966, Strandness and Bell (64) reported a normalization of ankle pressures in patients following endarterectomy or bypass surgery. Improvement was noted immediately after the surgery and was documented for 7 days. Performance capacity, however, was not measured.

More recently, Creasy et al. (65) compared exercise training with percutaneous transluminal angioplasty in a randomized trial. After 3 months, the angioplasty group had a better ankle blood pressure index and a greater walking distance to claudication. Maximum walking tended to be greater in the angioplasty group, but the advantage was not statistically significant. After 1 year, the distance to claudication as well as the maximum walking distance were significantly greater in the exercise group. These results indicate that regular exercise may be more effective than angioplasty for long-term improvement in functional capacity.

In another randomized trial, Lundgren et al. (56) compared training and surgical reconstruction. Three groups were involved in the study: trained (T), bypass surgery (S), and surgery plus training (S + T). Comparisons were made after 13 months. Symptom-free walking was greatest in the S + T group, and the S group performed better than the T group. Maximum calf blood flow was increased in all three groups, the changes being correlated with increases in performance. These results indicate that, for at least 13 months, surgery confers a greater benefit than exercise alone, but combining the two treatments gives the best results. This area needs more study, with a longer follow-up.

SPECIAL PRECAUTIONS, LIMITATIONS, AND PROBLEMS

There is no evidence to suggest that severe ischemia during exercise results in any tissue damage in the legs. This is important, as exercising to the point of near-maximum pain seems to result in the greatest improvement (42). This is different from the situation that exists in the heart, where prolonged ischemia may result in myocardial infarction. Since many patients with PVD also have coronary atherosclerosis, attention must focus on limitations to exercise that are dictated by the presence of concurrent coronary disease. We have seen a few cases in which PVD was the limiting factor for performance capacity on initial testing. After a few weeks of intensive walking therapy, a significant increase in performance capacity enabled the patients to work to a much higher heart rate during a standard treadmill test; they then exhibited an ischemic response in the electrocardiogram (31). Thus, regular treadmill testing is important.

DISEASE TREATMENT

Little attention has been focused on treating peripheral atherosclerosis by controlling risk factors. Whereas exercise can be effective for controlling many of the risk factors associated with atherosclerosis in healthier individuals, it is not known if the low-level activity undertaken by most patients with PVD has any significant impact on risk factors such as blood lipids, blood pressure, or diabetes mellitus. Two studies combined aggressive dietary modification with exercise in an attempt to modify risk factors significantly. Hall and Barnard (31) used a very low fat (<10% kJ), high–complex carbohydrate diet along with daily walking. In just 3 weeks, total serum cholesterol was reduced from 254 ± 18 to 182 ± 12 mg/dl (6.6 ± 0.5 to 4.7 ± 0.3 mmol/L) and serum triglycerides were reduced from 265 ± 60 to 180 ± 32 mg/dl (3.0 ± 0.7 to 2.1 ± 0.4 mmol/L). Blood pressure dropped from 139 ± 5 to 133 ± 7 mmHg for the systolic and from 81 ± 2 to 76 ± 2 mmHg for the diastolic reading. Although the decrease in blood pressure was not statistically significant, all four patients on antihypertensive drugs were able to discontinue medication. Three cardiac patients were initially taking propranolol (Inderal); one had the drug discontinued, one had the dosage reduced, and one patient's dosage was unchanged. Similar lipid results were reported by Hutchinson et al. (66) in a 1-year study. Thus, dietary modification combined with exercise can be effective for controlling risk factors associated with PVD.

In the past several years, aggressive treatment of hyperlipidemia has focused on the use of drugs. Several studies (40) have reported regression of lower limb atherosclerosis with treatment of hyperlipidemia by drugs combined with diet. Although regression of the disease was documented by serial angiograms, its effect on performance capacity was not evaluated. Thus, whereas exercise training can have a significant impact on performance, aggressive treatment of risk factors should be combined with exercise because of the progressive nature of atherosclerosis in PVD.

REFERENCES

1. Kannel, W.B., Skinner, J.J., Jr, Schwartz, M.J., et al., *Circulation* 41: 875–883, 1970.
2. Criqui, M.H., Coughlin, S.S., and Franek, A., *Circulation* 72: 768–773 (1985).
3. Davey Smith, G., Shipley, M.J., and Rose, G., *Circulation,* 82: 1925–1931 (1990).
4. Vogt, M.T., Wolfson, S.K., and Kuller, LH., *J. Clin. Epidemiol.,* 45: 529–542 (1992).
5. Friedman, S.A., in *Vascular Diseases: A Concise Guide to Diagnosis, Management, Pathogenesis, and Prevention* (S.A. Friedman, ed). J. Wright, PSG, Boston, pp. 1–30 (1982).
6. Murabito, J.M., D'Agostino, R.B., Silbershatz, H., and Wilson, P.W.F., *Circulation,* 96: 44–49 (1997).
7. Sytkowski, P.A., Kannel, U.B., and D'Agostino, R.B., *N. Engl. J. Med.,* 322: 1635–1641 (1990).

8. Mowat, B.F., Skinner, E.R., Wilson, H.M., Leng, G.C., Fowkes, F.G.R., Horrobin, D., *Atherosclerosis,* 131: 161–166 (1997).
9. Dry, T.J., Hines, E.A. Jr.,: *Ann. Intern. Med.* 14: 1893–1902 (1941).
10. Bell, E.T., *Arch Pathol.* 49: 469–473 (1950).
11. Barnhorst, D.A., and Barner, H.B., *N. Engl. J. Med.,* 278: 264–265 (1968).
12. Franklin, D.L., Schlegel, W., and Rushtner, R.F., *Science,* 134: 564–565 (1961).
13. Watson, N.W., and Rushmer, R.F., *Proc. San Diego Symp. Biomed. Eng.,* 3: 87–91 (1963).
14. Yao, S.T., Hobbs, J.T., and Irvine, W.T., *Br. Med. J.,* 4: 555–557 (1968).
15. Colt, J.D., *Am. J. Surg.,* 136: 198–201 (1978).
16. Strandness, D.E. Jr., *Peripheral Arterial Disease: A Physiologic Approach.* Little, Brown, Boston, p. 1 (1969).
17. Campbell, W.B., Skidmore, R., Woodcock, J.P., et al., *Cardiovasc. Res.,* 19: 206–211 (1985).
18. Carter, S.A., *N. Engl. J. Med.,* 287: 578–582 (1972).
19. Crigui, M.H., Franek, A., Barrett-Connor, E., et al., *Circulation,* 71: 510–515 (1985).
20. Leary, W.V., Allen, E.V.,: *Am Heart J* 22: 719–725, 1941.
21. Ejrup, B., *Acta. Med. Scand. (Suppl.).,* 211: 54 (1948).
22. Winsor, T., *Am. J. Med. Sci.,* 220: 117–126 (1950).
23. Carter, S.A., *Circulation,* 37: 624–637 (1968).
24. Yao, S.T., Hobbs, J.T., and Irvine, W.T., *Br. J. Surg.,* 56: 676–679 (1969).
25. Carter, S.A., *J.A.M.A.,* 207: 1869–1874 (1969).
26. May, A.G., DeWesse, J.A., and Rob, C.G., *Surgery,* 53: 513–524 (1963).
27. Carter, S.A., *N. Engl. J. Med.,* 287: 578–582 (1972).
28. Barnard, R.J., and Hall, J.A., in *Exercise in Modern* Medicine (B.A. Franklin, S. Gordon, and G.C. Timmis, eds.). Williams & Wilkins, Baltimore, pp. 107–117 (1989).
29. Hiatt, W.R., Marshall, J.A., Baxter, J., Sandoval, R., Hildebrandt, U., Kahn, L.R., and Hamman, R.F., *Clin. Epidemiol.,* 43: 597–606 (1990).
30. Ochard, T.J., and Strandness, D.E. Jr., *Diabetes Care,* 16: 1199–1209 (1993).
31. Hall, J.A., Barnard, R.J.,: *J. Cardiac. Rehabil.,* 2: 569–574 (1982).
32. Gardner, A.W., Skinner, J.S., Cantwell, B.W., and Smith, L.K., *Med. Sci. Sports Exerc.,* 23: 402–408 (1991).
33. Gardner, A.W., Skinner, J.S., and Smith, K.L., *Am. J. Cardiol.,* 68: 99–105 (1991).
34. Berglund, B., Eklund, B., *Clin. Physiol.,* 1: 253–256 (1981).
35. Alpert, J., del Rio H Garcia, Lassen, N.A.,: *Circulation,* 34: 849–855 (1966).
36. Lassen, N.A., Lindbjerg, J., and Munck, O., *Lancet,* 1: 686–689 (1964).
37. Tunis, S.R., Bass, E.B., and Steinberg, E.P., *N. Engl. J. Med.,* 325: 556–562 (1991).
38. Veith, F.J., Gupta, S.K., and Wengerten, K.R., *Ann Surg.,* 212: 402–414 (1990).
39. Coffman, J.D., *N. Engl. J. Med.,* 325: 577–578 (1991).
40. Barnard, R.J., in *Physical Activity, Fitness and Health* (C. Bouchard, R.J. Shephard, and T. Stephens, eds.). Human Kinetics, Champaign Illinois, pp. 622–632 (1994).
41. Regensteiner, J.G., and Hiatt, W.R., in *Exercise and Sport Sciences Reviews,* vol. 23 (J.O. Holloszy, ed.). Williams & Wilkins, Baltimore, pp. 1–24 (1995).
42. Gardner, A.W., and Poehlman, G.T., *J.A.M.A.,* 274: 975–980 (1995).

43. Larsen, O.A., Lassen, N.A., *Lancet,* 2: 1093–1095 (1966).

44. Hall, J.A., Dixson, G.H., Barnard, R.J., and Pritikin, N., *Phys. Sportsmed.,* 10: 90–101 (1982).

45. Foley, W., *Circulation,* 15: 689–700 (1957).

46. Jones, P.P., Skinner, J.S., Smith, L.K., John, F.M., Bryant, C.X., *J Cardiopulm. Rehabil.,* 16: 47–55 (1996).

47. Sanne, H., and Sivertsson, R., *Acta. Physiol. Scand.,* 73: 257–263 (1968).

48. Ernst, E.E., and Aartrai, A., *Circulation,* 76: 1110–1114 (1987).

49. Sorlie, D., Myhre, K., *Scand. J. Clin. Lab. Invest.,* 38: 217–222 (1978).

50. Zetterquist, Z., *Scand. J. Clin. Invest.,* 25: 101–111 (1970).

51. Yang, H.T., Dinn, R.F., and Terjung, R.L., *J. Appl. Physiol.,* 69: 1353–1359 (1990).

52. Mathien, G.M., and Terjung, R.L., *Am. J. Physiol. (Heart. Circ. Physiol, 19),* 250: H1050–H1059 (1985).

53. Ruell, P.A., Imperial, E.S., Bonar, F.J., and Thursby, P.F., *Eur. J. Appl. Physiol.,* 52: 420–425 (1984).

54. Saltin, B., and Gollnick, P.D., in *Handbook of Physiology: Skeletal Muscle.* American Physiological Society, Baltimore, pp. 555–631 (1983).

55. Lundgren, F., Dahllöf, A.-G., Scherstén, T., and Bylund-Fellinius, A.C., *Clin. Sci.,* 77: 485–493 (1989).

56. Lundgren, F., Dahllöf, A.-G., Lundholm, K., Scherstén, T., and Volmann, R., *Ann. Surg.,* 209: 346–355 (1989).

57. Terjung, R.L., Mathien, G.M., Erney, T.P., and Ogilvie, R.W., *Am. J. Cardiol.* 62: 15E–19E (1988).

58. Hiatt, W.R., Nawaz, D., and Brass, E.P., *J. Appl. Physiol.,* 62: 2382–2387 (1987).

59. Hiatt, W.R., Regensteiner, J.G., Hargarten, M.E., Wolfel, E.E., and Brass, E.P., *Circulation,* 81: 602–609 (1990).

60. Hiatt, U.R., Regensteiner, J.G., Wolfe, E.E., Carry, M.R., and Brass, E.P., *J. Appl. Physiol.,* 81: 780–788 (1996).

61. Hiatt, U.R., Wolfe, E.E., Meier, R.H., and Regensteiner, J.G., *Circulation,* 90: 1866–1874 (1994).

62. Poulin, M.J., Paterson, D.H., Govindasamy, D., and Cunningham, D.A., *J. Appl. Physiol.,* 73: 452–457 (1992).

63. Rosfors, S., Arnetz, B.B., Bygdeman, S., Sköldö, L., Lahnborg, G., Eneroth, P., *Scand. J. Rehab, Med.,* 22: 135–137 (1990).

64. Strandness D.E. Jr., and Bell, J.W., *Surgery,* 59: 514–516 (1966).

65. Creasy, T.S., McMillan, P.J., Fletcher, E.W.L., Collin, J., and Morris, P.J., *Eur. J. Vasc. Surg.* 4: 135–140 (1990).

66. Hutchinson, K., O'Berle, K., Crockford, P., Grace, M., Whyte, L., Gee, M., Williams, T., and Brown, G., *J.A.M.A.,* 249: 3326–3356 (1983).

19

Exercise and Cardiopulmonary Fitness in Individuals with Spinal Cord Injury

ROGER M. GLASER† and THOMAS W.J. JANSSEN
Wright State University School of Medicine
Dayton, Ohio

DAVID B. SHUSTER
Rehabilitation Institute of Ohio
Miami Valley Hospital
Dayton, Ohio

INTRODUCTION

Individuals with lower-limb paralysis due to spinal cord injury (SCI) typically use their arms for almost all activities of daily living (ADL), including wheelchair locomotion, as well as for exercise training and sports activities. However, several physiological factors including the relatively small muscle mass that is under voluntary control, deficient cardiovascular reflex responses, as well as inactivity of the skeletal muscle pump of the legs (potentially resulting in hypokinetic circulation), can markedly reduce the capacity for arm activity (39,54,74,78). Muscular weakness and the early onset of fatigue can discourage an active lifestyle, since ADL become relatively more stressful to perform (110) and limit the development of cardiopulmonary (aerobic) fitness. A sedentary lifestyle exacerbates this situation, since muscle strength and cardiopulmonary fitness progressively decrease, leading to a debilitative cycle that can be difficult to arrest or reverse (36,95). In addition, a number of secondary medical complications, which can

---

† Deceased.

cause much suffering and greatly increase the cost of medical care, tend to become more prevalent (19,86,134). Moreover, as a result of improvements in medical care, life expectancy of individuals with SCI has increased (41,42,166), with a concomitant increase in prevalence of cardiopulmonary disorders. Common long-term causes of death in the population with SCI are now a variety of cardiovascular and pulmonary disorders (9,42,123,177,184,185). The risk of coronary heart disease appears to be even higher than in the able-bodied (AB) population (42,62,123), which may be due in part to adoption of a sedentary lifestyle with consequent degenerative changes in the cardiovascular system (40, 90,121,184). The high risk of coronary heart disease among sedentary individuals with SCI is indicated by inferior blood lipid profiles, such as low high-density-lipoprotein cholesterol (HDL-C), high total and low-density-lipoprotein cholesterol, and high triglyceride concentrations relative to more active individuals with SCI, sedentary AB, and active AB individuals (30,40,90,112,121). Since activity level and cardiopulmonary fitness of those with SCI appear to be similarly related to coronary heart disease risk factors as in the AB population, it seems that (upper-body) exercise training may increase the health status and reduce cardiovascular risks of individuals with SCI just as leg exercise training benefits AB individuals.

Studies on wheelchair users with SCI indicated that those who maintain a more active lifestyle by regularly participating in exercise and sports programs can increase their muscle strength, cardiopulmonary fitness, and physical performance to levels well above those of their sedentary cohorts (34,46,78,81,95,186). In addition to fitness gains, habitual physical activity may also elicit improvements in health, psychosocial status, rehabilitation potential, functional independence, and quality of life (81,94,137,162). Therefore, studies have been performed to investigate whether exercise physiology principles could be utilized to develop specialized exercise testing and training techniques for individuals with SCI and to gain a better understanding of how their muscular, metabolic, and cardiopulmonary responses to various exercise modes differ from those elicited from AB individuals. This information may help elucidate how physical performance of individuals with paraplegia and tetraplegia can be optimally improved and how risks for secondary medical complications can be reduced. Upper-body exercise modes have traditionally been used for testing and training of individuals with SCI. However, physiological responses to arm exercise performed by individuals with SCI can be quite different than those for either arm or leg exercise by AB individuals. Therefore, this chapter discusses research related to the cardiopulmonary fitness and physiological responses to exercise of wheelchair users with SCI, the use of upper-body exercise techniques for cardiopulmonary fitness testing and training, and the use of training techniques that incorporate functional electrical stimulation (FES)-induced exercise of paralyzed leg muscles.

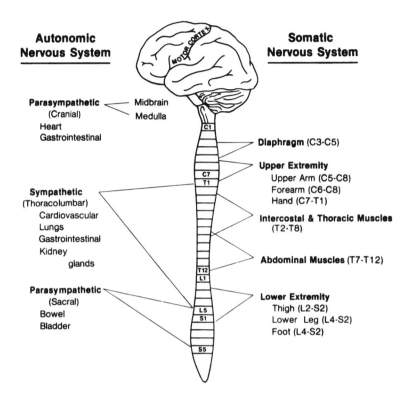

Autonomic Nervous System

Parasympathetic — Midbrain
(Cranial)   Medulla
Heart
Gastrointestinal

Sympathetic
(Thoracolumbar)
Cardiovascular
Lungs
Gastrointestinal
Kidney
        glands

Parasympathetic
(Sacral)
Bowel
Bladder

Somatic Nervous System

Diaphragm (C3-C5)

Upper Extremity
Upper Arm (C5-C8)
Forearm (C6-C8)
Hand (C7-T1)

Intercostal & Thoracic Muscles
(T2-T8)

Abdominal Muscles (T7-T12)

Lower Extremity
Thigh (L2-S2)
Lower Leg (L4-S2)
Foot (L4-S2)

FIGURE I   Schematic diagram of the central nervous system showing neural outflows from the somatic nervous system (providing skeletal muscle innervation) and autonomic nervous system (providing internal organ innervation). General innervations from each spinal cord level are indicated. (From Ref. 74.)

LIMITATIONS IN EXERCISE CAPABILITY OF INDIVIDUALS WITH SCI

The higher the level and more complete the SCI, the more widespread is the loss of somatic and autonomic nervous system function (Fig. 1) (74). Lesions in the thoracic and lumbar regions typically result in paraplegia with lower-limb and partial trunk muscle involvement. Lesions in the cervical region typically result in tetraplegia with lower-limb and trunk as well as upper-limb muscle involvement. The more skeletal muscles that are paralyzed, the lower will be the functional independence and the ability to perform voluntary exercise at sufficiently high metabolic rates to stimulate the cardiopulmonary system, and subsequently the lower will be the cardiopulmonary fitness level that may be achieved through exercise training. In individuals with higher-level SCI, paralysis of the intercostal muscles can severely limit pulmonary ventilation, which further reduces exercise capability and leads to secondary pulmonary problems. An additional effect of the skeletal muscle paralysis is the inability to activate the skeletal (or venous) muscle pump, which can lead to venous pooling in the paralyzed legs and a reduced venous return to the heart.

The aerobic exercise capability of individuals with SCI can also be limited by a diminished sympathetic outflow (see Fig. 1), since sympathetic stimulation is required for normal cardiovascular reflex responses to exercise. These reflexes normally augment blood flow to the metabolically active skeletal muscles by inducing vasoconstriction in relatively inactive tissues (such as the gut, kidneys, skin, and inactive muscles), vasodilation of arterioles in active skeletal muscle, venoconstriction (which facilitates venous return), and increases in heart rate, myocardial contractility, stroke volume and cardiac output (74,104). These reflexes are absent to varying degrees in most individuals with SCI, and those with lesions above T1 have lost central control of all sympathetic nerves that innervate the heart (from T1 to T4), markedly limiting cardioacceleration, myocardial contractility, and augmentation of stroke volume and cardiac output (59). Any cardioacceleration that occurs with exercise may be primarily due to withdrawal of vagal parasympathetic tone at the SA node. As a result, persons with tetraplegia usually have a peak exercise heart rate (e.g., 100–125 beat per minute) that is well below the age-predicted maximal. Compared to AB individuals, people with SCI, especially those with tetraplegia, respond to submaximal exercise with a lower stroke volume and a higher heart rate (34,102,105,116). The reduced venous return, resulting in chronic ventricular pressure and volume underloading, combined with the deficient myocardial contractility, can often lead to myocardial atrophy (114,133).

Thus, the loss of functional skeletal muscle mass and inactivity of the skeletal muscle pump in the lower extremities are compounded by diminished or nonexistent cardiovascular reflexes during exercise. Figure 2 schematically describes the various mechanisms for exercise and circulatory limitations for those with tetraplegia (54). The active arm muscles are fatigued quickly because of their relatively small mass, a potentially inadequate blood flow secondary to a hypokinetic circulation, a limited aerobic energy supply, and a greater component of anaerobiosis with the accumulation of metabolites in the muscles (37,39,54, 63,74). The early fatigue of the arm muscles during both wheelchair locomotion and exercise training can discourage many wheelchair users from leading active lives. Unfortunately, a sedentary lifestyle leads to a further decrement of physical fitness and an even greater reduction of functional capability. Aging further decreases cardiovascular, pulmonary, and muscular function, which can eventually lead to a loss of independence and an increase in medical complications (120).

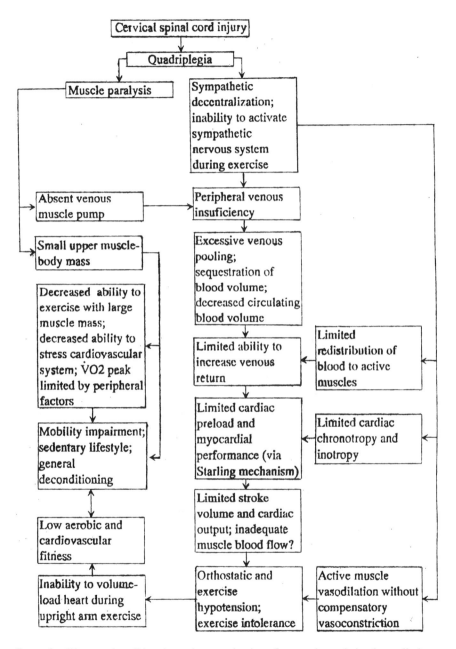

FIGURE 2   Diagram describing the various mechanisms for exercise and circulatory limitations for those with tetraplegia. (From Ref. 54.)

An active lifestyle, which incorporates specific exercise training and/or sports programs, is needed to break this debilitating cycle of *sedentary lifestyle—loss of fitness* and to enhance one's functional independence and quality of life (74, 78,95).

Special Exercise Precautions and Considerations

Individuals with SCI performing strenuous exercise are exposed to the usual risks known for AB individuals as well as additional risks due to their central nervous system damage and the resulting motor, sensory, and autonomic dysfunction. Generally, exercise guidelines recommended by the American College of Sports Medicine should be followed (1). Because of potential health risks, individuals with SCI should have a thorough medical examination [including a resting and stress test electrocardiogram (ECG)] prior to beginning a strenuous exercise program. Risks unique to individuals with SCI during exercise include exercise hypotension, orthostatic hypotension, autonomic dysreflexia (sudden and inappropriate blood pressure responses), thermoregulatory problems, trunk instability, pressure sores, muscle spasms, and ECG abnormalities (14,24,26,115,117, 142). In addition, many individuals with high-level (above T6) SCI lack the ability to perceive anginal pain as a result of disruption of ascending spinal cord afferents, which puts them at risk for unperceived cardiac (also called "silent") ischemia (10,175). Health care professionals involved with exercise for individuals with SCI should be aware of these risks and take appropriate safety precautions.

Blood pressure responses of individuals with SCI during exercise are quite different and inconsistent in comparison to those shown by AB individuals. Individuals with high-level SCI may exhibit a paradoxical drop in blood pressure as exercise progresses; this reflects a lowering of total peripheral resistance as blood vessels in active muscles dilate in response to hypoxia and increased concentrations of local metabolites, without a corresponding vasoconstriction in the inactive lower-body musculature and an increase in cardiac output (115). Exercise in an upright posture also causes blood pooling in the lower extremities, with an inadequate venous return and a low cardiac output, leading to orthostatic hypotension, with light-headedness or possible loss of consciousness. The risk may be reduced by regular orthostatic training (for example, head-up tilt, assisted standing, brace ambulation), maintenance of proper hydration, use of compression stockings and an abdominal binder, and physical conditioning.

Occasionally, some individuals with high-level SCI exhibit a sudden and inappropriate episode of extreme hypertension due to autonomic dysreflexia, caused by loss of central control (i.e., inhibition) of spinal reflexes and a subsequent exaggerated sympathetic response to noxious stimuli such as skin trauma, bowel impaction, and bladder overdistention. This situation is quite hazardous and can be fatal if not corrected in a timely manner (176). To help avoid this condition, the individual should follow proper health practices to eliminate noxious stimuli and seek medical treatment where appropriate. The bladder should be emptied just prior to exercise and during prolonged exercise bouts, and blood pressure should be monitored at regular intervals (at least during initial exercise sessions) (117). Exercise should be discontinued immediately if there are adverse reactions and appropriate action be taken to alleviate the problem (tilting up for hypertension and reclining for hypotension and syncope).

A security belt should be fitted around the individual's upper trunk during arm exercise to prevent falls if the individual has trunk instability and poor sitting balance. In addition, it is essential that pressure on weight-bearing tissues be minimized to prevent decubitus ulcers. Cushions should be placed under the ischial tuberosities and other weight-bearing areas, and pressure should be relieved periodically by raising the body off the cushion for 30–60 s every 20–30 min. Furthermore, many individuals with SCI experience occasional spasms in the paralyzed lower-limb muscles, ranging from mild to hazardous in their severity. So care must be taken to avoid damage to the lower limbs by strong spasms and rapid limb movements. Oral antispasmodic and muscle relaxant drugs help to control muscle spasms but may further limit exercise capability by reducing excitability not only of the paralyzed muscles but also of the nonparalyzed muscles. Potential side effects include light-headedness, ataxia, and depression (166).

Careful consideration also should be given to ambient temperature, relative humidity, and clothing worn as well as to exercise intensity and duration to prevent hyperthermia or hypothermia. Many individuals with SCI have a limited thermoregulatory capacity due to inadequate sweat secretion and impaired vasoregulation, so that overheating occurs more easily in this population than in the AB (57,102,157). This is especially true in a hot, humid environment, where prolonged strenuous exercise can cause severe dehydration, dangerously elevated body temperature, and possibly heat stroke and circulatory collapse. Under these conditions, frequent and adequate fluid replacement is essential. Exercise in cold environments may result in excessive heat loss, also exacerbated by impaired cardiovascular system control. If there are symptoms of either hyperthermia or hypothermia, exercise should be discontinued and clothing and environmental conditions should be appropriately adjusted.

PROBLEMS ASSOCIATED WITH ARM EXERCISE

Individuals with SCI use their relatively small and weak upper-body musculature for wheelchair propulsion and most other daily activities. This places them at a marked disadvantage on account of the limited peak oxygen uptake ($\dot{V}_{O_2}$) and power output (PO) capability for arm exercise, which is approximately two-thirds of leg exercise values for AB individuals who are not arm-exercise trained (4, 13,167,186). Arm-exercise capability may be further reduced by the disability as well as by diminished muscular and cardiopulmonary fitness resulting from a sedentary lifestyle and aging. Arm exercise is mechanically inefficient, and it is stressful to both the skeletal muscles and the cardiopulmonary systems compared with the same intensities of leg exercise (16,72,167,174). Indeed, when comparing wheelchair propulsion with walking and leg cycling, greater physiological stresses generally have been reported for hand-rim stroking (65,70,71,168, 183). The difference is more pronounced at the greater exercise intensities needed at high locomotive velocities and when negotiating architectural barriers such as carpeting and upward grades.

Compared to leg cycle ergometry for AB subjects at matched submaximal PO levels, arm exercise modes (arm cranking or wheelchair exercise) elicit greater metabolic stress, as indicated by the higher $\dot{V}_{O_2}$ and blood lactate values, a heavier cardiac load, with a higher heart rate, peripheral vascular resistance, intraarterial blood pressure, and stroke work and a greater demand on the pulmonary system (with a higher respiratory minute ventilation). A given absolute intensity of arm exercise also tends to elicit a lower cardiac output and ventricular stroke volume (5,12,16,65,66,159,167). The lower cardiac output and stroke volume may be due to a greater afterload on the heart on account of the higher peripheral vascular resistance and a lower end-diastolic volume due to an attenuated return of venous blood to the heart associated with inactivity of the skeletal muscle pump and disturbed vasoregulation in the paralyzed legs (74,78). Furthermore, the elevated intrathoracic pressure during hand-rim stroking might decrease the effectiveness of the thoracic pump (65). These factors together reduce the effective blood volume during wheelchair activity, limiting peak $\dot{V}_{O_2}$ and PO_{max} Therefore, wheelchair locomotion and arm-crank exercise, even at a low PO, can represent a relatively high exercise load with rapid onset of fatigue. Excessive cardiovascular and pulmonary stresses can hinder rehabilitation and impose risks upon certain individuals, including the elderly and those with cardiovascular or pulmonary impairments (65,74,78)

TECHNIQUES OF CARDIOPULMONARY FITNESS ASSESSMENT

Exercise stress testing enables assessment of cardiopulmonary fitness of individuals by evaluating exercise capacity and metabolic and cardiopulmonary responses. With AB individuals, leg exercise (treadmill walking/running or leg cycle ergometry) is typically used for stress testing and the large muscle mass that is contracted rhythmically in this way stimulates optimal (maximal) metabolic and cardiopulmonary responses for valid functional evaluation of these systems. The primary factor that limits maximal PO and $\dot{V}_{O_2}$ during these tests is *central circulatory* in nature, and the cardiovascular system is not able to deliver sufficient oxygen to the large exercising muscle mass (22,126, 152). In contrast, upper-body exercise (arm-crank and wheelchair exercise) activates a relatively small muscle mass. The primary limiting factors may be *peripheral* in nature, and local fatigue of the heavily stressed arm musculature can occur despite the delivery of sufficient blood and oxygen (6,64,76,91,156, 161). Another peripheral factor that may limit the performance of arm exercise is an inadequate venous return of blood to the heart owing to deficient skeletal muscle pump activity and impaired sympathetic vasoregulation. This can, in turn, limit cardiac output and the delivery of blood and oxygen to the arm muscles. Because of the lower PO capability and the early onset of fatigue, arm exercise may not provide sufficient stimulus to drive the metabolic and cardiopulmonary systems to full output, making valid functional evaluation of these systems difficult. Since the highest level of $\dot{V}_{O_2}$ that can be obtained for maximal effort arm exercise is somewhat lower than the true physiological maximum expected for leg exercise in AB individuals, the term *peak $\dot{V}_{O_2}$*, rather than *maximal $\dot{V}_{O_2}$*, is typically used.

Arm Exercise Modes

Clinical exercise stress testing as well as the training of wheelchair users with SCI typically involve arm-crank ergometers (ACE), since they are commercially available and the exercise intensity can be accurately set to desired levels. Wheelchair ergometers (WERG), which are stationary devices that enable close simulation of wheelchair locomotion, have also served these purposes (17,64,66,68, 180,182). Sophisticated WERGs that have been custom-designed and constructed for exercise physiological and biomechanical research studies can permit precise measurement of various operational torques, forces, and velocity for determining PO and propulsion characteristics (58,135). Although these devices are excellent for their intended purposes, wheelchair users may find them to have drawbacks, since they are relatively unavailable, expensive to construct, and do not permit the use of one's own wheelchair. However, another type of WERG, which may be advantageous for this population, consists of a person's own wheelchair mounted upon a commercially available roller system. To set exercise intensity accurately a roller system that permits measurement of propulsive force and velocity is necessary. Another wheelchair exercise mode that can be useful for exercise stress testing and training is operating a wheelchair on a motor-driven treadmill (45,60,89,107,171,173). Exercise intensity can be regulated by adjustment of velocity or grade or by applying additional resistive force via a pulley system (107,149,172). This system makes better simulation of actual wheelchair locomotion possible but is not practical for most wheelchair users.

Sawka et al. (154) compared WERG to ACE exercise at the same *submaximal* PO levels and found that WERG exercise generally elicited a higher oxygen uptake, respiratory minute volume, cardiac output, stroke volume, systolic blood pressure, and heart rate. Other studies found that *maximal* effort WERG and ACE exercise elicited similar peak oxygen uptake and respiratory minute volume but significantly lower maximal PO for WERG exercise (67,125). Due to similar maximal aerobic metabolic rates, it appears that both WERG and ACE can be used with similar results for exercise testing and training of wheelchair users. However, the concept of "exercise specificity" suggests that WERG exercise may be more appropriate than ACE exercise for individuals who propel their wheelchairs for sporting events or when wheelchair locomotion capability needs to be assessed, since it resembles more closely actual wheelchair locomotion (67,128). The lower metabolic rate and cardiopulmonary responses found for submaximal ACE exercise as well as the greater maximal PO achieved suggest that arm cranking may be superior to handrim stroking as a means of wheelchair locomotion. Indeed, Smith et al. (165) found a significantly lower oxygen uptake (−32%), respiratory minute volume (−30%) and heart rate (−19%) when operating an arm crank–propelled wheelchair relative to hand-rim propulsion under the same locomotive conditions, which has been confirmed by additional studies (125,170).

Stress Testing Protocols

The fundamental principles followed for lower-body exercise stress testing of AB individuals may be employed for upper-body exercise stress testing of individuals with SCI. Tests are usually progressive in exercise intensity and have well-defined *submaximal* or *maximal* effort endpoint criteria. Either *a continuous* or *discontinuous* protocol may be used. Discontinuous, submaximal protocols are preferable for stress testing of individuals with SCI, since they are relatively safe and comfortable. A suitable protocol would be to have exercise bouts that are 4–6 min in duration separated by 5–10 min of rest. For WERG and ACE tests, velocity is typically held constant (for example, a wheel velocity of 3 km/h and a crank rate of 50 rpm, respectively) while the resistance is increased. With WERG, 5 W appears to be an appropriate initial PO, as it is frequently encountered during daily wheelchair locomotion. PO increments of 5–10 W are appropriate for many individuals, and PO can be limited to 25–35 W for submaximal tests (64,65,122,154,155). For more fit individuals, the PO increment and maximal PO permitted can be greater. With ACE, the protocol can be the same, but the PO increments could be up to two times that for WERG. Steady-rate physiological responses can be determined during the last minute of each exercise bout. Criteria for exercise stress test termination include (a) voluntary cessation, (b) symptoms of cardiovascular or pulmonary abnormalities (e.g., chest discomfort, inappropriate ECG changes, marked hypertension or hypotension, dyspnea), (c) achievement of the maximal PO level required for the test, and (d) attainment of a predetermined heart rate (64). However, for individuals with high-level SCI, the heart-rate (HR) criterion may be less useful due to the interruption of sympathetic pathways to the heart and limited ability for cardioacceleration. Figure 3 illustrates metabolic and cardiopulmonary data of Glaser et al. (64) for a graded WERG test employing up to five 4-min exercise bouts, each followed by a 5-min rest. The subjects used for the development of this test protocol were AB and would be expected to exhibit physiological responses similar to those with paraplegia below T4, since sympathetic outflow to the heart would be intact. As PO was increased incrementally, $\dot{V}_{O_2}$ and HR responses increased linearly, analogous to the $\dot{V}_{O_2}$ and HR response patterns found for AB individuals during pro-

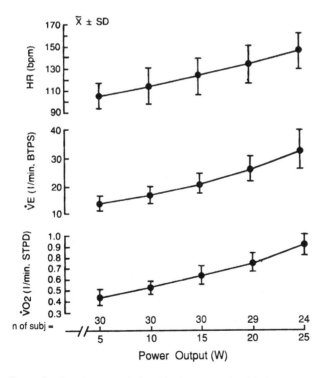

FIGURE 3   Steady-state relationships between wheelchair ergometer power output and oxygen uptake ($\dot{V}_{O_2}$), pulmonary ventilation (V_E), and heart rate (HR) for 30 able-bodied female subjects. (Modified from Ref. 64.)

gressive intensity treadmill running and leg cycling exercise. Maximal PO capability and peak $\dot{V}_{O_2}$ may be predicted from the submaximal data by extrapolating them to the estimated maximal HR level. In AB individuals, maximal HR during leg exercise is often estimated by using the formula 220 beats per minute minus age. However, this method would be less valid with those who have high-level SCI, since their cardioaccelatory mechanism can be markedly impaired, and the maximum HR achieved for arm exercise may be 10–20 beats per minute lower than for leg exercise (as found in AB individuals) owing to the smaller muscle mass. Thus, values obtained by using the formula 220 beats per minute minus age to estimate maximal HR may need to be reduced by 10–20 beats per minute for WERG and ACE exercise (154,167,181).

For accurate determination of peak metabolic and cardiopulmonary data, though, maximal exercise stress testing should be conducted to determine actual maximal PO and peak oxygen uptake. For this, the discontinuous, submaximal test can be extended to maximal effort by increasing the number of exercise bouts. However, drawbacks to this protocol are that much time would be required to complete the test, and the multiple bouts of exercise could lead to fatigue and underestimation of maximal PO and peak oxygen uptake. Therefore, if maximal testing is desired and submaximal data are not needed, a continuous maximal exercise protocol can be utilized. This shorter protocol begins at a low to moderate PO as a warm-up, and PO is then increased every 1–2 min until maximal effort is reached. By estimating fitness (possibly using previous submaximal testing), the initial PO level and the magnitude of increments can be set so that the individual will complete the test in several minutes (6,27,118,149,178,179).

Stress-testing fitness criteria are based upon the magnitudes of metabolic and cardiopulmonary responses elicited at given PO levels as well as the maximal PO achieved (64). At given submaximal PO levels, well-trained and more fit individuals typically exhibit lower heart-rate and pulmonary ventilation responses, indicating greater cardiopulmonary fitness, lower relative stress, and more functional reserve. In individuals with high-level SCI, however, care must be taken not to interpret the low exercise HR responses as an indication of superior cardiovascular fitness. As previously indicated, cardioacceleration in these individuals is limited by insufficient sympathetic stimulation, and most observed increases in HR are probably due to vagal withdrawal. Nevertheless, HR can still be used as an indicator of fitness in this population when expressed as a percentage of HR reserve (i.e., the functional range between resting and maximal HR) (108). For activities that do not require much skill (e.g., ACE), the submaximal $\dot{V}_{O_2}$ would be similar for both trained and untrained individuals. However, for activities requiring a greater degree of skill, a lower submaximal $\dot{V}_{O_2}$ response may be obtained from the trained individual, indicating lower aerobic energy expenditure and higher efficiency. At maximal-effort exercise, PO as well as peak values for $\dot{V}_{O_2}$, pulmonary ventilation, cardiac output, and stroke volume would be expected to be higher for fit individuals. But maximal HR may not be markedly different between more and less fit individuals, whereas it is reduced with age. Therefore, more fit individuals would possess greater metabolic and cardiopulmonary reserve, and specific submaximal tasks would be less stressful, since they are performed at a lower percentage of maximal PO, peak $\dot{V}_{O_2}$ pulmonary ventilation, and HR reserve.

EXERCISE TRAINING TECHNIQUES

Normal daily wheelchair activity may not provide sufficient exercise to train the muscular and cardiopulmonary systems; studies indicate that supplemental exercise training is necessary to improve physical fitness (92,109,117). Such training programs can increase cardiopulmonary fitness and reserve capability and make the activities of daily living (such as wheelchair locomotion and making transfers) less stressful, since they would be performed at lower percentages of maximal PO, peak oxygen uptake, and HR reserve (30,95,108,110). This could possibly contribute to an improved functional independence and rehabilitation outcome. Indeed, with wheelchair locomotion at 7 W, well-trained young wheelchair athletes are estimated to use less than 7% of their maximal PO and 18% of peak oxygen uptake. This is in contrast to older (50–60 year), sedentary wheelchair users who may utilize 44% of maximal PO and 51% of peak oxygen uptake, and to those aged 80–90 who may use 100% of their maximal PO and peak oxygen uptake for this routine locomotive task (71,155). In a 3-year study, Janssen, et al. (110) demonstrated that a decline of only 5–10 W in PO capability of sedentary wheelchair users with tetraplegia could result in a loss of independence. In contrast, however, their cohorts who regularly participated in sports activities and increased physical fitness generally maintained their independence and performed ADL with less stress. It is thus feasible that regular exercise training may reduce the stresses of wheelchair locomotion and other ADL, retard the decline in physical capability that typically accompanies aging, and lower some of the risks associated with secondary cardiovascular disabilities.

Arm-Exercise Training Protocols

To promote improved muscular and cardiopulmonary fitness as well as enhanced performance, arm exercise training for wheelchair users with SCI should, like leg exercise training, follow the fundamental principle of "overload" (74,78, 127). Exercise should be performed at intensities and/or durations that are beyond those normally encountered during daily life. Furthermore, exercise intensity and/ or duration should be progressively increased as performance improves until the desired fitness goals are reached. Regular exercise at the final intensity/duration levels is required to maintain the achieved fitness status. If exercise is discontinued, detraining will occur and fitness levels will diminish within several weeks. For optimal outcome, training should follow the "specificity of exercise" principle, where the mode of exercise used should be closely matched to the activity in which performance improvement is desired.

Arm-exercise training protocols may be either continuous or discontinuous in design. If enhanced cardiopulmonary fitness is the primary goal, PO should be adjusted to allow moderate levels of exercise of relatively long durations (15–60 min for continuous bouts, and 3–10 min for each of the several discontinuous bouts) without excessive fatigue or respiratory distress. Exercise sessions should occur two to five times per week (127). Traditionally, ACE exercise has been used for endurance training of wheelchair users with SCI. This exercise mode is readily available, and it has been shown to improve cardiopulmonary fitness (38, 93). Although wheelchair ergometer exercise elicits similar peak metabolic and cardiopulmonary responses, it has the advantage of more closely resembling actual wheelchair activity, so it may better enhance wheelchair locomotive performance. If enhancing muscular power is the primary goal, higher levels of PO would be used and exercise bouts would be of relatively short duration (e.g., from a few seconds to a few minutes). The large anaerobic energy component would result in a marked accumulation of blood lactate. This form of exercise would be useful for wheelchair athletes who want to improve sprinting performance as well as for most other wheelchair users, since many ADL (e.g., transfers, overcoming architectural barriers) require intense, short-duration efforts.

In developing an aerobic training protocol for leg exercise by AB individuals, an appropriate training intensity is typically established by having them exercise at between 60–90% of their maximal HR reserve, which usually corresponds to 50–85% of peak $\dot{V}_{O_2}$. The objective is to exercise at high enough intensity for a sufficient duration to permit cardiopulmonary adaptations to occur. But exercise intensity should be kept below the point where marked anaerobiosis occurs and a high concentration of lactate accumulates in the blood, which can severely shorten endurance and create discomfort. Actual measurement of HR during maximal-effort exercise for each individual would be preferred over prediction techniques to facilitate appropriate setting of training intensity. But for arm exercise by individuals with SCI, an effective training intensity may be more difficult to set, since it is more important that maximal-effort HR is known. Janssen et al. (108) showed that percentage of peak $\dot{V}_{O_2}$ and HR reserve were highly correlated during wheelchair exercise on a treadmill by individuals with paraplegia and tetraplegia. However, the absolute values for HR were lower in the individuals with the higher level lesions. Their regression equations predicted that exercise at 50–85% of peak $\dot{V}_{O_2}$ corresponded to HR reserve values of 40–85% for individuals with low-level paraplegia and 30–80% for those with high-level paraplegia and tetraplegia. Thus, HR response expressed either as a percentage of HR reserve or maximal HR can be a usable indicator of exercise stress in these populations, but the actual value used would be dependent upon the exercise response characteristics of the individual (99,108). Therefore, to set arm-exercise intensity for various individuals with SCI, direct determination of peak values for HR, PO, $\dot{V}_{O_2}$, pulmonary ventilation, and blood lactate concentration (during stress testing) would be desirable if the instrumentation is available. In individuals who do not exhibit a clear relationship among these variables (which is more common in those with tetraplegia), training at a percentage of maximal PO may be preferable (129). Where laboratory testing is not available, intensity criteria may be established according to the subjective feeling of stress and the actual exercise endurance capability. In most cases, it is likely that several trials will be needed for each individual to effectively set training intensity.

Physiological Adaptations to Arm-Exercise Training

Studies on individuals with SCI indicated that several weeks of endurance-type arm-exercise training can significantly increase the PO capability, peak oxygen uptake, and cardiopulmonary performance (43,117,130,145). Training with ACE in active wheelchair users increased their peak oxygen uptake by 12–19% in 7–20 weeks (136,145). Even greater gains in cardiopulmonary fitness were obtained when individuals with tetraplegia who had relatively low initial fitness levels were trained for only 5 weeks (43). Using WERG exercise, Miles et al. (130) reported that over 6 weeks of interval training (three times per week), eight wheelchair athletes increased their maximal PO capability by 31%, peak oxygen uptake by 26%, and peak respiratory minute volume by 32% (Table 1). These gains were even more remarkable considering that the athletic subjects had relatively high levels of fitness prior to training.

Although arm-exercise training limits the absolute level of aerobic fitness that can be achieved with training, some cardiopulmonary benefits can be expected for most individuals. However, the magnitudes by which aerobic fitness and exercise performance can be increased with training appear to be dependent upon the initial fitness level and the size of the muscle mass available for exercise. For instance, several studies on wheelchair athletes performing maximal effort ACE and WERG exercise indicated that their peak $\dot{V}_{O_2}$ is in the range of 2–3 L/min (25,60,74,97,130). This is approximately half of the maximal $\dot{V}_{O_2}$ that would be expected for healthy AB athletes performing maximal-effort leg exercise (e.g., cycling, running). Generally, greater gains in fitness may be expected from individuals with SCI who initiate training programs at relatively low fitness levels (depending upon pathological limitations) (74,78). It is plausible that many of the observed gains in arm-exercise performance are due to peripheral adaptations such as improved capillary density and/or metabolic capability within mus-

TABLE 1   Individual and Mean (±SD) Values for Pulmonary Ventilation ($\dot{V}_E$, L/min), Tidal Volume (V_T, L), Respiratory Frequency (R_f, Breaths per Minute) Power Output (W) and Peak Oxygen Uptake ($\dot{V}_{O_2}$, L/min), Attained During Maximal Wheelchair Ergometer Exercise Before (B) and After (A) 6 Weeks of Interval Training by 8 Wheelchair Athletes with SCI.

Subject	$\dot{V}_E$ B	$\dot{V}_E$ A	V_T B	V_T A	R_f B	R_f A	Power output B	Power output A	Peak $\dot{V}_{O_2}$ B	Peak $\dot{V}_{O_2}$ A
1	74.7	111.2	2.49	3.09	30	36	70	96	2.05	2.43
2	136.9	180.8	4.56	3.12	30	58	100	140	3.34	3.73
3	115.2	145.1	1.92	2.20	60	66	72	100	2.41	2.98
4	99.2	116.3	2.20	1.87	45	62	80	90	1.89	2.18
5	103.3	143.7	1.72	2.40	60	60	90	105	2.00	2.65
6	68.2	109.2	1.71	1.82	40	60	52	83	1.57	2.31
7	80.4	106.7	1.61	2.05	50	52	83	95	2.04	2.60
8	119.0	137.3	2.77	2.54	43	54	81	110	2.19	3.26
Mean	99.6	131.3	2.37	2.38	44.8	56	78.3	102.3	2.19	2.76
SD	22.4	23.8	0.91	0.47	10.9	8.6	14	16	0.49	0.49
	$p < 0.05$		NS		$p < 0.05$		$p < 0.05$		$p < 0.05$	

Source: Modified from Ref. 130.

cles (which would increase arteriovenous oxygen difference) rather than central circulatory adaptations (69,76,124,160,163). Nevertheless, regular arm-exercise training appears to increase maximal PO capability and peak oxygen uptake, and it may also decrease levels of physiological responses for given submaximal exercise tasks and ADL, including wheelchair locomotion (29,44,69,108,158, 178).

Exercise Training and Coronary Heart Disease Risk

Habitual arm-exercise training and sports participation may also reduce the risk for acquiring coronary heart disease (CHD). Cross-sectional studies on sedentary and physically active wheelchair users showed that the more active individuals had a superior blood lipid profile as indicated by a lower total cholesterol (TC), lower low-density-lipoprotein cholesterol (LDL-C), and greater high-density-lipoprotein cholesterol (HDL-C) (19,30,40,112). In a longitudinal study, Hooker and Wells (96) reported a decrease in TC (-8%), a significant increase in HDL-C ($+20\%$), and a decrease in LDL-C (-15%) in five men with SCI following 8 weeks of moderate-intensity WERG training (60–70% peak $\dot{V}_{O_2}$, 20 min per day, three times per week). These apparently beneficial alterations in the blood lipid profile extrapolated to a mean decrease of 20% in the group's future risk for CHD. Thus, if HDL-C does have a protective effect against coronary heart disease and TC and LDL-C increase its risk, these HDL-C, TC and LDL-C changes that may occur with increased physical activity suggest that the risk of CHD in individuals with SCI may be decreased with arm-exercise intervention in a similar fashion as leg exercise training benefits AB individuals. However, Davis et al. (33) showed that although a 16-week ACE training of untrained individuals with paraplegia resulted in a significant increase in peak oxygen uptake and stroke volume, left ventricular mass did not significantly change. More research is necessary to develop appropriate exercise modes and protocols and to document their efficacy for reducing the risk of cardiovascular disease in this population.

Body Position and Arm Exercise Capability

In some individuals with lower-limb paralysis, the etiology of upper-body muscle fatigue may be a central factor secondary to a peripheral factor. It is conceivable that inactivity of the skeletal muscle pump combined with impaired vasoregulation in the paralyzed lower limbs and abdominal region can limit venous return of blood from the lower body to the heart (a peripheral factor), thereby restricting the cardiac output capability during arm exercise (a central factor). Thus, pooling of blood in leg and abdominal vasculature can potentially lead to a hypokinetic circulation, reducing the availability of blood to the active upper-body musculature and limiting its exercise capability (74,76,78). Since individuals with SCI typically perform arm exercise in an upright, sitting position, this can elevate hydrostatic pressure and blood pooling in leg veins. It is plausible that arm exercise capability may be enhanced by placing the individual in a supine position. This can minimize the gravitational effects on blood, facilitate venous return, elevate cardiac output, and increase arm muscle blood flow to boost fatigue resistance.

In a preliminary study by Figoni et al. (50), subjects with tetraplegia performed maximal-effort ACE in a sitting and in a supine position on separate occasions. It was found that maximal-effort exercise in the supine position elicited significantly higher maximal PO as well as peak oxygen uptake, respiratory minute volume, stroke volume, and cardiac output. Similar results have been found in subjects with high-level paraplegia, but not to the same degree (100). The greater magnitudes of these responses suggest that cardiopulmonary training capability in individuals with SCI may be enhanced by using the supine position. Indeed, McLean and Skinner (129), who used ACE exercise to train subjects with tetraplegia in the sitting and supine positions, showed greater improvement in peak $\dot{V}_{O_2}$ (during testing in both the sitting and supine positions) when trained in the supine position. Although these studies suggest that the supine position can improve exercise outcome, more research is needed to determine advantageous protocols and long-term training effects.

Other techniques have been studied in an attempt to reduce the effects of gravity on venous return during arm exercise. Kerk et al. (113) used an abdominal binder with wheelchair athletes with high-level paraplegia during submaximal and maximal effort WERG exercise but found no differences in metabolic and cardiopulmonary responses or biomechanical characteristics compared to not using the abdominal binder. Hopman et al. (101) showed that use of a fighter pilot anti-G suit, which applied constant external pressure (52 mmHg) to the calves, thighs, and abdomen of men with paraplegia (below T5) during submaximal arm-crank exercise, can facilitate venous return and increase stroke volume. However, they did not show any improvement in maximal exercise capacity. Pitetti et al. (143) also used a fighter pilot anti-G suit, but fluctuated pressure every 2 min to simulate skeletal muscle pump activity; they found a significant increase in peak $\dot{V}_{O_2}$ during ACE and WERG exercise by individuals with predominantly high-level SCI. Although use of external compression to the lower limbs and abdomen may have some effect in facilitating venous return during arm exercise, use of electrical stimulation–induced rhythmic contractions of lower limb muscles may better activate the skeletal muscle pump for more effective results (75,146).

USE OF FUNCTIONAL ELECTRICAL STIMULATION–INDUCED EXERCISE OF THE PARALYZED LOWER-LIMB MUSCULATURE

During the past two decades, functional electrical stimulation (FES) research has been conducted with the goal of inducing exercise in paralyzed lower-limb muscles (28,132). Typically, electrical impulses from a stimulator are used in conjunction with skin-surface electrodes placed over motor points to induce tetanic contractions of controlled intensity. Therefore, FES-induced exercise of the paralyzed legs has the potential of utilizing a large muscle mass that otherwise would be dormant. In addition, this exercise augments the circulation by activation of the skeletal muscle pump. It is thus apparent that FES exercise modes can improve the health, cardiopulmonary fitness, and rehabilitation potential of individuals with SCI to levels higher than can be attained with arm exercise alone. Individuals with tetraplegia will most likely find this induced exercise mode particularly advantageous on account of the small muscle mass that is under voluntary control.

Special Considerations and Precautions

The primary requirement for FES use is that the muscles to be exercised are paralyzed because of upper motor neuron damage and that the motor units are intact and functional. The existence of stretch reflex activity and spasticity indicates that the individual is a potential candidate for FES exercise. However, if the individual retains some degree of sensate skin, FES may cause discomfort or pain and the high stimulation current that is required to induce forceful contractions may not be tolerated. Prior to initiating an FES exercise program, a thorough medical examination—including radiographs of the paralyzed limbs, range-of-motion testing, neurological examination, an ECG, and preferably evaluation of psychological status—is essential. The individual should be informed of the potential benefits and risks of FES exercise and clearly understand that FES *will not* regenerate damaged neurons or cure paralysis. It should also be understood that, as with voluntary exercise training, any health and fitness benefits derived from FES exercise training will be lost several weeks after this activity is discontinued.

Since the muscles, bones, and joints of the paralyzed lower limbs tend to be deteriorated, FES-induced contractions should be kept as smooth as possible and the contraction force generated should be limited to a safe level to prevent injury. Although FES exercise training can improve the strength and endurance of the paralyzed muscles and may *retard* osteoporosis progression, there is currently no evidence that osteoporosis can be markedly *reversed* by such activity

(11,88,164). Therefore, it is conceivable that the muscles will ultimately generate more force than the bones can withstand. In addition, FES may trigger severe spasms in some muscles, so it is important to observe the quality of the contractions to be certain that they are not hazardous (74,87). In individuals generally with lesions at or above T6, FES exercise may provoke autonomic dysreflexia, with episodic dangerously high blood pressure (3,74,87). Therefore, it is essential that blood pressure be monitored periodically, especially during the initial FES exercise sessions. Such exercise should be discontinued immediately if any response is observed that places the individual at risk.

Promoting Venous Return with FES During Voluntary Arm Exercise

Arm-exercise performance and the capability of developing high levels of cardiopulmonary fitness may both be limited by a hypokinetic circulation owing to an inadequate skeletal muscle pump activity. Although techniques to promote venous return, such as exercising in a supine position and use of external compression devices, may help alleviate this situation, another viable approach to promote venous return and enhance cardiac output and blood flow to the exercising upper-body muscles is FES-induced rhythmic contractions of the paralyzed leg muscles (75). Davis et al. (32,35) and Figoni et al. (48) showed that this FES technique can significantly augment the stroke volume and cardiac output during both rest and ACE exercise at various gravitational loads (sitting, supine, and head-up-tilt body positions). In addition, Phillips et al. (141) showed that leg blood flow was increased by 29% during arm cranking with concurrent FES-induced lower limb contractions compared to arm cranking alone. Thus, it appears that this technique can diminish venous stasis/pooling and alleviate the hypokinetic circulation in individuals with SCI, which can potentially enhance arm-exercise capability by increasing blood availability (82,98). Indeed, Glaser et al. (82) found significant increases in maximal PO (+9%), as well as peak oxygen uptake (+19%), pulmonary ventilation (+10%), stroke volume (+26%), and cardiac output (+37%) by subjects with paraplegia and tetraplegia when using this FES technique during ACE exercise. Thus far, however, long-term exercise training adaptations have not been determined using this technique. This same FES technique has been used during wheelchair locomotion by individuals with SCI in an attempt to reduce relative stress by increasing venous return (147). It was found that HR and ratings of perceived exertion were generally lower when using rhythmic FES-induced leg muscle contractions during locomotion at the three paced velocities tested. The FES technique may have several other clinical applications, including deep venous thrombus prophylaxis, reducing excessive edema, and alleviating orthostatic hypotension (54,75,146).

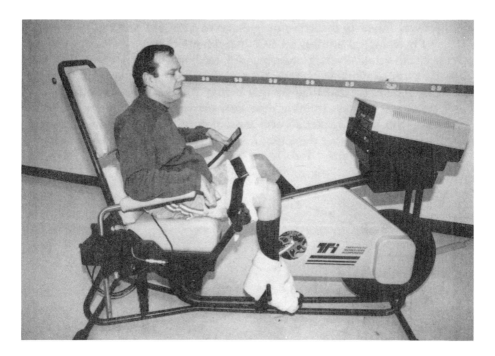

FIGURE 4   Functional electrical stimulation (FES) leg cycle ergometer exercise being performed by person with a spinal cord injury on an ERGYS I. (Therapeutic Alliances, Inc.)

Promoting Cardiopulmonary Fitness with FES-Induced Cycle Ergometry

To enhance cardiopulmonary fitness in individuals with SCI, a prototype leg cycle ergometer (LCE) propelled by computer-controlled FES-induced contractions of the paralyzed lower-limb muscle groups (quadriceps, hamstrings, and gluteus maximus) was designed and constructed by Petrofsky et al. (Fig. 4) (138). Studies indicate that FES-LCE exercise elicits relatively high magnitudes of aerobic metabolic and cardiopulmonary responses, as well as favorable central and peripheral hemodynamic responses from individuals with SCI (7,8,49,51,77,131,144, 148). Figure 5 provides data from Glaser et al. (77) depicting a steady-rate oxygen uptake, respiratory minute volume, and heart rate of 12 individuals with SCI during progressive-intensity FES-induced leg cycling indicating that relationships are quite linear. It is predicted from these data that a well-trained individual who can pedal at a PO of 43 W would have a peak oxygen uptake of about 2.0 L/

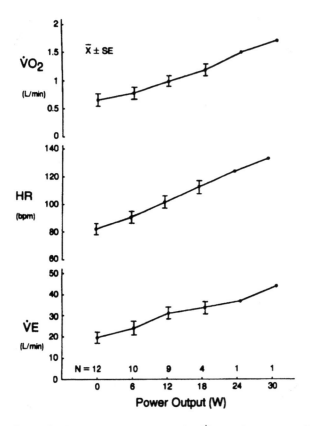

FIGURE 5   Steady-state oxygen uptake ($\dot{V}_{O_2}$), pulmonary ventilation ($\dot{V}_E$), and heart rate (HR) responses of individuals with spinal cord injury in relationship to power output for FES cycle ergometry. (Modified from Ref. 77.)

min with correspondingly high respiratory minute ventilation and HR responses. To put this in perspective, many AB individuals jog at oxygen uptake levels of 1.5–2.0 L/min (50–60% of their maximal oxygen uptake). Therefore, FES cycling offers individuals with SCI a potential means of training at a similar aerobic metabolic rate. However, individuals would have to be highly trained in FES-LCE exercise to achieve such high metabolic responses for long durations. Most individuals with SCI perform FES cycle ergometry at metabolic levels equivalent to walking (for example, an oxygen uptake of about 1 L/min). This can be quite beneficial for those with tetraplegia, as this metabolic rate is higher than they can achieve with arm exercise (21,108,129).

Another important advantage of FES cycle ergometry is that central hemo-

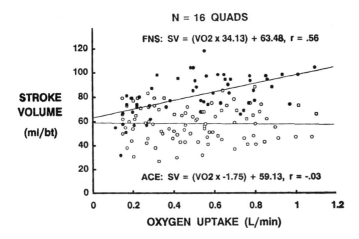

FIGURE 6   Individual data for stroke volume vs oxygen uptake of 16 individuals with tetraplegia during voluntary arm crank ergometer (ACE) and FES leg cycle ergometer exercise using progressive intensity power output levels. Linear regression equations and lines of best fit for ACE and FES cycling are provided. (From Ref. 53.)

dynamic responses for this exercise have been shown to be superior to those for voluntary arm exercise. Figoni et al. (49) found significantly higher stroke volume (92 versus 58 ml per beat) and cardiac output (8.0 versus 6.7 L/min) at the same oxygen uptake level of 1 L/min for six men with tetraplegia performing FES-LCE and arm-cranking exercise. Figure 6 illustrates individual data for stroke volume versus oxygen uptake in 16 individuals with tetraplegia during voluntary ACE and FES cycling exercise at an increasing PO (53). A probable mechanism for these responses is that FES-induced contractions of the paralyzed leg muscles activated the skeletal muscle pump and enhanced venous return, increasing cardiac preload and stroke volume (Frank-Starling mechanism). In addition, Bloomfield et al. (15) reported elevations in circulating catecholamines during acute FES-LCE exercise, which could also promote venous return as well as increase myocardial contractility. Also, Robergs et al. (153) found an increase in circulating endothelin after FES-LCE in individuals with SCI, which may influence baroreceptor function and therefore blood pressure control. Figoni et al. (49), moreover, found a 25% lower HR (87 versus 116 beats per min) and a 19% lower rate-pressure product during FES cycling, suggesting that the higher cardiac volume load was achieved with lower myocardial oxygen demands. Therefore, FES cycling is potentially more effective than arm cranking for cardiopulmonary training of individuals with tetraplegia and cause lower cardiovascular risk.

Studies on FES-LCE exercise training demonstrated several physiological adaptations, which probably reflected both peripheral (skeletal muscle) and cardiopulmonary benefits. Generally, significant improvements in PO capability and in peak oxygen uptake, pulmonary ventilation, stroke volume, and HR are seen after 6 weeks to 6 months of FES-LCE training (2,8,18,85,111,119,131,144, 153,164,169). Improved cardiopulmonary fitness resulting from FES-LCE training was also indicated by superior responses during submaximal exercise and rest. Under resting conditions, an increase in systolic blood pressure, heart rate, and cardiac index has been found in individuals with tetraplegia after FES-LCE training, which helped them to alleviate their chronic hypotension and improve cardiovascular stability (31,47,140). In contrast, for those with paraplegia, beneficial *reductions* in resting blood pressure and HR are commonly found (47,153). For a given submaximal oxygen uptake or PO level, lower HR, ventilatory equivalent for oxygen uptake, blood lactate concentration, and arterial blood pressure and faster oxygen uptake kinetics are among the improved responses found (8,47,139), similar to responses typically obtained for AB individuals following aerobic training. These data suggest that oxygen delivery to the muscle had improved and/or the aerobic capacity of the muscles was enhanced. Thus, as cardiopulmonary fitness increases, given submaximal FES-LCE exercise becomes relatively less stressful and higher PO levels are needed to further the training adaptations. Gains in cardiopulmonary fitness may ultimately translate into reduced risk for cardiopulmonary complications as well as less stressful performance of ADL tasks.

The relatively high magnitudes of metabolic and cardiopulmonary responses as well as advantageous peripheral and central hemodynamic responses obtained during FES-LCE exercise may provide benefits to decrease the risk for cardiovascular complications. Indeed, Danopulos et al. (31) detected increases in left ventricular mass (+4.1%) and left ventricular end-diastolic volume (+2.5%) in six subjects with tetraplegia after 12 weeks of training. More dramatically, Nash et al. (133) showed significant increases in left ventricular end-diastolic internal dimension (+6.5%), interventricular septal (+17.8%) and posterior wall (+20.3%) end-diastolic thicknesses, and in calculated left ventricular mass (+35%) in subjects with tetraplegia following 6 months of FES-LCE exercise training. These findings suggest that the left ventricular atrophy resulting from chronic volume underloading, commonly seen in those with tetraplegia (114), can be reversed with this induced exercise mode. With respect to blood lipid profile, Bremner et al. (18) did not find improvements in the lipid profile of six subjects with SCI after participating in a 24-week combined FES-LCE training program. In contrast, Brenes et al. (20) demonstrated a 6% increase in high-density lipoprotein-cholesterol following 4–5 months of FES-LCE training indicating reduced coronary heart-disease risks for persons with SCI.

Improving FES-LCE Exercise Responses

Although the original FES-LCE technology has been shown to be efficacious, a plateau in exercise performance is often reached after several months of training, which may be due to the person's inability to exercise at sufficiently high intensity levels to elicit continuous gains in performance. Recent research suggests that the efficacy of this original technology may be improved by appropriate modifications of FES parameters and the number of muscle groups activated. Data from Glaser et al. (83) indicated that increasing the maximal FES current from the original 140 to 300 mA resulted in recruitment of greater muscle mass and markedly increased PO and cardiopulmonary responses, and Figoni et al. (55) showed that additional activation of the gastro-soleus and anterior tibialis muscle groups could also augment metabolic and cardiopulmonary responses. Subsequently, Glaser et al. (84) showed that a system that combined these modified parameters provided markedly greater overload capability to enhance muscular and cardiopulmonary adaptations than the original system. Moreover, Janssen et al. (111) showed that only 6 weeks of training using this enhanced system in combination with a specially designed interval training program protocol elicited markedly improved PO capability and aerobic power in four men with SCI whose performance had plateaued during long-term (>6 years) training on the original FES-LCE. Therefore, this improved FES technology can increase training effectiveness and outcome.

To further activate more muscle mass and subsequently provide greater exercise responses to enhance cardiopulmonary fitness training capability, a hybrid mode of exercise is used, consisting of FES-induced lower-body exercise combined with voluntary upper-body exercise (Fig. 7). Several studies demonstrated that the addition of voluntary ACE exercise to FES-LCE exercise by individuals with tetraplegia and paraplegia resulted in significantly higher levels of $\dot{V}_{O_2}$, pulmonary ventilation, cardiac output, and stroke volume in comparison with performing either ACE or FES-LCE separately (23,32,52,56,73,80,98,119,151). Glaser (79) demonstrated this concept with a man with T8 paraplegia whose $\dot{V}_{O_2}$ was 0.25 L/min at rest; 0.75 L/min during FES leg cycling alone at 6.1 W; 0.75 L/min during voluntary arm cranking alone at 25 W; and 1.25 L/min during hybrid exercise at a total of 31.1 W. Thus, a $\dot{V}_{O_2}$ 0.5 L/min higher was achieved with this combined exercise. Subsequently, Hooker et al. (98) had eight subjects with tetraplegia perform this exercise and found significantly higher levels of oxygen uptake ($+55\%$, $+55\%$), pulmonary ventilation ($+53\%$, $+39\%$), heart rate ($+18\%$, $+33\%$), and cardiac output ($+47\%$, $+24\%$), and significantly lower total peripheral resistance (-34%, -21%) than for performing either ACE or FES-LCE separately, respectively. Climstein et al. (23) demonstrated that this hybrid exercise can produce similar response patterns in those with paraplegia.

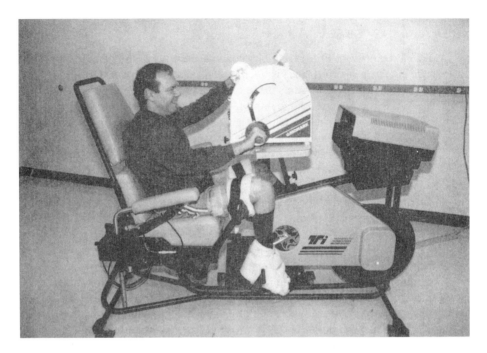

FIGURE 7 Hybrid (simultaneous FES-induced cycle ergometer and voluntary arm-crank ergometer) exercise being performed by a person with spinal cord injury. The adjustable stand supporting the arm crank ergometer was specially designed and constructed.

Figoni et al. (52) combined O-W (unloaded) FES-LCE with *maximal effort* ACE for nine subjects with tetraplegia and found significant increases in peak levels of oxygen uptake (+35%), stroke volume (+26%), cardiac output (+46%) and heart rate (+18%). Not all studies have been able to show an increase in heart rate with this hybrid exercise. Raymond et al. (151) showed that although the metabolic rate was higher during the hybrid exercise in individuals with paraplegia, heart rate was lower, which made them conclude that the cardiac stress is less for this mode of exercise. The higher magnitudes of metabolic and cardiopulmonary responses during the hybrid exercise indicated that maximal effort ACE by itself was not a sufficient stimulus to drive the cardiopulmonary system to full output. Hybrid exercise can apparently accomplish this due to the substantially larger muscle mass utilized and the enhanced peripheral and central hemodynamic responses that occur.

We find this combination exercise frequently elicits peak $\dot{V}_{O_2}$ levels of over 1.5 and 2.0 L/min from nonathletic persons with tetraplegia and paraplegia, respectively. Considering that maximal effort arm (i.e., ACE and WERG) exercise for aerobically trained wheelchair athletes had been reported to elicit peak oxygen uptake values in the range of 2–3 L/min, this hybrid exercise mode appears to be superior since similar peak oxygen uptake values can be obtained from the general population of persons with SCI. Indeed, a study by Krauss et al. (119) showed that a 6-week training program using this hybrid exercise improved peak levels of $\dot{V}_{O_2}$ for both ACE and hybrid exercises. Also, Raymond et al. (150) showed that a 10-week hybrid training program significantly increased peak oxygen uptake in individuals with paraplegia. Although this increase was not greater than with arm-crank training alone, significant improvements in submaximal cardiac output and stroke volume during arm exercise were observed, and this is where the major benefits may be located for those with paraplegia. Additionally, it is unlikely that arm exercise training by itself provides any marked improvements with respect to lower-limb circulation or integrity of the musculature. Therefore, the described hybrid exercise appears to provide more advantageous levels of metabolic and cardiopulmonary responses for aerobic conditioning of individuals with SCI while providing training benefits to both the upper- and lower-body musculature.

CONCLUSION

During the past 25 years, much research has been dedicated to developing exercise techniques that can be used to evaluate and to improve cardiopulmonary fitness of individuals with SCI. Traditionally, arm exercise modes have been used for these purposes and it has been shown that many physical and psychological benefits can be obtained by these exercise modes. However, recent innovations in FES techniques appear to be opening new avenues to more effective training. By utilizing FES to exercise paralyzed leg muscles, a greater muscle mass can be utilized and peripheral and central hemodynamic responses may be improved. The use of FES-induced cycle ergometer exercise can elicit aerobic metabolic and cardiopulmonary responses of sufficient magnitudes and durations to stimulate cardiopulmonary training effects. These responses seem superior to those elicited by voluntary ACE exercise, especially for individuals with tetraplegia. FES leg exercise is best used in conjunction with arm exercise (separately and combined) to optimize upper-body, lower-body and cardiopulmonary fitness. Hybrid-type exercise is the most promising exercise technique for promoting effective and efficient development of aerobic fitness in individuals with paraplegia and tetraplegia. Ultimately, FES exercise may contribute to improved health, cardiopulmonary fitness, and the rehabilitation potential of individuals with SCI.

ACKNOWLEDGMENTS

The authors wish to thank the Dayton Veterans Affairs Medical Center and the Rehabilitation Institute of Ohio at Miami Valley Hospital for enabling implementation of their research projects on individuals with spinal cord injuries. Most of the research projects from the authors' laboratory were supported by the Rehabilitation Research and Development Service of the U.S. Department of Veterans Affairs.

REFERENCES

1. American College of Sports Medicine, *ACSM's Guidelines for Exercise Testing and Prescription.* Williams & Wilkins, Baltimore (1995).
2. Arnold, P.B., McVey P., Farrell, W.J., Deurloo, T.M., and Grasso, A.R., *Arch Phys. Med. Rehabil.,* 73: 665–668 (1992).
3. Ashley, E.A., Laskin, J.J., Olenik, L.M., Bumham, R., Steadward, R.D., Cumming, D.C., and Wheeler, G.D., *Paraplegia,* 31: 593–605 (1993).
4. Astrand, P.-O., and Saltin, B., *J. Appl. Physiol.,* 16: 977–981 (1961).
5. Astrand, P.-O., Ekblom, B., Messin, R., Saltin, B., and Stenberg, J., *J. Appl. Physiol.,* 20: 253–256 (1965).
6. Bar-Or, O., and Zwiren, L.D., *J. Appl. Physiol.,* 38: 424–426 (1975).
7. Barstow, T.J, Scremin, A.M.E., Mutton, D.L., Kunkel, C.F., Cagle, T.G., and Whipp, B.J., *Med. Sci. Sports Exerc.,* 27: 1284–1291 (1995).
8. Barstow, T.J., Scremin, A.M.E., Mutton, D.L., Kunkel, C.F., Cagle, T.G., and Whipp, B.J., *Med. Sci. Sports Exerc.,* 28: 1221–1228 (1996).
9. Bauman, W.A., Spungen, A.M., Zhong, Y., Rothstein, J.L., Petry, C., and Gordon, S.K., *Paraplegia,* 30: 697–703. (1992).
10. Bauman, W., Raza, M., Chayes, Z. et al., *Arch. Phys. Med. Rehabil.,* 74: 740 (1993).
11. BeDell, K.K., Scremin, A.M.E., Perell, K.L., and Kunkel, C.F., *Am. J. Phys. Med. Rehabil.,* 75: 29–34 (1996).
12. Bevegard, S., Freyschuss, U., and Strandell, T., *J. Appl. Physiol.,* 23: 37–46 (1966).
13. Bergh, U., Kanstrup, I.-L., and Ekblom, B., *J. Appl. Physiol.,* 41: 191–196 (1976).
14. Blocker, W.P., Merrill, J.M., Krebs, M.A., et al., *Am. Correct. Ther. J.,* 37: 101 (1983).
15. Bloomfield, S.A., Jackson, R.D., and Mysiw, W.J., *Med Sci Sports Exerc.,* 26: 1213–1219 (1994).
16. Bobbert, A.C., *J. Appl. Physiol.,* 15: 1007–1014 (1960).
17. Brattgard, S.-O., Grimby, G., and Hook, O., *Scand J. Rehabil. Med.,* 2: 143–148 (1970).
18. Bremner, L.A., Sloan, K.E., Day, R.E., Scull, E.R., and Ackland, T., *Paraplegia,* 30: 647–655 (1992).
19. Brenes, G., Dearwater, S., Shapera, R., LaPorte, R.E., and Collins, E., *Arch. Phys. Med. Rehabil.,* 67: 445–450 (1986).

20. Brenes, G., *Proc. ASIA 15th Ann. Sci. Mtg.,* p.78 (1989).
21. Burkett, L.N., Chisum, J., Stone, W., and Fernhall, B., *Paraplegia,* 28: 512–521 (1990).
22. Clausen, J.P., Klausen, K., Rasmussen, B., and Trap-Jensen, J., *Am. J. Physiol.,* 225: 675–682 (1973).
23. Climstein, M., Fahey, A., Davis, G.M., and Sutton, J.R., *Med. Sci. Sports Exerc.,* 27(5 Suppl.): S83 (1995).
24. Cole, T.M., Kottke, F.J., Olson M., Stradal, L., and Niederloh, J., *Arch. Phys. Med. Rehabil.,* 14: 359–368 (1967).
25. Cooper R.A., Horvath S.M., Bedi J.F., Drechsler-Parks D.M., and Williams R.E., *Paraplegia,* 30: 573–581 (1992).
26. Corbett, J.L., Frankel, H.L., and Harris, P.J., *Paraplegia,* 9: 113–119 (1971).
27. Coutts, K.D., Rhodes, E.C., and McKenzie, D.C., *J. Appl. Physiol: Respir. Environ. Exerc. Physiol.,* 55: 479–482 (1983).
28. Cybulski, G.R., Penn, R.D., and Jaeger, R.J., *Neurosurgery,* 15: 132–146 (1984).
29. Dallmeijer, A.J., Hopman, M.T.E., Van As, H.J., and Van der Woude, L.H.V., *Spinal Cord,* 34: 729–735 (1996).
30. Dallmeijer, A.J., Hopman, M.T.E., and Van der Woude, L.H.V., *Arch. Phys. Med. Rehabil.,* 78: 1173–1176 (1997).
31. Danopulos, D., Kezdi, P., Stanley, E.L., Petrofsky, J.S., Stacy, R.W., Phillips, C.A., and Meyer, L.S., *J. Neurol. Orthop. Med. Surg.,* 7: 179–184 (1986).
32. Davis, G.M., Servedio, F.J., Glaser, R.M., Collins, S.R., Gupta, S.C., and Suryaprasad, A.G., *Proc. 10th Ann. RESNA Conf. Rehabil. Tech.,* pp. 591–593 (1987).
33. Davis, G.M., Shephard, R.J., and Leenen, F.H., *Eur. J. Appl. Physiol. Occup. Physiol.,* 56 (1): 90–96 (1987).
34. Davis, G.M., and Shephard, R.J., *Med Sci Sports Exerc.,* 20: 463–468 (1988).
35. Davis, G.M., Figoni, S.F., Glaser, R.M., Servedio, F.J., Gupta, S.C., and Suryaprasad, A.G., *Proc. Int. Conf. Assoc. Adv. Rehabil. Tech.,* pp. 326–327 (1988).
36. Davis, G.M., and Glaser, R.M., in *Physiotherapy: Foundations for Practice Series: Neurology* (Ada L, Canning C, eds.). Heinemann, London, pp. 155–195 (1990).
37. Davis, GM., Servedio, F.J., Glaser, R.M., Gupta, S.C., and Suryaprasad, A.G., *J. Appl. Physiol.,* 69: 671–677 (1990).
38. Davis, G.M., Plyley, M.J., and Shephard, R.J., *Can. J. Sport Sci.,* 16: 64–72 (1991).
39. Davis, G.M., *Med. Sci. Sports Exerc.,* 25: 423–432 (1993).
40. Dearwater, S.P., LaPorte, R.E., Robertson, R.J., Brenes, G., Adams, L.L., and Becker, D., *Med. Sci. Sports Exerc.,* 18: 541–544 (1986).
41. DeVivo, M.J., Fine, P.R., Maetz, H.M., and Stover, S.L., *Arch. Neurol.,* 37: 707–708 (1980).
42. DeVivo, M., Black, K., and Stover, S., *Arch. Phys. Med. Rehabil.,* 74: 248 (1993).
43. DiCarlo, S.E., Supp, M.D., and Taylor, H.C., *Phys. Ther.,* 63: 1104–1107 (1983).
44. DiCarlo, S.E., *Phys Ther.,* 62: 456–459 (1988).
45. Engle, P., and Hildebrandt, G., *Paraplegia,* 11: 105–110 (1973).
46. Eriksson, P., Löfström, L., and Ekblom, B., *Scand. J. Rehab Med.,* 20: 141–147 (1988).
47. Faghri, P.D., Glaser, R.M., and Figoni, S.F., *Arch Phys. Med. Rehabil.,* 73: 1085–1093 (1992).
48. Figoni, S.F., Davis, G.M., Glaser, R.M., Servedio, F.J., Gupta, S.C., Suryaprasad,

A.G., Rodgers, M.M., and Ezenwa, B.N., *Proc. Intl. Conf. Assoc. Adv. Rehabil. Tech.,* pp. 328–329 (1988).

49. Figoni, S.F., Glaser, R.M., Hendershot, D.M., Gupta, S.C., Suryaprasad, A.G., Rodgers, M.M., and Ezenwa, B.N., *Proc. 10th Ann. IEEE Conf. Eng. Med. Biol.,* pp. 1636–1637 (1988).

50. Figoni, S.F., Gupta, S.C., Glaser, R.M., et al., *Rehabil. R&D Prog. Rep.,* 25: 108 (1988).

51. Figoni, S.F., Glaser, R.M., Hooker, S.P., Rodgers, M.M., Ezenwa, B.N., Faghri, P.D., Suryaprasad, A.G., Gupta, S.C., and Mathews, T., *Proc 12th Ann. RESNA Conf. Rehab. Tech.,* pp. 97–98 (1989).

52. Figoni, S.F., Glaser, R.M., Rodgers, M.M., Ezenwa, B.N., Hooker, S.P., Faghri, P.D., and Gupta, S.C., *Med. Sci. Sports Exerc.,* 21: S96 (1989).

53. Figoni, S.F., Hooker, S.P., Glaser, R.M., Rodgers, M.M., Faghri, P.D., Ezenwa, B.N., Mathews, T., Suryaprasad, A.G., and Gupta, S.C., *Med. Sci. Sports Exerc.,* 22(2): S43, 1990.

54. Figoni, S.F., *Med. Sci. Sports Exerc.,* 25: 433–441 (1993).

55. Figoni, S.F., Rodgers, M.M., and Glaser, R.M., *Med. Sci. Sports Exerc.,* 26(5 Suppl): s77 (1994).

56. Figoni, S.F., Glaser, R.M., and Collins, S.R., *Clin. Kinesiol.,* 48: 94–95 (1995).

57. Fitzgerald, P.I., Sedlock, D.A., and Knowlton, R.G. *Med. Sci. Sports Exerc.,* 22: 629–635 (1990).

58. Forchheimer, F., and Lundberg, Å., *Scand. J. Rehab. Med.,* 18: 59–63 (1986).

59. Freyschuss, U., and Knuttson, E., *Life Sci.,* 8: 421–424 (1969).

60. Gass, G.C., and Camp, E.M., *Med. Sci. Sports,* 11: 256–259 (1979).

61. Gass, G.C., and Camp, E.M., *J. Appl. Physiol.,* 63: 1846–1852 (1987).

62. Geisler, W.O., Jousse, A.T., and Wynne-Jones, M., *Paraplegia,* 21: 364–373 (1983).

63. Glaser, R.M. *Med. Sci. Sports Exerc.,* 21: S149–S157 (1989).

64. Glaser, R.M., Foley, D.M., Laubach, L.L., Sawka, M.N., and Suryaprasad, A.G., *Paraplegia,* 16: 341–349 (1978–79).

65. Glaser, R.M., Laubach, L.L., Sawka, M.N., and Suryaprasad, A.G., in *Proceedings—International Conference on Lifestyle and Health, 1978: Optimal Health and Fitness for People with Physical Disabilities,* (A.S., Leon, and G.J. Amundson eds.). University of Minnesota Press, Minneapolis, pp. 167–194 (1979).

66. Glaser, R.M., Sawka, M.N., Laubach, L.L., and Suryaprasad, A.G., *J. Appl. Physiol. Respir. Environ. Exerc. Physiol.,* 46: 1066–1070 (1979).

67. Glaser, R.M., Sawka, M.N., Brune, M.F., and Wilde, S.W., *J. Appl. Physiol. Respir. Environ. Exerc. Physiol.,* 48: 1060–1064 (1980).

68. Glaser, R.M., Sawka, M.N., Young, R.E., and Suryaprasad, A.G., *J. Appl. Physiol. Respir. Environ. Exerc. Physiol.,* 48: 41–44 (1980).

69. Glaser, R.M., Sawka, M.N., Durbin, R.J., Foley, D.M., and Suryaprasad, A.G., *Am. J. Phys. Med.,* 60: 67–75 (1981).

70. Glaser, R.M., Sawka, M.N., Wilde, S.W., Woodrow, B.K., and Suryaprasad, A.G., *Paraplegia,* 19: 220–226 (1981).

71. Glaser, R.M., Simsen-Harold, C.A., Petrofsky, J.S., Kahn, S.E., and Suryaprasad, A.G., *Ergonomics,* 26: 687–697 (1983).

72. Glaser, R.M., Sawka, M.N., and Miles, D.S., *Proc. IEEE Nat. Aerospace Elect. Conf.,* 2: 946–953 (1984).

73. Glaser, R.M., Strayer, J.R., and May, K.P., *Proc. 7th Ann. IEEE Conf. Eng. Med. Biol. Soc.,* pp. 308–313 (1985).

74. Glaser, R.M., in *Exercise and Sports Sciences Reviews, Vol. 13* (R.L. Terjung, ed.). Macmillan, New York, pp. 263–303 (1985).

75. Glaser, R.M., Rattan, S.N., Davis, G.M., Servedio, F.J., Figoni, S.F., Gupta, S.C., and Suryaprasad, A.G., *Proc. 9th Ann. IEEE Conf. Eng. Med. Biol. Soc.,* pp. 615–617 (1987).

76. Glaser, R.M., *1988 Am. Assoc. EMG Electrodiag. Didactic Prog.,* pp. 21–26 (1988).

77. Glaser, R.M., Figoni, S.F., Collins, S.R., Rodgers, M.M., Suryaprasad, A.G., Gupta, S.C., and Mathews, T., *Proc. 10th Ann IEEE Conf. Eng. Med. Biol. Soc.,* pp. 1638–1640 (1988).

78. Glaser, R.M., and Davis, G.M., in *Exercise in Modern Medicine: Testing and Prescription in Health and Disease.* (B.A., Franklin, S. Gordon, and G.C. Timmis, eds.) Williams & Wilkins, Baltimore, pp. 237–267 (1989).

79. Glaser, R.M., in (Torg, J.S., Welsh, R.P., Shephard, R.J., eds): *Current Therapy in Sports Medicine—2.* B.C. Decker Toronto, pp. 166–170 (1989).

80. Glaser, R.M., in *Fitness for Aged, Disabled and Industrial Workers* (M. Kaneko ed.). Human Kinetics, Champaign, Illinois, pp. 127–134 (1990).

81. Glaser, R.M., in *Sports and Exercise in Mid-life* (S.L. Gordon, X. Gonzalez-Mestre, and W.E. Garrett, eds). American Academy of Orthopedic Surgeons Rosemont, Illinois, pp. 253–292 (1993).

82. Glaser, R.M., Figoni, S.F., Ponichtera-Mulcare, J.A., et al, *Proc. 16th Annu. RESNA Conf. Rehabil. Technol.,* pp. 416–418 (1993).

83. Glaser, R.M., Figoni, S.F., Couch, W.P., Collins, S.R., and Shively, R.A., *Med Sci Sports Exerc.,* 26(5 Suppl): s111 (1994).

84. Glaser, R.M., Couch, W.P., Janssen, T.W.J., et al., Proc. *RESNA 96 Annu Conf.,* p. 279–281 (1996).

85. Goss, F.L., McDermott, A, and Robertson, R.J., *Res. Q. Exerc. Sport.* 63: 76–79 (1992).

86. Graitcer, P.L., and Maynard, F.W. (Eds.) *Proceedings of the First Colloquium on Preventing Secondary Disabilities Among People with Spinal Cord Injuries.* Centers for Disease Control, Atlanta (1990).

87. Gruner, J.A., Glaser, R.M., Feinberg, S.D., Collins, S.R., and Nussbaum, N.S., *J. Rehabil. R & D,* 20: 21–30 (1983).

88. Hangartner, T.N., Rodgers, M.M., Glaser, R.M., and Barre, P.S., *J. Rehabil. Res. Dev.,* 31: 50–61 (1994).

89. Hartung, G.H., Lally, D.A., and Blancq, R.J., *Eur. J. Appl. Physiol.,* 66: 362–365 (1993).

90. Heldenberg, D., Rubinstein, A., Levtov, D., Werbin, B., and Tamir, I., *Atherosclerosis,* 39: 163–167 (1981).

91. Hjeltnes, N. *Scand. J. Rehabil. Med.,* 9: 107–113 (1977).

92. Hjeltnes, N., and Vokac, Z., *Scand. J. Rehab. Med.,* 11: 67–73 (1979).

93. Hjeltnes, N. *Scand. J. Soc. Med. Suppl.,* 29: 245–251 (1982).

94. Hjeltnes, N., and Jansen, T., *Paraplegia,* 28: 428–432 (1990).
95. Hoffman, M.D. *Sports Med.,* 3: 312–330 (1986).
96. Hooker, S.P., and Wells, C.L., *Med. Sci. Sports Exerc.,* 21: 18–22 (1989).
97. Hooker, S.P., and Wells, C.L., *Paraplegia,* 30: 428–436 (1992).
98. Hooker, S.P., Figoni, S.F., Rodgers, M.M., Glaser, R.M., Mathews, T., Suryaprasad, A.G., and Gupta, S.C., *J. Rehabil. Res. Dev.,* 29: 1–11 (1992).
99. Hooker, S.P., Greenwood, J.D., Hatae, D.T., Husson, R.P., Matthiesen, T.L., and Waters, A.R., *Med. Sci. Sports Exerc.,* 25: 1115–1119 (1993).
100. Hooker, S.P., Greenwood, J.D., Boyd, L.A., Hodges, M.R., McCune, L.D., and McKenna, G.E., *Eur. J. Appl. Physiol.,* 67: 563–566 (1993).
101. Hopman, M.T.E., Oeseburg, B., and Binkhorst, R.A., *Med. Sci. Sports Exerc.,* 24(9): 984–990 (1992).
102. Hopman, M.T.E., Oeseburg, B., and Binkhorst, R.A., *Med. Sci. Sports Exerc.,* 25: 577–583 (1993).
103. Hopman, M.T.E., Pistorius, M., Kamerbeek, I.C.E., and Binkhorst, R.A., *Eur. J. Appl. Physiol.,* 531–535 (1993).
104. Hopman, M.T.E., Verheijen, P.H.E., and Binkhorst, R.A., *J. Appl. Physiol.,* 75: 2079–2083 (1993).
105. Hopman, M.T.E., Monroe, M.B., Dueck, C.A., and Skinner, J.S., *Med. Sci. Sports Exerc.,* 26(5 Suppl): S77 (1994).
106. Huang, C.-T., McEachran, A.B., Kuhlemeier, K.V., DeVivo, M.J., and Fine, P.R., *Arch. Phys. Med. Rehabil.,* 64: 578–582 (1983).
107. Janssen, T.W.J., van Oers, C.A.J.M., Hollander, A.P., van der Woude, L.H.V., and Rozendal, R.H., *Med. Sci. Sports Exerc.,* 25: 863–870 (1993).
108. Janssen, T.W.J., van Oers, C.A.J.M., Veeger, H.E.J., Hollander, A.P., van der Woude, L.H.V., and Rozendal, R.H., *Paraplegia,* 32: 844–859 (1994).
109. Janssen, T.W.J., van Oers, C.A.J.M., van der Woude, L.H.V., and Hollander, A.P., *Med. Sci. Sports Exerc.,* 26: 661–670 (1994).
110. Janssen, T.W.J., van Oers, C.A.J.M., Rozendaal, E.P., Willemsen, E.M., van der Woude, L.H.V., and Hollander, A.P., *Med. Sci. Sports Exerc.,* 28: 551–559 (1996).
111. Janssen, T.W.J., Glaser, R.M., Almeyda, J.W., Pringle, D.D., and Mathews, T., *Proceedings of the RESNA '96 Annual Conference, Salt Lake City,* pp. 288–290 (1996).
112. Janssen, T.W.J., van Oers, C.A.J.M., van Kamp, G.J., TenVoorde, B.J., van der Woude, L.H.V., and Hollander, A.P., *Arch. Phys. Med. Rehabil.,* 78: 697–705 (1997).
113. Kerk, J.K., Clifford, P.S., Snyder, A.C., Prieto, T.E., O'Hagan, K.P., Schot, P.K., Myklebust, J.B., and Myklebust, B.M., *Med. Sci. Sports Exerc.,* 27: 913–919 (1995).
114. Kessler, K.M., Pina, I., Green, B., Burnett, B., Laighold, M., Bilsker, M., Palomo, A.R., and Myerburg, R.J., *Am. J. Cardiol.,* 58: 525–530 (1986).
115. King, M.L., Lichtman, S.W., Pellicone, J.T., Close, R.J., and Lisanti, P, *Chest,* 196: 1166–1171 (1994).
116. Kinzer, S.M., and Convertino, V.A., *Clin. Phys.,* 9: 522–533 (1989).
117. Knutsson, E., Lewenhaupt-Olsson, E., and Thorsen, M., *Paraplegia,* 11: 205–216 (1973).

118. Kofsky, P.R., Davis, G.M., Shephard, R.J., Jackson, R.W., and Keene, G.C.R., *Eur. J. Appl. Physiol.*, 51: 109–120 (1983).

119. Krauss, J.C., Robergs, R.A., DePaepe, J.L., Kopriva, L.M., Aisenbury, J.A., Anderson, M.A., and Lange, E.K., *Med. Sci. Sports Exerc.*, 25: 1054–1061 (1993).

120. Lammertse, D.P., and Yarkony, G.M. *Arch. Phys. Med. Rehabil.*, 72: s309–s311 (1991).

121. LaPorte, R.E., Adams, L.L., Savage, D.D., Brenes, G., Dearwater, S., and Cook, T., *J. Epidemiol.*, 120: 507–517 (1984).

122. Lasko-McCarthey, P., and Davis, J.A., *Eur J Appl Physiol.*, 63: 349–353 (1991).

123. Le, C.T., and Price, M., *J. Chronic Dis.* 35: 487–492 (1982).

124. Magel, J.R., McArdle, W.D., Toner, M., and Delio, D.J., *J. Appl. Physiol. Respir. Environ. Exerc. Physiol.*, 45: 75–79 (1978).

125. Martel, G., Noreau, L., and Jobin, J., *Paraplegia*, 29: 447–456 (1991).

126. McArdle, W.D., Glaser, R.M., and Magel, J.R., *J. Appl. Physiol.*, 30: 733–738 (1971).

127. McArdle, W.D., Katch, F., and Katch, V., *Exercise Physiology: Energy, Nutrition, and Human Performance.* Lea & Febiger, Philadelphia (1991).

128. McCafferty, W.F., and Horvath, S.M., *Res. Q. Am. Assoc. Health Phys. Educ. Recreat.*, 48: 358–371 (1977).

129. McLean, K.P., and Skinner, J.S., *Arch Phys Med Rehabil.*, 76: 139–150 (1995).

130. Miles, D.S., Sawka, M.N., Wilde, S.W., Durbin, R.J., Gotshall, R.W., and Glaser, R.M., *Ergonomics*, 25: 239–246 (1982).

131. Mohr, T., and Andersen, J.L., Biering-Sorensen, F., Galbo, H., Bangsbo, J., Wagner, A., and Kjaer, M., *Spinal Cord* 35: 1–16 (1997).

132. Mortimer, J.T., in *Handbook of Physiology: The Nervous System II* (J.M. Brookhart, V.B. Mountcastle, V.B. Brooks, S.R. Geiger, eds). American Physiological Society, Bethesda, Maryland, pp. 155–187 (1981).

133. Nash, M.S., Bilsker, M.S., Marcillo, A.E., Isaac, S.M., Botelho, L.A., Klose, K.J., Green, B.A., Rountree, M.T., and Shea, J.D., *Paraplegia*, 29: 590–599 (1991).

134. Nichols, P.J.R., Norman, P.A., and Ennis, J.R., *Scand. J. Rehab. Med.*, 11: 29–32 (1979).

135. Niesing, R., Eijskoot, F., Kranse, R., den Ouden, R., Storm, J., Veeger, H.E.J., and van der Woude, L.H.V., *Med. Biol. Eng. Comput.*, 28: 329–338 (1990).

136. Nilsson, S., Staff, P.H., and Pruett, E.D.R., *Scand. J. Rehabil. Med.*, 7: 51–56 (1975).

137. Noreau, L., and Shephard, R.J., *Sports Med. Training Rehab.*, 3: 165–181 (1992).

138. Petrofsky, J.S., Phillips, C.A., Heaton, H.H. III, and Glaser, R.M., *J. Clin. Eng.*, 9: 13–19 (1984).

139. Petrofsky, J.S., and Stacy, R., *Eur J Appl Physiol.*, 64: 487–492 (1992).

140. Phillips, C.A., Danopulos, D., Kezdi, P., and Hendershot, D., *Int. J Rehabil Res.*, 12: 147–157 (1989).

141. Phillips, W., Burkett, L.N., Munro, R., Davis, M., and Pomeroy, K., *Paraplegia*, 33: 90–93 (1995).

142. Pierce, D.S., and Nickel, V.H., *The Total Care of Spinal Cord Injuries.* Little, Brown Boston (1977).

143. Pitetti, K.H., Barrett, P.J., Campbell, K.D., and Malzahn, D.E., *Med Sci Sports Exerc.,* 26: 463–468 (1994).

144. Pollack, S.F., Axen, K., Spielholz, N. Levin, N. Haas, F., and Ragnarsson, K.T., *Arch. Phys. Med. Rehabil.,* 70: 214–219 (1989).

145. Pollock, M.L. Miller, H.S., Linnerud, A.C., Laughridge, E., Coleman, E., and Alexander, E., *Arch. Phys. Med. Rehabil.,* 55: 418–424 (1974).

146. Pompe van Meerdervoort, H.F., Hassani, S., Faghri, P.D., and Glaser, R.M., *Proceedings of the 18th Annual RESNA Conference on Rehabilitation Technology,* 396–398 (1995).

147. Ponichtera-Mulcare, J.A., Figoni, S.F., Glaser, R.M., Suryaprasad, A.G., and Gupta, S.C., *Proceedings of the 16th Annual RESNA Conference on Rehabilitation Technology,* 389–391 (1993).

148. Ragnarsson, K.T., O'Daniel, W., Edgar, R., Pollack, S., Jr., Petrofsky, J., and Nash, M.S., *Arch. Phys. Med. Rehabil.,* 69: 672–677 (1988).

149. Rasche, W., Janssen, T.W.J., van Oers, C.A.J.M., Hollander, A.P., and van der Woude L.H.V., *Eur. J. Appl. Physiol.,* 66: 328–331 (1993).

150. Raymond, J., Davis, G.M., Climstein, M., and Sutton, J.R., *Med. Sci. Sports Exerc.,* 29(5 Suppl): s85 (1997).

151. Raymond, J., Davis, G.M., Fahey, A., Climstein, M., and Sutton, J.R., *Spinal Cord,* 35: 680–685 (1997).

152. Reybrouck, T., Heigenhauser, G.F., and Faulkner, J.A. *J. Appl. Physiol.,* 38: 774–779 (1975).

153. Robergs, R.A., Appenzeller, O., Qualls, C., et al. *J. Appl Physiol.,* 75: 2400–2405 (1993).

154. Sawka, M.N., Glaser, R.M., Wilde, S.W., and von Luhrte, T.C., *J. Appl. Physiol Respir. Environ. Exerc. Physiol.,* 49: 784–788 (1980).

155. Sawka, M.N., Glaser, R.M., Laubach, L.L., Al-Samkari, O., and Suryaprasad, A.G., *J. Appl. Physiol: Respir. Environ. Exerc. Physiol.,* 50: 824–828 (1981).

156. Sawka, M.N. in *Exercise and Sport Sciences Reviews,* Vol. 14 (K.B. Pandolf, ed.). Macmillian, New York, pp. 175–210 (1986).

157. Sawka M.N., Latska, W.A., and Pandolf, K.B., *Med. Sci. Sports Exerc.,* 21: S132–S140 (1989).

158. Sedlock, D.A., Knowlton, R.G., and Fitzgerald, P.I., *Eur. J. Appl. Physiol.,* 57: 55–59 (1988).

159. Schwade, J., Blomqvist, C.G., and Shapiro, W., *Am. Heart J.,* 94: 203–208 (1977).

160. Shenberger, J.S., Leaman, G.J., Neymyer, M.M., Musch, T.I., and Sinoway, L.I., *Med. Sci. Sports Exerc.,* 21: 96–101 (1990).

161. Shephard, R.J., Bouhlel, E., Vandewalle, H., and Monod, H., *J. Appl. Physiol.* 64: 1472–1479 (1988).

162. Shephard, R.J., *Scand. J. Rehab. Med.,* 23: 51–59 (1991).

163. Simmons, R., and Shephard, R.J., *Int. Z. Angew. Physiol.,* 30: 73–84 (1971).

164. Sloan, K.E., Bremner, L.A., Byrne, J., Day, R.E., and Scull, E.R., *Paraplegia,* 32: 407–415 (1994).

165. Smith, P.A., Glaser, R.M., Petrofsky, J.S., Underwood, P.D., Smith, G.B., and Richards, J.J., *Arch. Phys. Med. Rehabil.,* 64: 249–254 (1983).

166. Stauffer, E.S., in *The Total Care of Spinal Cord Injuries* (D.S. Pierce and V.H. Nickel, eds). Little, Brown, Boston pp. 81–102 (1978).

167. Stenberg, J., Astrand, P-O., Ekblom, B., Royce, J., and Saltin, B., *J. Appl. Physiol.,* 22: 61–70 (1967).

168. Traugh, G.H., Corcoran, P.J., and Reyes, R.L., *Arch. Phys. Med. Rehabil.,* 56: 67–71 (1975).

169. Twist, D.J., Culpepper-Morgan, J.A., Ragnarsson, K.T., Petrillo, C.R., and Kreek, M.J., *Am. J. Phys. Med. Rehabil.,* 71: 156–163 (1992).

170. van der Woude, L.H.V., de Groot, G., van Ingen Schenau, G.J., and Rozendal, R.H., *Ergonomics,* 29: 1561–1573 (1986).

171. van der Woude, L.H.V., Veeger, H.E.J., Rozendal, R.H., van Ingen Schenau, G.J., Rooth, F., and van Nierop, P., *Med. Sci. Sports Exerc.,* 20: 492–500 (1988).

172. Veeger, H.E.J., van der Woude, L.H.V., and Rozendal, R.H., *J. Rehab. Res. Dev.,* 26: 37–46 (1989).

173. Voigt, E.-D., and Bahn, D., *Scand. J. Rehabil. Med.,* 1: 101–106 (1969).

174. Vokac, Z., Bell, H., Bautz-Holter, E., and Rodahl, K., *J. Appl. Physiol.,* 39: 54–59 (1975).

175. Walker, W., and Khokhar, M., *Arch. Phys. Med. Rehabil.,* 73: 91 (1993).

176. Wheeler, G., Cumming, K., Burnham, R. et al., *Paraplegia,* 32: 292–299 (1994).

177. Whiteneck, G.G., Charlifue, S.W., Frankel, H.L., Fraser, M.H., Gardner, B.P., Gerhard, K.A., Krishnan, K.R., Menter, R.R., Nuseibeh, I., Short, D.J., and Silver, J.R., *Paraplegia,* 30: 617–630 (1992).

178. Whiting, R.B., Dreisinger, T.E., and Abbott, C., *South. Med. J.,* 76: 1225–1227 (1983).

179. Wicks, J.R., Lymburner, K., Dinsdale, S.M., and Jones, N.L., *Paraplegia,* 15: 252–261 (1977–78).

180. Wicks, J.R., Oldridge, N.B., Cameron, B.J., and Jones, N.L., *Med. Sci. Sports Exerc.,* 15: 224–231 (1983).

181. Wilde, S.W., Glaser, R.M., Sawka, M.N., Miles, D.S., and Fox E.L., *Fed. Proc.,* 39: 289 (1980).

182. Wilde, S.W., Miles, D.S., Durbin, R.J., Sawka, M.N., Suryaprasad, A.G., Gotshall, R.W., and Glaser, R.M., *Am. J. Phys. Med.,* 60: 277–291 (1981).

183. Wolfe, G.A., Waters, R., and Hislop, H.J., *Phys. Ther.,* 57: 1022–1027 (1977).

184. Yekutiel, M., Brooks, M.E., Ohry, A., Yarom, J., and Carel, R., *Paraplegia,* 27: 58–62 (1989).

185. Young, J.S., Burns, P.E., Bowen, A.M., and McCutcheon, R. *Spinal Cord Injury Statistics: Experience of the Regional Spinal Cord Injury Systems.* Good Samaritan Medical Center, Phoenix, (1982).

186. Zwiren, L.D., and Bar-Or, O., *Med. Sci. Sports,* 7: 94–98 (1975).

20

The Effect of Cardioactive Drugs on Exercise Testing and Training

NANETTE KASS WENGER
Emory University School of Medicine
Atlanta, Georgia

INTRODUCTION

The spectrum of patients with cardiovascular disease currently considered candidates for exercise training has broadened considerably (1). Patients arbitrarily excluded from exercise rehabilitation in former years—i.e., elderly individuals, patients with angina or exercise-induced ischemia, those with serious ventricular arrhythmias, and patients with cardiac enlargement, ventricular dysfunction, or compensated heart failure, among others—now constitute an increasing proportion of individuals for whom exercise training has been documented to provide benefit (2). These medically complex cardiac patients typically receive multiple drugs, many of which have the potential to alter, favorably or adversely, the determinants of exercise performance and the capacity for physical work. As well, there has been a sizable increase in the application of exercise-based testing for diagnosis, assessment of functional capacity, risk stratification (3), evaluation of therapeutic interventions, and exercise prescription. The impact of cardioactive drugs on exercise testing and training as well as knowledge about exercise-drug interactions has thus assumed compelling importance.

EXERCISE: PATHOPHYSIOLOGICAL ALTERATIONS WITH MYOCARDIAL ISCHEMIA AND ISCHEMIC VENTRICULAR DYSFUNCTION

Exercise and Myocardial Oxygen Demand

The major determinants of myocardial oxygen demand include ventricular systolic wall tension, heart rate, and the contractile state of the myocardium. Left ventricular wall tension is determined by both left ventricular pressure and volume. Elevation of the systemic arterial pressure (left ventricular pressure) or ventricular dilatation (increased ventricular volume) increases left ventricular wall tension, with a resultant increase in myocardial oxygen demand.

Dynamic exercise results in an increase of all the determinants of myocardial oxygen demand—heart rate (generally proportional to the intensity of exercise), myocardial contractility, and ventricular wall tension—and thus can elicit cardiac abnormalities not present at rest (2). In the normal heart, virtually the maximal amount of available oxygen is extracted by the myocardium at rest; thus, in contrast to skeletal muscle, myocardium cannot respond to an increase in oxygen demand by the extraction of additional oxygen from its perfusing blood. An increase in myocardial oxygen demand can be met only by an increase in coronary blood flow, rendering this the determining factor for increasing oxygen delivery to the myocardium. A decrease in coronary vascular resistance normally occurs in response to an increase in myocardial oxygen demand. In young, healthy subjects, this decrease in coronary vascular resistance enables an augmentation of coronary blood flow from 60 ml/100 g of left ventricular myocardium at rest to as much as 300 ml/100 g of myocardium at peak exercise.

Exercise-induced tachycardia not only augments myocardial oxygen demand (the cardiac work rate per minute increases with the increase in the heart rate) but may also limit myocardial oxygen delivery. Rapid heart rates encroach on the percentage of the cardiac cycle allotted to diastole, the predominant period for coronary and myocardial perfusion. Thus, tachycardia concomitantly engenders a progressive increase in myocardial oxygen demand and a lessened time for the delivery of blood and oxygen to the myocardium.

In addition to its effects on myocardial oxygen demand, exercise may also induce arrhythmias; exercise is associated with a progressive lessening of vagal tone and an increase in circulating catecholamines and in sympathetic nervous system activity. The latter two factors can enhance myocardial automaticity and late potentials while shortening myocardial conduction time and refractory periods (4).

Response to Exercise of the Coronary Patient: Factors in the Genesis of Myocardial Ischemia

Atherosclerotic obstruction of the coronary arteries limits their ability to increase coronary blood flow in response to an increase in myocardial oxygen demand. Inadequate delivery of oxygen to the working myocardium results in a variety of pathophysiological responses that underlie the clinical presentations of coronary atherosclerotic heart disease.

As discussed above, myocardial oxygen supply is determined primarily by coronary blood flow, and, to a lesser extent, by the arteriovenous oxygen difference. In addition to the duration of diastole (a function of the heart rate), coronary blood flow is affected by coronary vascular resistance (whose determinants are a combination of fixed and dynamic coronary arterial obstructive lesions) and by the gradient between the aortic diastolic pressure and the left ventricular end-diastolic pressure (the latter increasing with ventricular dysfunction).

The increase in coronary blood flow and the resultant oxygen supply are typically insufficient to meet increased myocardial oxygen demand when atherosclerotic obstruction of the coronary arterial luminal diameter exceeds 50–70%. The manifestations of myocardial ischemia: angina pectoris, ventricular dysfunction with a depressed ejection fraction and a compensatory increase in systolic ventricular volume, and abnormalities of cardiac rhythm are consequences of the discrepancy between myocardial oxygen supply and demand and the inability to supply the metabolic demands of the myocardium.

The ischemic threshold in patients with chronic stable angina can vary with the type of exercise, particularly when dynamic changes in coronary vasomotor tone occur at the site of stenosis. Isometric hand-grip may worsen ischemia, and this can be reversed by intracoronary nitrates. In other patients, warm-up exercise can increase the ischemic threshold and abrupt onset of exercise can decrease it (5).

In patients with atherosclerotic obstruction of the coronary arteries, a number of factors influence the balance between myocardial oxygen supply and demand. Some of these variables have diagnostic value in that exercise-based procedures (exercise testing with and without radionuclide studies or echocardiographic imaging) accentuate the discrepancy between myocardial oxygen supply and demand, enabling confirmation of the likelihood of coronary heart disease. Conversely, a variety of medical interventions used in the management of patients with symptomatic coronary heart disease—pharmacotherapy and prescriptive exercise training—favorably alter the myocardial oxygen supply/demand equation by decreasing myocardial oxygen demand. They limit or control one or more of the factors that increase myocardial oxygen requirements: increased heart rate, increased blood pressure, and increased myocardial contractility. Alternatively, blood supply to the myocardium can be increased and myocardial oxygen supply improved by revascularization procedures that either reduce or bypass the obstructing lesions in the coronary arteries: percutaneous transluminal coronary angioplasty (PTCA) or other transcatheter revascularization techniques and coronary artery bypass graft surgery (CABG). Both categories of therapy, PTCA and CABG, restore coronary blood flow and improve myocardial oxygen supply, limiting the difference between the myocardial oxygen supply and demand and thereby decreasing or eliminating the resultant clinical ischemic syndromes. Improvement in contractile function characteristically occurs in areas of previously ischemic myocardium following revascularization. The degree of residual ventricular dysfunction is determined by the extent of prior myocardial infarction and scarring.

Manifestations of Myocardial Ischemia

The most common symptomatic manifestations of myocardial ischemia are angina pectoris and myocardial infarction. Symptoms and signs of ischemic ventricular dysfunction may also occur.

Myocardial glucose and free fatty acids are metabolized by oxidative mechanisms to support the mechanical activity of the heart when adequate blood supply is present. With an inadequate oxygen supply, an anaerobic glycolytic pathway is used for energy production. Because of the lesser efficiency of anaerobic glycolysis, ischemic myocardium may evidence inadequate mechanical activity (poor contractility). Finally, myocardial ischemia may result in electrical instability of the heart, with resultant electrocardiographic abnormalities and disturbances of cardiac rhythm.

The workload required to precipitate manifestations of myocardial ischemia is a reasonable predictor of subsequent proximate coronary events and is the basis for risk stratification procedures (2). Thus, exercise testing (with and without radionuclide or echocardiographic imaging) is used to categorize high-risk patients following a coronary event or as preoperative evaluation for non-cardiac surgery (6). Evidence of myocardial ischemia at a low workload, even in asymptomatic patients recovered from myocardial infarction, defines a population with a high risk of recurrent myocardial infarction or sudden cardiac death. This subgroup requires prompt coronary arteriography and subsequent appropriate therapy (7–10). In recent years, risk stratification has assumed particular importance in myocardial infarction patients following successful coronary thrombolysis. Patients with substantial residual myocardial ischemia at exercise testing require evaluation for revascularization procedures designed to salvage ischemic myocardium (11). Atherosclerosis of the coronary arteries may result in the loss of the endothelium-dependent vasodilation with exercise, such that exercise-induced vasoconstriction occurs at the site of atherosclerotic plaques.

MECHANISMS BY WHICH ANTIANGINAL (ANTI-ISCHEMIC) DRUGS LIMIT MYOCARDIAL OXYGEN DEMAND: IMPLICATIONS FOR EXERCISE TESTING AND EXERCISE TRAINING

Nitrate Drugs

Nitrate drugs, the oldest class of antianginal drugs, given acutely, uniformly improve exercise tolerance, so that an increased duration and/or intensity of exercise can be performed prior to the onset of symptoms or signs of myocardial ischemia. Based on these data, physicians traditionally recommend the prophylactic use of nitroglycerin; for example, advising a patient unable to walk a flight of steps without developing angina to use a sublingual nitroglycerin tablet before attempting to do so. The stairs are then typically negotiated without difficulty. Exercise testing confirms that the administration of sublingual nitroglycerin can improve treadmill exercise capacity by as much as 1 metabolic equivalent (MET) (12). Comparable benefit is provided by new formulations, such as long-acting nitrate tablets, nitroglycerin ointments, long-acting patch preparations, and oral sprays. However, a nitrate-free interval is required to prevent the development of nitrate tolerance when long-acting formulations are used (13). The action of nitrate drugs in improving exercise tolerance reflects not only an alleviation of the symptoms of myocardial ischemia but also an improvement in activity-precipitated ischemic ventricular wall-motion abnormalities; enhancement of the ventricular ejection fraction and thereby of cardiac output further increases the exercise capacity (14,15). Some reports refute the improvement in exercise tolerance with chronic nitrate use (16).

The beneficial effect of nitrate drugs involves a number of mechanisms that operate concomitantly to decrease the myocardial oxygen demand. Nitrate drugs relax vascular smooth muscle. The predominant effect is venodilation, with a resultant decrease in left ventricular filling pressure and volume (reduction of myocardial oxygen demand by reduction of preload). By decreasing left ventricular end-diastolic volume and pressure, nitrate drugs favor coronary collateral flow. Coronary collateral vessels are thin-walled conduits located predominantly in the subendocardium and are vulnerable to compression when intraventricular pressures are raised during diastole (the major interval for coronary blood flow). Nitrate drugs limit the elevation of left ventricular diastolic pressure that is associated with exercise-related angina and probably with spontaneous angina. Nitrate drugs are also arteriolar vasodilators; they decrease peripheral vascular resistance (with resultant lowering of the systemic arterial pressure), and thereby reduce left ventricular workload. They improve left ventricular function during isometric exercise in coronary patients with left ventricular dysfunction, presumably by reduction of both ventricular preload and ventricular afterload (15).

Nitrate-related coronary vasodilation can increase myocardial oxygen supply. Although nitrate drugs administered to normal subjects result in vasodilation of the epicardial coronary arteries, the role of vasodilation in patients with coronary atherosclerotic obstruction is uncertain. Whereas coronary vasodilation may contribute to an increase in exercise performance prior to the onset of signs or symptoms of myocardial ischemia, nitrates are unlikely to induce coronary vasodilation in already ischemic areas of myocardium. Myocardial ischemia per se is such a potent stimulus to vasodilation that maximal local vasodilation may have already been induced by the ischemia. Because nitrate drugs have substantial peripheral effects, they remain beneficial for patients with severe coronary arterial obstruction who cannot dilate their coronary arteries.

Nitrate drug use decreases ST-segment depression at exercise electrocardiographic (ECG) testing (17). In patients with only a modest severity of angina and myocardial ischemia, administration of nitrates may be sufficient to reduce or eradicate both the symptomatic and the ECG manifestations of myocardial ischemia at exercise testing (14).

The typical instruction to patients to sit down when using sublingual nitroglycerin has particular importance during exercise training. The patient who takes several sublingual nitroglycerin tablets following substantial exercise-induced vasodilation may experience nitrate-related hypotension and syncope if not seated. Additionally, the combination of drug and exercise-related vasodilation may initiate baroreceptor-mediated reflex tachycardia; the resultant increase in myocardial oxygen demand may increase the angina, despite some concomitant coronary vasodilation. Further, a seated patient is immediately identifiable to the exercise supervisor(s) as a person requiring attention.

β-Adrenergic Blocking Drugs

β-Blocking drugs are frequently administered to patients following myocardial infarction to decrease the risk of both reinfarction and cardiac death (18,19). β-blockade continues to impart survival benefit following coronary thrombolysis (20).

Both cardioselective and noncardioselective β-blocking drugs improve exercise tolerance and decrease the signs and symptoms of myocardial ischemia by reducing the response to catecholamine stimulation. The major effect is a decrease in the exercise-related increases in heart rate and systolic blood pressure; that is, a decrease in the exercise rate-pressure or double product. There is less diminution in the resting heart rate and systemic arterial blood pressure. Myocardial contractility decreases concomitantly because β-blocked myocardium is less responsive to catecholamine stimulation. Thus, this class of compounds enables patients to exercise to a greater intensity and for a longer duration before they reach the rate-pressure product that previously evoked myocardial ischemia.

The decrease in heart rate seems a more important contributor to the decrease in myocardial oxygen demand than the decreases in systemic arterial pressure and myocardial contractility. This is clinically evident as a more dramatic response to β-blockade among patients whose resting heart rates are initially high. The prolongation of diastolic time, attendant on a slowing of the heart rate, allows improvement in myocardial perfusion, with particular enhancement of subendocardial coronary collateral flow. If β-blockade leads to an excessive depression of myocardial contractility, as may occur with preexisting ventricular dysfunction at rest, paradoxical worsening of activity tolerance and increased angina pectoris may occur. Depression of myocardial contractility results in an increase in left ventricular filling pressure and volume, with an increase in pulmonary capillary pressure. With the compensatory cardiac dilatation, an increase in myocardial wall tension is required to initiate contraction; this increases the myocardial oxygen demand, with resultant activity-related myocardial ischemia. Noncardioselective β-blocking drugs may precipitate bronchoconstriction in patients with reactive airway disease, limiting the ability to exercise.

Because β-blockade so effectively reduces the myocardial oxygen demand in patients for whom its application is appropriate, patients who undergo exercise testing for risk stratification while receiving β-blocking drugs may not develop the manifestations of myocardial ischemia (angina and ST depression) that would occur at lower intensities of exercise in the absence of such drug therapy. Therefore, the predictive accuracy of risk stratification by exercise testing is decreased in patients who are receiving β-blocking or other anti-ischemic drugs. The early appearance of adverse features retains an unfavorable prognostic significance (21), but some patients may not show exercise intolerance and/or evidence of myocardial ischemia until moderate levels of exercise are reached (21,22). This pharmacotherapy-modified exercise tolerance may preclude the recognition of some patients at increased risk of recurrent coronary events. Data from serial exercise tests performed for up to 36 months following myocardial infarction in patients with and without metoprolol therapy showed a significantly higher maximal heart rate in the placebo-treated group throughout the study. Termination of exercise due to angina pectoris or ST-segment depression on the ECG occurred more frequently in the placebo group (23).

Exercise training is both feasible and effective in patients of all ages who train while being treated with β-blocking drugs (24). Functional improvements of as much as 30% have been described with both cardioselective and noncardioselective β-adrenergic blocking drugs in coronary patients as well as in healthy subjects (25,26). The presumed basis for the increased workload and increased duration of activity achieved prior to myocardial ischemia is that β-blockade does not alter the adaptive responses of cardiac, peripheral vascular, or skeletal muscle to exercise training: an increase in oxidative enzymes, an increase in capillary supply, and a decrease in exercise-induced blood lactate levels (27,28) (see below). The lack of change in the anaerobic (lactate) threshold with both selective and nonselective β-blocking drugs suggests that the blood flow to exercising muscles is unaltered by these therapies. This suggests that peripheral vasoconstriction is not an important adverse effect of such drugs. β₁-selective drugs may offer advantage with regular aerobic exercise in that they have less of an adverse effect on substrate metabolism than does a nonselective β-blocker (29).

Calcium Channel–Blocking Drugs

Calcium channel–blocking drugs selectively block calcium-dependent excitation-contraction coupling, both in the myocardium and in vascular smooth muscle; they inhibit calcium entry into the conduction system as well. The predominant anti-ischemic effect is due to potent peripheral arteriolar vasodilation and a resultant decrease in myocardial oxygen demand (30,31). The decrease in afterload substantially decreases cardiac work. Despite potent coronary vasodilation, there is only a limited increase in the myocardial oxygen supply following the oral administration of diltiazem. Intracoronary administration of diltiazem decreases the exercise-induced vasoconstriction of stenotic coronary arteries. The vasodilator effect on stenotic vessel segments of diltiazem and nitroglycerin seems additive (32), although the precise mechanisms underlying the vasodilation remain uncertain. For heart rate–limiting calcium blocking drugs, the increased diastolic time permits increased myocardial perfusion.

The calcium channel–blocking drugs currently available for clinical use are characterized by different chemical formulations and differing negative inotropic and electrophysiological properties. Verapamil, which is also an effective agent to correct supraventricular tachyarrhythmias, is most likely to depress atrioventricular conduction. Short-acting nifedipine characteristically induces considerable tachycardia secondary to profound vasodilatation, an adverse effect not seen with long-acting preparations. And diltiazem appears to cause fewer problems with heart rate than do the other drugs. All except amlodipine may worsen preexisting ventricular dysfunction. In the CASIS trial (33), silent ischemia during exercise testing was more effectively suppressed by amlodipine, whereas ischemia during ambulatory ECG recording was more effectively suppressed by atenolol; combination therapy was more effective in both settings.

The T-type calcium channel blocker mibefradil increases exercise tolerance and time to ST-segment depression at exercise testing comparably to diltiazem; heart rate and blood pressure were reduced by this therapy at each stage of exercise testing (34).

Because this class of compounds so effectively decrease myocardial oxygen demand, exercise test risk stratification has less predictive accuracy for patients thus treated (35). As with the β-blocked patient, calcium-blocking drug therapy may increase exercise tolerance and reduce or delay evidence of myocardial ischemia until moderate levels of exercise (higher workloads) have been accomplished, owing to the decrease in heart rate and systolic blood pressure response to any given level of exercise. Patients may thus not be recognized as being at high risk, although this would have been evident prior to the institution of pharmacotherapy. It remains uncertain whether the deferring of an abnormal response to moderate levels of exercise suggests a more favorable outcome while the patient is receiving pharmacotherapy.

This class of drugs interacts with a number of aspects of exercise training. When verapamil or diltiazem is given, the occurrence of atrioventricular conduction abnormalities may alter the heart rate and require reassessment of the exercise prescription.

The profound peripheral vasodilatation resulting from the administration of calcium-antagonist drugs may cause ankle edema, at times sufficiently pronounced to limit the use of this class of agents. Such edema is due to local factors; it may be more prominent in elderly patients with poor tissue turgor, but should not be misconstrued as evidence of heart failure. If this error is made and diuretic drugs are administered, inappropriately, to reduce ankle edema, they concomitantly reduce the circulating blood volume. When additional exercise-induced vasodilatation occurs, symptomatic hypotension and occasionally syncope may result. The use of support hose is recommended to limit ankle edema. If the dosage of a calcium channel–blocking drug has been increased or a diuretic drug has been added to a calcium–blocking drug regimen, it is wise to check the patient's weight prior to the initiation of exercise. Patients whose weight is lower than usual should have their blood pressure assessed in the sitting and standing positions prior to exercise to be sure that hypovolemic postural hypotension is not present.

This emphasizes the importance of volume status as a determinant of hemodynamic competence in patients who are receiving drugs with major arteriolar vasodilator effects. Patients who are taking calcium–blocking drugs should be cautioned that any viral or other illness characterized by nausea, vomiting, and diarrhea may result in hypovolemia, with adverse effects on the ability to exercise. In such circumstances, it is prudent to assess body weight and postural changes in blood pressure prior to the initiation of exercise.

MECHANISMS BY WHICH EXERCISE TRAINING FAVORABLY AFFECTS THE MYOCARDIAL OXYGEN SUPPLY:DEMAND RATIO

Individualized prescriptive exercise training is the hallmark of rehabilitative physical activity for the coronary patient. Its major goal is the improvement of cardiorespiratory fitness, with resultant lessening of symptoms and enhancement of functional capacity.

Dynamic exercise training lessens myocardial oxygen demand by decreasing the heart rate and systolic blood pressure responses to any given submaximal workload. There is a decreased myocardial workload and oxygen demand at any level of total body work and oxygen demand. The main mechanisms for functional improvement and a lessening of ischemic symptoms after dynamic exercise training appear to be regulatory changes in the peripheral circulation, adaptations that allow exercise to be performed more efficiently. These include an increase in overall arteriovenous oxygen extraction, a decrease in systemic vascular resistance, and an improved distribution of the cardiac output during exercise; all these responses decrease the demand for oxygen transport. Specific adaptive changes in skeletal muscle include an increased percentage of type I (slow-twitch) fibers, an increase in mitochondrial oxidative enzymes, an increase in the capillary density around muscle fibers, and an increase in the myoglobin content. The combination of increased oxygen extraction, increased vagal tone, lessened catecholamine release, and a number of other factors may decrease the rate-pressure product and other determinants of myocardial oxygen demand by as much as 18%. An added favorable effect of exercise training is an increase in maximal oxygen uptake of about 20%, with even more benefit evident in previously sedentary or physically unfit patients.

As a result, the symptoms and signs of myocardial ischemia in the exercise-trained coronary patient appear at a greater workload and/or a longer work duration than prior to training (1). Trained coronary patients function further from their ischemic threshold during usual daily activities; any submaximal task is perceived as requiring a lessened intensity of exertion because it requires a lesser percentage of their now increased work capacity. The improvement in functional capacity after exercise training reflects a decreased myocardial oxygen demand for any submaximal task. The patient shows (a) an increase in the maximal oxygen consumption, (b) a lower heart rate and systolic blood pressure at rest, (c) a lesser increase in the heart rate and systolic blood pressure at any submaximal workload, (d) a more rapid return to normal of the heart rate following exercise, (e) lessened or absent angina at workloads that previously induced this symptom, and (f) decreased or absent ST-segment changes on the exercise ECG at workloads that previously precipitated these changes (36–38).

There is little or no evidence that the moderate-intensity, short-term exercise training typically undertaken by middle-aged or older adults following myocardial infarction or myocardial revascularization procedures improves either myocardial contractility or ventricular systolic function. Prolonged, high-intensity exercise training has been reported to improve cardiac function in selected coronary patients (38–40). The effects of exercise training on ventricular diastolic function in coronary patients have been less well studied. Further, there is little or no evidence that the coronary collateral circulation or myocardial function improves as a result of dynamic exercise training. Training favorably affects systemic vascular resistance; the increase in systemic vasodilation that occurs with training is an important contributor to the improved stroke volume and cardiac output.

EXERCISE TRAINING OF THE PATIENT WITH VENTRICULAR SYSTOLIC DYSFUNCTION AND HEART FAILURE

Exercise training can improve both exercise tolerance and symptoms in patients with compensated heart failure and with moderate to severe left ventricular systolic dysfunction. Skeletal muscle adaptations appear to mediate the improvement in exercise tolerance. Improvement in measures of functional capacity occurs without deterioration of the ventricular ejection fraction. The effect of exercise training on the improvement of symptomatic and functional status is additive to that accomplished by the use of ACE inhibitor therapy (1,41–43). The lack of correlation of improvement in functional capacity with an improvement in ventricular ejection fraction supports the concept that the favorable effect of exercise training reflects adaptations in the peripheral circulation and skeletal musculature rather than adaptations in the cardiac musculature. In ambulatory patients awaiting cardiac transplantation, a combination of pharmacotherapy and exercise training improved peak oxygen uptake and exercise performance in 38 of 68 patients so treated; 31 of these 38 patients improved to the extent that they could be removed from the transplantation list with excellent early survival (44).

β-blocking drugs have also been shown to decrease symptoms and increase exercise tolerance in patients with heart failure (left ventricular systolic dysfunction) as well as to improve left ventricular function. This improvement in exercise tolerance was evident with metoprolol (a β_1-selective blocker) but not with bucindalol (a nonselective β-blocker) or carvedilol (a nonselective β-blocker and α_1-blocker) owing to their blunting of the exercise heart rate.

INTERACTIONS OF COMMONLY USED CARDIOVASCULAR DRUGS WITH EXERCISE TESTING AND TRAINING

There has been a progressive increase in the use of exercise testing and training in the management of patients with coronary atherosclerotic heart disease, most of whom are likely to be prescribed a variety of cardiovascular drugs.

The exercise-related features of the antianginal (anti-ischemic) drugs—nitrate preparations, β-adrenergic-blocking drugs, and calcium channel–blocking drugs—have been discussed above. It appears appropriate to review the drug-exercise interactions of antihypertensive drugs, antiarrhythmic drugs, digitalis, and other pharmaceuticals used to treat heart failure. Nonetheless, the effect of drugs and/or the presence of systemic arterial hypertension had small effect on the sensitivity and specificity of the exercise ECG as compared with the effects of angiographic criteria (17).

Most evaluations of functional capacity and of coronary risk status that involve exercise testing address the heart rate and blood pressure responses to graded intensities of exercise and the resultant symptomatic, ECG, or other objective abnormalities (including those demonstrated by radionuclide and echocardiographic imaging). Typically, both symptomatic and objective responses relate prominently to changes in the rate-pressure product. Cardiovascular drugs that alter the balance between myocardial oxygen supply and demand by influencing any of its determinants—but particularly the heart rate and systolic blood pressure—are likely to modify the results obtained at exercise testing and the ability to perform exercise.

Changes in the exercise ECG associated with pharmacotherapy may reflect hemodynamic changes, direct effects of the drug on the myocardium, or both. Because the exercise test response and the exercise capacity of many patients with coronary disease are substantially altered by a number of the commonly used cardiovascular drugs, alone or in combination, the effects of pharmacotherapy must be considered when evaluating the results of an exercise test (as discussed above), as well as when prescribing exercise training. Exercise testing that is undertaken to derive an exercise prescription should be performed with the patient on an optimal medical regimen.

Subsequently, any major change in pharmacotherapy requires repetition of the exercise test and revision of the exercise prescription; this is not only because of the specific consequences of the altered drug therapy but also because alterations in drug treatment usually reflect an alteration in clinical status. Nonetheless, patients receiving virtually all cardiovascular drugs can undergo exercise testing and the treated individuals retain their capability and suitability for exercise training.

Diuretic Drugs

The potassium-wasting diuretics, predominantly thiazide preparations and loop diuretics, may factitiously suggest myocardial ischemia on the exercise ECG if hypokalemia has been induced. Hypokalemia-related abnormalities of the ST segment and T wave may appear both at rest and with exercise. Diuretic-induced hypomagnesemia may also contribute to an abnormal ECG. Even if serum potassium levels are normal, intracellular potassium levels may be inadequate with magnesium deficiency, since adequate magnesium levels are needed to transport potassium ions across the cellular membrane into the myocytes.

Further, hypokalemia may lead to skeletal muscle weakness and fatigue;

the latter may be misinterpreted as a consequence of myocardial ischemia or other causes of cardiac dysfunction, particularly if fatigue limits exercise tolerance. In the patient who is receiving digitalis, hypokalemia may induce arrhythmias both at rest and with exercise. Serum potassium levels increase with vigorous exercise if total body potassium is not depleted, so that an excessive risk of arrhythmia with exercise should not be anticipated.

Exercise diuresis may reduce the circulating blood volume. When exercise-induced vasodilation also occurs, symptomatic hypotension may result from the hypovolemic state.

Antihypertensive Drugs

The ability of the previously hypertensive patient to exercise is improved by virtually all categories of antihypertensive drugs owing to a reduction in both the resting and the exercise induced cardiac workload when the blood pressure is controlled (45). Antihypertensive drugs lessen the increase in blood pressure induced by both dynamic and isometric exercises.

For patients participating in an exercise regimen, the response to antihypertensive therapy should be checked both at rest and with exercise. Many antihypertensive drugs—including β-adrenergic-blockers, heart rate–limiting calcium channel–blocking drugs, reserpine, and prazosin, among others—limit the heart rate or autonomic responses or effect significant vasodilation. If excessive, these changes may result in exercise-related symptomatic hypotension, dizziness, and even syncope. Alternatively, when there is inadequate control of the blood pressure during exercise, the increased myocardial oxygen demand of the exercise-related hypertension may limit the ability to exercise.

Despite their hemodynamic effects, the β-blocker atenolol and the α_1-selective blocker doxazosin, given in moderate doses, did not adversely affect exercise performance in male hypertensive runners (46).

Vasodilator Drugs

Vasodilator drugs have been discussed as therapy for myocardial ischemia and for hypertension, but they also figure prominently in the therapy of cardiac failure. Various vasodilator drugs act on different vascular beds; although they produce prompt symptomatic and hemodynamic improvement in the patient with heart failure at rest, their effect on exercise tolerance is variable. Many effect little or no immediate objective improvement of exercise tolerance in such individuals. Exercise tolerance, as documented objectively by exercise testing, may improve later; this is postulated to be due in part to alterations in regional blood flow and in part to a "spontaneous" training effect as the previously sedentary patients, now with an improved symptomatic status, undertake reasonable levels of physical activity.

Vasodilator therapy, administered to the patient with heart failure, is designed to overcome the excessive vasoconstriction that attempts to compensate for the limited cardiac output; "compensatory" vasoconstriction imposes an increased workload on the failing left ventricle. The improvement in exercise capacity attendant on vasodilator therapy, particularly in the patient with myocardial dysfunction and cardiac failure, depends in part on the type of vasodilator agent that is used (47), because the various vasodilator drugs act on different vascular beds and involve different mechanisms of vasodilation.

Vasodilator drugs such as hydralazine and the calcium channel–blocking drugs act directly on arteriolar smooth muscle, independently of the mechanism or mechanisms causing the vasoconstriction, to counteract the compensatory vasoconstriction of heart failure and decrease the workload of the left ventricle. However, they may not improve exercise tolerance even when the symptoms and hemodynamic abnormalities of heart failure are improved. With exercise, vasoconstriction normally occurs in the renal and splanchnic vascular beds, diverting blood flow to exercising skeletal muscles. In patients treated with hydralazine or calcium channel–blocking drugs, these changes in regional blood flow cannot occur because of the direct vasodilator action of the drug on smooth muscle, with resultant suboptimal delivery of blood to exercising muscle. The most important mechanism effecting the redistribution of blood flow with exercise appears to be an α-adrenergic–mediated vasoconstriction of the vasculature. When α-adrenergic blockers such as prazosin are used to overcome the vasoconstriction of heart failure, they result in generalized vasodilation without diversion of blood flow to exercising muscle, creating the need for an excessive increase in cardiac output. Energy output is "wasted" in perfusing the viscera during exercise; therefore, improvement of the exercise capacity is either absent or is substantially limited if the patient with heart failure is so treated.

Vasodilator drugs such as the angiotensin-converting enzyme inhibitors counteract the excessive vasoconstriction of heart failure by decreasing angiotensin II, vasopressin, and/or norepinephrine but permit normal sympathetic regulation of the vascular tone during exercise; the resultant vasoconstriction of the renal and splanchnic vascular beds decreases the blood flow to the viscera and permits an increase in blood flow to exercising muscle. This in part explains the early improvement in exercise tolerance when angiotensin-converting enzyme inhibitor preparations are administered to patients with heart failure (48). Data are limited for angiotensin II receptor antagonists.

Digitalis Glycosides

There is a minimal increase in myocardial oxygen demand when digitalis is administered to normal individuals, owing to the increase in myocardial contractility. In contrast, when digitalis is administered to patients with heart failure, the beneficial effect on the ventricular dimensions, heart rate, and wall tension de-creases the net cardiac workload and myocardial oxygen demand despite the increase in myocardial contractility (49,50). The exercise-induced increase in ventricular end-diastolic pressure in the patient with heart failure is at least par-tially corrected after treatment with digitalis. Digitalis is described to increase the exercise capacity in patients with heart failure (51).

Digitalis typically accentuates any underlying repolarization abnormalities on the ECG and may produce repolarization abnormalities both at rest and with exercise. Exercise-induced ST-segment changes may occur even 1–2 weeks after digitalis is discontinued. Although ST-segment and T-wave changes are dose-dependent, repolarization abnormalities may be present even with subtherapeutic dosages of digitalis and occur both in normal subjects and in patients with coro-nary disease. Because of these repolarization abnormalities, the predictive accu-racy of ST-segment changes with exercise is lessened in patients who are receiv-ing digitalis glycosides, and imaging techniques are usually added to the exercise test. However, the amplitude of digitalis-induced repolarization abnormalities is greatest at heart rates between 110 and 130 beats per minute and does not progress with increasing exercise intensity, as is characteristic of the ST-segment abnor-malities of myocardial ischemia (52). Severe exercise-induced ST segment de-pression (> 2 mm) suggests myocardial ischemia even in patients receiving digi-talis. As well, ST-segment depression associated with a decreased QT duration suggests digitalis effect, whereas ischemic ST-segment depression is usually as-sociated with prolongation of the corrected QT (53).

As previously noted, a combination of digitalis therapy and diuretic-related hypokalemia increases the likelihood of exercise-related arrhythmias.

Antiarrhythmic Agents

All patients who are receiving antiarrhythmic drugs must be considered at in-creased risk of arrhythmic complications because of the characteristics of their underlying clinical problem. Ventricular ectopic beats pose a greater risk of pro-gression to ventricular tachycardia or ventricular fibrillation when they are associ-ated with myocardial ischemia and/or myocardial dysfunction.

All type IA antiarrhythmic agents—quinidine, procainamide, disopyra-mide—may, paradoxically, be proarrhythmic by virtue of their prolongation of the QT interval of the ECG.

Quinidine depresses sinus node function, slowing the heart rate. It also has a vagolytic effect that increases the heart rate, and blocking effect upon α-recep-tors; the resultant vasodilation and reflex increase in sympathetic activity further increase the heart rate. The net result is an increased heart rate at rest and at low levels of activity, but quinidine has little effect on the heart rate or blood pressure with moderate- to high-level exercise (54). Quinidine QT prolongation may favor the occurrence of ventricular arrhythmias. Neither procainamide nor disopyramide produces significant alterations of the resting or exercise heart rate and blood pressure (55). However, disopyramide substantially depresses myocardial contractility; patients who are receiving this preparation require careful surveillance for exercise-induced ventricular dysfunction.

Amiodarone decreases the maximal exercise heart rate by as much as 20 beats per minute. QRS prolongation with exercise is also described.

Postmenopausal Estrogen Therapy

The acute administration of sublingual estrogen (estradiol-17β) to postmenopausal women with coronary disease is described to improve exercise tolerance and increased the time to ST-segment depression. Importantly, this study involved supraphysiological doses of hormone. Postulated mechanisms include direct coronary vasodilation, peripheral vasodilation, or a combination of these mechanisms (58). In another study, women with stable angina receiving postmenopausal estrogen (Premarin) exhibited no beneficial effect on exercise-induced myocardial ischemia (57).

Psychotropic Drugs: Cardiovascular Effects and Interaction with Cardiovascular Drugs

Many patients with coronary disease have associated emotional problems; they may thus be prescribed phenothiazine drugs or tricyclic antidepressant compounds. Many psychotropic drugs produce repolarization abnormalities during exercise testing and may also cause orthostatic hypotension. Further, many tricyclic antidepressant drugs may be arrhythmogenic, as their effect on cardiac conduction resembles that of type 1A antiarrhythmic drugs; they may also depress myocardial contractility.

Tricyclic antidepressants (TCAs) block the synaptic reuptake of norepinephrine and may also block the synaptic uptake of clonidine, interfering with blood pressure control; conversely, withdrawal of TCAs may cause serious hypotension because there is no longer antagonism to the clonidine. Tricyclic antidepressants also impair the hepatic metabolism of warfarin, causing excessive anticoagulation in patients receiving the drug. At least in early reports, a newer TCA, alprazolam, appears to have little or no cardiotoxicity or adverse drug-drug interactions.

Lithium carbonate is used to treat affective disorders. Although it does not interfere with exercise tolerance (58), abnormalities of sinus node and AV conduction have been described (59), as has potentiation of heart failure. Sodium restriction and/or administration of thiazide diuretics can precipitate lithium toxicity.

Phenothiazine tranquilizers may decrease myocardial contractility, induce heart failure and arrhythmias, produce cardiac conduction abnormalities, and cause a variety of ECG changes (predominantly QT prolongation and ST-T abnormalities) both at rest and with exercise (60).

ACKNOWLEDGMENT

With appreciation to Jeanette Zahler and Julia Wright for assistance in preparation of the manuscript.

REFERENCES

1. Wenger, N.K., Froelicher, E.S., Smith, L.K., Ades, P.A., Blumenthal, J.A., Certo, C.M.E., Dattilo, A.M., Davis, D., DeBusk, R.F., Drozda, J.P., Jr, Fletcher, B.J., Franklin, B.A., Gaston, H., Greenland, P., McBride, P.E., McGregor, C.G.A., Oldridge, N.B., Piscatella, J.C., and Rogers, F.J., *Cardiac Rehabilitation. Clinical Practice Guideline No. 17*. AHCPR Publication No. 96–0672, U.S. Department of Health and Human Services, Public Health Service, Agency for Health Care Quality and Research and the National Heart, Lung, and Blood Institute, Rockville, Maryland (1995).
2. Fletcher, G.F., Balady, G., Froelicher, V.F., Hartley, L.H., Haskell, W.L., and Pollock, M.L., *Circulation* 91: 580–615 (1995).
3. Ryan, T.J., Anderson, J.L., Antman, E.M., Braniff, B.A., Brooks, N.H., Califf, R.M., Hillis, L.D., Hiratzka, L.F., Rapaport, E., Riegel, B.J., Russell, R.O., Smith, E.E., III, and Weaver, W.D.,: Circulation 94: 2341–2350 (1996).
4. Podrid, P.J., Venditti, F.J., Levine, P.A., and Klein, M.D., *Am. J. Cardiol.,* 62: 24H–33H (1988).
5. Pupita, G., Kaski, J.C., Galassi, A.R., Vejar, M., Crea, F., and Maseri, A., *Am. Heart J.,* 118: 539–544 (1989).
6. Eagle, K.A., Brundage, B.H., Chaitman, B.R., Ewy, G.A., Fleisher, L.A., Hertzer, N.R., Leppo, J.A., Ryan, T., Schlant, R.C., Spencer, W.H., III, Spittell, J.A. Jr., and Twiss, R.D., Committee Members; Ritchie, J.L., Cheitlin, M.D., Eagle, K.A., Gardner, T.J., Garson, A., Jr, Lewis, R.P., Gibbons, R.J., O'Rourke, R.A., and Ryan, T.J., Task Force Members, *Circulation,* 93: 1278–1317 (1996).
7. DeBusk, R.F., Blomqvist, C.G., Kouchoukos, N.T., Luepker, R.V., Miller, H.S., Moss, A.F., Pollock, M.L., Reeves, T.J., Selvester, R.H., Stason, W.B., Wagner, G.S., and Willman, V.L., *N. Engl. J. Med.,* 314: 161–166 (1986).
8. Hamm, L.F., Stull, G.A., and Crow R.S., *Prog. Cardiovasc. Dis.,* 28: 463–476 (1986).
9. Stone, P.H., Turi, Z.G., Muller, J.E., Parker, C., Hartwell, T., Rutherford, J.D., Jaffee, A.S., Raabe, D.S., Passamani, E.R., Willerson, J.T., Sobel, B.E., Robertson, T.L., Braunwald, E., and the MILIS Study Group, *J. Am. Coll. Cardiol.,* 8: 1007–1017 (1986).
10. Wenger, N.K., Learning Center Highlights, American College of Cardiology, 1: 14–19 (1986).

11. Melin, J.A., DeCoster, P.M., Renkin, J., Detry, J.M.R., Beckers, C., and Col, J., *Am. J. Cardiol.,* 56: 705–711 (1985).
12. Markis, J.E., Gorlin, R., Mills, R.M., Williams, R.A., Schweitzer, P., and Ransil, B.J., *Am. J. Cardiol.,* 43: 265–271 (1979).
13. Schaer, D.H., Buff, L.A., and Katz, R.J., *Am. J. Cardiol.,* 61: 46–50 (1988).
14. Glancy, D.L., Richter, M.A., Ellis, E.V., and Johnson, W., *Am. J. Med.,* 62: 39–46 (1977).
15. Flessas, A.P., and Ryan, T.J., *Am. Heart, J.,* 105: 239–242 (1983).
16. Sullivan, M., Savvides, M., Abouantoun, S., Madsen, E.B., and Froelicher, V., *J. Am. Coll. Cardiol.,* 5: 1220–1223 (1985).
17. Backman, C., Jacobsson, K.–A., Linderholm, H., and Osterman, G., *Clin. Physiol.,* 14: 475–485 (1994).
18. Frishman, W.H., Furberg, C.D., and Friedewald, W.T., *Curr. Probl. Cardiol.,* 9: 1–51 (1983).
19. Pedersen, T.R., for the Norwegian Multicenter Study Group, *N. Engl. J. Med.,* 313: 1055–1058 (1985).
20. The TIMI Study Group, *N. Engl. J. Med.,* 320: 618–627 (1989).
21. Murray, D.P., Tan, L.B., Salih, M., Weissberg, P., Murray, R.G., and Litter, W.A., *Br. Heart. J.,* 60: 474–479 (1988).
22. Ho, S.W.C., McComish, M.J., and Taylor, R.R., *Am. J. Cardiol.,* 55: 258–262 (1985).
23. Olsson, G., Rehnqvist, N., Freyschuss, U., and Zetterquist, S., *Am. J. Cardiol.,* 61: 519–523 (1988).
24. Hare, T.W., Lowenthal, D.T., Hakki, H.H., and Goodwin, M., *Clin Pharmacol. Ther.,* 33: 206 (1983).
25. Pratt, C.M., Welton, D.E., Squires, W.G. Jr, Kirby, T.E., Hartung, G.H., and Miller, R.R., *Circulation,* 64: 1125–1129 (1981).
26. Sweeney, M.E., Fletcher, B.J., and Fletcher, G.F., *Am. Heart J.,* 118: 941–946 (1989).
27. Wolfel, E.E., Hiatt, W.R., Brammell, H.L., Carry, M.R., Ringel, S.P., Travis, V., and Horwitz, L.D., *Circulation,* 74: 664–674 (1986).
28. Vanhees, L., Fagard, R., and Amery, A., *Am. Heart J.,* 108: 270–275 (1984).
29. Head, A., Kendall, M.J., and Maxwell, S., *Clin. Cardiol.,* 18: 335–340 (1995).
30. Moskowitz, R.M., Piccini, P.A., Nacarelli, G.V., and Zelis, R., *Am. J. Cardiol.,* 44: 811–816 (1979).
31. Bonow, R.O., Leon, M.B., Rosing, D.R., Kent, K.M., Lipson, L.C., Bacharach, S.L., Green, M.V., and Epstein, S.E., *Circulation,* 65: 1337–1350 (1982).
32. Nonogi, H., Hess, O.M., Ritter, M., Bortone, A., Corin, W.J., Grimm, J., and Krayenbuehl, H.P., *J. Am. Coll. Cardiol.,* 12: 892–899 (1988).
33. Davies, R.F., Habibi, H., Klinke, W.P., Dessain, P., Nadeau, C., Phaneuf, D.C., Lepage, S., Raman, S., Herbert, M., Foris, K., Linden, L., and Buttars, J.A., *J. Am. Coll. Cardiol.,* 25: 619–625 (1995).
34. Davies, G.J., Kobrin, I., Caspi, A., Reisin, L.H., de Albuquerque, D.C., Armagnijan, D., Coelho, O.R., and Schneeweiss, A., *Am. Heart J.,* 134 (2 Pt 1): 220–228 (1997).
35. Mukharji, J., Kremers, M., Lipscomb, K., and Blomqvist, C.G., *Am. J. Cardiol.,* 55: 267–270 (1985).
36. Saltin, B., *Ann. N.Y. Acad. Sci.,* 301: 244–251 (1977).

37. Clausen, J.P., *Prog. Cardiovasc. Dis.,* 18: 459–495 (1976).
38. Paterson, D.H., Shephard, R.J., Cunningham, D., Jones, N.L., and Andrew, G., *J. Appl. Physiol.,* 47: 482–489 (1979).
39. Hagberg, J.M., Ehsani, A.A., and Holloszy, J.O., *Circulation,* 67: 1194–1199 (1983).
40. Ehsani, A.A., Martin, W.W. III, Heath, G.W., and Coyle, E.F., *Am. J. Cardiol.,* 50: 246–254 (1982).
41. Coats, A.J., Adamopoulos, S., Meyer, T.E., Conway, J., and Sleight, P., *Lancet,* 335: 63–66 (1990).
42. Meyer, T.R., Casadei, B., Coats, A.J., Davey, P.P., Adamopoulos, S., Radaelli, A., and Conway, J., *J. Intern. Med.,* 230: 407–413 (1991).
43. Giannuzzi, P., Tavazzi, L., Temporelli, P.L., Corra, U., Imparato, A., Gattone, M., Giordano, A., Sala, L., Schweiger, C., and Malinverni, C., *J. Am. Coll. Cardiol.,* 22: 1821–1829 (1993).
44. Stevenson, L.W., Steimle, A.E., Fonarow, G., Kermani, M., Kermani, D., Hamilton, M.A., Moriguchi, J.D., Walden, J., Tillisch, J.H., Drinkwater, D.C., and Laks, H., *J. Am. Coll. Cardiol.,* 25: 163–170 (1995).
45. Virtanen, K., Janne, J, and Frick, M.H., *Eur. J. Clin. Pharmacol.,* 21: 275–279 (1982).
46. Fahrenbach, M.C., Yurgalevitch, S.M., Zmuda, J.M., and Thompson, P.D., *Am. J. Cardiol.,* 75: 258–263 (1995).
47. Tan, L.B., *Cardiovasc. Res.,* 21: 615–622 (1987).
48. Creager, M.A., Massie, B.M., Faxon, D.P., Friedman, S.D., Kramer, B.L., Weiner, D.A., Ryan, T.J., Topic, N., and Melidossian, C.D., *J. Am. Coll. Cardiol.,* 6: 163–170 (1985).
49. Gross, G.J., Warltier, D.C., Hardman, H.F., and Somani, P., *Am. Heart, J.,* 93: 487–495 (1977).
50. Parker, J.O., West, R.O. Jr, Ledwich, J.R., and DiGiorgi, S. *Circulation,* 40: 453–462 (1969).
51. Sullivan, M, Atwood, J.E., Myers, J., Feuer, J., Hall, P., Kellerman, B., Forbes, S., and Froelicher, V., *J. Am. Coll. Cardiol.,* 13: 1138–1143 (1989).
52. Sundqvist, K., Atterhog, J.H., and Jogestrand, T., *Am. J. Cardiol.,* 57: 661–665 (1986).
53. Ellestad, M.H., *Cardiol,Clin.,* 11: 241–252 (1993).
54. Fenster, P.E., Dahl, C., Marcus, F.I., and Ewy, G.A., *Am. Heart. J.,* 104: 1244–1247 (1982).
55. Fenster, P.E., Comess, K.A., and Hanson, C.D., *Cardiology,* 69: 366–370 (1982).
56. Rosano, G.M., Sarrel, P.M., Poole-Wilson, P.A., and Collins, P. *Lancet,* 342: 133–136 (1993).
57. Sbarouni, E., Kyriakides, Z.S., Nikolaou, N., and Kremastinos, D.T., *Am. J. Cardiol.,* 79: 87–89 (1997).
58. Tilkian, A.G., Schroeder, J.S., Kao, J., and Hultgren, H., *Am. J. Cardiol.,* 38: 701–708 (1976).
59. Hagman, A., Arnman, K., and Ryden, L., *Acta. Med. Scand.* 205: 467–471 (1979).
60. Grant, D., Crawford, M.H., and O'Rourke, R.A., *Am. Heart. J.,* 102: 465–466 (1981).

21

The Psychosocial Benefits of Exercising

Sotile Psychological Associates
Winston-Salem, North Carolina

The various short-term psychological benefits of exercise training are well documented in both healthy populations and those with heart disease (1). Heart patients who exercise regularly generally show enhanced well-being (2) and improvements in overall psychosocial adjustment (3). However, the mechanism by which this benefit is derived and the long-range effects of regular exercise on psychosocial functioning remain to be assessed.

The purpose of this chapter is to provide a brief overview of six areas of positive psychosocial changes that have been found to be associated with regular physical exercise: reduced anxiety and depression; diminished stress responsivity; enhanced self-efficacy; improved cognitive functioning; enhanced marital and sexual functioning; and modification of the type A behavior pattern (TYABP). Practical implications for clinical work are emphasized, followed by a brief discussion of salient caveats and controversies in the literature.

REDUCED ANXIETY AND DEPRESSION

Evidence that regular aerobic exercise acutely enhances management of anxiety and depression can be found in research with both healthy and cardiac populations. Peronnet et al. (4) reported that an extended period of aerobic exercise (2 h at 53% $\dot{V}_{O_2 max}$) buffered epinephrine responses to mental stress. Hayden and Allen (5) studied active versus sedentary college students and noted a reduction in anxiety scores with regular exercise. A 3-month exercise program led to significant improvement in anxiety scores in a study of Danish men (6). In a meta-analysis of published studies, Petruzello et al., (7) concluded that, irrespective of the intensity or the duration of the exercise, an acute bout of aerobic exercise led to reduced tension and anxiety levels for up to 30 min following activity.

While the acute beneficial effects of aerobic exercise on anxiety states is seldom questioned, research has yielded mixed results regarding the crucial question of whether acute exercise buffers psychological responses to subsequent stressors and challenges. In a thoughtful review of this topic, Rejeski et al. (8) pointed out that various researchers (e.g., Refs. 9 and 10) have reported that as little as a 10-min bout of exercise led to reduced tension and anxiety levels in subsequent exposure to a digit-backward task employed as a stressor. Sime (11) reported that a 10-min bout of aerobic exercise led to a lowered state of anxiety. However, similar studies (e.g., Refs. 12 and 13) reported null findings.

In an effort to clarify this issue, Rejeski and colleagues (8) compared the effects of an attention control condition and a 40-min bout of aerobic exercise at 70% heart rate reserve on 24 white and 24 black female subjects of low to moderate fitness levels. Results yielded clear evidence that exercise reduced both the frequency and intensity of anxiety-related thoughts that occurred in anticipation of interpersonal threat and challenge.

While it remains for future researchers to determine the length of time that specific psychological functions are enhanced following an acute bout of aerobic exercise (8), astute clinicians typically prescribe exercising as a means of enhancing emotional control in rehabilitating cardiac patients. The importance of managing emotional distress in this population is underscored by three factors. First is the fact that both morbidity and mortality rates for recovering cardiac patients become elevated in the presence of depression (18). Second, cardiac patients who struggle with anxiety or depression are more difficult to manage clinically (19). For example, a recent study of 58 patients indicated that those with depressed mood had greater perception of anginal pain than nondepressed patients (20). Finally, the sheer number of cardiac patients who struggle with anxiety or depression suggests that attending to these issues should be a part of standard cardiac care. Specifically, between 30 and 50% of myocardial infarction (MI) patients experience elevated levels of anxiety or depression in hospital and throughout the first 6 months of recovery (21); up to 33% of patients may remain chronically depressed or anxious despite recovery of functional capacity (22). A meta-analysis of 28 relevant studies found that exercise programs should not be the only treatment for anxiety and depression in coronary patients but can be beneficial as an additional treatment component (23).

The benefits of regular exercise on mood states is noteworthy. For example, in a randomly assigned and controlled study of exercise training versus psychotherapy, Greist et al. (14) showed that regular exercise can be as efficacious as psychotherapy for the treatment of clinical depression. Diminution of anxiety and depression levels may result from exercise-related increases in brain levels of catecholamines and β-endorphins and from enhanced endorphins in the peripheral bloodstream (15). Exercising also typically leads to enhanced feelings of mastery and self-efficacy (16). Improvement in mood may also come from the distraction from negative mood that comes during exercise and the social support that accompanies participating in group exercise classes (17).

Participating in a regular exercise program undoubtedly conforms to the various components of a cognitive/behavioral approach to treatment of emotional distress. In cognitive/behavioral treatment, depressed or anxious patients are coached to monitor and disrupt distressing cognitions and are encouraged to each day engage in various behaviors that yield three outcomes: a sense of accomplishment, fulfillment of certain obligations, and pleasurable sensations. Clinical experience suggests that even highly anxious or depressed individuals who exercise regularly do report, at minimum, brief periods of pride in their accomplishment and diminution of their psychological distress. These positive experiences and outcomes can lead to enhanced self-perceptions that serve as a foundation for motivating the patient to engage in further antianxiety or antidepressant treatment strategies (24).

DIMINISHED STRESS RESPONSIVITY

An impressive research literature has documented the importance of regular aerobic exercising as a stress-management tool. In addition to the aforementioned antianxiety and antidepressant effects, regular physical exercise in nonmedical populations has been shown to diminish muscular tension and increase overall stress-management ability and general feelings of well-being and self-esteem. In addition, regular exercise has been found to reduce the cardiovascular impact of emotional stressors (25).

In clinical practice, combination approaches to stress management are most often employed (19). Sime et al. (26) proposed that because aerobic exercise of moderate intensity and duration decreases muscle tension acutely, exercise should be recommended as a prelude to relaxation training. These same researches pointed out that training in relaxation can even enhance responses to exercise. For example, Benson et al. (27) found that oxygen consumption at a fixed workload was significantly lower (4%) when subjects used a relaxation-response technique during exercise on a bicycle ergometer.

It has also been proposed that pairing relaxation training with exercise enhances the physical and psychic outcomes of rehabilitation. The benefits of incorporating relaxation therapy consisting of systematic breathing therapy into formal cardiac rehabilitation was convincingly demonstrated by VanDixhoorn and colleagues (28). These researchers showed that relaxation training and behavior therapy decreased failure rates by as much as 50% in cardiac rehabilitation populations. Stress-management interventions that emphasize physical exercise have also been found to enhance control of arrhythmias and overall psychosocial functioning (29).

As was pointed out by Sotile (19), prescribing regular exercise is a crucial component of the standard of care in stress management counseling. Exercise can provide a tangible modality for stressed individuals to distract themselves from worries, release tension, and rejuvenate otherwise depleted coping energies. Regular exercise can also serve as a positive coping tool when modifying various risk factors (e.g., smoking cessation). Exercising is also a way of creating an area of control over a tangible factor, a process that enhances coping in the face of uncontrollable stressors. Furthermore, this taking of control seems to generalize to enhance self-efficacy for coping in general and for specific tasks.

ENHANCED SELF-EFFICACY

Self-efficacy refers to an individual's appraisal of his or her ability to perform a specific behavior or accomplish a certain task (30). Self-efficacy is not a global psychological trait; it is thought to be task-specific. This cognitive variable has been shown to affect both behavioral and health outcomes. Ewart (31) argued that physical exertion, self-efficacy, and emotion are causally related and that exercise training is useful in promoting psychological adjustment and enhanced quality of life because of its effects on self-efficacy.

Bandura (30) claimed that self-efficacy can be influenced by four sources of information: enactive information, vicarious information, persuasive communication, and internal feedback. Each of these sources of self-efficacy can be used to bolster psychosocial functioning in response to exercise.

Enactive information is derived from the individual's actual performance—the most reliable and effective source of confidence for a given activity and for activities similar to it. Based on this principle, individuals should be instructed to expect that confidence in exercise ability will grow with practice, and that, as exercise confidence grows, activities that entail similar levels of exertion (e.g., sexual relations) will also be approached with more efficacy.

Vicarious information comes from observing others. Participation in formal exercise group programs can be a potent source of vicarious information. Here, individuals benefit from observing others exercising and concluding that they can achieve similar success through their own efforts.

Persuasive communication is the form of efficacy influence most often used by health care professionals in their delivery of clinical care. Unfortunately, this is the least potent source of efficacy information. The effectiveness of this mode of influence is dependent upon the patient's belief in what is being communicated. Patients filled with self-doubt may doubt messages of reassurance and efforts to persuade them.

Internal feedback from one's physiological state directly affects feelings of efficacy regarding one's capabilities. Here, it is important to remember that the efficacy effect is most often specific to the activity being performed. If generalization of self-efficacy is to occur, the individual must be helped to pair the demonstrated area of performance cognitively with a desired target of performance enhancement. For example, a treadmill testing experience can be a teachable moment to enhance self-efficacy for activities of daily living.

An individual's perceived physical and cardiac efficacy reliably predicts post-MI activity levels, and research has shown that controlled exercise can enhance such self-efficacy (32). For example, Ewart et al. (33) showed that treadmill exercise testing soon after an MI led to improved self-efficacy gains in patients who were extremely fearful of physical exertion. These researchers used treadmill performance and medical counseling to boost efficacy and demonstrated that higher efficacy led to greater effort on the treadmill, which, in turn, led to further enhanced efficacy. Employing a mixed group of recovering MI patients and patients who had undergone coronary artery bypass grafting (CABG) Oldridge and Rogowski (34) demonstrated that both a ward ambulation program and a dedicated exercise center program were effective in enhancing self-efficacy for walking time and overall exertion.

Finally, there appears to be a circular interplay among cognitions, moods, and self-efficacy judgments. Kavanagh and Bower (35) reported that inducing positive moods by having an individual recall a pleasant interpersonal experience led to increased self-efficacy for a variety of tasks, including athletic performance.

IMPROVED COGNITIVE FUNCTIONING

Recovering cardiac patients, especially those who are elderly, often complain of diminished short-term memory, problem-solving difficulties, and slowed psychomotor reaction time (36). The facts that exercise has been found to immediately facilitate attention (37) and that physically fit individuals generally perform better on measures of cognitive function than less fit individuals (38,39) suggest that exercising may be a way to improve cognitive functioning for cardiovascular patients. Clinical claims often support this notion. However, a recent review of the literature (40) concluded that there is no definitive proof that exercise improves reaction time (41) or memory (42).

When exercise does result in cognitive improvements, the exact mechanism of change is difficult to discern. It may be that aerobic exercise helps replenish otherwise depleted neurochemical activity that mediates the cognitive process. The anxiety relief that comes with physical exertion may also eliminate an emotional factor that otherwise interferes with encoding of information and thereby proves to be disruptive of memory, concentration, and/or attention.

ENHANCED MARITAL AND SEXUAL FUNCTIONING

The importance of marital and family harmony in promoting risk-factor management and overall psychosocial adjustment in recovering cardiac populations has been well documented (43–46). Participating in regular exercise can help soothe anxieties of loved ones concerned about the effects of exertion on a recovering heart patient—an important aspect of rehabilitation. In a noteworthy study, Taylor et al. (47) demonstrated that a wife's confidence in her husband's exercise capacity may be significantly enhanced by having the wife not only observe but also experience walking on a treadmill for 3 min at the same peak work rate that was achieved by her husband just 3 weeks post-MI. By encouraging the couples to generalize these treadmill experiences to their at-home behaviors, the researchers were able to lessen marital tensions regarding the recovering patient's physical capabilities. This study found that the combined perception of the patient and his wife concerning the patient's exercise capacity was the most consistent predictor of the patient's later exercise performance 11 and 26 weeks post-MI.

Exercise-based, comprehensive rehabilitation programs have also been found to lead to diminished dependency on social support from others (e.g., Ref. 48). In addition, several studies reported that exercise training led to increased frequency of sexual activity among cardiac patients (3,49). Grief et al. (50) reported that even short-term (1-week) supervised exercise soon after MI led to improved sexual functioning 1 month post-MI in 62 male and female patients as compared with a no-exercise group. Similar results were reported in a study of 8 male and 4 female MI or heart surgery patients who participated in a 2-week fitness course post-MI or heart surgery (51).

MODIFICATION OF THE TYPE-A BEHAVIOR PATTERN

The effects of exercise on the various components of type A behavior pattern (TYABP) are not clear from the existing literature. In general, there appears to be a positive but not consistent correlation between regular exercise and reduced type A scores, especially in the area of hostility (52).

In a review of the relevant literature, Schmeid et al. (53) proposed that regular aerobic exercise could significantly enhance attempts to modify the TYABP. This notion is supported by the work of Blumenthal and colleagues (29), who found significant reductions in cardiovascular responses to mental arithmetic challenges in healthy type-A men who underwent aerobic exercise training but not in a strength-training group. On the other hand, Saraganian et al. (54) reported that neither exercise nor stress management interventions altered psychophysiological reactivity in type-A men.

In clinical practice, prescribing regular exercise as a means of helping highly hostile type-A patients control stress and anger reactions is commonplace. It appears that aerobic exercise accomplishes several important tasks for such patients: it enhances parasympathetic calming capabilities, diminishes hyperreactive sympathetic arousal tendencies, and leads to discharge of muscular tension (55). The net effect is better control of acute bouts of stress and anger.

CAVEATS AND CONTROVERSIES FROM THE LITERATURE

The short-term benefits of exercising have been well documented in each of the areas discussed above. However, several questions in this literature remain unanswered or bogged in controversy.

How Long Do the Benefits of Exercise Last?

The question remains whether regular exercise promotes lasting changes in psychosocial functioning. A national exercise study of 651 male MI patients failed to find any long-term psychosocial benefits of exercise (49)—a finding consistent with other investigations (e.g., Ref. 56). For example, a review of 10 studies that assessed changes in mood and personality functioning among patients with coronary heart disease exposed to organized exercise programs reported that the literature showed relatively few consistent improvements in any aspect of psychological functioning (40). On the other hand, a randomly assigned and controlled study of moderate-intensity exercise (57) found an improved sense of well-being in the exercising group.

When Exercising Does Work to Enhance Psychosocial Functioning, What Is the Mechanism of Change?

It has been argued that the enhanced well-being that comes with regular participation in exercise programs may not have to do with increased levels of physical fitness. For example, Blumenthal et al. (58) showed that changes in emotional functioning among participants in aerobic exercise classes occurred independently of actual change in fitness. Furthermore, in a study of 129 patients randomly allocated to usual care, usual care plus advice sessions, or exercise training, Mayou (59) found no difference in any psychosocial variables after 3 months. Mayou hypothesized that the psychosocial benefits that come from many exercise interventions may stem from nonspecific variables such as social support.

How Much Exercise Is Enough to Enhance Psychosocial Functioning?

The confusing association between exercise intensity and psychosocial factors raises interesting questions regarding the desired exercise target. In healthy, sedentary populations, high-intensity exercise has been found to increase tension and anxiety levels (60). Moses et al. (61) reported that while moderately intense exercise led to diminished levels of anxiety for middle-aged subjects, a more intense exercise program was associated with increased anxiety. On the other hand, a study of younger subjects found that high-intensity exercise was more effective in reducing psychological stress than was moderate exercise (62).

Bennet and Carol (63) concluded that such findings suggest that the level of exercise per se may not be the critical factor mediating psychological distress. "Rather, it may be accompanying changes on psychological variables such as self-efficacy or mastery associated with success in achieving and maintaining a prescribed or recommended level of exercise that is crucial" (p. 177). Such notions underscore the importance of tailoring an exercise program to the individual abilities and goals of participants rather than using predetermined norms in structuring exercise programs.

What Are the Shortcomings of the Existing Research Literature?

Bennett and Carroll (63) pointed out that a sufficiently large study to allow subgroup analyses of the psychosocial effects of exercise with recovering heart patients has yet to be conducted. The authors proposed that, because patients included in exercise programs are among the most physically able MI patients, they may also be the least anxious or depressed. Furthermore, highly anxious patients may select themselves out of participation in an organized, exercise-based rehabilitation program. As a result, the scope of psychosocial changes noted in exercise programs may be limited by the sample of patients being studied. Emory et al. (40) echoed these concerns, pointing out that existing studies are sorely lacking adequate nonexercise control-group comparisons, suffer from small sample sizes, and typically are nonrandom experimental designs.

Finally, until recently, most exercise research conducted with healthy and cardiac patient populations tended to focus on younger subjects. A recent investigation by Lavie and Milan (64) was a noteworthy exception to this trend. These researchers reported that even elderly patients over age 75 with coronary heart disease (CHD) evidenced marked improvements in quality-of-life parameters after participating in cardiac rehabilitation exercise training.

CONCLUSIONS

Clearly, exercise is not a panacea for promoting psychosocial well-being, and whether or not exercise leads to lasting psychosocial improvement remains for future researchers to discern. But a wealth of anecdotal and clinical data have touted the psychosocial benefits of regular exercising, and very few studies have suggested any harmful psychosocial effects from regular exercise. In general, it appears that health care providers would be remiss not to recommend exercising as a means of enhancing overall psychosocial functioning for both healthy and cardiac populations.

REFERENCES

1. Shephard, R.J., *J. Sports Med. Phys. Fit.,* 34: 91–98 (1994).
2. McPherson, B., Paivio, A., and Yhasz, M., *J. Sports. Med. Phys. Fit.,* 7: 95–102 (1967).
3. Rovario, S., Holmes, D.S., and Holsten, R.D., *J. Behav. Med.,* 7: 61–81 (1984).
4. Peronnet, F., Massicotte, D., Paquet, J., Brisson, B., and Champlain, J. de, *Eur. J. Appl. Physiol.,* 58: 551–558 (1989).
5. Hayden, R., and Allen, G., *J. Sports Med.,* 24: 69–74 (1984).
6. Fasting, K., and Gronningsaeter, H., *Scand. Jo. Sports Sci.,* 8: 99–103 (1986)
7. Petruzzello, S.J., Landers, D.M., Hatfield, B.D., Kubitz, K.A., and Salazar, W. *Sports Med.,* 11: 143–182 (1991).
8. Rejeski, W.J., Thompson, A., Brubaker, P.H., and Miller, H.S., *Health Psychol.,* 11: 355–362 (1992).
9. Roth, D.L., *Psychophysiology,* 26: 593–602 (1989).
10. Roth, D.L., Bachtler, S.D., and Fillingim, R.B., *Psychophysiology,* 27: 694–701 (1990).
11. Sime, W.E., *Med. Sci. Sports Exerc.,* 9: 55 (1977).
12. Duda, J.L., Sedlock, D.A., Melby, C.L., and Thaman, C., *Int. J. Sport Psychol.,* 19: 119–133 (1988).
13. Fillingim, R.B., Roth, D.L., and Cook, E.W., *Psychophysiology,* 26: S24, (1989).
14. Greist, J.H., Jefferson, J.W., and Marks, I.M., *Anxiety and Its Treatment.* Warner Books, New York (1986).
15. Harber, V.J., and Sutton, J.R., *Sports Med.* 1: 154–171 (1984).
16. deCoverley Veale, D.M.W., *Acta Psychiatr, Scand.* 76: 113–120 (1987).
17. Stein, R.A., in *Heart & Mind: The Practice of Cardiac Psychology* (R. Allan and S. Scheidt, eds.). American Psychological Association, Washington, D.C. (1996).
18. Frasure-Smith, N., and Prince, R., *Psychosom. Med.,* 51: 485–513 (1989).
19. Sotile, W.M., *Psychosocial Interventions for Cardiopulmonary Patients: A Guide for Health Professionals.* Human Kinetics, Champaign, Illinois (1996).
20. Krittayaphong, R., Light, K.C., Golden, R.N., Finkel, J.B., and Sheps, D.S., *Clin. J. Pain,* 12 (2): 126–133 (1996).
21. Trelawney-Ross, C., and Russell, O., *J. Psychosom. Res.,* 31: 125–130 (1987).
22. Stern M.J., and Pascale, L., *J. Psychosom. Res.,* 23: 83–87 (1979).
23. Kugler, J., Seelbach, H., and Kruskemper, G.M., *Br. J. Clin. Psychol.,* 33: 401–410 (1994).
24. Pierce, T.W., Madden, D.J., Siegel, W.C., and Blumenthal, J.A., *Health Psychol.,* 12: 286–291,(1993).

25. Lake, B.W., Suarez, E.C., Schneiderman, N., and Tocci, N., *Health Psychol.*, 4: 169 (1985).

26. Sime, W.E., McGahan, M., Eliot, R.S., in *American College of Sports Medicine: ACSM's Resource Manual for Guidelines for Exercise Testing and Prescription.* Lea & Febiger, Philadelphia, pp. 489–506 (1993).

27. Benson, H., Dryer, T., and Hartley, H., *Human Stress*, 4: 38 (1978).

28. VanDixhoorn, J., Duivenvoorden, H.J., Pool, J., and Verhage, F., *J. Psychosom. Res.*, 34: 327–337, (1990).

29. Blumenthal, J.A., Emery, C.F., Walsh, M.A., Cox, D.R., Kuhn, C.M., Williams, R.B., and Williams, R.S., *Psychosom. Med.*, 50: 418–433 (1988).

30. Bandura, A., *Psychol. Rev.* 84: 191–215 (1977).

31. Ewart, C.K., in *Self-Efficacy, Adaptation, and Adjustment: Theory, Research, and Application* (J.E. Maddux, ed.). Plenum Press, New York, pp. 203–226 (1995).

32. O'Leary, A., *Behav. Res. Ther.*, 23: 437–451 (1985).

33. Ewart, C.K., Taylor, C.B., Reese, L.B., and DEBusk, R.F., *Am. J. Cardiol.*, 51: 1076–1080 (1983).

34. Oldridge, N.B., and Rogowski, B.L., *Am. J. Cardio.* 66: 362–365 (1990).

35. Kavanagh, D.J., and Bower, G.H., *Cog. Ther. Res.* 9: 507–525 (1985).

36. Barclay, L.L., Weiss, E.M., Mattis, S., Bond, O., and Blass, J.P., *J. Am. Geriatr. Soc.* 36: 22–28 (1988).

37. Tomporowski, P.D., and Ellis, N.R., *Psychol. Bull.* 99: 338–346 (1996).

38. Gultin, B., *Res. Q.* 37: 211–220 (1966).

39. Weingarten, G., and Alexander, J.F., *Percept. Motor Skills*, 31: 371–378 (1970).

40. Emery C.F., Pinder, S.L., and Blumenthal, J.A., *J. Cardiopulm. Rehab.*, 9: 46 (1989).

41. Dustman, R.E., Ruhling, R.O., Russell, E.M., Shearer, D.E., Bonekat, W., Shigeoka, J.W., Wood, J.S., and Bradfort, D.C., *Neurobiol. Aging*, 5: 35–42 (1984).

42. Molloy, D.W., Beerschoten, D.A., Borrie, M.J., Crilly, R.G., and Cape, R.D.T., *J. Am. Geriatr. Soc.*, 36: 29–33, (1988).

43. Sotile, W.M., *J. Cardiopulm. Rehab.*, 13: 237 (1993).

44. Sotile, W.M., *Heart Illness and Intimacy: How Caring Relationships Aid Recovery.* Johns Hopkins University Press, Baltimore, (1992).

45. Sotile, W.M., Sotile, M.O., Ewen, G.S., and Sotile, L.J., *Sports Med. Training Rehab.* 4: 115 (1993).

46. Sotile, W.M., Sotile, M.O., Sotile, L.J., and Ewen, G.S., *Sports Med. Training Rehab.*, 4: 217 (1993).

47. Taylor, C.B., Bandura, A., Ewart, C.K., Miller, N.H., and DeBusk, F., *Am. J. Cardiol.*, 55: 635–638 (1985).

48. Burgess, A.W., Lerner, D.J., D'Agostino, R.B., Vokonas, P.S., Hartman, C.R., and Gaccione, P., *Soc. Sci. Med.* 24: 359–370 (1987).

49. Stern, M.J., and Cleary, P., *Arch Intern. Med.*, 142: 1093–1097 (1982).

50. Greif, H., Kreitler, S., Kaplinsky, E., Behar, S., and Scheinowitz, M., *Behav. Med.*, 21(2): 75–85 (1995).

51. Solcova, I., Maly, O., Sykora, J., and Jakoubek, B., *Activ. Nerv. Sup.*, 32(3): 189–190 (1990).

52. Shaeffer, M., Krantz, D.S., and Weiss, S.M., *J. Cardiol. Rehab.*, 10: 371–377 (1988).
53. Schmied, L.A., Steinberg, H., Moss, T., and Sykes, E.A., *J. Sports Sci.*, 12: 433–445 (1994).
54. Seganian, P., Roskies, E., Hanley, J.A., Oseasohn, R., and Collu, R., *Psychol. Health*, 1: 195–213 (1987).
55. Williams, R.B., *The Trusting Heart: Great News about Type A Behavior and Your Heart.* Time Books, New York (1989).
56. Naughton, J., Bruhn, J., Lategola. M., *Arch. Phys. Med. Rehab.*, 49: 131–137 (1968).
57. Moses, J., *J. Psychosom. Res.*, 33: 47–61 (1989).
58. Blumenthal, J., Williams, R.S., Needels, T., and Wallace, A. *Psychosom. Med.*, 44: 529–536 (1982).
59. Mayou, R.A., *J. Cardiac Rehab.*, 3: 397–402 (1983).
60. Steptoe, A., and Cox, S., *Health Psychol.*, 7: 329–340 (1988).
61. Moses, J., Steptoe, A., Mathews, A., and Edwards, S., *J. Psychosom. Res.*, 33: 47–61 (1989).
62. Norris, R., Carroll, D., and Cochrane, R., *J. Psychosom. Res.*, 36: 55–65 (1992).
63. Bennett, P., and Carroll, D., *J Psychosom. Res.* 38(3): 169–182 (1994).
64. Lavie, C.J., and Milani, R.V., *Am. J. Cardiol.*, 78: 675–677 (1996).

22

The Costs and Benefits of Exercise Programs in Secondary and Tertiary Rehabilitation*

ROY J. SHEPHARD
University of Toronto
Toronto, Ontario, Canada

INTRODUCTION

Major U.S. corporations now spend 48% of their after-tax profits on medical care for employees and their dependents (121), and this expense has been rising steeply year by year. Companies have reacted to this trend by containing costs through a shift to managed health care (50,55). Currently, 16% of the total U.S. population and 19% of those who are insured receive managed forms of medical coverage. Objectives of the managed schemes include the delivery of medical services in an integrated and cost-effective manner and the benchmarking of minimum treatment needs in various clinical conditions, so that optimal low-cost providers of necessary services can be identified (160). Providers of managed health care also recognize that many of the conditions for which insurance claims are made (for instance, atherosclerotic heart disease and its complications) could have been avoided through an increase in physical activity and other changes of

---

* *Secondary rehabilitation* is used here in its epidemiological sense—the prevention of clinical manifestations in a person who already has subclinical disease. *Tertiary rehabilitation* refers to exercise prescribed with a view to controlling existing symptoms or preventing a recurrence of disease.

lifestyle. In consequence, there is a correspondingly strong interest in analyzing the costs and benefits associated with secondary and tertiary rehabilitation programs.

ISSUES AFFECTING COSTS AND BENEFITS OF SECONDARY AND TERTIARY REHABILITATION

Physical inactivity is now widely accepted as a costly luxury for the individual, the employer, and society as a whole, but accurate estimation of potential human and economic gains from secondary and tertiary rehabilitation remain elusive for several reasons (147,148,152,156).

Environmental Influences

It is unclear how far personal efforts to maintain health through increased physical activity and an improved lifestyle may be offset by adverse influences from an unfavorable social environment (3,15,16,82). The major focus of health promotion has been on the behavior of the individual, but data such as the dramatic decrease of Russian life expectancy with collapse of the Soviet system (25) suggest that the overall social environment also has a major influence on cardiovascular health.

Type of Activity

There is little agreement on the relative effectiveness of various types, intensities, and amounts of physical activity in secondary and tertiary prevention.

"Lumping" of Diagnoses, Ages, and Gender

Estimates of societal costs have commonly lumped, as a single composite item, direct expenses incurred from all forms of chronic cardiovascular disease, whereas the duration of hospitalization, necessary medications, surgical interventions, and other treatment costs differ substantially between ischemic heart disease, hypertension, congestive heart failure, and other cardiovascular diagnoses (132).

Most analyses also consider costs and benefits independently of the individual's age and gender, but this is plainly fallacious. The incidence of ischemic heart disease rises steeply with age, and hospital treatment is generally much shorter for a cardiac patient who is under the age of 45 years than for an older individual. A comparison of costs and benefits thus makes it easier to justify an exercise program for the older adult (165) than for a younger individual [where some European studies suggest that the injuries incurred during strenuous and adventurous sports generate costs that offset any benefit from a small reduction in cardiac problems (5,104,143,175)].

Likewise, there are substantial differences in both the risk of cardiac disease and the approach to physical activity between men and women. In general, women exercise more cautiously and are correspondingly less vulnerable to injury, although the activities that they select may also be less effective in reducing the risk of cardiac disease.

Social Contribution from Extended Survival

Much of the imputed expense of chronic cardiovascular disease relates not to direct medical costs but rather to a reduction in the individual's quality of life and the broader social consequences of the productivity which is lost through illness, early retirement, and premature death.

If a physically active adult survives and continues working through to a normal age of retirement, there is disagreement as to whether one should calculate the resulting benefit as the full additional salary that the person earns (81) or merely the added amount the individual can contribute to society, that 25–50% of annual income which is distributed to others through taxation and the support of dependents (132).

Russell (142) has taken the extreme position that if outcomes for healthy individuals and those with chronic disease are compared in terms of years of survival, or quality-adjusted survival, then any additional allowance made for differences in earning power between the two categories of subject is an erroneous form of "double counting."

Changing Roles of Participation in the Labor Force

Most classical analyses of costs and benefits assume that 95% or even 100% of those of employable age have an opportunity to work. However, patterns of labor-force participation have changed quite rapidly in recent years. Most women of working age have now moved into full-time employment outside of the home, but unemployment rates have also risen steeply among their male peers. Among those who are currently most vulnerable to ischemic heart disease (poorly educated young adults who are heavy smokers), the real unemployment rate in North America may now be as high as 30%.

Automation and displacement of labor-intensive work to the "third world" seem likely to worsen the employment prospects of such individuals still further in the near future. It is thus unrealistic (152,156) to assume that everyone who is protected against premature cardiac disease will find full-time salaried employment through to an age of 65 or 70 years.

Care and Support of Relatives

Calculations of the social costs of cardiovascular disease should allow for the losses of production that arise from caring for the sick and experiencing the grief of bereavement. However, in the absence of better information, most economists have merely ascribed an arbitrary percentage of total costs to losses from this source (see, for example, Ref. 80).

Need for Discounting

There is a long and uncertain lag period between the development of "silent" cardiovascular disease and the appearance of significant clinical manifestations, with their associated personal and socioeconomic costs. Many of the anticipated benefits from secondary and tertiary preventive programs are similarly distant. Estimates of costs and benefits thus become highly susceptible to assumptions about the discount rate (the device that economists use to assess the willingness of an individual or of society to sacrifice now for a future good).

The discount rate may be regarded as the true (inflation-corrected) return on current investment. Russell (142) has argued for a figure of 5%. Accepting such a rate, if a physical activity program yields a benefit of $1000 after an average of 20 years, then the corrected benefit diminishes to $1000 \times (0.95)^{20}$, or $358. In the example of Field et al. (43), a discounting of all anticipated benefits from a secondary preventive program almost doubled the costs per added year of life relative to a similar calculation that was made without without discounting.

In some recent years, the inflation-corrected return on conservative investments has been 3% rather than 5%. Plainly, if costs or benefits are not anticipated until after an interval of 10 to 20 years, even small differences in the assumed discount rate have a major impact upon the likely balance sheet (140). A further problem in such analyses is that whereas all economists are agreed on the need to discount the cost side of the equation, there is less agreement concerning the need to discount future health benefits (134). Some authors maintain that health is not a tradeable resource that can be invested in various ways, and thus it should not be discounted; they find no evidence that people view future health less highly than their current condition (119). Others point to continued heavy smoking and drinking as proof that many of the population do indeed discount future health relative to current unhealthy indulgences.

Terminal Disability

The adoption of an active lifestyle may delay by 10 to 20 years the day when aerobic power, muscle strength, flexibility, and other important functional characteristics drop below the threshold values that together permit independent living (161) (Chapter 5). However, if the costs and benefits of an active lifestyle are being analyzed for a young adult, institutionalization is 40 or 50 years distant, even for a sedentary person. The socioeconomic impact of delaying a very costly loss of independence is thus highly susceptible to the assumptions that are made regarding the discount rate.

Quality of Life

A full economic model should include appropriate allowances for the personal and social benefits of an enhanced quality of life among active individuals (161). Unfortunately, retrospective analyses of hospital records rarely provide useful information on quality of life (91). Furthermore, there is lack of agreement as to how the various factors that limit quality of life can be integrated in a given person, compared from one person to another, or converted to an overall dollar cost.

The perceived health associated with a given degree of disability varies enormously from one person to another, depending on the individual's interests socioeconomic situation, and personality (Table 1). Nevertheless, a reduction in quality of the residual life span is one major consequence of chronic illness.

Despite methodological problems, there is widespread agreement that the total costs of chronic cardiovascular disease are very high in both personal and

Table I Factors to Be Considered in Calculating an Overall Score for Quality of Life, with Associated Ratings (shown in parentheses)

Mobility	Physical activity	Social activity
Drove car and used bus or train without help (5)	Walked without physical problems (4)	Did work, school, or housework and other activities (5)
Did not drive or had help to use bus or train (4)	Walked with physical limitations (3)	Did work, school, or housework but other activities limited (4)
In house (3)	Moved own wheelchair without help (2)	Limited in amount or kind of work in school or housework (3)
In hospital (2)	In bed or chair (1)	Performed self-care but did no work, school, or housework (2)
		Had help with self-care (1)

Note: Each year of survival is multiplied by a time-specific quality-of-wellness score, which is integrated (in terms of utility, relative desirability, and social preference). Typical items considered in reaching an appropriate multiplier at any given time point are listed in the table.
Source: From Ref. 74.

societal terms. Klarman (81) set the expense to the overall economy at $11,000 per worker per year (81), although a more realistic figure is probably $3000–$6000; all estimates have been approximated to 1998 U.S. dollars, adjusting earlier published figures by means of the general consumer price index, or, in the case of medical items, by the medical inflation rate.

COST-BENEFIT, COST-EFFECTIVENESS, AND COST-UTILITY ANALYSIS

The principles governing cost-benefit, cost-effectiveness, cost-utility, and cost-minimization analyses in general and the use of such methodologies in the evaluation of secondary and tertiary rehabilitation programs are discussed in several recent monographs and review articles (35,109,133–136,140,142,147,148,152, 156,157,160). However, it is useful to summarize the main characteristics and limitations of each of these approaches.

Cost-Benefit Analysis

In our present context, a cost-benefit analysis (133) attempts to express all the costs associated with cardiac disease and all the benefits anticipated from an increase in habitual physical activity in dollar terms (Tables 2 and 3). The hope is that benefits will exceed costs. If this is not the case, then the question becomes how much should an individual, a company, or a society pay to achieve a given improvement in cardiac health?

Problems of Expressing Costs in Dollar Terms

Many items important to a cost-benefit analysis—such as a poor quality of survival, grief among relatives, and the time required to participate in an exercise program—are very difficult to express in dollar terms.

Russell (142) has discussed the traditional assessment of time commitments in terms of an average working wage. One can debate such nice points as the availability of equivalent paid work in an era of high unemployment; the likely personal and social costs of an alternative use of leisure time, such as a trip to the theater (a point largely ignored by Russell) (142); and the pleasure that would result if currently ''free'' time were allocated to earning extra taxes for the government. If a given type of physical activity is enjoyed, then the personal cost of participation may be much less than the corresponding marginal earning power. On the other hand, if exercise is imposed by some external agency (a physician, an employer, or the government) and is heartily disliked, then the individual may equate the opportunity foregone with an equivalent amount of paid work (58).

Table 2   Annual Cost of Cardiovascular Disease to the U.S. and Canadian Economies

	Annual cost, billions of dollars[a]	
	United States ischemic heart disease	Canada, all CV disease
Direct costs	25.1	7.1
Personal services and supplies (hospital care, services of physicians and nurses, provision of drugs)	21.1	
Nonpersonal items (research, training, public health, capital construction, and insurance)	4.0	
Indirect costs	144.6	12.5
Premature death	101.7	
Loss of output from illness	15.7	
Intangible effects on productivity (pain, suffering, orphanhood)	27.2	
Total costs	169.7	19.6

[a] Data approximated to 1998 U.S. dollars, based on current exchange rates and changes in the general cost of living, with the exception of the item for direct medical costs, where an inflation rate 1.55 times greater than that for the general cost of living has been assumed.
Sources: From Refs. 81 and 184.

The Ethical Dilemma of Costing Lost Productivity

Minimization of the costs of illness is an important and sometimes highly ethical function of the government and other health maintenance organizations. However, it should not become the only goal of a health professional, a health-care system, or society as a whole (37). Indeed, in some circumstances it can justify bizarre policies.

Particular problems arise when estimates of lost production are included in a cost-benefit comparison. It then becomes easier to justify the provision of an exercise program (and, indeed, other costly forms of medical treatment) to a highly paid executive than to a production-line worker. Perhaps for this reason some companies restrict the use of their exercise facilities to senior executives. By a further extension of such totalitarian logic, there is no good economic reason to rehabilitate a severely disabled patient who is unlikely to return to work. Moreover, once the age of retirement is passed, no one has any social value as a source of paid work. Inevitably, a rigid cost-benefit approach thus argues against allocating resources to an improvement of health among senior citizens.

The policies inspired by such calculations are not only ethically unacceptable, but they also ignore the real contributions that elderly and disabled individuals can bring to their communities.

Table 3   Costs to the Canadian Economy (millions of dollars) from Cardiovascular Disease, with Comparable Costs[a] for Coronary Vascular Disease Where Available

	Cardiovascular disease	Coronary disease
Direct costs		
Personal items		
Hospital care	4512 million	1068 million
Medical care	792	
Drugs	955	244
	6259	
Nonpersonal items		
Research	55	11.6
Disability pensions	256	
Survivors pensions	359[b]	
Death benefits	43[b]	
Orphans pensions	35[b]	
Children of disabled	21[b]	
Sickness benefits	65[b]	
Other health expenditures[b]	4858	
	5692	
Total direct costs	11.95 billion	
Indirect costs		
Loss of future income	8529 million	5520 million
Short-term disability	168	
Chronic disability	3425	
Intangibles not included	——	
Total indirect cost	12.12 billion	
Total cost	24.07 billion	

[a]All costs approximated to 1998 U.S. dollars, using current exchange rates and consumer price index or medical cost inflation rate as appropriate
[b]Assessed at proportion of total expenditures (26%).
Source: Health and Welfare Canada, Economic burden of illness in Canada, 1986, in Chronic Diseases in Canada. 12 (3 Suppl.): (3) (1991).

Cost-Effectiveness Analysis

The cost-effectiveness approach generally starts from the assumption that some form of treatment will be offered to a patient. The analyst thus seeks to make an objective choices between competing options. Plainly, an appropriate measure of effectiveness is critical to the success of this approach.

In the early stages of secondary rehabilitation, process variables may be chosen—for example, the investment in equipment and advertising needed to attract 100 participants. However, in the context of cardiac health, patient outcomes are more suitable indices of effectiveness. The dollar costs of clinical treatments such as the use of β-blockers, angioplasty, bypass surgery, and cardiac transplant operations can be compared with preventive and rehabilitative programs in terms of the unit cost per year of productive work, per complication avoided, per year of pain-free life, per added year of life expectancy, or (ideally) per added year of quality-adjusted life (7,44,53,74,96,141,186).

To reduce the expense of analysis, conclusions are usually based on existing records (134). Cost-effectiveness analysis avoids some of the pitfalls of cost-benefit analysis and is commonly used in the context of managed health care. However, costs and outcomes still require careful discounting, particularly if they do not occur in the immediate future.

Cost-minimization analysis (136) is a variant of cost-effectiveness analysis. As its name implies, cost-minimization seeks to find the cheapest method of treating a given condition. It is ethically appropriate only when the outcomes of alternative programs are either the same or very similar.

Checking Medical and Surgical Claims

The quality of outcome is usually evaluated by a biased observer—the physician or surgeon who is directly involved in treatment. It is therefore salutary to look at the change in outcome caused by the "delisting" of a supposedly "effective" medical or surgical treatment. Levine et al. (88) reduced overall costs by $2.2 million ($122,222 per patient) when 18 patients were withdrawn from a cardiac transplant waiting list; furthermore, this benefit was apparently realized with no adverse effect upon clinical outcome!

Drastic treatments such as cardiac transplantation may extend a person's life span by a couple of years, but even where such an operation is warranted and the claim of added calendar life span is substantiated, the patient's quality of life is severely restricted because a substantial part of the added life span is taken up by special investigations and treatments. The extension of lifespan thus requires heavy discounting in terms of quality-adjusted life years (QALYs) (74).

Checking Effectiveness in the Community

Poor compliance reduces the effectiveness of both health-promotion initiatives and many traditional forms of medical therapy on moving from the clinical laboratory to the community (Table 4). Surgery largely escapes such strictures, since it is a once-only event, undertaken in a hospital or an outpatient facility. However, medication produces much poorer results in the "real world" than in the laboratory, because the patient may fail to follow the recommended treatment. Likewise, if exercise is taken in the community rather than the laboratory, the propor-

TABLE 4   Arbitrary Data Illustrating the Attenuation of Benefits from an Exercise Program Designed to Reduce the Risk of Ischemic Heart Disease on Moving from the Clinical Laboratory to the Community

Fraction of population	Fraction of population	Risk of cardiac disease	Contribution to population risk
Prior to program			
Active	0.2	1R	0.2R
Sedentary	0.8	2R	1.6R
Total population risk		1.8R	
Effect of program			
Initially active	0.2	1R	0.2R
Initially sedentary			
Participants	0.16		
(respondents)	0.144	1R	0.144R
(nonrespondents)	0.016	2R	0.032R
Nonparticipants	0.64	2R	1.28R
Total population risk		1.656R	
Reduction of risk to community = (1.8R − 1.656R)/1.8R = 8%			

Note: It is assumed that initially 20% of the population are taking adequate physical activity for cardiovascular health. The risk of cardiac disease in this group is 1R, and in the sedentary population it is 2R. It is further assumed that 20% of those initially inactive become active as a result of program, and that 90% of those who become active respond by the expected halving in their risk of future cardiovascular disease.

tion of patients who meet their exercise prescriptions declines exponentially with time (85,146).

The effectiveness of any program thus depends on both therapeutic response as observed under controlled laboratory conditions and anticipated compliance with the prescribed regimen (Table 4). Haskell et al. (57) have suggested that compliance can be enhanced by substituting moderate exercise and appropriate medication for a more rigorous regimen based on exercise alone.

Time as an Element in Effectiveness Calculations

A successful comparison of alternative treatments depends very much on the completeness of costing.

Exercise rehabilitation programs often fare badly in cost-effectiveness analyses (for example, Ref. 142), because account is taken of the personal or company time that participants invest in exercise programs. In contrast, many analyses of clinical treatment consider only the immediate costs of surgery, medication, and hospital bed use, neglecting the time invested by the patient in traveling to and from the hospital or clinic and in waiting for attention once he or she has arrived.

Table 5   The influence of a Substantial Weekly Dose of Physical Activity[a] upon the Years of Added Life to an Age of 80 Years

Age of starting physical activity, years	Calendar years gained [b]	
	Relative to <2.1 MJ/week	Relative to <8.4 MJ/week
35–39	2.51	1.50
40–44	2.34	1.39
45–49	2.10	1.10
50–54	2.11	1.20
55–59	2.02	1.13
60–64	1.75	0.93
65–69	1.35	0.67
70–74	0.72	0.44
75–79	0.42	0.30
35–79[c]	2.15	1.25

[a]An added weekly energy expenditure of 8.4 MJ (2000 kcal), as estimated from an activity questionnaire. Items considered include the walking of city blocks, the climbing of stairs, and sports play, with gains of calendar life expectancy expressed relative to subjects with lower levels of leisure energy expenditure (<2.1 MJ/week or <8.4 MJ/week).
[b]Data adjusted to allow for the effects of cigarette smoking, hypertension, low gain of body mass since attending university, and history of early mortality in parents.
[c]Weighted average for specified period.
Note: Estimates of years of added life based upon the mortality experience of Harvard alumni, 1962–1978.
Sources: From Refs. 112 and 115.

An exercising patient may invest much of any added survival time in either the prescribed activity or in travel to and from an exercise facility. Paffenbarger (112) and Paffenbarger et al. (115) estimated that an optimal program of increased physical activity could extend the life span of a middle-aged adult by as much as 2.2 years (Table 5). But even if we ignore travel time, the physical activity itself (perhaps 5 h/week, continued over 50 years of adult life) would occupy more than 2 years of 16-h waking days. If the exercise sessions and associated travel are enjoyed (as in much rural recreation), the participant may accept physical activity as a good investment of leisure time, and there is no need to include an equivalent opportunity cost in the final balance sheet. But if an exercise program involves tedious urban driving to a distant recreational facility and the prescribed activity is perceived as burdensome, then the time that is occupied, or the "opportunity foregone," must be costed at the equivalent marginal wage rate ($12–$15/h).

For some people, family involvement in a community exercise program can be a very positive social experience, reducing opportunity costs and increasing overall effectiveness. But for other households, regular attendance of a family member at a worksite fitness class, a rehabilitation center, or even a community-based exercise program is disruptive, to the point that a substantial opportunity cost should be attributed to such participation.

Implications of Opportunity Costs for Effective Programming

The opportunity costs associated with secondary and tertiary rehabilitation are difficult to evaluate because of interindividual differences in attitudes toward habitual physical activity and differences in perceptions of time. Nevertheless, such differences are important determinants of both the attributed cost and the effectiveness of exercise programs.

The investment of time is perceived as more costly by a time-conscious (type A) personality than by a relaxed (type B) individual. The type A person is attracted to short bouts of intensive exercise, hoping that these will yield results similar to those that could have been accomplished in a longer period of more moderate physical activity. The type A participant may also perceive an interval training program as less cost-effective than continuous exercise and will be anxious to ensure that nominal class time is devoted to physical conditioning rather than to ancillary goals such as social interaction. Finally, a time-oriented individual is tempted to exceed the prescribed ceiling of exercise intensity or duration in an attempt to hasten the training process (Chapter 4).

Rudman and Lipping (138) suggest that time is a particularly important barrier to regular physical activity in women of low socioeconomic status, possibly owing to the competing claims of child care.

Irrespective of personality, socioeconomic status, or gender, a large proportion of adults report "lack of time" as their main reason for not undertaking the recommended amount of physical activity per week. It is thus helpful to incorporate as much as possible of the recommended energy expenditure into the vigorous pursuit of everyday activities such as walking to work and climbing stairs (18) (the "active living" approach; see below), rather than insisting upon regular attendance at a formal exercise class in some distant location.

Cost-Utility Analysis

Economic studies conducted for government, industry, or health maintenance organizations properly use cost-benefit and cost-effectiveness analyses to compare potential treatments. However, studies that examine and evaluate consumer choices are best considered as cost-utility analyses (135). The consumer is supposed to derive a certain satisfaction or "utility" from each of a variety of options. He or she then seeks to maximize utility within the limits imposed by external constraints such as income or time. For example, a treatment that costs $20,000 may be regarded as an appropriate use of disposable income if it extends good quality life by a year. Likewise, a variety of pastimes are pursued until all "free" time is occupied. The marginal cost of undertaking physical activity is then equal to the benefit foregone in not pursuing some other type of activity, less any perceived rewards that accrue from exercising (such as "feeling better" or an enhancement of personal appearance).

One immediate flaw in cost-utility analyses is the assumption that everyone makes rational decisions in order to optimize benefit "at the margin." In fact, a poor socioeconomic environment may sap self-esteem and the sense of self-efficacy, limiting the individual's perceived range of choices. There are also many powerful social forces, both overt and hidden persuaders, that encourage people to make less than optimal decisions. Large investments in both social engineering and health promotion are thus required to counter undesirable social norms and facilitate appropriate choices for health (52).

Valuing Human Life

Whether treatment is purchased by government, an insuring agency, or the individual, it is necessary to set a value on human life. Estimates vary widely depending on the risk under consideration. In terms of the safety of air travel, figures may be as high as $22 million, but for the expense associated with the introduction of a coronary care unit it may drop to only $100,000 (7).

In general, any treatment can be regarded as unequivocally "effective" if the cost per QALY is less than $30,000, "ineffective" if it exceeds $150,000, and debatable if it lies between $30,000 and $150,000.

Quality of Survival

The quality of survival (Table 1) is rarely included in either cost-benefit or cost-effectiveness calculations, in part because such information cannot usually be ascertained from retrospective analysis of hospital records (91). However, it is an important element of cost-utility analyses. Conclusions based on quality-adjusted survival sometimes differ markedly from those that are based on mere survival.

For instance, the discounted cost of treatment by intravenous tissue plasminogen activator following myocardial infarction was estimated at $32,000 per added life year (92), but a prospective trial found that the cost per added QALY was only $1060 (87). In quality-adjusted terms, many traditionally recommended medical and surgical treatments of cardiovascular disease are quite expensive. For example, a main vessel coronary bypass operation costs a health insurer between $7600 (170) and $10,000 (109, 141) per QALY in North America and $3780 per QALY in the United Kingdom (186,187). If the patient still suffers from mild angina, survival is less pleasant, and the cost rises to $86,000 per QALY (109).

Because the prognosis without surgery is better for single-vessel than for main-vessel disease, the utility of surgical treatment is lower for single-vessel disease, and the cost of a bypass operation rises to about $76,000 per added QALY

JUSTIFICATION OF CARDIAC FOCUS

Regular physical activity has the potential to bring important dividends in many areas of secondary and tertiary prevention (23,24). Nevertheless, we will illustrate issues of cost-benefit, cost-effectiveness, and cost-utility analysis with specific reference to the secondary and tertiary prevention of ischemic heart disease for several reasons:

1. *Availability of data.* Several countries have already made serious attempts to estimate the direct and indirect costs attributable to cardiac disease (Tables 2 and 3) (81,131,132,139,184).

2. *Known safety.* An increase of physical activity is a very safe recommendation for the patient with cardiovascular disease. Noakes (107) estimated that a year of supervised exercise was six times less risky than the immediate chances of dying from coronary bypass surgery. In the context of cardiac disease, there is thus little chance that the adverse health effects of an increase in physical activity will outweigh its potential health benefits, leaving no "effectiveness" to evaluate.

3. *Known efficacy.* There is now good community-based evidence concerning the therapeutic efficacy of regular physical activity in both the secondary (114,127,149) and tertiary (111,129,151) prevention of ischemic heart disease.

4. *Patient acceptance.* A physical activity or exercise prescription is pleasant and positive advice relative to the dour list of medical prohibitions commonly associated with the treatment of cardiac disease, and there is a need to explore this advantage in terms of quality-adjusted life expectancy. Given a well-designed physical activity prescription and effective methods of reinforcing this recommendation, long-term compliance is better than for many other forms of prolonged medical treatment (146).

5. *Need to weigh the effectiveness of exercise relative to surgical alternatives.* Surgery has the advantage that in general it is targeted upon that segment of the population most in need of treatment (141). Thus, its overall cost-effectiveness is sometimes greater than might be anticipated from the cost of a single operation.

In contrast, it is difficult to target preventive programs (43). For example, if an exercise program is launched, this is usually available not only to the sedentary and the diseased but also to those who are already fit; indeed, the latter are commonly its major users.

Nevertheless, if costing is restricted to the immediate societal expenses of personnel and serviced space, a tertiary rehabilitation program compares quite favorably with targeted surgical alternatives; Noakes (107) equated the costs of coronary vascular bypass surgery (currently about $35,000 per person in the United States, with the prospect that angina may recur after 2–3 years) with 74 years of participation in a supervised phase 3 tertiary exercise program; on the same scale, an angioplasty ($17,000) would equate to 37 years of phase 3 exercise.

6. *Attitude of health maintenance and insurance schemes.* The need to practice ''defensive medicine'' has caused a substantial escalation in costs, both for preexercise clearance and the subsequent supervision of exercise programs, particularly in the United States. Perhaps as a reaction to this trend, many health maintenance and medical insurance schemes currently refuse to reimburse the costs of medically supervised exercise programs for all except a few categories of patient (46, 68). Other insurers contain costs by providing only a limited phase 2 service following myocardial infarction (for example, a total of 12 rehabilitation sessions, irrespective of the patient's risk profile, 55). In consequence, only a disappointing 15–20% of eligible patients are referred to cardiac rehabilitation programs (50).

Present patterns of secondary and tertiary rehabilitation thus need critical reevaluation (50). The commonly recommended scale of rehabilitation dates from an era when a prolonged hospital stay led to a substantial deterioration in physical fitness following myocardial infarction. Successful rehabilitation was thus thought to require repeated sessions of intensive exercise in order to restore aerobic power (50).

The time is now ripe to make a critical analysis of the cost-effectiveness of both initial medical clearance and the continued close supervision of physical activity programs.

OBSTACLES TO DETAILED ECONOMIC ANALYSIS OF EXERCISE PROGRAMS

We have already noted some major difficulties in estimating the costs of chronic cardiovascular disease and the likely benefits from secondary and tertiary rehabilitation. Medical costs are commonly cited for the broad category of ''cardiovascular diseases'' rather than for specific diagnoses such as ischemic heart disease or myocardial infarction (note the impact of the lumping of diagnoses upon cost comparisons between Canada and the United States, Table 2 and 3). Again, it is generally assumed that the direct costs of cardiovascular disease are independent of age, whereas a large fraction of current medical expenditures reflects inappropriate treatment of the frail elderly during the final weeks of life (47,48,179). Further, because of differences in the method of calculation, the sum allowed for the dominant cost (lost productivity from premature death) varies fourfold from Klarman (80,81) to Roberts (132).

Additional obstacles to a detailed economic analysis of exercise programs arise from variations in the proposed treatment and its social setting. There are major disagreements about methods of program evaluation and discount rates, uncertainties about the economic value of prolonged survival, and a need to attribute fiscal benefits between various segments of the economy.

Variations of Treatment and Social Setting

The costs of augmenting habitual physical activity vary widely, depending on the type of regimen that is recommended and its social setting.

Intensity of Activity

The main personal cost of exercising is the time committed by the participant. A high-intensity, short-duration program might thus seem cheaper than more prolonged bouts of lower-intensity activity. However, immediate consequences of a high-intensity program are demands for rigorous medical screening, elaborate exercise equipment, and sophisticated professional monitoring. A substantial period of moderate-intensity activity may thus be more cost-effective provided that the intensity reaches the threshold for health benefit (Chapter 1).

Potential of "Active Living"

Many exercise scientists now maintain that a simple program of "active living" can provide sufficient physical activity to maintain health. The concept of active living emphasizes the incorporation of vigorous physical activity into ordinary daily life through commuting (walking or cycling to and from the place of employment), work (use of the stairs rather than the elevators) and a physical approach to domestic chores (the use of manual rather power equipment) (31).

As discussed below, this approach minimizes the cost to the consumer (in terms of both time and the purchase of special clothing). The costs to society and the employer are also low (possibly provision and maintenance of sidewalks and cycle paths, or the installation of showers at work).

Advantages and Disadvantages of Specialized Exercise Facilities

Attendance at a custom-built exercise facility or a specialized rehabilitation center has the advantage that it allows better-supervised and more intensive bouts of exercise. On the other hand, if the center is located at the opposite end of a large city, the patient may gain no more than a nominal half hour of exercise for 2 h of driving and a half-hour of changing into and out of special clothing. Unfortunately, if managed health care plans are prepared to contribute to the costs of supervised rehabilitation, they usually insist that patients attend a specified center, mainly because this center has contracted a favorable rate for its rehabilitation services. Patients are denied the option of membership in an alternative program, even if it is much more conveniently located (55). In part because of these problems, King et al. (79) found that compliance was much better for home-based exercise programs than for classes organized at specialized centers.

Exercise is the sole form of intervention at some facilities, but more commonly a specialized fitness and health promotion center offers a modular program that includes counseling on many important aspects of personal lifestyle (159). In the case of tertiary rehabilitation, a structured and closely supervised program has the further advantage that the underlying medical condition is monitored on a regular basis. Supervision allows adjustment of both exercise and drug prescriptions whenever the patient's clinical condition changes.

Commercial Exploitation of Formal Programs

Unfortunately, both the medical profession and the fitness industry have added a great deal of expense to many exercise programs and other active pursuits. Doctors have sometimes recommended very expensive and ineffective procedures for the immediate medical clearance and subsequent supervision of those who intend even a modest increase in their habitual physical activity. Likewise, the fitness industry has created expensive fads and fashions in the type of activity to be pursued, the clothing to be worn, and the equipment supposedly needed for optimal enjoyment of a given pursuit (142,154).

Although the major part of such expense is unwarranted, it is often included in estimates of the costs of exercising. Currently, it is a significant barrier to participation and an important limitation upon the effectiveness of exercise programs.

Diversity of Social Settings

At the macrolevel, the social setting in which an active lifestyle must be pursued ranges from the highly technological free-enterprise system of North America through the social democracies and centralized state economies of Europe to developing societies with very limited resources.

Many sports sociologists overlook the breadth of this diversity, accepting a myopic focus upon issues of gender, color, or sexual orientation at a national or regional level. However, the social context has a major impact on personal attitudes, costs, and access to various types of physical activity and alternative treatments.

In North America, adults have been conditioned by the media, commercial interests, and even physical education professionals to equate "exercise" with attendance at a professionally supervised fitness center; they expect expensive preliminary testing and access to elaborate exercise equipment. In contrast, the physicians of Dunedin, New Zealand, have advocated moderate hill walking as an acceptable low-cost source of physical activity for both the coronary-prone and "postcoronary" patients. Again, in some developing societies, cycling to work and other physical demands of daily activity still provide an adequate energy expenditure for health.

The Canadian program of "Active Living," "Exercise Lite" in the United States, and "Life—Be in it" in Australia have recently attempted to reclaim a low-cost, uncomplicated approach to physical activity (31). The vigorous pursuit of daily activities is seen to offer renewed health, empowerment, and self-actualization largely unshackled by such constraints as poverty, gender, or membership of a minority group.

Diversity of Costs

Economic analyses of exercise and health face a diversity of costs from one country to another. The fees for standard medical and surgical treatments differ two or threefold, even between the United States and commonwealth countries such as Canada and New Zealand. For example, coronary bypass operations may cost $35,000 in the United States (121) but (on published exchange rates) only $12,000 in New Zealand (54). In developing societies, both available therapeutic options and their costs differ even more radically from what has become the accepted norm in North America.

Objective Evaluation

As in many branches of science, the evaluation of equivocal data on costs and benefits tends to be colored by the wishes of the investigator. It is thus important to recognize that just as surgeons tend to evaluate the results of surgery, so many analyses of the costs and benefits of exercise have been commissioned by the operators of fitness programs. Further, the individuals collecting and interpreting the data have commonly had a strong emotional if not a personal financial interest in demonstrating positive outcomes. Thus problems of limited recruitment, poor compliance and a lack of therapeutic response (Table 5) have sometimes been downplayed.

Need to Discount Benefits

Some of the psychosocial benefits of increased physical activity can be demonstrated within a few weeks of joining an appropriate exercise program—"feeling better" and an improved self-image, for example. If enhancement of mood state improves a person's quality of life by 10%, beginning at the age of 30 years, then there is a very substantial immediate increase in that individual's quality-adjusted life expectancy (161). Such benefits are incurred more or less concurrently with program expenditures and thus need little discounting.

However, much of the health benefit imputed to a well-designed physical activity program reflects the prevention of chronic disease. If the exerciser is a young adult, disease is avoided only after a long and uncertain lag period. Fiscal estimates then become highly susceptible to assumptions about the discount rate. Some investigators have assumed a figure equal to the inflation-corrected return on government bonds or industrial investments (for instance, 5%). Others have applied an artificially high discount rate, attempting to compensate for what they regard as an overstatement of the benefits of exercise. Others, again, undertake a sensitivity analysis, using several potential discount rates ranging from 0 to 10% (140,152).

Eventually, a steady state is reached. Uncertainties caused by an inappropriate choice of lag-time or discount rate should then disappear. The immediate program costs incurred by one cohort of the population are offset by the health and social benefits reaped in an earlier cohort of the same population.

Costs and Benefits of Extended Survival

Avoidance of Premature Death

Most analyses assume that avoidance of premature death has economic as well as personal benefits. Such assessments suppose that all survivors are willing to work through to a fixed normal age of retirement and to find appropriate employment.

This argument may be appropriate in secondary rehabilitation, but empirical data suggest that return to work following a nonfatal myocardial infarction depends more on social and psychological factors than on exercise-generated improvements in general health and physical work capacity (147,155). For example, the cardiac program of the Toronto Rehabilitation Centre, an outpatient facility, serves a predominantly white-collar population. In this setting, the physical demands of employment are low, and most class members have a strong motivation to return to work. The 3-year compliance with our exercise prescription is 82% (164), and 86% of the group return to their normal work within 6 months. Other cardiac rehabilitation programs treat patients from lower socioeconomic groups; they report 6-month exercise compliance rates as low as 50% (33,110).

Perk and Hedback (122) found that in a rural area of Sweden, where the main occupation was the cutting of lumber, the climate was cold, and governmental social benefits were easily obtained, only 50–55% of patients had returned to work 6 months after sustaining a myocardial infarction.

Social Need for Work

A further imponderable is the *need* for everyone to work in our highly automated postindustrial society. Many analyses have estimated the costs of chronic illness and premature mortality by assuming that 95% of the labor force normally work through to an age of 65 or even 70 years. However, there has been a progressive displacement of labor-intensive industries from North America to the third world during the latter half of the twentieth century, and employment opportunities for older individuals have been correspondingly reduced in developed countries. A growing personal wealth has also encouraged a reduction in the average age of retirement. An increasing proportion of patients thus remain outside the paid labor force after recovery from myocardial infarction.

Pension Costs and Chronic Disability

Some actuaries have expressed a concern that an exercise-induced lengthening of the life span could increase the load on overburdened health care plans and pension funds (140,156,160,181,182).

There are several weaknesses in such arguments (Table 6). In fact, both the personal and the social impact of extended survival depends very much upon the quality of any added years. Will health be good, or will there be gross incapacitation from angina and heart failure? Although not included in the calculations of Table 6, the person who remains in good health often retires later than the person who is in poor health (39,173), and a 1- to 2-year extension of working life in itself may be sufficient to meet other costs associated with an increase in the average age of death.

Moreover, the enormous societal costs of supporting our elders reflect medical and institutional needs during the final months of life (48,54,125,179) rather than the expense of feeding and clothing individuals who remain fit (47, 147,161). Canadian studies suggest that the average sedentary adult spends 8–9 years with some degree of disability and a final year of total dependency (27, 150). Women survive longer than men, but they also experience a longer period of dependency (19). In contrast, seniors who have remained active retain sufficient aerobic power, muscle and bone strength, and flexibility to live independent lives; they do not require a long period of institutional support (114,161).

Finally, the main effect of exercise is to avoid premature rather than late mortality. In old age, the curves of calendar survival for active and sedentary individuals come together (114,120) (Fig. 1). Vigorous physical activity may

TABLE 6   The Costs and Benefits of a 2-Year Extension of Life Span Induced by Starting Exercise at Age 35

Costs	
Pension payment	= $20,000/year
Extension of payments	= 2 years
Gross addition to pension	= $40,000
Tax recovered at 30%	= $12,000
Net cost	= $28,000
Added medical costs at $1,000/year	= $2,000

Total social cost = $30,000, commencing at death of inactive person (age 75 years, 40 years distant).

Benefits

Reduced institutional costs ($1,000/year: for 11 years, commencing at age 65) = $11,000

Comparison of costs (C) and benefits (B) at selected discount rates (D):

		2%	5%	10%
Costs $\times$ (D)^{40}	=	$13,454	$4,161	$575
Benefits $\times$ (D)^{30}	=	5,512	2,018	372
Net cost	=	7,942	2,143	203

Note: The net cost quickly becomes a benefit if the active person is able to continue his or her productive life for a longer period.

even shorten life slightly among the very old (90). Actuarial fears that an increase of physical activity will generate social costs by extending survival are thus unwarranted.

Attribution of Costs and Benefits

Cost-benefit analyses usually take a broad social view, seeking to maximize national wealth and ignoring any temporary transfer of costs or benefits to one particular sector of the economy (140,142,152). Likewise, cost-effectiveness analyses rarely consider who makes the investment needed to achieve a given outcome. Policy decisions should usually be determined without regard to attribution of costs or benefits. Nevertheless, there are exceptions.

Worksite programs promoting fitness and health promotion commonly increase productivity (72,158), and the distribution of any resulting economic gains between the employer and the employed may become an issue of hot debate. Moreover, if management is asked to sponsor and support an exercise facility, they will want to know the impact of that program on the corporate rather than the national balance sheet.

Likewise, if an insuring agency is considering a scale of reimbursement

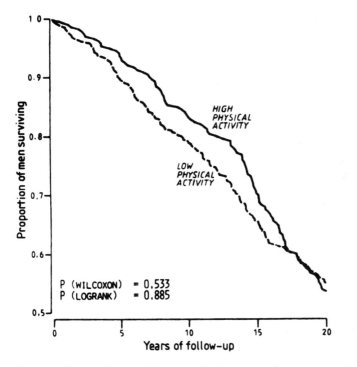

FIGURE I   Cumulative mortality curves for inactive and active populations living in Finland. Note that the survival curves for the two groups come together in old age. (From Ref. 120.)

for tertiary rehabilitation, their focus will be upon costs and effectiveness within a narrow sector of the economy (46,62,68,77). They will have a strong interest in both the shortening of immediate disability and the potential to avoid a second cardiac incident, with its attendant work loss and medical costs, but they may show much less concern about the opportunity costs incurred by the patient through participation in a specific type of program.

DIRECT COSTS OF AN EXERCISE PROGRAM

The most obvious direct costs of a formal exercise class are expenditures on personal services and supplies. Salaries are typically the main item (12). A physician may provide initial medical clearance, regular follow-up, and ongoing supervision (38), with appropriate treatment of any complications. An exercise professional commonly prescribes exercise and provides immediate supervision of activity classes. To these expenditures must be added the patient's opportunity and travel costs, charges for the purchase of any clothing and equipment that safety, fashion or social convention dictate as necessary for a particular pursuit, and a variety of less readily determined nonpersonal items—including the capital construction, equipment, and maintenance of an exercise or sport facility by the municipality or private enterprise, the insurance of program operators against exercise-related accidents (63), investment in the training of sports physicians and exercise supervisors, research in the sport sciences, and the promotion of regular physical activity either by mass advertising (government sponsored health promotional agencies such as ParticipACTION in Canada and the President's Council on Physical Fitness in the U.S.), or through individual counseling by physicians, nurses, and other health professionals.

Secondary Rehabilitation

Program Costs

The direct cost of a secondary rehabilitation program for the middle-aged, coronary-prone individual depends greatly upon the scale of intervention that is contemplated. Possible options range from a gradual increase in normal daily activity (''Active Living'') through the enhanced use of existing community sport and fitness facilities to the development of specific worksite exercise and health promotional programs.

"Active Living"

Both U.S. and Canadian governments are currently attracted by the concept that an increase in normal, daily physical activities such as vigorous walking can enhance endurance fitness and prevent various ''diseases of inactivity'' in middle-aged and older people (100–102,114,162). In surveys of the Harvard Alumni, Paffenbarger and associates (113–115) found a substantial association between deliberate walking and stair climbing and protection against fatal heart attacks. Likewise, Morris et al. (101–102) found that British executive-grade civil servants were protected against various manifestations of ischemic heart disease by what they termed *vigorous getting about* (rapid walking, gardening, and other activities that generated peaks of energy expenditure higher than 31 kJ/min, or 7.5 kcal/min). Interest was promoted by initial personal instruction, continuing support, and recommendation of a moderate-intensity regimen that could be maintained without attending a specialized center (65).

The societal costs of activities such as walking, stair climbing, and gardening are quite limited. Certainly, there is no reason for the patient to seek an extensive preliminary medical clearance. Such clearance can be an important source of expense, since the resolution of false-positive stress tests brings the cost of an exercise electrocardiogram to about $1100 per patient (94). Day-by-day supervision is also unnecessary for the usual moderate walking program. Finally, there is no need for costly facilities.

Municipalities may face a call for the paving (and in Canada and the northern United States of snow-ploughing) sidewalks. However, in some communities people have simply formed walking clubs that exploit the extensive climate-controlled space of major shopping centers. This is an attractive option in cities with very hot or very cold climates.

National and regional governments may spend some money in promoting this type of activity through various forms of advertising (18), but if walking and cycling become significant components of commuter transportation, there are also economic savings because of a reduced demand for parking spaces and/or feeder buslines and a lessening of vehicle-related air pollution.

The individual who deliberately increases his or her weekly walking distance may need to purchase additional shoes, socks, and food (a total expenditure of perhaps $400/year) (147), but if the required activity is built into the daily schedule, the opportunity cost is surprisingly small.

Relative Costs of Walking and Jogging

It is interesting to contrast the costs of rapid walking and other forms of active living with a regimen built around deliberate jogging. Because the legs of the jogger are subjected to a substantial impact stress, the risks of mechanical injury and associated orthopedic costs are much greater than for the walker.

Most joggers are also persuaded to buy quite costly running shoes and clothing. At least one jogging suit is purchased, and if there are wide seasonal extremes of climate, the exerciser may be tempted to buy several uniforms appropriate to different weather conditions.

Jogging causes the body temperature to rise sufficiently that it is necessary to take a shower, and except in rare instances where such facilities are available at work, it is difficult to adopt jogging as a method of commuting. Instead, jogging becomes a charge upon the individual's leisure time, and it thus has a much higher opportunity cost than walking. Finally, because jogging demands a relatively high intensity of physical activity, many middle-aged individuals find it prudent to request periodic medical evaluations, with specific prescription of an appropriate jogging pace.

Worksite Fitness and Health Promotion Programs

It has been argued that worksite fitness classes are the most cost-effective of organized exercise programs (147,148). The overhead costs encountered in a commercial or a community exercise program are reduced or avoided at the worksite. The closeness of the facility eliminates most of the opportunity cost of exercise-related travel (147,148), and normal office staff may be willing to be trained as volunteer leaders of exercise classes. Promotional costs are also low, since publicity channels and peer-support networks are already established within a large corporation.

On the other hand, the quality of the recreational experience in a renovated office basement or a corner of the shop floor may be less than could have been found in the alternative setting of a rural resort. If a worker devotes an hour of "free" time to exercise, this may thus be seen as a time-consuming duty rather than as a pleasure, and an equivalent opportunity cost must be calculated. Some companies grant release time so that employees can participate in a worksite fitness program; the cost of such arrangements must also be included in the final balance sheet.

Economic analyses of worksite programs sometimes take little account of the costs of serviced space; it is argued that the area allocated to an exercise class was previously underused or unused. However, if a specially designed health promotional facility is constructed, this can be very expensive, particularly if it is located in a downtown office tower. Further, unless the schedule of the employee and/or the hours of operation of the center are very flexible, problems of commuting and child care may leave the facility empty for a large part of both day and night.

Depending on the size of the company (Table 7) and the scale of the program, total costs for staff, equipment, and serviced space range from $800 to $3200 per participant-year, or (with a typical 20% participation rate) $160–640 per worker per year. Unfortunately, such expenditures currently attract mainly that 20% of employees who enjoy exercising. Many of these people were previously active elsewhere (85), although they find it more convenient to exercise at the worksite. The marginal cost of persuading lazier employees to exercise is likely to be high, and the worksite program is unlikely to attract that 20% of adults who declare that "nothing" would make them more active. Further, the standard worksite program fails to reach such important target groups as the retired elderly, women with young children, the disabled, and the unemployed. Finally, worksite initiatives are not available to the self-employed and those working in very small companies (who together account for a large and growing fraction of the total labor force).

Community Initiatives

The construction and operating costs are often lower for community exercise facilities than for comparable worksite initiatives, because the costs of land and occupied space are much smaller in the suburbs than in the centers of large cities. Nevertheless, the necessary acreage for facility, parking and access roads is still

TABLE 7 Costs of Possible Tactics for the Delivery of Worksite Exercise Programs and Applicability to Corporations of Various Sizes

Expected number of participants	Recommended approach	Cost per participant-year
<400	Campuswide[a] facility with full-time supervisor	$500–$800
5–50	Minimal on-site facility, testing and exercise prescription only	$250–$800
75–250	150–300 m² facility with part- or full-time supervisor	$600–$800
400–850	600–1200 m² facility[b] with full-time supervisor	$500–$800

[a]It is assumed that several companies are located on a single industrial campus and that they cooperate to provide the needed facility
[b]If participation rate reaches the anticipated level (20% of a 2000-member work force), a facility of 600 m² provides a standard space allowance of 0.3 m² per worker
Note: All costs have been approximated to 1998 U.S. dollars.
Source: Based in part on R.S. Wanzel, Rationale for employee fitness programs, in *Employee Fitness: the How To* (K.S. Wanzel, ed). Ontario Ministry of Culture and Recreation, Toronto, pp. 1–16 (1979).

a substantial expense (147,148). In order to keep the per-participant expense low, the facility must be used for a large part of the day throughout much of the year. Swimming lakes and cross-country ski trails have great esthetic appeal, thus reducing the opportunity costs to users, but such facilities fare poorly on a cost-effectiveness calculation because they are only used for a few weeks in each season. The costs of more heavily used municipal recreational facilities such as ice-skating/roller rinks lie in the range $60–$350 per citizen per year (147,148).

Farquhar et al. (42) have studied the effectiveness of broadly based communitywide health promotional initiatives. Their "Five City Study" was effective in reducing blood cholesterol, blood pressure, pulse rate, cigarette smoking, and heart disease. Similar encouraging findings have emerged from the Minneapolis Heart Health Project, the Pawtucket Heart Health Project, and the North Karelia project (121).

Promotional Costs

In Britain, individual motivation to a change of lifestyle has been attempted in general practice using a lifestyle questionnaire, a health check, and a follow-up by nurses among those with significant cardiac risks. The cost is about $49 per patient, or $2.40 to $3.75 for a 1% reduction in coronary risk (84). Such an initiative would be cost-effective only if the change in behavior persisted for several years (188).

In North America, the main thrust of promotion has been through mass advertising. Nevertheless, when the expenditures on government motivational programs are expressed in per capita terms, they seem small, particularly as compared with the budgets of other groups influencing personal lifestyle, such as cigarette manufacturers. In Canada, the annual cash investment of government and private sponsors together totals only about $1.5 million, or 5 cents per citizen, although this figure is augmented by donations of "free" advertising time and space. There is little evidence that such investment alters exercise behavior; indeed, stronger campaigns which have focused on specific medium-sized cities for periods of up to 6 months have had only limited success in increasing physical activity among local residents (69). Nevertheless, the organizations concerned have claimed some success in that people's awareness of the need for exercise has been increased through their personal promotional efforts.

Tertiary Rehabilitation

The close supervision of exercise programs during the first 3 months after myocardial infarction (phase 1 and phase 2 programs) can be very expensive, particularly if the physician insists upon continuous electrocardiographic (ECG) monitoring of exercise responses (34,41,45,99,168). Health maintenance organizations and other agencies that offer medical insurance are thus scrutinizing the direct costs of tertiary rehabilitation ever more closely (12,46,68).

The optimal solution probably lies in a careful gradation of risk, with a corresponding stratification of supervision and monitoring procedures (97,118, 174) (Table 8).

Phase 1 and Phase 2 Treatment

Debate continues on the merits of ECG and/or medical surveillance of postcoronary patients (168).

Froelicher et al. (50) point out that in the early days of postcoronary rehabilitation, programs did not include telemetric monitoring. The "need" for such equipment was generated as sicker patients began exercising, and intensive-care technology was repackaged into an outpatient format. Telemetry became an insurance provider's standard that was required for the reimbursement of exercise sessions. Currently, many third-party payers prefer telemetry ECG-monitored home exercise programs to the greater expense of continued attendance at supervised exercise classes (46).

Regular structured telephone contact is another option for phase 2 (32,57, 98,105). Wasson et al. (182a) claimed that telephone contacts were 28% cheaper than regular clinic visits, and this saving could be achieved without adverse consequences for the patient. DeBusk et al. (32) noted that patients who received regular telephone calls returned to work sooner; they also had fewer subsequent problems and lower overall treatment costs.

In the United States, costs for the early phases of treatment can amount to $7000–$9000 per patient, and because of limited reimbursement by insurers, many patients have strong financial incentives to noncompliance (50). Agencies such as Blue Cross and Blue Shield currently consider low-risk patients as ineligible for formal cardiac rehabilitation once they have been discharged from hospital. Moderate-risk patients are candidates for 8–12 weeks of thrice-weekly phase 2 rehabilitation, and high-risk patients are reimbursed for more intensive surveillance (46).

Phase 3 Rehabilitation

The total cost of phase 3 rehabilitation varies widely with the extent of exercise testing, medical supervision, and counseling. Some economic analyses have ignored the use of serviced space. If the gymnasium at a rehabilitation center is occupied uniquely by a single group of cardiac patients, meeting one to three times per week, an annual cost of $550–650 per patient should be assessed for this serviced space. In the example of Berra and Hall (12), the more economic option of renting appropriate space accounts for some 15% of the operating budget.

Home Programs

A home program is the most economical arrangement during phase 3. Regular telephone contact can sustain compliance, and reinforcing visits can be made to a supervising clinic every 1–2 months (or sooner if untoward symptoms appear). Some training is possible when using such a plan, but both the intensity of effort and the resultant conditioning response are less than that which is obtained from more closely supervised activity sessions (75). Moreover, the risk of sudden death (although still less than 1 in 100,000 h of physical activity) is several times higher at home than with exercise in a clinic (167).

Supervised Programs

Phase 3 programs are often operated by community agencies such as the YMCA. The main expenses arise in the supervision of stress testing and programs. All other costs, including property rental, account for less than a quarter of the total budget (12). Assuming two stress tests per patient ($600 each) and a thrice-weekly program ($600, or about $2.75 per patient session), the cost of a 21-month phase 3 program in the United States is about $1850 (12,128,190).

In Sweden, a typical outpatient program operated by a small hospital involves a salaried physician, two physiotherapists, and one trainee physiotherapist who together supervise a group of 16 postcoronary patients. A total of 27 rehabilitation sessions are provided over a period of 2 years, and after adding an arbitrary 10% allowance for materials and equipment (but apparently no charge for facilities), an operating cost of about $8 per patient session is estimated (60,122).

In Australia, a typical combination of two exercise tests and a thrice-weekly phase 3 conditioning program costs a total of about $1135 per patient (131).

In Canada, the medically supervised Toronto Rehabilitation Centre program continues throughout phase 3 of treatment. The service includes one salaried physician, a physiotherapist, and three student assistants per class of 50 patients. The personal cost of a single 1-h class amounts to about $4 per participant. The main advantage of having a physician present at testing and exercise sessions is not the occasional need for cardiac resuscitation (paramedical professionals can undertake this just as effectively as a medically qualified doctor). Rather, the physician has the opportunity to examine the reactions of the patient to exercise, to evaluate any symptoms that have been reported, and to match the objective conditioning response against the extent of training that has been noted in the patient's diary records. Johanna Kennedy (administrator of the Toronto Rehabilitation Centre) has estimated the total cost of their 4-year tapered phase 3 program at $2360 per participant. This figure includes five routine exercise tests per patient, medically supervised exercise sessions held once weekly for the first year and monthly for a further 6 months, telemetry during exercise sessions, a 24-h ambulatory monitoring of the ECG when required, further exercise tests when required, telephone or personal access to the exercise supervisor, and psychological screening. Although the cost of the program is quite high, it compares favorably with briefer U.S. programs that provide only paramedical supervision of exercise classes. The high cost of some programs in the United States reflects extensive surveillance by fee-for-service medical staff, attempts to recoup the costs of expensive test equipment, and the major costs of insurance against contingency litigation (63).

Overall Assessment

In terms of operating cost, supervised exercise sessions are good value. It remains more debatable whether repeated stress tests are cost-effective, given the day-to-day variability in such signs as ST-segment depression (8), although if a range of parameters are observed, a useful stratification of risk and thus of treatment may be obtained (Table 8).

The patient usually bears the institutional costs of phase 3 rehabilitation in the United States. But opportunity costs are a much greater expense in a large city. If 2 h is invested in travel time to and from the rehabilitation center, the total opportunity cost of a 60-min exercise class is 3 h, $36–$45 per visit. Two years of thrice weekly attendance thus demands a total opportunity investment

TABLE 8 Potential Guidelines for the Stratification of Risk Following Myocardial Infarction

---

Low Risk: Exercise capacity 7 METs or greater, cardiac ejection fraction >50%, no significant PVCs, no evidence of residual myocardial ischemia.

Moderate risk: Myocardial ischemia (exercise ST-segment depression >0.2 mV or perfusion abnormalities on thallium imaging), cardiac ejection fraction 35–50%, no "dangerous" forms of PVC.

High risk: Recurrence of angina following infarction, symptoms and signs of congestive cardiac failure, exercise capacity 5 METs or less, limited by angina, ST-segment depression or fall of blood pressure, cardiac ejection fraction <35%, dangerous PVCs (polyfocal, runs of PVCs, R-on-T phenomenon) or ventricular fibrillation, persistence of angina or ST-segment depression following exercise.

Key: MET = metabolic unit; PVC = premature ventricular contraction.

of $10,800–$13,500. Even the simplified, tapered Toronto plan generates an opportunity cost of $2160–$2700 over 4 years, matching the direct operating costs of the program.

CALCULATING THE ECONOMIC BENEFITS OF INCREASED PHYSICAL ACTIVITY

There are important ethical objections to basing treatment decisions on a rigid cost-benefit analysis, but nevertheless there is interest in calculating the likely savings from participation in a secondary or tertiary program of preventive exercise.

Economic Benefits of Secondary Prevention

There are both acute and chronic potential benefits from secondary prevention. In the short term, exercise enhances mood state, and the active individual "feels better." She or he is thus more productive at work and makes fewer demands for the medical treatment of minor complaints. In a longer-term perspective, the exerciser also has a reduced risk of incurring the direct personal and nonpersonal costs of chronic illness and the indirect social costs of lost production, premature death, and intangible items such as pain, suffering, and care as an invalid.

Benefits to the Employer

In the North American economy, acute gains accrue mainly to the employer; this provides a strong economic incentive for the introduction of worksite fitness and lifestyle programs (72,73,147,148,152,156–158,160). Potential benefits in-

TABLE 9   Estimate of the Financial Benefits Accruing from a Worksite Fitness and
Health Promotion Program: Example from a Life Insurance Company Head Office

Type of Benefit	Amount of benefit
Company image	Enhanced by in-house program (particularly if marketing a health-related product)
Greater worker satisfaction	Higher-quality production—less customer complaints
Increased productivity	Up to 2.7% advantage over control ($200 per worker-year)
Reduced absenteeism	Up to 1 day/year (replacement cost 1.75 days/year) = $42 per worker-year
Decreased employee turnover	Up to 16.2% difference relative to control group (cost of training replacement $550 per worker-year)
Reduced industrial injuries	$73/year
Reduced demand for medical services	Reduced (32% decrease of costs for medical and hospital services relative to controls, saving of $288 per worker-year)
Employment in fitness facility	Labor-intensive, contributes to reduction of unemployment
Total saving: $1153 for costed items in life insurance company example	

Note: It is assumed that 20% of employees participate in the program. Benefits are calculated per worker-year and have been approximated to 1998 U.S. dollars. Based in part on Refs. 147 and 148.

clude an improvement of corporate image with recruitment of premium employees (11,171), a lesser rate of employee turnover (156,171), greater productivity (158), reduced absenteeism (73,160,180), and fewer industrial injuries [in heavy physical work, but not in office staff, (14,29,172,183)]. Depending on the employee participation rate, the costs of training workers, the state of the labor market, and the availability of analogous incentives at other potential employers, the cumulative benefit to the company may be as large as $850 per worker-year (Table 9).

One survey of 12 major U.S. companies (73) suggested an average cost/benefit ratio of 2.89:1.00 from investment in health promotion programs. Only one of the twelve companies that were surveyed estimated that they had incurred a loss on their investment, and this was seen only in the first year of a 2-year program.

The largest gain in the worked example (Table 9) comes from a reduction in employee turnover and the training of replacement employees. The cost of

TABLE 10 To Illustrate the Economic Consequences of Exercise-Induced Reduction of Coronary Disease During Working Life

Reduction in fatal myocardial infarctions
  Average annual incidence of fatal myocardial infarctions in sedentary population 20/
    10,000 over period 35 to 65 years.
  If exercise reduces deaths to 15/10,000 for first 5 years of program, and to 10/
    10,000 for remaining 25 years of program, 275 premature deaths per 10,000 are
    prevented which otherwise would have occurred an average of 16 years after
    inception of the program (age 51 yr).
  If salary = $40,000/year, and social contribution is 50% of this, or $20,000/year,
    benefit = $(65 - 51) \times (275/10,000) \times \$20,000 = \$7,700$

Benefit B discounted at rates D shown below:

	2%	5%	10%
Benefit $\times$ D^{16} =	$5,425	$3,103	$1,386

Note: Gains shown here must be set against any costs incurred from longer survival (Table 6).

this item varies widely with the state of the labor market; in our current economy, human capital depreciates rapidly as traditional skills become obsolete. Moreover, once competing companies have developed equivalent health promotion programs, a given program probably does little to reduce employee turnover. There thus remain many uncertainties in such balance sheets.

Reduced Medical Costs

Empirical data (147,148,152,156) show that in North America, the introduction of a worksite fitness and health promotion program reduces the demand for medical services. In consequence, the sponsoring company can negotiate a more favorable contract with the agency that is providing medical insurance (152,156). Furthermore, moderate aerobic activity causes no significant increase in the demand for orthopedic treatment (165), and unless an extensive preliminary medical clearance is required, exercisers show no increase in the number of cardiac consultations.

In contrast, some European studies of young adults (5,6,89,104) have found a substantial injury cost from sports such as rugby football, soccer, and skiing (in Britain, an annual total of some $600 million, or $10 per capita).

North American programs show a reduction of medical costs among program participants within a few months of initiating an exercise program. Presumably, this reflects an enhancement of immune function (163), an improvement of perceived health (4,64), a greater sense of self-efficacy (67), or a lessening of depression (26) rather than the prevention of chronic illness. Additional benefits may develop later from the prevention of conditions such as ischemic heart disease.

Several well-designed studies with random allocation of workers to control and experimental programs have found early reductions in medical claims of up to $800 per worker-year (20). One negative report came from a reanalysis of the Blue Cross of Indiana data (144). The authors admitted that potential intergroup differences may have been obscured by contamination of supposed nonpartici- pants with an interest in exercise; they also used a conservative, nonparametric analysis, comparing medical costs for individual subjects with the costs incurred by these same individuals over the preceding 2 years. Bell and Blanke (9) also found no reduction in health care utilization when they compared participants and nonparticipants over the first 8 months of operation of a trucking company's wellness program; however, in this study, the exercisers had greater access to costly (and probably unnecessary) diagnostic investigations.

In addition to the commonly observed reduction in medical claims, the active individual enjoys the dividend of enhanced personal health. The latter ben- efit is difficult to express in dollar terms, but it is one of the most important reasons why many people engage in regular physical activity.

Avoidance of Lost Production

In a long-term perspective, the avoidance of chronic illness and premature death are the most important economic benefits that stem from regular exercise (Table 2). Attributing a social cost of 100% to lost earnings, Klarman (80) set the total indirect costs of cardiac disease at $27.6 billion in the U.S. economy of 1962, about $145 billion, or $1400 per worker-year, in 1998 dollars.

Australian estimates of long-term costs (131,132) are only about a quarter as large, partly because the global term *cardiac disease* has been broken down into specific diagnostic categories such as myocardial infarction, hypertension, and congestive heart failure but largely because the allowance for lost production has been set at 25% rather than 100% of the individual's anticipated income (147, 148). The Australian investigators have argued that if survival is extended, a person works for a longer period, but their personal consumption of goods and services is also increased, so that only a fraction of increased earnings is contrib- uted to society as a whole.

Empirical Tests of Secondary Prevention

To what extent might regular physical activity curb the long-term costs of chronic disease? Studies of both worksite and community programs suggest that regular vigorous physical activity can decrease the ''coronary'' death rate by 50% or more (17,101–102,112–116,127,149). Indeed, some of the best-designed stud- ies show a threefold difference between active and inactive groups (127). However, given that the average age of employees in many companies is around 40 years, the immediate direct and indirect costs of cardiovascular disease may be less than suggested by either Klarman (80) or Roberts (132). Yen et al. (189) suggested that cardiovascular disease accounted for only 14% of medical costs in the company that they examined.

The intensity of effort needed for protection against cardiovascular disease is also hotly debated (113). Most North American investigators now believe that protection can be derived from a moderate intensity of physical activity that causes only small increments in aerobic fitness; moreover, medical savings are greatest when such a regimen is implemented (2). On the other hand, some authorities in the United Kingdom still maintain that the prevention of cardiac disease requires vigorous physical activity (peaks of up to 31 kJ/min, 7.5 kcal/min) (102).

Potential Attenuation of Benefits

The imputed economic benefit from an increase in habitual physical activity depends greatly on the assumptions made, including the societal impact of a prolonged loss of production (25% or 100% of the salary that is no longer earned?), the effectiveness of the activity program that is undertaken (a 25%, 50%, or 67% decrease in the incidence of ''cardiac'' deaths), and the anticipated long-term compliance with the proposed regimen (10 or 20% of employees) (33,66,146). Heirich et al. (61) compared three different types of programs in a population of automotive workers. The presence of a fitness facility alone had little influence upon cardiac risk factors, but effectiveness was greatly increased by one-to-one counseling, plus organization of the worksite to encourage peer support and mutual involvement in exercise. Applying the most optimistic of these assumptions to Klarman's estimated cost of $1400 (80), the benefits from an exercise program would amount to ($1400 × 100% × 67% × 20%), or $188 per worker-year, but on the most conservative set of assumption ($1400 × 25% × 25% × 10%) it would drop to $8.75 per worker-year (Table 4). Keeler et al. (76) made a theoretical comparison of the expected life expectancy for active and inactive segments of the population. Assuming an annual discount rate of 5%, they calculated that the active group would subsidize their sedentary peers by some $2400 per person over their life course.

Whichever of these calculation proves correct, the economic benefits associated with the avoidance of premature death do not in themselves provide financial justification for more than a modest exercise program. However, we can add to these social benefits the more substantial gains that arise from improvements in perceived health. The resulting decreases in medical consultations and usage of hospital beds alone have yielded documented economies of $240–$850 per worker-year (152,156). As already noted, improvements of mood state also have a positive effect on work performance, which may yield benefits as large as $850 per worker-year.

Conclusion

A sophisticated exercise or health promotion program cannot always be justified in terms of its impact on the costs of cardiac disease, but "Active Living" and other low-cost initiatives are economically attractive, particularly if the balance sheet reflects the short-term benefits of an enhanced mood state to the individual and society.

Tertiary Prevention

Economic justification for tertiary prevention may be sought in a prolongation of calendar or quality-adjusted life span, a decrease in the recurrence of life-threatening events such as myocardial infarction, and an earlier return to work following the initial illness (88), with fewer and less costly readmissions to hospital (1).

Prolongation of Life

Endurance exercise programs reduce the incidence of fatal reinfarctions by 20–30%, although many randomized trials find little change in the number of nonfatal reinfarctions (Table 11) (21,51,95,108,111,129,151,153). A cumulative analysis involving almost 6000 patients shows only one major trial where deaths were more frequent in the exercised than in the control group (130). The control subjects in this experiment received a dose of exercise that was supposedly homeopathic, but in fact there was a substantial crossover of actual behavior between exercised and control groups, so that after 3–4 years there was little difference of fitness between the two groups. Both groups had a very low mortality, but when death rates were reanalyzed in terms of gains in aerobic fitness rather than initial group assignment (30), a benefit of the order observed in other trials became apparent.

The typical mortality rate of control subjects in most exercise trials was around 4% per year, although this figure has since decreased with advances such as increased use of β-blocking drugs. The economic impact of a 30% decrease in mortality rate among exercisers (Table 12) can be estimated as follows. Let us assume the patient has an average age of 45 years, as in the Toronto Rehabilitation Centre cardiac population, and the individual's societal contribution is 100% of an annual income of $26,000. Over the residual career span of 20 years, the total likelihood of death is $[1 - (0.96)^{20}]$, or about 55%. The typical case fatality loses about a half of his or her 20-year residual working career (an income of $26,000 \times 10$), and averaged over the total sample, the loss is ($260,000 \times

TABLE 11 Results of Major Randomized Trials of Exercise in the Tertiary Prevention of Myocardial Infarction

Author	Sample size	Entry post-M I	Follow-up time, years	Treatment type	Exercise group			Control group			Therapeutic benefit
					N	Deaths	%/year	N	Deaths	%/year	
Kentala (1972)	298	6–8 weeks	1	Individual supervised 2–3 times/week	152	26	17.1	146	32	21.9	0.81
	165[a]				77[c]	11	7.2	81[c]	11	6.9	1.04
Kallio (1981)	375 (74F, 301M)	Hospital discharge (2 weeks)	3	Exercise + health education	188	41	7.3	187	56	9.9	0.73
Kallio et al. (1988)	375 (74F, 301M)	Hospital discharge (2 weeks)	10	Exercise + health education (3-year progress)	188[c]	82	8.2	187[c]	97	9.7	0.85
Hamaleinen et al. (1988)	456	Hospital discharge (2 weeks)	6	Exercise + health education (3/12); controls received community program	228	45[d]	7.5	228	55[d]	9.2	0.82
Palatsi (1976)	380	2–3 months	1	Daily home program (non-randomized allocation based on time of recruitment)	180	18	4.1	200	28	5.8	0.64
Wilhelmsen et al. (1975)	315 (35F, 280M)	3 months	4	Individually supervised 3 times/week hospital-based	158	28	4.4	157	35	5.6	0.80
Shaw (1981)	651	2–36 months	3	Individually supervised 3 times/week	323	15	1.3	328	24	2.1	0.63

Study	N										
Rechnitzer et al. (1983)	751 (731 retained)	2–12 months	3–4	Partially supervised (2–4 times/week); controls received homeopathic exercise	379	15[d]	0.98	354	13[d]	0.91	1.08
Vermeulen et al. (1983)	98	—	5	—	47	2	0.85	51	5	1.90	0.45
Marra et al. (1985)	161	2 months	4–5	Individually supervised, increasing to four times/week (controls received homeopathic exercise)	81	6	1.35	80	5	1.90	0.45
Roman (1985)	193	2 months	Up to 9	Individually supervised	93	16	3.6	100	27	5.8	0.59
Carson et al. (1982)	303	6 weeks	25/12	Individually supervised	151	12	3.9	152	21	7.9	0.57
Lamm et al. (1982)[b]	1360	4–12 weeks	3	Individually supervised 3 times/week for 6 weeks	705	105	5.0	655	105	5.3	0.93
Bengtsson (1983)	171	1.5 months	1	Exercise + counseling for 3 months	81	8	9.9	90	6	6.7	1.48
Froelicher et al. (1984)	146	4 months	1	Supervised exercise for 8 weeks versus usual care	74	0		76	1		
Levin et al. (1991)	305[c]	1.5 months	5		147	43	29.3	158	50	31.6	0.93
TOTAL	5947					421			504		0.835

[a]Numbers suitable for long-term follow-up.
[b]Excluding (1) data of Kallio, (2) centers with low-level of follow-up, and (3) centers with significant baseline differences (see Ref. 111 for details)
[c]Same subjects as previous sample
[d]Coronary deaths + assuming 4-year follow-up of all subjects
[e]Nonrandom assignment.

0.55), or $143,000. Let us assume that 50% of patients sustain an appropriate volume of training to influence recurrence of the infarct. In these individuals, the salary loss is reduced by 30%, giving a saving of ($143,000 × 0.5 × 0.3), or $21,450. However, the benefit is on average 10 years distant, so at a 5% discount rate, the true economic benefit is [$21,450 × $(0.95)^{10}$], or $12,842; when the discounted benefit is averaged over 20 years, the yield is $642 per patient per year.

On less optimistic assumptions, the initial age of the patient may be 55 years, and the residual career span 10 years. The probability of death is [1 − $(0.96)^{10}$], or 0.336, after an average of 5 years. If 25% of earnings are contributed to society, the cumulative loss is ($26,000 × 0.25 × 0.336 × 5), or $10,920. If the exercise program reduces the fatal recurrence rate by 20% and 25% of patients maintain an appropriate dose of training, the estimated benefit would drop to ($546); discounting at 5% over an average of 5 years, this decreases further to $422, a benefit of $42.20 per patient per year.

Earlier Return to Work

Exercise programs may yield quite substantial benefits in terms of an earlier return to full-time work and a lesser likelihood of premature retirement (Table 12).

A work assessment in itself may be cost-beneficial (126). Differences in the number of patients working both 6 months and 5 years after myocardial infarction generally favor exercise programs by a margin of 5–10% (36,87,124), 14% (80), 17% (106), 27% (176) or 30% (40). All survivors are consumers, whether they work or not. On an optimistic assumption (50% of patients participate effectively in the exercise program, with a resulting 30% increase in their work-force participation), the economic impact might be ($26,000 × 0.50 × 0.30), or $3900 per year, whereas on a more conservative assumption (25% effective exercise participation, 10% increase in work-force participation), the benefit would drop to ($26,000 × 0.25 × 0.1), or $650 per patient-year.

Detailed observations of blue-collar workers in a rural area of southeastern Sweden support the order of benefit indicated by these calculations; a rehabilitated group earned an average of $3100 per year more than controls over a 5-year period (87,122), with a substantially (20%) lower incidence of sick leave in the more active group. Likewise, a Russian study (106) noted that over the first year of operation, an exercise rehabilitation program yielded dividends of 805 rubles per patient, about U.S. $1775 at official exchange rates for the period; this benefit was derived mainly from gains in productivity. A benefit of $4.30 per $1.00 invested was suggested, putting the cost of the Russian exercise program at $413 per patient-year. Other analyses from Lithuania (40) have reported an economic loss that was 94% greater with the standard patterns of treatment than with exercise rehabilitation; this would correspond, for instance, with a return to work of 61 and 80% in the two groups of patients.

Table 12   Costs and Benefits of Exercise Rehabilitation Following Myocardial Infarction

---

Gain from earlier return to work
  3 months at full salary of $40,000 = $10,000
Reduction of work loss from premature death
  Assuming average age at death = 55 years, initial annual mortality 40/10,000, and median age of death after nonfatal infarction at 68 years; approximately one-third of sample die before normal age of retirement (65 years).
  Annual mortality among exercise participants decreases by 25%, to 30/10,000, so that some 8% of sample are spared premature death.
  Loss from premature death = 50% of annual salary of $40,000 for an average of 5 years = $100,000.
  Benefit from exercise program = $100,000 × 0.33 × 0.25 = $8,250 realized on average 5 years after start of exercise program.

Benefits discounted (D) at rates shown

	2%	5%	10%
Earlier return to work	$10,000	$10,000	$10,000
Premature death × D^5	7,910	6,498	4,795
Total benefit	17,910	16,498	14,795
Benefit per year	1,791	1,649	1.480

Variables modifying the above estimates plainly include the average age of the person when disability is first incurred, the success of the physician and exercise specialist in maintaining enthusiasm for the physical activity program, the extent of social benefits and other negative incentives to resumption of full-time work following rehabilitation, opportunities for employment of the older worker, and (in industries that still have a heavy physical demand) the potential to modify the employee's job description to allow lighter work. Over the first year following myocardial infarction, it may be quite difficult to justify a phase 3 program in terms of greater productivity, although in a 5- to 10-year perspective, the cumulative impact of a greater likelihood of return to work and continued productivity could well match program costs.

Reduced Demands for Treatment Postinfarction

Ades et al. (1) found that participants in a 12-week tertiary prevention program incurred $870 less in subsequent hospital costs than their nonparticipating peers. Bondestam et al. (22) found that in the first 3 months following myocardial infarction, patients assigned to a rehabilitation program had a lower incidence of rehospitalization and paid fewer visits to the emergency department than controls;

after 12 months, days of hospitalization were similar for the two groups, but the exercisers still showed benefit in terms of a reduced use of emergency services.

Likewise, Perk et al. (124) noted that the percentage of patients who required readmission to hospital following coronary bypass grafting was lower for exercisers than for controls (14 versus 32%); there were also fewer episodes of readmission among those that did need additional hospital treatment (1.1 versus 2.9 visits), the demand for anxiolytic drugs was lower, and self-perceptions of physical work capacity were enhanced. An improvement of perceived health, and in particular a lightening of depression, is likely to be of particular importance after the onset of clinical illness, greatly influencing the value of each year of survival.

Overall Cost-Effectiveness

Finally, it may be asked how the overall cost-effectiveness of tertiary rehabilitation compares with that of alternative treatments.

Oldridge (109,110) estimated the cost of an 8-week cardiac rehabilitation program at $10,750 per QALY, as compared with $10,000 per QALY for a bypass operation in left-main vessel disease and $86,300 per QALY for a bypass to treat single vessel disease with mild angina. Data from the United Kingdom (53) provide rather similar estimates for alternative treatment: $6500 per QALY for coronary artery bypass graft in patients with left main vessel disease and severe angina, and $58,000 per QALY for one-vessel disease with moderate angina.

Hatziandreu et al. (58) analyzed the cost-effectiveness of exercise in terms of gains in quality-adjusted life expectancy. On this index, regular exercise was more effective than the correction of hypertension, but (in part because of the targeting of surgery), their calculations suggested that it was less effective than coronary bypass surgery.

CONCLUSIONS

If conservative assumptions are made about the likely fiscal benefits from an increase of physical activity, it is difficult to justify sophisticated programs for either secondary or tertiary rehabilitation simply in terms of a reduction in economic losses from continuing illness and premature death. However, regular physical activity also has a marked effect on mood state and perceived health. In the symptom-free adult, a secondary preventive program may thus lead to a substantial enhancement of industrial performance and a decrease in the acute demand for incidental medical services. After myocardial infarction, such benefits are even more important, and in a 5- to 10-year perspective these items can more than repay the costs of a comprehensive phase 3 cardiac rehabilitation program.

Nevertheless, the primary reason for advocating an increase of physical activity is not to save money. Rather, regular moderate exercise is a pleasant, readily accepted form of therapy, which is better received than most medical or surgical alternatives. It is on such grounds that we should commend it to our patients, both those who are ostensibly healthy and those who have already developed cardiovascular disease.

ACKNOWLEDGMENT

Dr. Shephard's studies are currently supported in part by a research grant from Canadian Tire Acceptance Limited.

REFERENCES

1. Ades, P.A., Huang, D., and Weaver, S.O., *Am. Heart J.,* 123: 916–921 (1992).
2. Anderson, D.R. and Jose, W.S., *Fitness in Business,* 1: 173–174 (1987).
3. Anderson, V., and Draper, P., in *Health Through Public Policy: the Greening of Public Health.* Green Press, London, pp. 169–180 (1991).
4. Andersson, G., The Importance of Exercise for Sick Leave and Perceived Health, Ph.D. dissertation, Linköping University, Linköping, Sweden (1987).
5. Andersson, G., Malmgren, S., and Ekstrand, J., *Int. J. Sports Med,* 7: 222–225 (1986).
6. Asikainen, P., Lüthje, P., Järvinen, M., Avikainen, V., and Koskinen, I., *Scand. J. Med. Sci. Sports,* 1: 228–231 (1991).
7. Avorn, J., *N. Engl. J. Med.,* 310: 1294–1301 (1984).
8. Bailey, D.A., Shephard, R.J., and Mirwald, R.L., *Can. J. Appl. Sport Sci.,* 1: 67–78 (1974).
9. Bell, B.C., and Blanke, D.J., *Health Values,* 16: 3–13 (1992).
10. Bengtsson, K., *Scand. J. Rehabil. Med.,* 15: 1–9 (1983).
11. Bernacki, E.J. and Baun, W., *J. Occup. Med.,* 26: 529–531 (1984).
12. Berra, K., and Hall, L.K., in *Heart Disease and Rehabilitation* (M.L. Pollock and D.H. Schmidt, eds.), Human Kinetics, Champaign, Illinois, pp. 187–200 (1995).
13. Berlin, J.A., and Colditz, G.A., *Am. J. Epidemiol.* 132: 612–628 (1990).
14. Biering-Sorensen, F., Bendix, T., Jorgensen K., Manniche, C., Nielsen, H., in *Physical Activity, Fitness and Health* (C. Bouchard, R. J. Shephard, and T. Stephens, eds.). Human Kinetics, Champaign, Illinois, pp. 737–748 (1994).
15. Black, D., *Inequalities in Health: Report of a Research Working Group,* Department of Health and Social Services, London (1980).
16. Black, D., *A Doctor Looks at Health Economics,* Office of Health Economics, London (1994).

17. Blair, S.N., Kohl, H.W., Paffenbarger, R.S., Clark, D.G., Cooper, K.H., and Gibbons, L.W., *J.A.M.A.,* 262: 2395–2401 (1989).
18. Blamey, A., Mutrie, N., and Aitchison T., *Br. Med. J.,* 311: 289–290 (1995).
19. Blanchet, M., in *Exercise, Fitness and Health* (C. Bouchard, R.J. Shephard, T. Stephens, J. Sutton, and B. McPherson, eds.), Human Kinetics, Champaign, Illinois, pp. 127–132 (1990).
20. Bly, J.L., Jones, R.C., and Richardson, J.E., *J.A.M.A.,* 256: 3235–3240 (1986).
21. Bobbio, M., in *Proceedings, IVth World Congress of Cardiac Rehabilitation, Brisbane,* p. 92 (1988).
22. Bondestam, E., Breikss, A., and Hartford, M., *Am. J. Cardiol.,* 75: 767–771 (1995).
23. Bouchard, C., Shephard, R.J., Stephens, T., Sutton, J., and McPherson, B., *Exercise, Fitness and Health.* Human Kinetics, Champaign, Illinois (1990).
24. Bouchard, C., Shephard, R.J., and Stephens, T., *Physical Activity, Fitness and Health.* Human Kinetics, Champaign, Illinois (1994).
25. British Medical Journal, *Br. Med. J.,* 308: 553 (1994).
26. Broadhead, W.E., Blazer, D.G., and George, L.K., *J.A.M.A.,* 264: 2524–2528 (1990).
27. *Canada Health Survey,* Health Canada, Ottawa (1982).
28. Carson, P., Phillips, R., Lloyd, M. et al., *J. R. Coll. Phys. Surg.,* 16: 141–147 (1982).
29. Chenoweth, D., *Second National Symposium on the Economic Impact of Worksite Health Promotion Programs,* Buffalo, New York (1993).
30. Cunningham, D.A., Rechnitzer, P.A., Andrew, G.M., Kavanagh, T., Parker, J.O., Shephard, R.J., Sutton, J.R., and Oldridge, N.B., *Sports Training Med. Rehabil.,* 2: 131–139 (1991).
31. Curtiss, J.E., and Russell, S.J., *Physical Activity in Human Experience: Interdisciplinary Perspectives.* Human Kinetics, Champaign, Illinois, pp. 1–286 (1997).
32. DeBusk, R.F., Miller, N.H., Superko, H.R., Dennis, C.A., Thomas, R.J., Lew, H.T., Berger, W.E., Heller, R.S., Rompf, J., Gee, D. et al., *Ann. Intern. Med.,* 120: 721–729 (1994).
33. Dishman, R. *Exercise Adherence,* 2nd ed. Human Kinetics, Champaign, Illinois (1995).
34. Dolatowski, R.P., Squires, R.W., Pollock, M.L., Foster, C.R., and Schmidt, D.H., *Med. Sci. Sports Exerc.,* 15: 281–286 (1983).
35. Drummond, M.F., and Jefferson, T.O., *Br. Med. J.* 313: 275–283 (1996).
36. Dwyer, T., and Rutherford, R., *Proceedings of IVth Congress of Cardiac Rehabilitation, Brisbane,* p. 87 (1988).
37. Ekins, P., Hillman, M. and Hutchinson, R., *Wealth Beyond Measure: An Atlas of New Economics.* Gala Books, London, 1992.
38. Erfurt, J.C., Foote, A., and Heirich, M.A., *Am. J. Health Prom.* 5: 438–448 (1991).
39. Eskelinen, L., Kohvakka, A., Merisalo, T., Hurri, H., and Wägar, G., *Scand. J. Work Environ. Health,* 17 (Suppl. 1): 40–47 (1991).
40. Estany, E.R., de Leon, O.P., Chesa, C.S., Duenas, A., and Canero, A.H., *Proceedings of the IVth World Congress of Cardiac Rehabilitation, Brisbane,* p. 145 (1988).
41. Fardy, P.S., Doll, N., Taylor, J., and Williams, M., *Phys. Sportsmed.,* 10 (6): 145–154 (1982).

42. Farquhar, J., Fortmann, S., Flora, J., Taylor, B., Haskell, W.L., Williams, P., Maccoby, N., and Wood, P., *J.A.M.A.,* 264: 359–365 (1990).
43. Field, K., Thorogood, M., Silagy, C., Normand, C., O'Neill, C., and Muir, J., *Br. Med. J.,* 310: 1109–1112 (1995).
44. Fineberg, V., Scadden, D., and Goldman, L., *N. Engl. J. Med.,* 310: 1301–1307 (1984).
45. Fletcher, G.F., and Cantwell, J.D., *Chest,* 71: 27–32 (1977).
46. Franklin, B.A., Bonzheim, K., Berg, T., and Bonzheim, S., in *Heart Disease and Rehabilitation* (M.L. Pollock and D.H. Schmidt, eds.). Human Kinetics, Champaign, Illinois, pp. 209–227 (1995).
47. Frics, J., *Aging Well.* Addison-Wesley, Reading, Massachusetts (1980).
48. Fries, J.F., Bloch, D.A., Harrington, H., Richardson, N., and Beck, R., *Am. J. Med.,* 94: 455–462 (1993).
49. Froelicher, V.F., Jensen, D., and Sullivan, M., *J.A.M.A.,* 252: 1291–1297 (1984).
50. Froelicher, V.F., Herbert, W., Myers, J., and Ribisl, P., *J. Cardiopulm. Rehabil.,* 16: 151–159 (1996).
51. Furberg, D., *Am. J. Cardiol.,* 60: 28A–32A (1987).
52. Godin, G. and Shephard, R.J., *Sports Med.,* 10: 103–121 (1990).
53. Gudex, C. *QALYs and Their Use by the Health Service.* Centre for Health Economics, University of York, York, England (1986).
54. Hadorn, D.C., and Holmes, A.C., *Br. Med. J.,* 314: 135–138 (1997).
55. Hall, L.K., *J. Cardiopulm. Rehabil.,* 14: 228–231 (1994).
56. Hamalainen, H., Kallio, V., and Arstila, M. *Proceedings of IVth World Congress of Cardiac Rehabilitation, Brisbane,* p. 93 (1988).
57. Haskell, W.L., Alderman, E., Fair, J., Maron, D., Mackey, S., Superko, R., Williams, P., Johnstone, I., Champagne, M., Krauss, R., and Farquhar, J., *Circulation,* 84: II–140 (1991).
58. Hatziandreu, E.L., Koplan, J.P., Weinstein, M.C., Caspersen, C.J.L., and Warner, K.J., *Am J Public Health,* 78:1417–1421 (1988).
59. Hedbäck, B., and Perk, J., *Scand. J. Rehabil. Med.,* 22: 15–20 (1990).
60. Hedbäck, B., Perk, J., and Engvall, J., *Proceedings of the 4th World Congress of Cardiac Rehabilitation, Brisbane,* p. 93 (1988).
61. Heirich, M.A., Foote, A., Erfurt, J.C., and Konopka, B., *J. Occup. Med.,* 35: 510–517 (1993).
62. Herbert, D.L. *Exerc. Stand. Malpract. Rep.,* 2 (1): 1–6 (1988).
63. Herbert, W.G., and Herbert, D.L., in *Heart Disease and Rehabilitation* (M.L. Pollock and D.H. Schmidt, eds.). Human Kinetics, Champaign, Illinois, pp. 433–444 (1995).
64. Herzlich, C., *Health and Illness.* Academic Press, London (1973).
65. Hillsdon, M., Thorogood, M., Anstiss, T., and Morris, J., *J. Epidemiol. Commun. Health,* 49: 448–453 (1995).
66. Hollander, R.B., and Lengermann, J.J., *Soc. Sci. Med.,* 26: 491–501 (1988).
67. Holman, H., Manzonson, P., and Lorig, K., *Trans. Assoc. Am. Phys.,* 102: 204–208 (1989).
68. Humphrey, R., *J. Cardiopulm. Rehab.,* 8: 276–278 (1988).
69. Jackson, J.J., Diffusion of an Innovation: An Explanatory Study of Sport Participa-

tion's Campaign at Saskatoon. Ph.D. Dissertation, University of Saskatchewan, Saskatoon, Canada (1975).

70. Kallio, V., in *Physical Conditioning and Cardiovascular Rehabilitation* (L.S. Cohen, M.B. Mock, and I. Ringqvist, eds.). Wiley, New York, pp. 257–270 (1981).

71. Kallio, V., Hamalainen, H., Hakkila, J., Luurila, O., Knuts, L-R., and Arstila, M., *Proceedings, IVth World Congress of Cardiac Rehabilitation, Brisbane,* p. 67 (1988).

72. Kaman, R., *Worksite Fitness and Wellness Programs.* Human Kinetics, Champaign, Illinois (1995).

73. Kaman, R., and Patton, R.W., in *Physical Activity, Fitness and Health* (C. Bouchard, R.J. Shephard, and T. Stephens, eds.). Human Kinetics, Champaign, Illinois, pp. 134–1144 (1994).

74. Kaplan, R.M., in *Behavioral Epidemiology and Disease Prevention* (R.M. Kaplan and M.H. Criqui, eds.). Plenum Press, New York, pp. 31–56 (1985).

75. Kavanagh, T., and Shephard, R.J., *Arch. Phys. Med. Rehabil.* 61: 114–118 (1980).

76. Keeler, E.B., Manning, W.G., Newhouse, J.P., Sloss, E.M., and Wasserman, J., *Am. J. Publ. Health,* 79: 975–981 (1989).

77. Kelly, J.J., *Cardiac Rehabilitation Guidelines.* Blue Cross and Blue Shield of Virginia, Richmond, Virginia (1986).

78. Kentala, E., *Ann. Clin. Res.,* 4 (Suppl. 9): 1–84 (1972).

79. King, A.C., Haskell, W.L., Taylor, C.B., Kraemer, H.C., and DeBusk, R.F., *J.A.M.A.,* 266: 1535–1542 (1991).

80. Klarman, H.E., in *The Heart and Circulation. Second National Conference on Cardiovascular Disease: Vol. 2, Community Services and Education* (E.C. Andrus, ed.). U.S. Public Health Service, Washington, D.C. (1964).

81. Klarman, H.E., in *Preventive and Community Medicine* 2nd Ed. (D.W. Clark and B. MacMahon, eds.). Little, Brown, Boston, pp. 603–615 (1981).

82. Labonté, R., *Policy Options,* 3: 54–55 (1982).

83. Lamm, G., Denolin, H., and Dorossiev, D., *Adv. Cardiol.,* 31: 107–111 (1982).

84. Langham, S., Thorogood, M., Normand, C., Muir, J., Jones, L., and Fowler, G., *Br. Med. J.* 312: 1265–1268 (1996).

85. Leatt, P., Hattin, H., West, C., and Shephard, R.J. *Can. J. Public Health,* 79: 20–25 (1988).

86. Levin, L.A., in *Assessment of Health Care Techniques: Case Studies, Key Concepts and Strategic Issues* (A.K. Szczepura and J. Kankaanpää, eds.). Wiley, Chichester, England, pp. 199–214 (1996).

87. Levin, L.A., Perk, J., and Hedbäck, B., *J. Intern. Med.,* 230: 427–434 (1991).

88. Levine, T.B., Levine, A.B., Goldberg, A.D., Tobes, M., Narins, B., and Lesch, M., *Am. Heart J.,* 132: 1189–1194 (1996).

89. Lindblad, B.E., Hoy, K., Helleland, H.E., and Terkelsen, C.J., *Scand. J. Med. Sci. Sports,* 1: 221–224 (1991).

90. Linsted, K.D., Tonstad, S., and Kuzma, J.W., *J. Clin. Epidemiol.,* 44: 355–364 (1991).

91. McNeill, B.J., *Ann. N.Y. Acad. Sci.,* 703: 63–73 (1993).

92. Mark, D.B., Naylor, D., Nelson, C.I., Joilis, J.G., Clapp-Channing, N., and Hlatky, M.A., *Cost-Effectiveness of Tissue Plasminogen Activator Relative to Streptokinase*

in Acute Myocardial Infarction: Results from the GUSTO Trial. American Heart Association Conference, Atlanta, 8–11 November (1993).

93. Marra, S., Paolillo, V., Spadaccini, E., and Angelino, P.F., *Eur. Heart J.,* 6: 656–663 (1985).

94. Marwick, T.H., Anderson, T., Williams, M.J., Haluska, B., Melin, J.A., Pashkow, F., and Thomas, J.D., *J. Am. Coll. Cardiol.,* 26: 335–341 (1995).

95. May, G.S., Eberlein, K.A., Furberg, C.D., Passamani, E.R., and DeMets, D.L., *Prog. Cardiovasc. Dis.,* 24: 331–352 (1982).

96. Maynard, A., *Br. Med. J.* 295: 1537–1541 (1987).

97. Miller, H.S. and Fletcher, G.F., in *Heart Disease and Rehabilitation* (M.L. Pollock and D.H. Schmidt, eds.), Human Kinetics, Champaign, Illinois, pp. 229–242 (1995).

98. Miller, N.H., *J. Cardiopulm. Rehabil.,* 16: 349–352 (1996).

99. Mitchell, M., Franklin, B., Johnson, S. and Rubenfire, M., *Arch. Phys. Med. Rehabil.,* 65: 463–466 (1984).

100. Morris, J.N. *Res. Quart.* 67: 216–220 (1996).

101. Morris, J.N., Everitt, M.G., Pollard, R.L., Chave, S.P.W., and Semmence, A.M., *Lancet,* 2: 1207–1210 (1980).

102. Morris, J.N., Clayton, D.G., Everitt, M.G., Semmence, A.M., and Burgess, E.H., *Br. Heart J.,* 63: 325–334 (1990).

103. McNeil, B.J., *Ann. N.Y. Acad. Sci.,* 703: 63–73 (1993).

104. Nicholl, J.P., Coleman, P., and Williams, P.T., *Injuries in Sport and Exercise.* Sports Council, London (1993).

105. Nicklin, W.M., *Heart Lung,* 15: 268–272 (1986).

106. Nikolaeva, L.F., Karpova, G.D., Rubanovich, A., Evdakov, V.A., Aronov, D.M., Aleshin, O.I., Modorova, A.A., Zhydko, N.I., and Deev, A.D., *Proceedings of IVth World Congress of Cardiac Rehabilitation, Brisbane,* p. 118 (1988).

107. Noakes, T.D., *S. Afr. Med. J.,* 62: 238–240 (1982).

108. O'Connor, G.T., Buring, J.E., Yusuf, S., Goldhaber, S.Z., Olmstead, E.M., Paffenbarger, R.S., and Hennekens, C.H., *Circulation,* 80: 234–244 (1989).

109. Oldridge, N.B., *J. Cardiopulm. Rehabil.,* 15: 9–13, 1995.

110. Oldridge, N.B., in *Heart Disease and Rehabilitation* (M.L. Pollock and D.H. Schmidt, eds.), Human Kinetics, Champaign, Illinois, pp. 393–404 (1995).

111. Oldridge, N.B., Guyatt, G.H., Fischer, M.E., and Rimm, A.A., *J.A.M.A.,* 260: 945–950 (1988).

112. Paffenbarger, R., *Med. Sci. Sports Exerc.,* 20: 426–438, 1988.

113. Paffenbarger, R. and Min-Lee, I., *Res. Q.,* 67(Suppl.): S11–S28 (1996).

114. Paffenbarger, R., Hyde, R.T., Wing, A.L., and Hsieh, C.C., *N. Engl. J. Med.,* 314: 605–613 (1986).

115. Paffenbarger, R., Hyde, R.T., and Wing, A.L., in *Exercise, Fitness and Health* (C. Bouchard, R.J. Shephard, T. Stephens, J. Sutton and B. McPherson, eds.). Human Kinetics, Champaign, Illinois, pp. 33–48 (1990).

116. Paffenbarger, R., Hyde, R., Wing, A., Jung, D., and Kampert, J., *Med. Sci. Sports Exerc.,* 23: S82 (1991).

117. Palatsi, I., *Acta Med. Scand.,* 599 (Suppl): 7–84 (1976).

118. Parmley, W.W., *Cardiology,* 15: 4–5 (1986).

119. Parsonage, M., and Neuberger, H., *Health Economics,* 1: 71–76 (1992).
120. Pekkanen, J., Marti, B., Nissinen, A., Tuomilehto, J., Punsar, S. and Karvonen, M., *Lancet,* 1 (8548): 1473–1477 (1987).
121. Pelletier, K.R., *Am. J. Health Prom.,* 8: 50–62 (1993).
122. Perk, J., and Hedbäck, B., *Proceedings of the Fourth World Congress of Cardiac Rehabilitation,* Brisbane, p. 110 (1988) (Abstr.).
123. Perk, J., Hedbäck, B., and Jutterdal, S., *Scand. J. Rehabil. Med.,* 21: 13–17 (1989).
124. Perk, J., Hedbäck, B., and Engvall, J., *Scand. J. Soc. Med.,* 18: 45–51 (1990).
125. Phillips, S., Fox, N., Jacobs, J., and Wright, W.E., *Bone,* 9: 271–279 (1988).
126. Picard, M.H., Dennis, C., Schwartz, R.G., Ahn, D.K., Kraemer, H.C., Berger, W.E., Blumberg, R., Heller, R., Lew, H., and DeBusk, R.F., *Am. J. Cardiol.,* 63: 1308–1314 (1989).
127. Powell, K.E., Thompson, P.D., Caspersen, C.J., and Kendrick, J.S., *Annu. Rev. Public Health,* 8: 253–287 (1987).
128. Pyfer, H.R., and Doane, B.L., in *Exercise Testing and Exercise Training in Coronary Heart Disease* (J.P. Naughton, H.K. Hellerstein, and I.C. Mohler, eds.). Academic Press, New York, pp. 365–369 (1973).
129. Quaglietti, S., and Froehlicher, V.F., in *Physical Activity, Fitness and Health* (C. Bouchard, R.J. Shephard, and T. Stephens, eds.). Human Kinetics, Champaign, Illinois, pp. 591–608 (1994).
130. Rechnitzer, P.A., Cunningham, D.A., Andrew, G.M., Buck, C.W., Jones, N.L., Kavanagh, T., Oldridge, N.B., Parker, J.O., Shephard, R.J., Sutton, J.R., and Donner, A., *Am. J. Cardiol.,* 51: 65–69 (1983).
131. Reznik, R., *Proceedings of the Fourth World Congress of Cardiac Rehabilitation,* Brisbane, p. 86 (1988) (Abstr).
132. Roberts, A.D., *The Economic Benefits of Participation in Regular Physical Activity.* Recreation Ministers' Council of Australia, Canberra, Australia, pp. 1–32 (1982).
133. Robinson, R., *Br. Med. J.,* 307: 924–926 (1993).
134. Robinson, R., *Br. Med. J.,* 307: 793–795 (1993).
135. Robinson, R., *Br. Med. J.,* 307: 859–862 (1993).
136. Robinson, R., *Br. Med. J.,* 307: 736–738 (1993).
137. Roman, O., *J. Card. Rehabil.* 5: 93–96 (1985).
138. Rudman, W.J., and Lipping, A., *Am. J. Health Prom.,* 6: 250 (1992).
139. Russell, D., *The Cost of Doing Nothing.* University of Otago, Dunedin, New Zealand (1987).
140. Russell, L.B., *Is Prevention Better than Cure?* Brookings Institute, Washington, D.C., pp. 1–129 (1986).
141. Russell, L.B., *Science,* 246: 892–896 (1989).
142. Russell, L.B., in *Physical Activity in Human Experience: Interdisciplinary Perspectives* (J.E. Curtiss and S.J. Russell, eds.). Human Kinetics, Champaign, Illinois, pp. 163–185 (1997).
143. Sandelin, J., Santavirta, S., Lättila, R., Vuolle, P., and Sarna, S., *Int. J. Sports Med.,* 9: 61–66, 1988.
144. Sciacca, J., Seehafer, R., Reed, R., and Mulvaney, D., *Am. J. Health Prom.,* 7: 374–383, 395 (1993).
145. Shaw, L.W., *Am. J. Cardiol.,* 48: 39–46 (1981).

146. Shephard, R.J., *Phys. Sportsmed.*, 13(7): 88–101 (1985).

147. Shephard, R.J., *The Economic Benefits of Enhanced Fitness.* Human Kinetics, Champaign, Illinois (1986).

148. Shephard, R.J., *Fitness and Health in Industry.*, Karger, Basel, Switzerland (1986).

149. Shephard, R.J., *Sports Med.*, 3: 26–49 (1986).

150. Shephard, R.J., in *International Perspectives in Adapted Physical Activity* (M. Berridge and G. Ward, eds.). Human Kinetics, Champaign, Illinois, pp. 235–242 (1987).

151. Shephard, R.J., *Physician Sportsmed.*, 16(6): 116–127 (1988).

152. Shephard, R.J., *Sports Med.*, 7: 286–309 (1989).

153. Shephard, R.J., *Can. J. Sport Sci.*, 14: 74–84 (1989).

154. Shephard, R.J., in *Sports, Medicine and Health* (G.P.H. Hermans and W.L. Mosterd, eds.). Excerpta Medica, Amsterdam, pp. 97–106 (1990).

155. Shephard, R.J., *Fitness in Special Populations.* Human Kinetics, Champaign, Illinois (1990).

156. Shephard, R.J., *Med. Sci. Sports Exerc.*, 24: 354–370 (1992).

157. Shephard, R.J., *Med. Exerc. Nutr. Health,* 3: 268–284 (1994).

158. Shephard, R.J., in *Worksite Fitness and Wellness Programs* (R. Kaman, ed.). Human Kinetics, Champaign, Illinois, pp. 147–173 (1995).

159. Shephard, R.J., *Am. J. Health Prom.,* 10: 436–452 (1996).

160. Shephard, R.J., in *Workplace Health: Employee Fitness and Exercise* (J. Kerr, A. Griffiths, and T. Cox, eds.). Taylor and Francis, London, pp. 29–54 (1996).

161. Shephard, R.J., *Quest,* 48: 354–365 (1996).

162. Shephard, R.J., in (A. Leon, ed.). Human Kinetics, Champaign, Illinois, pp. 76 86 (1997).

163. Shephard, R.J., *Physical Activity and Immune Function,* Cooper Publications, Carmel, Indiana (1997).

164. Shephard, R.J., Corey, P., and Kavanagh, T., *Med. Sci. Sports Exerc.* 13: 1–5 (1981).

165. Shephard. R.J., Corey, P., Renzland, P., and Cox, M.H., *Can. J. Public Health,* 73: 259–263 (1982).

166. Shephard, R.J., Corey, P., and Cox, M., *Can. J. Public Health,* 73: 183–187 (1982).

167. Shephard, R.J., Kavanagh, T., Tuck, J., and Kennedy, J., *J. Cardiac Rehabil.,* 3: 321–329 (1983).

168. Simoons, M., Lap, C., and Pool, J., *Am. Heart J.,* 100: 9–14 (1988).

169. Sullivan, S., and Flynn, T.J., *The Revolution at Hand.* National Committee for Quality Health Care, Washington, D.C., pp. 3–65 (1992).

170. Torrance, G.W., *J. Health Economics,* 5: 1–30 (1986).

171. Tsai, S.P., Baun, W.B., and Bernacki, E.B., *J. Occup. Med.,* 29: 572–575 (1987).

172. Tsai, S.P., Bernacki, E.B., and Baun, W.B., *Prev. Med.,* 17: 475–482 (1988).

173. Tuomi, K., Ilmarinen, J. Eskelinen, L., Järvinen, E., Toikkanen, J., and Klockars, M., *Scand. J. Work Environ. Health,* 17 (Suppl. 1): 67–74 (1991).

174. Van Camp, S.P., in *Heart Disease and Rehabilitation* (M.L. Pollock and D.H. Schmidt, eds.). Human Kinetics, Champaign, Illinois, pp. 423–432 (1995).

175. Van Galen, W.C.H.W., and Diedericks J., *Sports Injuries in the Netherlands.* Institute of Sports Medicine, Limburg, Netherlands (1988).

176. Vasilauskas, D., Krisciunasx, A., and Lazaravicius, A., *Proceedings of IVth World Congress of Cardiac Rehabilitation, Brisbane,* p. 144 (1988).

177. Vermeer, F., Simoons, M.L., De Zwaan, C., Van, E.S., Verheugt, F.W.A., Van Der Laarse A., et al., *Br. Heart J.,* 59: 527–534 (1988).

178. Vermeulen, A., Lie, K.I., and Durrer, D., *Am. Heart J.,* 105: 798–801 (1983).

179. Wachtel, T.J., *Am. J. Med.,* 94: 451–454 (1993).

180. Walker, J., Cox, M., Thomas, S., Gledhill, N., and Salmon, A., *Canada Life 10: Corporate Fitness Ten Years After.* Ontario Ministry of Tourism and Recreation, Toronto, Ontario (1991).

181. Warner, K.E., *Health Educ. O.,* 14: 39–55 (1987).

182. Warner, K.E., Wickizer, T.M., Wolfe, R.A., Schidroth, J.E., and Samuelson, M.H., *J. Occup. Med.,* 30: 106–112 (1988).

182a. Wasson, J., Gaudette, C., Whaley, F., Sauvigne, A., Baribeau, P., and Welch, H.G., *J.A.M.A.,* 267: 1788–1793 (1992).

183. Whitmer, W., *Business Health,* cited by W. Whitmer, In: Worksite Health Promotion Economics, R.L. Kaman, ed. Human Kinetics Publisher, Champaign, IL, 1995, pp. 79–95: 60–66 (1992).

184. Wigle, D.T., Mao, Y., Wong, T., and Lane, R., *Economic Burden of Illness in Canada, 1986.* Health and Welfare Canada, Ottawa, Ontario (1990).

185. Wilhelmsen, L., Sanne, H., Elmfeldt, D., Grimby, G., Tibblin, G., and Wedel, H., *Prev. Med.,* 4: 491–508 (1975).

186. Williams, A., *Br. Med. J.,* 291: 326–329 (1985).

187. Williams, A., *Screening for Risk of Coronary Heart Disease* (M. Oliver, M. Ashley-Miller, and D. Wood, eds.). Wiley, London (1986).

188. Wonderling, D., Langham, S., Buxton, M., Normand, C., and McDermott, C., *Br. Med. J.,* 312: 1274–1278 (1996).

189. Yen, L.T., Edington, E.W., and Witting, P., *Am. J. Health Prom.,* 6: 46–54 (1991).

190. Zohman, L.R., in *Exercise Testing and Exercise Training in Coronary Heart Disease* (J.P. Naughton, H.K. Hellerstein, and I.C. Mohler, eds.). Academic Press, New York, pp. 329–336 (1973).

About the Editors

Roy J. Shephard is Professor Emeritus of Applied Physiology, Faculty of Physical Education and Health and Department of Public Health Sciences, Faculty of Medicine, University of Toronto, Ontario, Canada. He is also a Consultant to the Toronto Rehabilitation Centre. The author or coauthor of over 1300 journal articles, book chapters, and abstracts, he is also the author or coauthor of about 50 books. He is a past president of the American College of Sports Medicine and the Canadian Society of Exercise Physiology, an Honorary Fellow and Vice-President of the British Association of Sport and Medicine, an Honorary Fellow of the Belgian Society of Sports Medicine, and a Fellow of the American Academy of Physical Education. Dr. Shephard received the B.Sc. degree (1949) in physiology, the M.B.B.S. degree (1952) with distinction in forensic medicine and public health, the Ph.D. degree (1954) in physiology, and the M.D. degree (1959) from the University of London, England. He also holds honorary doctorates from the University of Ghent, Belgium, and the University of Montreal, Quebec, Canada.

Henry S. Miller, Jr. is Professor of Internal Medicine/Cardiology and Medical Director, Cardiac Rehabilitation Program, Wake Forest University School of Medicine, Winston-Salem, North Carolina. The author or coauthor of nearly 70 journal articles, book chapters, and abstracts, he is a past president and current member of the American College of Sports Medicine and a Fellow of the American College of Physicians, the American College of Cardiology, and the Council on Clinical Cardiology. He is a member of the Council on Epidemiology and the American Association of Cardiovascular and Pulmonary Rehabilitation, which also presented him with its 1997 Award of Excellence. Dr. Miller received the B.S. degree (1950) in medical science and the M.D. degree (1954) from Wake Forest University.